P
COMPANI

TEXT

D1235226

SURGERY

POCKET COMPANION TO SABISTON

TEXTBOOK *of* SURGERY

17*th* EDITION

COURTNEY M. TOWNSEND, JR., M.D.
Professor and John Woods Harris Distinguished Chairman
Department of Surgery, The University of Texas Medical Branch
Galveston, Texas

R. DANIEL BEAUCHAMP, M.D.
J. C. Foshee Distinguished Professor of Surgery
Chairman, Section of Surgical Sciences
Vanderbilt University School of Medicine; Surgeon-in-Chief
Vanderbilt University Hospital Nashville, Tennessee

B. MARK EVERS, M.D.
Professor and Robertson-Poth Distinguished Chair in General Surgery
Department of Surgery
The University of Texas Medical Branch Galveston, Texas

KENNETH L. MATTOX, M.D.
Professor and Vice Chairman
Department of Surgery, Baylor College of Medicine
Chief of Staff and Chief of Surgery
Ben Taub General Hospital, Houston, Texas

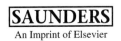

SAUNDERS
An Imprint of Elsevier

ELSEVIER
SAUNDERS

The Curtis Center
170 S Independence Mall W 300 E
Philadelphia, Pennsylvania 19106

POCKET COMPANION TO SABISTON TEXTBOOK
OF SURGERY, SEVENTEENTH EDITION   ISBN 07216-0482-X

NOTICE

Previous editions copyrighted

Library of Congress Cataloging-in-Publication Data
Pocket companion to Sabiston textbook of surgery.--17th ed. / [edited by]
Courtney M.Townsend Jr.
  p.; cm.
 ISBN 0-7216-0482-X
  1. Surgery--Handbooks, manuals, etc. I. Townsend, Courtney M. II. Sabiston,
David C., 1924- III. Sabiston textbook of surgery.
 [DNLM: 1. Surgical Procedures, Operative--Handbooks. 2. Surgery--Handbooks.
WO 39 P7386 2004]
RD31.T4732 2004
617--dc22   2004046836

Acquisitions Editor: Judith Fletcher
Developmental Editor: Kim J. Davis
Production Manager: Mary B. Stermel

Printed in the United States of America

Last digit is the print number: 9 8 7 6 5 4 3 2 1

Preface

The *Pocket Companion* provides an immediate source of key information on topics covered in the 17th edition of the *Sabiston Textbook of Surgery: The Biological Basis of Modern Surgical Practice.* It can be carried in a coat pocket and will provide medical students and residents readily available pertinent information. This condensed version has been prepared from the material in the chapters of the 17th edition. The *Pocket Companion* is not meant to supplant the textbook and, in all instances, the reader is referred to the 17th edition of the textbook for complete coverage of the topic.

Courtney M. Townsend, Jr., M.D.

Contents

CHAPTER 1

ETHICS IN SURGERY

- Ethics is about thinking through what we believe is good or bad, right or wrong, and why we think that way.
- The ethical precepts of the medical profession have traditionally been summarized in various oaths and codes.
- The American College of Surgeons Statements on Principles contains a fellowship pledge that includes a promise to maintain the College s historical commitment to the ethical practice of medicine.
- Responsibility to the patient in contemporary clinical ethics entails maximum patient participation, permitted by the patient s condition, in decisions regarding the course of care.
- Consent is permission, granted by the patient to the surgeon, to make a diagnostic or therapeutic intervention on the patient s behalf.
- The ultimate goal is to achieve the best outcome, not only in terms of adherence to ethical principles of practice but also in keeping with patients moral values, with what matters most to patients in their relationships and their lives. Achieving this goal entails the provision of information and the granting of consent, but this exchange must take place in the context of a conversation about how the proposed intervention will affect a particular patient s life.
- In addition to enhancing mutuality and promoting understanding, meaningful conversation contributes to better health outcomes and to patients satisfaction with their care.
- Contemporary clinical ethics is evolving toward a relational understanding of interactions between doctors and patients. In the parlance of ethics, this means that ethical principles are being supplemented by moral virtues.

CHAPTER 2

MOLECULAR AND CELL BIOLOGY

HUMAN GENOME

Structure of Genes and DNA

- DNA is composed of four types of deoxyribonucleotides containing the bases adenine (A), cytosine (C), guanine (G), and thymine (T).
- The nucleotide sequences of the opposing strands of DNA are complementary to each other.
- Human genome contains 3×10^9 nucleotide pairs.
- Messenger RNA (mRNA) encodes proteins or structural RNA.
- DNA molecule that directs the synthesis of a functional RNA molecule is called a *gene*.
- Human genome contains 24 different DNA molecules.
  - Each DNA has 10^8 bases and is packaged in a separate chromosome.
  - 22 different autosomes.
  - 2 different sex chromosomes.
- Each somatic cell contains two copies 46 chromosomes.
- DNA replication and segregation each chromosome is packaged into a compact structure with the aid of special proteins including histones.

DNA Replication and Repair

- DNA replication must occur rapidly but with extremely high accuracy.
- Both strands contain identical genetic information and serve as templates.
- Fidelity of DNA replication is of critical importance because any mistake, called a *mutation,* will result in wrong DNA sequences being copied to daughter cells.
- Change in a single base pair is called a *point mutation.*
- A single amino acid change as the consequence of the point mutation is called a *missense mutation.*

- If the point mutation results in the replacement of an amino acid codon with a stop codon, it is called a *nonsense mutation*.
- If there is an addition or deletion of a few base pairs, it is called *frameshift mutation*.
- Several proofreading mechanisms are used to eliminate mistakes during DNA replication.

RNA and Protein Synthesis

- The transfer of information from DNA to protein proceeds through the synthesis of an intermediate molecule known as RNA.
- RNA differs from DNA in two respects:
  - Its sugar-phosphate backbone contains ribose instead of deoxyribose sugar.
  - Thymine (T) is replaced by uracil (U), a closely related base that pairs with adenine (A).
- RNA molecules are synthesized from DNA by a process known as *DNA transcription*.
- RNA is synthesized as a single-stranded molecule.
- RNA synthesis is a highly selective process.
- One percent of the entire human DNA nucleotide sequence is transcribed into functional RNA sequences.
- Exons are the DNA nucleotide sequences that code for proteins.
- Exons are separated by introns, the noncoding sequences.
- RNAs are translated into amino acid sequences.
- Each triplet of nucleotides forms a codon that specifies one amino acid.
- The rule by which different codons are translated into amino acids is called the genetic code.

Control of Gene Expression

- Gene expression can be controlled at six major steps.
  - The first and most important step is gene transcription.
  - RNA processing.
  - RNA transport control.
  - mRNA stability control.
  - Translation control.
  - Protein activity control.
- RNA synthesis begins with the binding and assembly of the *general transcription machinery* to the *promoter* region of a gene.

- Rate of transcription is regulated by gene regulatory proteins that bind to specific DNA sequences called regulatory elements.
- The balance between transcriptional activators and repressors determines the rate of transcription.

RECOMBINANT DNA TECHNOLOGY

Restriction Nucleases

- Restriction nucleases cut DNA at specific sequences.
- Each restriction nuclease will cut a DNA molecule into a series of specific fragments.
- These fragments have either cohesive ends or blunt ends.

Polymerase Chain Reaction

- Polymerase chain reaction (PCR) can enzymatically amplify a segment of DNA a billion-fold.
- To amplify a segment of DNA, two single-stranded oligonucleotides, or *primers,* must be synthesized.
- The PCR reaction mixture consists of the double-stranded DNA sequence (the template), two DNA oligonucleotide primers, heat-stable DNA polymerase, and four types of deoxynucleotide triphosphate.

DNA Sequencing

- Sequencing DNA is based on an enzymatic method requiring *in vitro* DNA synthesis.

DNA Cloning

- DNA cloning techniques allow identification of a gene of interest from the human genome.
- DNA fragments are joined to a self-replicating genetic element (a virus or a plasmid).
- Virus or plasmids are small circular DNA molecules that occur naturally and can replicate rapidly.

DNA Engineering

- DNA engineering the ability to generate new DNA molecules of any sequence.

- One powerful application of DNA engineering is the synthesis of large quantities of cellular proteins for medical application.
- Using DNA engineering techniques, it is now possible to alter the coding sequence of a gene.

Transgenic Animals

- The ultimate test of the function of a gene is to either
  - Overexpress the gene in an organism and see what effect it has.
  - Delete it from the genome.
- To overexpress a gene, the DNA fragment encoding the gene of interest, or the *transgene,* must be constructed using recombinant DNA techniques.
- The transgene DNA fragments are then introduced into the male pronucleus of a fertilized egg.
- Analyzing these animals has provided important insights into the functions of many human genes and has provided animal models of human diseases.
- A major disadvantage of using transgenic animals is that they will only reveal dominant effects of the transgene, because these animals still retain two normal copies of the gene in their genome.
- Knockout animals animals that do not express both copies of the gene of interest.
- Heterozygous males and females are generated and can then be bred to produce animals that are homozygous for the mutated gene.
- Knockout animals can be studied to determine which cellular functions are altered.

RNA Interference

- RNA interference (RNAi) is a novel technology that silences specific genes by double-stranded RNA (dsRNA).
- RNAi requires synthesis of a dsRNA that is homologous to the target gene.
- Once taken up by the cells, the dsRNA is cleaved into 21- to 23-nucleotide long RNAs called short interfering RNAs (siRNAs).
- The antisense strand of the siRNA binds to the target mRNA leading to its degradation by an RNAi silencing complex.

CELL SIGNALING

- Cells must be coordinated to form specific tissues.

- Both neighboring and distant cells influence the behavior of cells through intracellular signaling mechanisms.

Ligands and Receptors

- Cells communicate with one another by means of multiple signaling molecules.
- These signaling molecules, also called *ligands,* bind to specific proteins, called *receptors.*
- The receptor becomes activated and generates a cascade of intracellular signals.
- Cell surface receptors are divided into three classes:
  - Ion channel-coupled receptors that are involved in rapid synaptic signaling between electrically excitable cells.
  - G protein-coupled receptors that regulate G proteins.
  - Enzyme-coupled receptors that act either directly as enzymes or are associated with enzymes.
- Some extracellular signals are small hydrophobic molecules, such as steroid hormones, thyroid hormones, retinoids, and vitamin D.
  - Communicate with target cells by diffusing across the plasma membrane and binding to intracellular receptors.

G Protein-Coupled Receptors

- G protein-coupled receptors are the largest family of cell surface receptors.
- The receptors share an intracellular domain that binds to a specific trimeric G protein.
- Activated trimeric G protein alters the concentrations of one or more small intracellular signaling molecules, referred to as *second messengers.*
- Two major second messengers regulated by G protein-coupled receptors are cyclic AMP (cAMP) and calcium.

Enzyme-Coupled Receptors

- Enzyme-coupled receptors are a diverse family of transmembrane proteins with similar structure.
- Each receptor has an extracellular ligand-binding domain and a cytosolic domain that either has intrinsic enzyme activity or is associated directly with an enzyme.
- Some receptors have guanylyl cyclase activity.
- Others have tyrosine kinase activity.
- Some enzyme-coupled receptors have serine and threonine kinase activities.

- Receptors for most known growth factors belong to the tyrosine kinase receptor family.
- Activated receptor kinase initiates an intracellular relay system.
- The Ras proteins serve as crucial links in the signaling cascade.

CELL DIVISION CYCLE

- Cell division cycle is the fundamental means by which organisms propagate and by which normal tissue homeostasis is maintained.
- The cell division cycle is divided into four distinct phases.
  - Replication of DNA occurs in the S phase (S = synthesis).
  - Nuclear division and fission occur in the mitotic phase, or M phase.
  - Intervals between the two phases are called the G_1 and G_2 phases (G = gap).

Cyclin, Cyclin-Dependent Kinase (Cdk), and Cdk Inhibitory Protein (CKI) Regulate Cell Division Cycle

- The progression of the mammalian cell cycle through specific phases is governed by the sequential activation and inactivation of a highly conserved family of regulatory proteins, cyclin-dependent kinases (Cdks).
- Cdk activation requires binding of cyclin.
- Cdk activities are inhibited by Cdk inhibitory proteins (CKIs).

Cell Cycle Checkpoints

- Two key checkpoints G_1/S and the G_2/M transitions.
- G_1 is dependent on Cdk4 and Cdk6, which are activated by association with one of the D-type cyclins: D1, D2, or D3.
- Cdk1 (cdc2) is essential for the transition from G_2 into the M phase.
- There are two families of Cdk inhibitory proteins: the CIP/KIP family and the INK family.
- A key target of the G_1 Cdks is the retinoblastoma tumor suppressor protein (pRb).

Oncogenes and Tumor Suppressor Genes

- Cell cycle regulatory proteins are often targets of mutations.
- If the mutated gene is cancer causing, it is referred to as an *oncogene* and its normal counterpart is called a *proto-oncogene*.

- *Tumor suppressor genes* prevent excess and uncontrolled cellular proliferation and these genes are inactivated in some forms of cancer.

Apoptosis

- Physiologic cell death is a genetic program pathway and is called *apoptosis*.

Biochemical and Morphologic Features of Apoptosis

- Apoptosis is a highly regulated energy-requiring form of cell death that is genetically programmed.
- In the early phase of apoptosis, cells exhibit a shrunken cytoplasm.
- One of the earliest biochemical features of apoptotic cells is the externalization of phosphatidyl serine residues on the plasma membrane.
- Middle events include chromatin condensation with resultant crescent-shaped nuclei and subsequent nuclear fragmentation.
- Late in apoptosis, the cells begin to fragment into discrete plasma membrane-bound vesicles termed *apoptotic bodies,* which are then phagocytized by neighboring cells and macrophages without inducing an inflammatory response.
- The molecular machinery that governs apoptosis can be divided into three parts:
  - Signaling of apoptosis by a stimulus.
  - Regulation by proapoptotic and antiapoptotic factors.
  - Activation of the cell s execution (i.e., death) pathways.

Apoptotic Stimuli

- Many stimuli activate the process of apoptosis:
  - DNA damage through ionizing radiation.
  - Growth factor and nutritional deprivation.
  - Activation of certain death receptors (e.g., Fas receptor [FasR] and tumor necrosis factor receptor [TNF-R1]).
  - Metabolic or cell cycle perturbations.
  - Oxidative stress.
  - Many chemotherapeutic agents.

Bcl-2 Family

- Apoptosis is regulated by the expression of certain intracellular proteins belonging to the *Bcl-2* family of genes.

- Bcl-2 is a potent inhibitor of apoptosis.
- Bcl-x_s, Bax, Bak, and Bad function as proapoptotic regulators.

Caspases

- Caspases, or *c*ysteine *aspa*rtate protea*ses*, are proteolytic enzymes synthesized as inactive proenzymes requiring cleavage for activation.
- Activated caspases results in the destruction of cytoskeletal and structural proteins, nuclear structural components, and cell adhesion factors.

HUMAN GENOME PROJECT

- Identification and sequencing of the entire human genome.
- Human Genome Project has provided new information on the genetic variations in the human population by identifying DNA variants such as single nucleotide polymorphisms.
- Single nucleotide polymorphisms are thought to serve as genetic markers for identifying diseased genes by linkage studies in families.
- Assess an array of genes that may change (either increase or decrease) over time or with treatment.
- DNA chips provide for one of the most promising approaches to large-scale studies of genetic variations.

Transplantation

- Significant impediment remains the availability of suitable organs.
- Human Genome Project may enable transplant investigators to genetically engineer animals.
- Pluripotent stem cells have the ability to divide without limit and to give rise to many types of differentiated and specialized tissues with a specific purpose.

Oncology

- The results of the Human Genome Project will have far reaching effects on diagnostic studies, treatment, and counseling of cancer patients and family members.
- Screening for high-risk groups.
- Prophylactic surgery may soon become more prevalent as a first-line treatment in the fight against cancer.
- For example, the discovery of the association between mutations of the *ret* proto-oncogene and hereditary medullarly

thyroid carcinoma has allowed surgeons to identify patients who will eventually develop medullary thyroid cancer.
- Another area of controversy is in the treatment of patients with mutations of the breast cancer susceptibility genes, *BRCA-1* and *BRCA-2*.

Pediatric and Fetal Surgery

- Prenatal diagnostic testing and screening.

NOVEL TREATMENT STRATEGIES

Gene Therapy

- Genetic makeup of the patient s cells.
- Two strategies: germline and somatic cell gene therapy.
- A wide array of somatic cell gene therapy protocols designed to treat single-gene diseases, a variety of cancers, or human immunodeficiency virus (HIV) are currently under development with some gene therapy protocols in clinical trials.
- Goals:
  - To repair or compensate for a defective gene.
  - To enhance the immune response directed at a tumor or pathogen.
  - To protect vulnerable cell populations.
  - To kill tumor cells.
- Many protocols for the treatment of cancer are under evaluation:
  - Alteration of cancer cells.
  - Host cells to produce cytokines.
- A repertoire of viral-based vectors has been analyzed:
  - Retroviruses.
  - Nonviral systems.
  - Liposomes.
  - DNA-protein conjugates.
  - DNA-protein-defective virus conjugates.

Drug Design

- Based on information from the fields of genomics and structural biology, rational drug design can be devised to treat a host of diseases.
- The identification of human genetic variations will eventually allow clinicians to subclassify diseases and adapt therapies that are appropriate to the individual patient.

- These observations have spawned the field of pharmacogenomics, which attempts to use information regarding genetic variations in patients to predict responses to drug therapies.

Genetic Engineering of Antibodies

- Genetic engineering has allowed for the modification of mouse monoclonal antibodies to reduce the immune response directed against them.

ETHICAL, PHYSIOLOGIC, AND LEGAL IMPLICATIONS

- Genetic-based medicine.
- Ethical, psychologic, and legal implications.
- Ownership of the genetic information.
- Access to information.
- Counsel both the patient and other family members.

CHAPTER 3

THE ROLE OF CYTOKINES AS MEDIATORS OF THE INFLAMMATORY RESPONSE

- Inflammation is fundamentally a protective response.
- Inflammation connotes not only localized effects, such as edema, hyperemia, and leukocytic infiltration, but also systemic phenomena, for example, fever and increased synthesis of certain acute-phase proteins.
- Septic shock is the clinical manifestation of a systemic inflammatory response run amok.

BASIC DEFINITIONS AND CLASSIFICATION SYSTEMS

- Cytokines are small proteins or glycoproteins secreted for the purpose of altering the function of target cells in an endocrine, paracrine, or autocrine fashion.
- Many cytokines are pleiotropic (Table 3–1).

INTERFERON-γ

- The immune response to infection has two broad components.
- The innate responses, which occur early and are not antigen specific, depend largely on the proper functioning of natural killer (NK) cells.
- The acquired responses, which develop later after antigen processing and the clonal expansion of T- and B-cell subsets, are antigen specific.
- A number of cytokines, including transforming growth factor-β (TGF-β), tumor necrosis factor (TNF), interleukin (IL)-1, IL-6, IL-10, IL-12, and IL-18, are synthesized by cells of the innate immune system and contribute to the ability of the host to mount an early, innate immune response to an infectious challenge (Fig. 3–1).

TABLE 3–1. Cellular Sources and Important Biologic Effects of Selected Cytokines

Cytokine	Abbreviation	Main Source(s)	Important Biologic Effect(s)
Tumor necrosis factor	TNF	Mφ*, others	See Table 3-3
Lymphotoxin-α	LT-α	T$_H$1†,NK‡	Same as TNF
Interferon-α	IFN-α	Leukocytes	Increases expression of cell-surface class I major histocompatibility complex (MHC) molecules; inhibits viral replication
Interferon-β	IFN-β	Fibroblasts	Same as IFN-α
Interferon-γ	IFN-γ	T$_H$1	Activates Mφ; promotes differentiation of CD4⁺ T cells into T$_H$1 cells; inhibits differentiation of CD4⁺ T cells into T$_H$2 cells
Interleukin-1α	IL-1α	Keratinocytes, others	See Table 3-3
Interleukin-1β	IL-1β	Mφ, NK, PMN§, others	See Table 3-3
Interleukin-2	IL-2	T$_H$1	In combination with other stimuli, promotes proliferation of T cells; promotes proliferation of activated B cells; stimulates secretion of cytokines by T cells; increases cytotoxicity of NK cells
Interleukin-3	IL-3	T cells	Stimulates pluripotent bone marrow stem cells, increasing production of leukocytes, erythrocytes, and platelets
Interleukin-4	IL-4	T$_H$2	Promotes growth and differentiation of B cells; promotes differentiation of CD4⁺ T cells into T$_H$2 cells; inhibits secretion of proinflammatory cytokines by Mφ
Interleukin-5	IL-5	T cells, mast cells	Induces production of eosinophils from myeloid precursor cells
Interleukin-6	IL-6	Mφ, T$_H$2, enterocytes, others	Induces fever; promotes B-cell maturation and differentiation; stimulates hypothalamic-pituitary-adrenal axis; induces hepatic synthesis of acute-phase proteins
Interleukin-8	IL-8	Mφ, endothelial cells, others	Stimulates chemotaxis by PMN; stimulates oxidative burst by PMN
Interleukin-9	IL-9	T$_H$2	Promotes proliferation of activated T cells; promotes immunoglobulin secretion by B cells

Interleukin-10	IL-10	T$_H$2, Mφ	Inhibits secretion of proinflammatory cytokines by Mφ
Interleukin-11	IL-11	Neurons, fibroblasts, others	Increases production of platelets; inhibits proliferation of enterocytes
Interleukin-12	IL-12	Mφ	Promotes differentiation of CD4+ T cells into T$_H$1 cells; enhances IFN-γ secretion by T$_H$1 cells and NK cells
Interleukin-13	IL-13	T$_H$2, others	Inhibits secretion of proinflammatory cytokines by Mφ
Interleukin-18	IL-18	Mφ, others	Co-stimulation with IL-12 of IFN-γ secretion by T$_H$1 cells and NK cells
Monocyte chemotactic protein-1	MCP-1	Mφ, endothelial cells, others	Stimulates chemotaxis by monocytes; stimulates oxidative burst by macrophages
Granulocyte-macrophage colony-stimulating factor	GM-CSF	T cells, Mφ, endothelial cells, others	Enhances production by the bone marrow of granulocytes and monocytes; primes Mφ to produce proinflammatory mediators after activation by another stimulus
Granulocyte colony-stimulating factor	G-CSF	Mφ fibroblasts	Enhances production by the bone marrow of granulocytes
Erythropoietin	EPO	Kidney cells	Enhances production by the bone marrow of erythrocytes
Transforming growth factor-β	TGF-β	T cells, Mφ, platelets, others	Stimulates chemotaxis by monocytes and fibroblasts; induces synthesis of extracellular matrix proteins by fibroblasts; inhibits secretion of cytokines by T cells; inhibits immunoglobulin secretion by B cells; downregulates activation of NK cells

*Cells of the monocyte-macrophage lineage.
†T$_H$1 subset of differentiated CD4+ T helper cells.
‡Natural killer cells.
§Polymorphonuclear neutrophils.
¶T$_H$2 subset of differentiated CD4+ T helper cells.

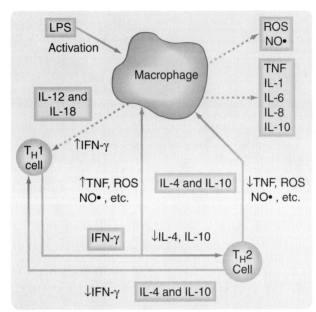

■ **FIGURE 3–1.** Simplified representation of the responses of three important cell types (macrophages, T helper cells with a T_H1 phenotype, and T helper cells with a T_H2 phenotype) involved in the inflammatory response to an archetypical proinflammatory stimulus, namely exposure to lipopolysaccharide (LPS), a component of the outer cell wall of Gram-negative bacteria. In response to stimulation by LPS, macrophages secrete the cytokines, IL-12 and IL-18. IL-12 promotes the differentiation of naive $CD4^+$ T cells (T_H0 cells) into T_H1 cells capable of producing IFN-γ following activation, and together IL-12 and IL-18 stimulate secretion of IFN-γ by T_H1 cells. IFN-γ, in turn, further upregulates the production of proinflammatory cytokines (e.g., TNF, IL-1, IL-6, and IL-8) and other pro-inflammatory mediators (e.g., reactive oxygen species [ROS] and nitric oxide [NO]) by LPS-stimulated macrophages. IFN-γ also downregulates production of anti-inflammatory cytokines (IL-4 and IL-10) by T_H2 cells. IL-4 and IL-10 act to downregulate production of IFN-γ by T_H1 cells and production of proinflammatory cytokines and other proinflammatory mediators by macrophages. IL-10 is not only produced by T_H2 cells, but it is also secreted by stimulated macrophages as well, creating an autocrine negative feedback loop.

- Interferon (IFN)-γ has a central role in the innate immune response to microbial invasion, particularly by intracellular pathogens.
- Signaling induced by binding of IFN-γ to its receptor results in signal transduction via activation of a protein tyrosine phosphorylation cascade known as the JAK-STAT pathway.

INTERLEUKIN-1 AND TUMOR NECROSIS FACTOR

- IL-1 and TNF are structurally dissimilar pluripotent cytokines.
- Although these compounds bind to different cellular receptors, their multiple biological activities overlap considerably.
- Many of the biological effects of either IL-1 or TNF are greatly potentiated by the presence of the other cytokines (Tables 3–2 and 3–3).

Interleukin-1

- IL-1 is an extremely potent mediator and is synthesized by a wide variety of cell types, including monocytes, macrophages, B lymphocytes, T lymphocytes, NK cells, keratinocytes, dendritic cells, fibroblasts, neutrophils, endothelial cells, and enterocytes.

TABLE 3–2. Partial List of the Physiologic Effects Induced by Infusing Human Subjects IL-1 or TNF

Effect	IL-1	TNF
Fever	+	+
Headache	+	+
Anorexia	+	+
Increased plasma ACTH level	+	+
Hypercortisolemia	+	+
Increased plasma nitrite/nitrate levels	+	+
Systemic arterial hypotension	+	+
Neutrophilia	+	+
Transient neutropenia	+	+
Increased plasma acute-phase protein levels	+	+
Hypoferremia	+	+
Hypozincemia		+
Increased plasma level of IL-1RA	+	+
Increased plasma level of TNF-R1 and TNF-R2	+	+
Increased plasma leve of IL-6	+	+
Increased plasma level of IL-8	+	+
Activation of coagulation cascades	-	+
Increased platelet count	+	-
Pulmonary edema	-	+
Hepatocellular injury	-	+

TABLE 3–3. Partial List of the Effects of IL-1 and TNF on Various Target Cells

Cell Type	Important Effects	IL-1	TNF
T cell	IL-2 synthesis	↑	↑
	IL-2R expression	↑	↑
Monocyte/macrophage	IL-1 synthesis	↑	
	TNF synthesis	↑	
	IL-6 synthesis	↑	↑
	IL-10 synthesis	↑	
	GM-CSF synthesis	↑	→
	G-CSF synthesis	↑	↑
	Prostaglandin synthesis	↑	→
	Tissue factor expression	↑	↑
Neutrophils	Complement receptor 3 expression	→	↑
	IL-8 synthesis	↑	↑
	Priming for increased oxidant production	↑	↑
Endothelial cells	GM-CSF synthesis	↑	↑
	G-CSF synthesis	↑	↑
	Prostacyclin synthesis	↑	↑
	E-selectin expression	↑	↑
	VCAM-1 expression	↑	↑
	ICAM-1 expression	↑	↑
	Tissue factor expression	↑	↑
Hepatocytes	Albumin synthesis	↓	↓
	C-reactive protein synthesis	↑	↓
	Insulin-like growth factor-1 synthesis	↓	↓
	Complement component 3	↑	↑
	Inducible nitric oxide synthase expression	↑	→
Fibroblasts	Hepatocyte growth factor synthesis	↑	↑
	Vascular endothelial growth factor	↑	→

- Many IL-1-induced physiologic effects occur as a result of enhanced biosynthesis of other inflammatory mediators, including prostaglandin E_2 (PGE_2) and nitric oxide; thus, IL-1 increases expression of the enzyme cyclooxygenase-2 (COX-2).

Tumor Necrosis Factor

- TNF is a pivotal mediator of endotoxic shock in animals.
- Although cells of the monocyte/macrophage lineage are the major sources of TNF, other cell types, including mast

cells, keratinocytes, T cells, and B cells, are also capable of releasing the cytokine (Box 3–1).

- The soluble form of TNF exists as a homotrimer, a feature that is important for the cross-linking and activation of TNF receptors.

- Members of the TNF family of ligands are primarily involved with the regulation of cellular proliferation or the converse process, programmed cell death (apoptosis).

- The downstream events leading to caspase activation (apoptosis) or gene transcription (inflammation) after recruitment of TNF-receptor-associated death domain (TRADD) are exceedingly complex; a deliberately oversimplified model is depicted in Figure 3–2.

Interleukin-1 and/or Tumor Necrosis Factor as Targets for Anti-Inflammatory Therapeutic Agents

- In view of the central importance of IL-1 and TNF as mediators of the inflammatory response, investigators have regarded blocking the production or the actions of these cytokines as a reasonable strategy for treating a variety of

---

Box 3–1. Partial List of Stimuli Known to Initiate Release of Tumor Necrosis Factor

Endogenous Factors
Cytokines (TNF-α, IL-1, IFN-γ, GM-CSF, IL-2)
Platelet-activating factor
Myelin P2 protein
HMGB1
HSP70
HSP60

Microbe-Derived Factors
Lipopolysaccharide
Zymosan
Peptidoglycan
Streptococcal pyrogenic exotoxin A
Streptolysin O
Lipoteichoic acid
Staphylococcal enterotoxin B
Staphylococcal toxic shock syndrome toxin-1
Bacterial (CpG) DNA
Flagellin

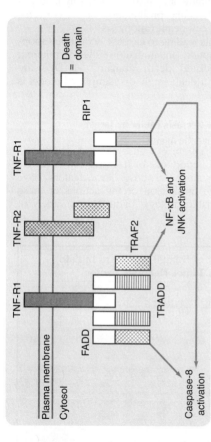

■ **FIGURE 3–2.** Simplified view of intracellular signal transduction events initiated by binding of TNF to its cellular receptors. There are two TNF receptors, called TNF-R1 and TNF-R2. Both receptors are homodimeric transmembrane proteins. Although both TNF-R1 and TNF-R2 are capable of initiating signal transduction, different pathways are involved. After TNF binds to TNF-R1, a number of proteins, including receptor interacting protein (RIP), Fas-associated death protein (FADD), and TNF-receptor-associated death domain (TRADD), associate with the receptor. The intracytoplasmic tail of TNF-R1 and portions of these other signaling molecules share a highly conserved sequence of about 80 amino acids, which is called the "death domain." Homotypic interactions among the death domains of these various proteins are essential for formation of the functional signaling complex. After docking to the receptor complex, TRADD recruits other proteins (e.g., TRAF2 and MADD), which, in turn, initiate protein kinase pathways, leading to activation of the transcription factor, NF-kB, and the protein kinase, c-JUN N-terminal kinase (JNK). TRAF2 also can interact with TNF-R2. Association of FADD with the TNF-R1 receptor complex leads to activation of the proteolytic enzyme, caspase-8, which is the proximal element in a signaling cascade leading to apoptosis ("programmed cell death").

conditions associated with excessive or poorly controlled inflammation.

- At least two agents designed to neutralize the effects of secreted TNF have been shown to have significant clinical efficacy in other important inflammatory conditions, such as Crohn's disease and rheumatoid arthritis.
- Infliximab, a monoclonal anti-TNF antibody, has been approved by the U.S. Food and Drug Administration for the treatment of enteric fistulas secondary to Crohn's disease.

INTERLEUKIN-6 AND INTERLEUKIN-11

- IL-6 is a pluripotent cytokine that is produced not only by immunocytes (e.g., monocytes, macrophages, and lymphocytes) but also by many other cell types, including endothelial cells and intestinal epithelial cells.
- Factors known to induce expression of IL-6 include IL-1, TNF, platelet activating factor, LPS, and reactive oxygen metabolites.
- Physiologic effects of IL-6 are diverse and include induction of fever, promotion of B-cell maturation and differentiation, stimulation of T-cell proliferation and differentiation, promotion of differentiation of nerve cells, stimulation of the hypothalamic-pituitary-adrenal axis, and induction of synthesis of acute phase proteins (e.g., C-reactive protein) by hepatocytes.
- IL-11 is expressed in a variety of cell types; expression of IL-11 can also be upregulated by IL-1, TGF-β, and other cytokines or growth factors.
- IL-11 is a hematopoietic growth factor, having particular activity as stimulator of megakaryocytopoiesis and thrombopoiesis.
- Activation of target cells via the IL-6 or IL-11 receptor complexes requires the cooperation of two distinct proteins.
- For both receptors, a distinct protein, called gp130, is required for signal transduction.
- Signal transduction involves the association of the IL-6/IL-6R complex or the IL-11/IL-11R complex with gp130.
- Dimerization of gp130 leads to downstream signaling via members of the JAK family of protein tyrosine kinases.
- JAK kinase activation leads, in turn, to phosphorylation and activation of STAT3, a member of the STAT family of signaling proteins.
- Elevated plasma levels of IL-6 are consistently observed in patients with sepsis or septic shock.

- IL-11 is under active investigation as a therapeutic agent for a number of indications, including stimulation of thrombopoiesis in patients receiving cytotoxic chemotherapy for malignancies and treatment of Crohn's disease.

INTERLEUKIN-8 AND OTHER CHEMOKINES

- The ability to recruit leukocytes to an inflammatory focus by promoting chemotaxis is the primary biological activity of a special group of cytokines called chemokines.
- Each chemokine contains about 70 to 80 amino acids, including three or four conserved cysteine residues.
- The four chemokine subgroups are defined by the degree of separation of the first two NH_2-terminal cysteine residues: the CXC or α-chemokines and the CC or β-chemokines.
- CXC chemokines, exemplified by IL-8, contain a characteristic amino acid sequence (glutamate-leucine-arginine); these chemokines act primarily on polymorphonuclear neutrophils.
- Other chemokines, including the CC chemokines and members of CXC subgroup not containing the glutamate-leucine-arginine sequence, act, for the most part, on monocytes, macrophages, lymphocytes, or eosinophils.
- Many different cell types are capable of secreting chemokines; cells of monocyte/macrophage lineage and endothelial cells are particularly important in this regard.

INTERLEUKIN-12 AND INTERLEUKIN-18

- IL-12 is a cytokine produced primarily by antigen-presenting cells.
- The most important biological activity associated with Il-12 is to promote Th1 responses by T helper cells; IL-12 promotes the differentiation of naïve T cells into Th1 cells capable of producing IFN-γ after activation.
- IL-12 also has been implicated in the pathogenesis of inflammatory bowel disease.
- IL-18 is structurally related to IL-1β and functionally a member of the Th1-inducing family of cytokines.
- The main biological activity of IL-18 is to induce production of IFN-γ by T cells and NK cells.
- IL-18 acts most potently as costimulant in combination with Il-12.
- IL-18 has also been shown to induce production of CC and CXC chemokines from human mononuclear cells.

INTERLEUKIN-4, INTERLEUKIN-10, AND INTERLEUKIN-13

- IL-4, Il-10, and Il-13 can be regarded as inhibitory, anti-inflammatory, or counter-regulatory cytokines.
- All three of these cytokines are produced by Th2 cells and, among other roles, serve to modulate the production and effects of proinflammatory cytokines like TNF and IL-1.
- IL-4 inhibits the production of TNF, IL-1, IL-8, and PGE$_2$ by stimulated monocytes or macrophages and downregulates endothelial cell activation induced by TNF.
- IL-10 is an 18-kD protein that is produced primarily by Th2 cells but is also released by activated monocytes and other cell types.
  - IL-10 acts to downregulate the inflammatory response through numerous mechanisms.
  - IL-10 inhibits production of numerous proinflammatory cytokines, including IL-1, TNF, IL-6, IL-8, IL-12, and GM-CSF, by monocytes and macrophages.
  - IL-10 downregulates the proliferation and secretion of IFN-γ primarily by inhibiting the production of IL-12 by macrophages.
- In trauma and burn patients, increased production of IL-10 has been associated with a greater risk of serious infection, and in patients with sepsis, a greater risk of mortality or shock.
- These findings support the view that whereas excessive production of proinflammatory mediators may be deleterious in trauma and sepsis, the development of the Th2 phenotype, characterized by markedly increased production of IL-10 and IL-4, may lead to excessive immunosuppression and may deleteriously affect outcome on this basis.
- IL-13 is a 12-kD protein closely related to IL-4.
- Binding of either IL-4 or IL-13 to their respective receptors induces signaling by activating the same JAK kinases, JAK1 and Tyk2; IL-4, but not IL-13, also activates JAK3.
- IL-13 downregulates production of proinflammatory cytokines (e.g., IL-1, TNF, IL-6, IL-8, IL-12, G-CSF, GM-CSF, and macrophage inflammatory protein-1α).

INDUCIBLE NITRIC OXIDE SYNTHASE AND CYCLOOXYGENASE-2

- Downstream actions of the proinflammatory cytokines occur as a result of increased expression of two key enzymes, iNOS (NOS-2) and COX-2.
- Biological actions of nitric oxide (NO), including vasodilatation, induction of vascular hyperpermeability, and inhibition

of platelet aggregation, are mediated through activation of the enzyme soluble guanylyl cyclase (sGC).

- Excessive production of NO as a result of iNOS induction in vascular smooth muscle cells is thought to be a major factor contributing to the loss of vasomotor tone and the loss of responsiveness to vasopressor agents ("vasoplegia") in patients with septic shock.

- COX-1 and COX-2 catalyze the stereospecific oxidation of arachidonate to form the cyclic endoperoxide PGG_2.

- The prostaglandins, including PGE_2 and PGI_2 (prostacyclin), and thromboxane A_2 (TxA_2) are lipid mediators derived from the unstable intermediate compound PGG_2.

- Both of these reactions are major regulatory steps in the formation of prostaglandins and TxA_2.

- COX-1 is expressed constitutively in a variety of tissues, and mediators produced by this isoform are thought to be important in a variety of homeostatic processes, such as regulating renal perfusion and salt and water handling, maintaining hemostasis by modulating platelet aggregation, and preserving gastrointestinal mucosal integrity.

- COX-2, however, is an inducible enzyme like iNOS; COX-2 expression is induced by a number of stimuli, including various growth factors and proinflammatory cytokines.

- Interestingly, the functional activity of COX-2 depends on activation of the enzyme.

- Activation of COX-2 is thought to be mediated by the powerful oxidant $ONOO^-$, thereby providing a tight functional linkage between the NO and the prostaglandin mediator systems.

- Pharmacologic inhibition of cyclooxygenase activity is the basis for the anti-inflammatory actions of the class of compounds known as nonsteroidal anti-inflammatory drugs.

- Some adverse side effects of these agents (e.g., gastric mucosal ulceration) are thought to be mediated by inhibition of COX-1.

- Identification of COX-2 as the "inflammatory" isoform of cyclooxygenase led to intense efforts to develop drugs selective for the inducible enzyme.

- The recent introduction into clinical practice of COX-2 selective agents represents a potential advance in pharmacology and holds the promise of a safer approach.

CHAPTER 4

SHOCK, ELECTROLYTES, AND FLUID

INTRODUCTION

- In health, an individual maintains physiologic balance termed "homeostasis." The body is divided into compartments separated by membranes of variable permeability characteristics. Each compartment has a different composition, and within each is a directed flow of fluid and movement of solutes. The physiologic balance of homeostasis controls the exchange of water and solutes between these compartments. In a healthy individual a wide range of physiologic systems are coordinated and in equipoise.
- Homeostasis is maintained only if there is adequate delivery of energy, fuels, and oxygen to cells.
- Shock is a circumstance in which homeostasis is disrupted. A universal physiologic threat to the patient in shock is deficient oxygen delivery to the mitochondria of cells. As a consequence, aerobic metabolism cannot be sustained at the rate needed to maintain cell function. The cell cannot recover from sustained interruption of aerobic metabolism.
- An emphasis on therapy that measurably influences whole organ function should not deflect the appreciation that patient survival will ultimately be determined by events within cells.

BODY WATER AND SOLUTE COMPOSITION

Total Body Water

- In most adults, water accounts for 45% to 60% of the total body weight.
- The proportion of the body weight made up of fat is associated with the variance of total body water (TBW) per kilogram of body weight in both genders.
- Investigators have measured TBW in humans using indicator dilution methods with deuterium oxide (D_2O—an isotope of

water), tritium and nonradioactive water enriched with the heavy isotope ^{18}O.

- Predicting the body composition of an individual patient should be done with models that include age, gender, and race (as independent predictor variables), as well as the standard measures of stature such as height and weight.

Compartments of Total Body Water

- TBW largely distributes in two compartments, the intracellular water (ICW) and extracellular water (ECW) spaces.
- ECW accounts for 20% of the total body weight.
- Movement of solutes—particularly sodium and potassium—across the cell membrane is both tightly controlled and energy-dependent. In contrast, water moves passively and quickly across the cell membranes separating the ECW and ICW. Water moves to establish osmotic equilibrium between these two compartments.
- Several methods can be used to measure the size of ECW and ICW in humans.
- TBW can be measured via indicator dilution methods, most commonly with deuterium oxide (D_2O).
- ECW can be measured as the distribution volume of bromide (administered as NaBr) or sulfate ($^{35}SO_4$), although new methods using heavy isotopes of sulfate have been reported that have the advantage of avoiding patient exposure to radioactive isotopes.
- Bioimpedance spectroscopy has been reported as a useful and clinically practical method of measuring ECW and ICW.
- Most potassium in the human body is found within the cells, and measures of the entire body potassium content can be used to indicate ICW.
- A patient with a smaller intracellular space compared with normal controls is a patient with measurable deficits in lean body mass and functional reserve.

Filtered Plasma Forms Interstitial Fluid

- The ECW is subdivided into the plasma and interstitial compartments. Fluid and solutes circulate from the plasma compartment to the interstitial compartments and back to the plasma compartment via lymphatics.
- The plasma volume is measured by indicator dilution methods, which depend on intravenous injection of a large molecule that can be easily assayed. Considerable experience has been reported using radioactive-labeled albumin.

- Clinical investigators have also used Evans Blue dye (which preferentially binds albumin) or indocyanine green dye as alternatives to radioactive-labeled albumin.

EXTRACELLULAR WATER AND ELECTROLYTES

Control of Extracellular Sodium

- Sodium is the predominant cation in ECW and associates with the anions chloride and bicarbonate. These three electrolytes constitute more than 90% of the active osmoles in the ECW. The predominant cation in ICW is potassium, which is electrochemically balanced primarily by organic phosphates.
- The difference in electrolyte composition between ICW and ECW is sustained because the normally functioning cell membrane, predominantly composed of lipids, acts as a barrier to sodium.
- The ubiquitous enzyme Na^+/K^+-ATPase, for example, plays a key role in sustaining the difference in electrolyte composition of the ECW and ICW. Na^+/K^+-ATPase, also known as the "sodium pump," moves sodium across the cell membrane by undergoing molecular conformational changes that consume energy. The pump binds three sodium ions in the ICW, and then energy provided by hydrolysis of ATP to ADP changes the conformation within the Na^+/K^+-ATPase enzyme. The bonded intracellular sodium is then moved across the membrane and released into the extracellular fluid. Two potassium ions enter the cell in association with the three sodium ions leaving the cell in active transport by Na^+/K^+-ATPase. With three cations out and two cations into the cell, the electrochemical consequence is a net negative intracellular charge termed the "resting membrane potential." Most anionic molecules in the cell are large, cannot diffuse across the cell membrane, and thus are restricted to ICW; these negatively charged macromolecules contribute to resting membrane potential. Voltage of the resting membrane potential is essential for cell function and is the basis for nerve cell conduction and muscle cell contraction.
- The substantial difference between potassium concentration in ICW and ECW favors diffusion of potassium along a concentration gradient to the ECW. The transport of potassium along this gradient is passive, meaning no energy is required. However, the negative charge of the resting membrane potential powerfully favors potassium to remain intracellular.

Total Body Sodium Mass Determines the Size of the Extracellular Water Compartment and Is Regulated by Renal Function

- The nephron is the basic functional unit of renal function. Patients with normal renal function have glomerular filtration rates in excess of 100 mL per minute.
- Renal tubular function varies along the path of the nephron, and four regions of distinct function have been defined:
    - The proximal convoluted tubule.
    - The thin descending and thick ascending limbs of the loop of Henle.
    - The distal convoluted tubule.
    - The medullary collecting duct, which transverses the renal medulla and drains urine into the renal pelvis.
- At the luminal surface of cells in the proximal convoluted tubules 60% to 70% of the filtered sodium and water is absorbed into cells.
- Most filtered bicarbonate is absorbed in the proximal convoluted tubule through specific pores on the luminal surface of the cell.
- This movement of solute in the loop of Henle's countercurrent structure produces the hypertonic environment within the medullary section essential for the reabsorption of water from the collecting ducts.
- In the distal convoluted segment, aldosterone and natriuretic peptides influence sodium absorption from the filtrate.
- The final segment of the nephron is the collecting duct, which passes through the hypertonic interstitial fluid of the medullary portion of the kidney. Water absorption from the filtrate, which enables the production of concentrated urine and thus when the individual is threatened by dehydration preserves TBW, is accomplished in the collecting duct under the control of the hormone arginine vasopressin.

Extracellular Water Homeostasis in Pathologic Circumstances

- In circumstances of shock, serious infection, burn, or pathologic loss of body fluids, the mechanisms that maintain the homeostasis of the ECW and its solutes can be overwhelmed.
- Reflex mechanisms of survival advantage in these circumstances include both short-term depletion of ICW to preserve ECW size and shifts of interstitial fluid to the plasma volume. These mechanisms preserve blood volume and especially the flow of blood to vital organs.

- After an episode of shock and resuscitation, patients have a substantial perturbation in composition, including an expanded ECW space and excess sodium. Multiple homeostatic mechanisms lead to a restoration of normal ECW size and composition. These include intrinsic renal function.

- Natriuretic peptides are a family of at least three molecules, named atrial natriuretic peptide (ANP), brain natriuretic peptide (BNP), and C-type natriuretic peptide.

- Both ANP and BNP are elevated in patients with hypertension, expanded blood volume, congestive heart failure, and other forms of heart disease. Compensatory cardiovascular actions of ANP and BNP include arterial smooth muscle relaxation and vasodilation and increased microvascular membrane permeability. These latter actions result in a shift of plasma fluid and proteins into the interstitium that, combined with venous capacitance vessel dilation, reduces cardiac preload.

- C-type natriuretic peptides have been identified in vascular smooth muscle cells as well as endothelial cells, and are hypothesized to act locally to produce paracrine or autocrine vasodilation.

- Control of the ECW size is influenced by a second major physiologic mechanism that influences the ECW osmolality. Arginine vasopressin (AVP) is a peptide synthesized in the hypothalamus and is released when ECW osmolality exceeds 280 mOsm/L. This molecule increases the absorption of water from the distal tubule in the nephron. As more water is absorbed and urine osmolality exceeds ECW osmolality, the net result is gain in ECW.

- In summary, the body has two parallel but separate groups of physiologic mechanisms for control of ECW. Sodium balance is determined by renal function, which is regulated by hormones. As osmolality exceeds its threshold, a second and independent mechanism dependent upon AVP becomes activated, resulting in a net gain of body water.

- In normal conditions, osmolality and sodium balance are modulated within a narrow range. In shock caused by acute depletion of ECW through hemorrhage, these compensatory mechanisms are stressed to produce a rapid correction.

BIOCHEMISTRY AND PHYSIOLOGY OF ACID-BASE REGULATION

- With its single positive charge and the lowest elemental molecular weight, the ubiquitous proton influences all vital biochemical reactions. The molar concentration of protons in ECW, $[H^+]$, is normally 40 ± 2 nmol/L. Proton concentration is maintained in a narrow range by multiple regulatory pathways.

- In clinical practice, [H^+] is measured as pH, the logarithm to the base 10 of 1/[H^+, nmol/L]. The normal plasma pH value is 7.40. Patients with excess protons in arterial blood have an acidemia. Patients with an arterial pH below 7.40 have an alkalemia. Patients with acid-base disorders that produce a pH less than 7.00 or a pH greater than 7.70 have low rates of survival; therefore, homeostasis of pH is critical.
- An adult consuming a standard Western diet generates 50 to 100 mEq of protons daily from absorbed nutrients. Renal function principally eliminates the excess protons as the urinary solutes NH_4^+ and $H_2PO_4^-$.
- Two physiologic functions protect the body against substantial falls in pH following the sudden release of a large number of protons: the neutralizing capacity of buffers and the exhalation of CO_2 by the lungs.
- Bicarbonate is the predominate buffer in ICW and ECW. Protons and one bicarbonate reversibly combine to form carbonic acid (H_2CO_3). Carbonic acid can further disassociate into water and the gas CO_2. In pulmonary capillaries, the CO_2 in blood readily diffuses into alveoli. This loss of CO_2 drives the conversion of more carbonic acid into CO_2 to be exhaled as a respiratory gas. As CO_2 is exhaled, the body achieves a net proton loss.
- Bicarbonate acts as a major buffer in ICW and ECW, but proteins are important buffers only in ICW. Hydrogen ions can bind the imidazole site in the amino acid histidine present in cell proteins; however, as a consequence, bound protons can adversely alter the protein's charge and function. The third major system for intracellular buffering involves inorganic phosphates.
- The inorganic phosphate buffer system accounts for less than 10% of intracellular buffer capacity and makes only a minimal contribution to control of extracellular pH.
- The ICW pH is 7.10, substantially lower than the normal ECW pH of 7.40.
- Although the transport of ions across the cell membrane is restricted, the neutral gas CO_2 readily crosses cell membranes. As CO_2 builds in the ECW, the bicarbonate buffer system shifts toward protons. The enzyme carbonic anhydrase accelerates the kinetics of carbonic acid hydrolysis to carbon dioxide and water and vice versa.
- Cells principally depend on the high-energy terminal phosphate bond in ATP to do this work.

- Using oxygen and fuels, oxidative phosphorylation occurs in cells, and in the mitochondria in particular, to convert ADP back to ATP. In oxidative phosphorylation, the high-energy phosphate bond and proton are recaptured.

Renal Function and Control of pH

- The kidney plays an essential role in control of the body acid-base balance, because the excess protons produced through daily dietary intake are eliminated through the urine in a tightly regulated manner. The DCT segment is critical to the control of acid-base balance.
- Aldosterone released from the adrenal gland in response to the renin-angiotensin-aldosterone axis increases tubular absorption of filtered sodium in the DCT by increasing its exchange for protons; as a result, more bicarbonate is released by the tubule cells into ECW even if the pH is greater than 7.40.

Clinical Practice and Measurement of Acid-Base Status

- Clinicians depend on analysis of arterial blood composition to assess total body acid-base balance. Three components of the arterial blood gas are used: the pH, the partial pressure of carbon dioxide ($PaCO_2$), and the bicarbonate concentration. The pH is a measure of $[H^+]$ concentration in ECW and indicates whether the ICW is acidotic or alkalotic. $PaCO_2$ provides the clinician a measure of pulmonary alveolar ventilation. Electrodes in blood gas machines enable immediate measure of the pH and $PaCO_2$, and these values can help define the patient's acid-base status using the Henderson-Hasselbalch equation.
- The Henderson-Hasselbalch equation implies the concept that two factors, bicarbonate and $PaCO_2$, are principal determinants of a patient's acid-base status. Assuming the blood sample temperature is 37°C, the Henderson-Hasselbalch equation describes normal arterial blood gas as follows:

$$pH = 7.40 = 6.1 + \log_{10}(24/1.33)$$

- The Henderson-Hasselbalch based blood gas analysis carries the advantage that a change in proton concentration is linearly proportional to changes in the two most important extracellular buffers: the bicarbonate concentration, which is influenced by renal function, and partial pressure of carbon dioxide, which is influenced by alveolar ventilation.

Acidosis and Alkalosis

- The four paradigms of acid-base disorder are metabolic acidosis, metabolic alkalosis, respiratory acidosis, and respiratory alkalosis.
- Acidemia is an increase in $[H^+]$ in ECW. The pH in arterial blood of patients with acidemia falls from the normal value of 7.40.
- Metabolic acidemia is presented in the Henderson-Hasselbalch equation as a decline in bicarbonate buffer, the numerator in the right side of the equation. Impaired alveolar ventilation causes increased partial pressure of carbon dioxide and a respiratory acidemia that is demonstrated in the Henderson-Hasselbalch equation as an increase in the denominator. A decrease in $[H^+]$ in an arterial blood sample—an increased pH, or alkalemia—occurs as a result of added bicarbonate buffer or because the $PaCO_2$ is decreased by hyperventilation.
- In most clinical situations, physiologic compensatory adjustments have already taken place in response to the sudden pathologic change in acid-base status.
- A calculated base deficit using information reported in the arterial blood gas provides a method to assess a patient's status. Calculation of base deficit is based on the mass balance implicit in the Henderson-Hasselbalch equation. The pH and $PaCO_2$ are used to predict what the bicarbonate would be if that same sample of arterial blood had a normal pH of 7.40 and a normal $PaCO_2$ of 40 mm Hg. If the predicted bicarbonate is less than the normal value of 24 mEq/L, this indicates a base deficit and the patient has a component of metabolic acidosis. If a patient's arterial blood gas sample has a predicted bicarbonate that exceeds 24 mEq/L, this indicates a negative base deficit, or "metabolic alkalosis."
- Stewart proposed an alternative approach to the interpretation laboratory data regarding acid-base status. In contrast to the Henderson-Hasselbalch approach, the Stewart method is based quantitatively on buffer and acid concentrations.
- The strong ion difference is the sum of sodium, potassium, calcium, and magnesium concentrations minus lactate and chloride concentrations. The concentration of weak acids (proteins and phosphates—also called the nonvolatile buffers to contrast these with bicarbonate) is a defining aspect of the Stewart approach.
- The Henderson-Hasselbalch equation indicates the pH status of the extracellular fluid environment where the bicarbonate buffer system dominates. The Henderson-Hasselbalch

equation does not reliably inform the clinician regarding the acid-base status of the intracellular environment, where pH is lower and buffer systems other than bicarbonate influence pH.

- In circumstances of a rapid change in proton concentration, the pH of the ECW and ICW may not change in parallel.
- To avoid this paradoxical ICW acidosis, intravenous bicarbonate therapy should be infused slowly in patients with profound metabolic acidemia.

Clinical Patterns of Acid-Base Disorders

Metabolic Acidosis

- Lactic acidosis is a common problem in seriously ill and injured patients who suffer impaired delivery of oxygen. In mitochondria, oxidative phosphorylation uses chemical energy derived from oxygen and fuels to transform ADP to ATP.
- The arterial blood gas analysis of a patient with lactic acidosis from shock typically demonstrates a base deficit and a decrease in pH that—in patients who are spontaneously breathing—is usually associated with compensatory hyperventilation to reduce $PaCO_2$.
- Calculating the anion gap is an alternative but less specific method to determine the presence of lactic acidosis.
- Successful treatment of a patient with lactic academia of any etiology is determined more by the capacity of the clinician to correct the primary clinical problem than by infusion of buffer to reverse acidosis.
- The indications for intravenous infusion of bicarbonate in patients with lactic academia are debated, but most authors conclude that patients with a pH less than 7.20 benefit from slow sodium bicarbonate infusions.
- Levy et al proposed that lactic acidosis in septic patients is a multifactorial process consistent with reduced mitochondrial oxygen availability and dysfunction of normal biochemical processes in the cytosol.
- A specific pathophysiologic mechanism for lactic acidosis is thiamine deficiency, a clinical problem commonly seen in alcoholics who consume a diet deficient in vegetables. Thiamine deficiency leads to lactic acidosis because pyruvate dehydrogenase requires thiamine as a critical cofactor.
- Therefore, lactic acidosis can occur because of impaired clearance or overproduction. Type A lactic acidosis encompasses any mechanism resulting in excessive production of lactate from pyruvate. Type B lactic acidosis occurs in patients with impaired hepatic clearance of lactate.

- Not all patients resuscitated from shock have acidemia resulting from lactic acid. Dilution metabolic acidemia occurs in situations in which large volumes of isotonic sodium chloride solutions have been rapidly infused.
- Patients with gastrointestinal (GI) fistula drainage or diarrhea exceeding 4 liters per day can experience enough bicarbonate loss to induce acidemia. Duodenal, proximal small bowel, and pancreatic fistulae can produce large volumes of fluid rich in sodium bicarbonate.
- In patients with diabetes mellitus, insulin deficiency leads to dysfunction of two major biochemical pathways, and diabetic ketoacidosis may result. Depressed insulin levels trigger lipolysis, in which triglycerides are converted into glycerol and free fatty acids. These free fatty acids are released to the circulation and are taken up by the liver, where they are converted into two-carbon ketoacids, beta hydroxybutyric acid and acetoacetic acid. These ketoacid fuels can support oxidative phosphorylation in brain and kidney cells. However, oxidative phosphorylation of ketoacids in mitochondria is slowed in patients without sufficient insulin to maintain glucose transport across cell membranes.
- Acidemia develops in ketoacidosis as protons are generated during hepatic ketone production and as ADP and protons accumulate because of impaired oxidative phosphorylation.
- Proper treatment of diabetic ketoacidosis involves insulin infusion, which repletes the intracellular supply of glucose and enables the excess ketones to be used as fuels.
- In addition to ordering sufficient insulin to lower blood sugar, the clinician must anticipate a need to infuse several liters of balanced electrolyte and substantial amounts of supplemental potassium chloride to avoid precipitous hypokalemia.
- Alcoholics develop a ketoacidosis syndrome, but the pathophysiologic mechanism is not insulin deficiency. Alcoholics who binge drink large amounts of ethanol (ETOH) over days and fail to consume a normal diet experience a fall in insulin because of starvation and, consequently, undergo lipolysis and hepatic conversion of free fatty acids to ketones.
- Ketoacidosis should be suspected in alcoholic patients with acidemia if they exhibit an increased anion gap.
- Acidemia is a hallmark of renal failure.
- Renal tubular acidosis syndromes are rare causes of mild to moderate acidemia. The acidosis is caused by impaired tubular cell capacity to excrete protons and synthesize bicarbonate.

Metabolic Alkalosis

- Metabolic alkalosis develops as excess bicarbonate accumulates in the ECW. Clinicians can produce this problem by infusing large amounts of bicarbonate to treat patients with acute lactic acidosis, especially when the acidosis is successfully and promptly cleared. Similarly, mechanical ventilation of patients with chronic hypoventilation syndromes—as occurs in restrictive lung disease or morbid obesity—can also produce a metabolic acidosis.
- If these patients are intubated for surgery or to treat acute respiratory failure and a normal $PaCO_2$ is rapidly achieved (with mechanical ventilation), the excess bicarbonate causes a metabolic alkalosis. This complication can be avoided if mechanical ventilation is modulated to achieve a slow return to normal $PaCO_2$.
- Hypokalemic, hypochloremic metabolic alkalosis is a pattern of acid-base disorder that occurs in patients with prolonged vomiting or sustained high gastric fluid drainage.
- This situation is best corrected by the intravenous infusion of isotonic fluids with sufficient KCl to replete deficits of these ions. As ECW expands and KCl levels correct, aldosterone levels decline and the nephron produces an alkaline urine to correct the alkalemia.
- Diuretic therapy can also produce a metabolic alkalemia.

Respiratory Alkalosis

- Regulatory centers in the brain normally respond to fluctuations in arterial $PaCO_2$ levels by either increasing or decreasing minute ventilation to keep $PaCO_2$ in the range of 40 ± 2 mm Hg. In circumstances of fear, stress, sepsis, fever, or pain, patients can experience an abrupt increase in alveolar ventilation that results in a decline in $PaCO_2$ and an associated alkalemia.
- Respiratory alkalemia, also termed hypocapnia, can be a serious complication of mechanical ventilation when a patient with pharmacologic paralysis is inadvertently overventilated.

Respiratory Acidosis

- Acute onset of respiratory acidosis is most commonly the consequence of an abrupt decline in alveolar ventilation. A patient who has a normal arterial blood gas and suddenly stops ventilating will double his or her $PaCO_2$ from 40 to 80 mm Hg within minutes.

- Central chemoreceptors in the brainstem provide primary control over ventilation and respond to higher proton concentrations by stimulating increased respiratory rates. However, in situations of chronic hypercarbia, renal compensation blunts the capacity of chemoreceptors to respond to further increases in $PaCO_2$ by increasing bicarbonate concentration in ECW. Therefore, these patients depend on the second reflex mechanism to stimulate ventilatory drive: chemoreceptors in the carotid bodies that are stimulated by decreased arterial oxygen saturation. Patients with chronic hypercarbia who are given supplemental oxygen to maintain high oxygen saturations are at high risk for sudden death from a hypoventilation-induced critical increase in $PaCO_2$; such an increase may induce carbon dioxide narcosis that suppresses even chemoreflex-driven ventilation.

HYPONATREMIA AND HYPOTONICITY

- Sodium, with the corresponding anions chloride and bicarbonate, normally determines more than 95% of the osmolality of ECW. Thus, the diagnosis and management of disorders in sodium concentration and ECW osmolality are linked.
- Mild hyponatremia exists when serum [Na^+] lies between 130 to 138 mEq/L.
- Moderate hyponatremia exists when serum [Na^+] measures between 120 to 130 mEq/L.
- Severe hyponatremia is defined as a serum [Na^+] less than 120 mEq/L. As serum [Na^+] declines, risk of seizure increases and patients become comatose. Patients are at risk for death from cerebral swelling if serum [Na^+] drops below 110 mEq/L.
- Acute hyponatremia evolves over a few hours and poses a risk of cerebral swelling as TBW osmolality declines. Chronic hyponatremia develops over days, allowing solute transport out of cells and decreasing the amount of cell swelling. It is clinically important to differentiate acute from chronic hyponatremia because rates of correction should differ substantially.

Acute Hyponatremia Syndromes

Postoperative Hyponatremia

- The special risk to menstruating women for the development of postoperative hyponatremia was reported by Ayus and colleagues.

- Surgeons can reduce the risk of postoperative hyponatremia by always ordering isotonic intravenous fluids. Furthermore, patients—particularly small-statured women—who develop lethargy, headache, and altered mental status in the postoperative period should have serum sodium concentrations checked.
- Steele and coworkers proposed the concept of desalination to account for hyponatremia in postoperative patients.
- Elevated arginine vasopressin (AVP) levels were associated with the increase in urine osmolality. These authors concluded that pain, apprehension, or stresses related to surgery can cause a sustained release of AVP during the first 1 to 2 days after surgery. Because of the production of a large amount of concentrated urine, desalination led to acute hyponatremia.
- Acute hyponatremia can complicate a diuretic-induced, forced diuresis.
- In each of these situations, the ECW space becomes dehydrated; if replacement fluids in the form of intravenous solutions, enteral tube feedings, or a liquid diet are hypotonic fluids, hyponatremia will result.
- Cerebral salt wasting is a cause of hyponatremia most commonly reported in neurosurgical patients. Patients with a brain lesion develop hyponatremia associated with sustained, elevated urine sodium concentrations in the setting of a normal creatinine clearance.
- Berendes, et al correlated markedly elevated brain natriuretic peptide levels that persisted for 8 days with salt wasting in these patients and hypothesized that this peptide, rather than elevated AVP, accounted for the onset of low serum sodium concentrations. Treatment of patients with cerebral salt wasting requires administration of sufficient daily sodium to sustain normal total body sodium balance.
- Acute water intoxication is s rare cause of hyponatremia.

Chronic Hyponatremia

- The syndrome of inappropriate antidiuretic hormone (SIADH) release has been a carefully studied cause of chronic hyponatremia. The diagnosis of SIADH can only be made in euvolemic patients. Patients should have serum osmolalities less than 270 mOsm/kg H_2O along with an inappropriately concentrated urine osmolality, defined as a urine osmolality greater than 100 mOsm/kg H_2O.
- Patients with indisputable SIADH are those with an AVP-secreting tumor, usually a carcinoid or small cell carcinoma of the lung.

- Patients with chronic renal disease may develop an impaired capacity to retain sodium and subsequently develop hyponatremia.

Treatment of Hyponatremia

- Surgeons must differentiate between patients with acute and chronic hyponatremia. Patients who suffer the acute onset of serum $[Na^+]$ below 110 mEq/L and develop neurologic symptoms should be corrected to a $[Na^+]$ of about 120 mEq/L over the first 24 hours of therapy. In contrast, patients who present with a chronically reduced serum $[Na^+]$ of less than 110 mEq/L will not commonly exhibit neurologic symptoms. Rapid correction in patients with chronic hyponatremia can lead to central pontine myelinolysis, a severe, permanent neurologic disorder characterized by spastic quadriparesis, pseudobulbar palsy, and depressed levels of consciousness.
- Safe corrective treatment requires the surgeon to monitor the patient's physical examination and serial checks of serum sodium concentration over the first 48 hours of treatment. Patients with profound acute hyponatremia who manifest signs of severe encephalopathy—lethargy, seizures, or coma— should undergo prompt therapy that accomplishes a slow increase in the ECW $[Na^+]$. To avoid the complications of central pontine myelinolysis, the maximum rate of sodium correction should not exceed 0.25 mEq/L per hour. Thus, the rate of increase in serum $[Na^+]$ should not exceed 8 mOsm/kg H_2O per day.
- Patients with chronic hyponatremia are less likely to have encephalopathy or other neurologic symptoms; thus, there is less urgency to bring about a correction of serum sodium.

Hypernatremia and Syndromes of Hypertonicity

- Hypernatremia is the most common cause of hypertonicity. Patients have moderate hypernatremia if serum $[Na^+]$ lies between 146 to 159 mEq/L and severe, life-threatening hypernatremia if serum $[Na^+]$ exceeds 160 mEq/L.
- The danger of hypernatremia is brain shrinkage and consequently neurologic dysfunction. Brain cell dehydration manifests clinically as altered levels of consciousness, seizures, and coma.
- As a normal response to increased serum $[Na^+]$ and osmolality, the kidney produces a concentrated urine.

- Nephrons accomplish antidiuresis by responding to AVP, which the hypothalamus releases in amounts proportional to the extent that the serum osmolality exceeds a threshold of approximately 280 mOsm/kg H_2O.
- ETOH suppresses AVP release. Intoxicated patients with hypernatremia may produce large volumes of hypo-osmolar urine, and, consequently, renal water losses inappropriately further increase serum [Na^+].
- Typically, as blood ETOH levels fall, urine outputs decline and urine specific gravity approaches 1.030, leading to a renal correction of hypernatremia.

Causes of Hypernatremia

- Diabetes insipidus is a syndrome of excessive excretion of greater than 500 mL/hr of hypotonic urine and results in TBW contraction and hypernatremia if the patient does not drink water at rates that exceed urine flow rates.
- Central diabetes insipidus is characterized by a decline or loss in the ability of the hypothalamus to produce and excrete AVP. The acute onset of diabetes insipidus occurs in patients with brain injury, intracerebral hemorrhage, skull base or pituitary surgery, or cerebral infection.
- Nephrogenic diabetes insipidus is defined as an impaired capacity of renal tubules to respond to AVP and concentrate urine. Patients with nephrogenic diabetes insipidus have elevated levels of circulating AVP and polyuria and can develop moderate hypernatremia.
- Lithium, glyburide, demeclocycline, and amphotericin B can all induce nephrogenic diabetes insipidus via direct effects on tubular cells.
- Hypernatremia can also emerge rapidly in patients because of excessive and uncontrollable losses of hypotonic fluids.
- Hypernatremia is rarely caused by ingestion or intravenous infusion of a large sodium load.
- Two populations at particular risk for dehydration and hypernatremia are very young children and the infirm elderly.

Treatment of Hypernatremia

- Treatment of patients with hypernatremia resulting from dehydration involves intravenous or oral administration of water. Hypernatremic patients typically have significantly reduced blood volumes.
- Postural hypotension, low central venous pressure, and poor skin turgor are signs of significant dehydration. Evaluation

may also involve measurement of urine characteristics to categorize the problem as either a nonrenal water loss or diabetes insipidus. Patients produce small volumes of maximally hyperosmolar urine if their hypernatremia is a consequence of nonrenal water loss. In contrast, urine osmolality is inappropriately less than serum osmolality in patients with diabetes insipidus. Hypernatremic patients with either mechanism of hypernatremia require rehydration; the key difference is that patients with central diabetes insipidus should be given AVP or a synthetic analog, desmopressin.

- To correct an elevated serum [Na^+], the surgeon orders either an intravenous infusion or enteral intake of sufficient solute-free water to achieve a positive water balance. Correction of a sustained hypernatremia should be cautious because a rapid decline in ECW osmolality can lead to cerebral injury resulting from rapid cytosol swelling. Serum [Na^+] should be corrected at a rate of no more than 10 mEq per day, unless the patient is symptomatic from severe acute hypernatremia.
- Patients with hypernatremia may also have deficits in total body potassium related to the shrinkage of the ICW.
- Patients with hypernatremia resulting from central diabetes insipidus should be treated with antidiuretic hormone. AVP may be continuously infused in patients and adjusted to achieve desired urine flow rates.
- Desmopressin (1-desamino-8-D-argine vasopressin [DDAVP]) is a synthetic analog of AVP that has a half-life of several hours following intravenous injection. DDAVP is the agent of choice for treating patients with central diabetes insipidus because it effectively induces renal tubular water reabsorption without acting as a vasopressor.
- Rarely has a gain in total body sodium been identified as the cause of hypernatremia. Intravenous infusions of hypertonic sodium bicarbonate during aggressive treatment of severe acidemia and infusion of hypertonic saline during resuscitation of hypovolemic patients can increase serum [Na^+].

Pathophysiology of Potassium

- An increase or decrease of potassium concentration greater than 3 mmol/L can lead to death.
- The kidney controls the concentration of potassium in the ECW by adjusting potassium excretion in urine.
- A normal ECW [K^+] is maintained at 4 mmol/L largely because renal function in the DCT segment of the nephron excretes excess potassium.

- The more negative the charge produced in the tubule by the electrogenic reabsorption of sodium, the more moles of potassium enter the tubule fluid.
- The hormone aldosterone controls potassium excretion by increasing the activity of the enzyme responsible for electrogenic reabsorption of sodium.
- Patients on a normal diet with an elevated serum [K+] are capable of excreting more than 400 mmol of potassium per day. Patients with a depressed serum [K+] should produce less than 20 mmol of potassium per day.

Hyperkalemia

- Hyperkalemia is defined as a [K+] greater than 5.0 mmol/L. As extracellular potassium concentration exceeds 6 mmol/L, alterations occur in the resting cell membrane potential that impair normal depolarization and repolarization.
- Hyperkalemia in the range of 6 to 7 mmol/L may be associated with tall T-waves. Symmetrically peaked T-waves indicate dangerous hyperkalemia, particularly if T-waves are higher than the R-wave in more than one lead.
- As the [K+] level exceeds 8 mmol/L, suddenly, lethal arrhythmias ensue, such as asystole, ventricular fibrillation, or a wide pulseless idioventricular rhythm.
- Rapid-onset hyperkalemia is most commonly due to renal dysfunction or failure.
- Precipitous hyperkalemia should be anticipated in patients who experience sudden reperfusion of a vascular bed that had been ischemic for hours.
- Precipitous hyperkalemia can be a complication of intravenous injection of succinylcholine—a depolarizing paralytic agent—when used in patients who have muscle atrophy from disuse, neurologic denervation syndromes, severe burns, direct muscle trauma, or rhabdomyolysis syndromes or have required prolonged bed rest.

Treatment of Acute Hyperkalemia

- Several interventions are useful in patients at risk from cardiac arrhythmias from hyperkalemia. Intravenous calcium can immediately reduce the risk of arrhythmia in hyperkalemic patients with characteristic electrocardiogram changes.
- Sodium bicarbonate infusion buffers ECW protons and allows net transfer of cytosol protons across the cell membrane via carbonic acid. The shift of protons out of the cell is associated with a shift of potassium into the cell.

- Insulin and glucose infusions prompt increased Na^+/K^+-ATPase activity and a decline in ECW potassium concentration as the ECW potassium is pumped into the ICW.
- In the patient with acute renal failure, definitive reduction of $[K^+]$ can only be accomplished by renal replacement therapy; hemodialysis can be used to achieve a negative potassium balance in minutes, whereas continuous filtration methods clear potassium at a much slower rate.

Hypokalemia

- Patients with hypokalemia have a serum $[K^+]$ less than 3.5 mmol/L. Generalized symptoms commonly associated with depressed serum $[K^+]$ include fatigue, weakness, and ileus.
- Hypokalemia is a common problem among hospitalized patients and can usually be attributed to GI or renal losses.
- The combination of catecholamines and aldosterone alters function in the DCT segment of the nephron, and the consequence is greater renal excretion of potassium.
- Long-term diuretic therapy can reduce ICW $[K^+]$, with the consequence of impaired conduction and electrical automaticity leading to arrhythmias.
- The risk of hypokalemia-associated arrhythmia is higher in patients treated with digoxin, even when potassium concentrations are in the "low normal" range.

Clinical Syndromes of Acute Hypokalemia

- Diuretic administration is a common iatrogenic mechanism of reducing serum $[K^+]$. Thiazide and loop diuretics, as well as osmotic diuresis produced by mannitol infusion, increase delivery of sodium to the DCT segment of the nephron. In the presence of elevated aldosterone, sodium is absorbed while potassium enters the filtrate and is lost in urine.

Treatment

- Hypokalemic patients require potassium replacement. Because being serum $[K^+]$ poor reflects ICW deficits, patients should be closely monitored during replacement therapy.
- Hypokalemic patients with concurrent acidemia should have delayed correction of ECW pH.
- Diabetics in ketoacidosis may present with normal serum $[K^+]$ but rapidly develop hypokalemia as insulin is administered and glucose shifts into cells.

- If the patient is on a diuretic that wastes potassium, he or she should either receive supplemental potassium or be given an additional drug that spares potassium, such as triamterene or spironolactone. Hypokalemic patients may also need magnesium, which is an important cofactor for potassium uptake and maintenance of intracellular potassium levels.

Calcium and Magnesium

- Calcium, a divalent cation, is a critical component of many extracellular and intracellular reactions. It is an essential cofactor in the coagulation cascade, and intracellular ionized calcium participates in regulation of neuronal, myocardial, and renal tubular functions. Calcium is assayed in a serum sample as total serum calcium concentration (normally 8.5 to 10.5 mg/dL).
- Ionized calcium, $[Ca^{2+}]_i$, is the biochemically active species that constitutes approximately 45% of the total serum calcium.
- The serum calcium concentration is controlled by the interaction of the hormone parathormone (PTH), the hormone calcitonin, and vitamin D. Vitamin D is not one molecule but a mixture of sterols with antirachitic activity. The ICW $[Ca^{2+}]_i$ is substantially lower than ECW $[Ca^{2+}]_i$.
- Turnover of calcium salts in bone is constant and integral to maintaining a stable $[Ca^{2+}]_i$ in ECW. Receptors in the membranes of parathyroid cells can identify low or falling $[Ca^{2+}]_i$, which rapidly stimulates the release of PTH.
- The hormone also works with vitamin D to enhance absorption of calcium from the lumen of the gut. Increased extracellular $[Ca^{2+}]_i$ suppresses the release of PTH, and as hormone levels fall, osteoblasts use calcium to synthesize new bone.
- Magnesium is an essential cation in the enzymatic activity that enables ATP conversion to ADP and energy release. Less than 1% of the total body magnesium content is found in the extracellular fluid.
- Hypomagnesemic patients exhibit central nervous, muscular, and cardiovascular signs and symptoms similar to those of depressed ECW calcium concentration; in actuality, symptoms are often the net result of deficiencies in both cations.

Hypercalcemia

- Hypercalcemia can be suspected when serum calcium levels exceed the normal range (9 to 11 mg/dL, 2.2 to 2.7 mmol/L).

Confirmation of the diagnosis of hypercalcemia requires that $[Ca^{2+}]_i$ exceed 1.4 mmol/L.

- Calcium levels greater than 15 mg/dL produce symptoms of weakness, stupor, and other central nervous dysfunction.
- Hyperparathyroidism—or unregulated PTH secretion—is a common cause of significant hypercalcemia.
- PTH induces phosphaturia and depresses serum phosphate concentrations, and these laboratory findings corroborate the diagnosis of primary hyperparathyroidism.
- Patients with malignancies can develop hypercalcemia independent of the hormone PTH. Selected tumors have been demonstrated to produce a PTH-related peptide that shares 8 of its first 13 amino acids with PTH, which induces calcium release from bone and reduces calcium loss in urine.
- Patients with hyperparathyroidism resulting from a parathyroid adenoma or hyperplasia are cured of hypercalcemia by excision of the diseased parathyroid tissue. Hypercalcemic patients on thiazide drugs should be converted to alternative therapies. Patients with a malignancy and hypercalcemia may respond to surgical excision, radiation therapy, or chemotherapy.
- Severe hypercalcemia related to release of calcium from bone can be successfully managed by bisphosphonate treatment.
- Calcitonin is the calcium-lowering hormone produced by parafollicular cells of the thyroid gland. Administration of exogenous calcitonin effectively induces renal excretion of calcium and suppresses osteoclast bone reabsorption.

Hypocalcemia

- Acute hypocalcemia can be a life-threatening event. This condition impairs transmembrane depolarization, and $[Ca^{2+}]_i$ below 0.8 mEq/L can lead to central nervous system (CNS) dysfunction. Hypocalcemic patients complain of paresthesias and muscle spasms (including tetany) and develop seizures.
- Cardiac dysfunction also occurs in patients with hypocalcemia. Low plasma $[Ca^{2+}]_i$ is associated with impaired cardiac contractility, and intravenous infusion of calcium can improve cardiac output in these patients.
- Acute hypocalcemia can also be a complication of severe pancreatitis and is speculated to be the consequence of ionized extracellular calcium becoming linked to fats in the peripancreatic inflammatory phlegmon.
- Infusion of 10 mL of a 10% $CaCl_2$ solution provides 272 mg of calcium (equivalent to 13.6 mmol of ionized calcium), whereas the same volume of 10% calcium gluconate

contains only 90 mg of calcium (equivalent to 4.5 mmol of ionized calcium).

Hypermagnesemia and Hypomagnesemia

- Hypermagnesemia is an electrolyte abnormality most often seen in patients with renal failure. Hypermagnesemia can be exacerbated by ingestion of magnesium-containing drugs, particularly antacids, and such agents should be avoided.

CONTROL OF PLASMA VOLUME AND THE CIRCULATION OF INTERSTITIAL FLUID

- Blood flow delivers oxygen to the arterioles, capillaries, and venules, which together form the microcirculation.
- The flow of lymph—a filtrate of plasma—is a second circulation of fluid and solutes that also plays a vital role in sustaining a viable cell environment.
- Several factors are critical to the control of the second circulation. Driving forces in the capillary move water and solute across the microvascular membrane. The permeability characteristics of the microvascular membrane determine the proportion of plasma proteins blocked from entry into the interstitium. The compliance of the interstitial matrix modulates the extent to which pressures change as the matrix contracts or swells and the interstitial pressure drives fluid into lymphatics.
- An important function of the second circulation is the unidirectional flux of soluble proteins from plasma to the interstitium and through lymphatics back to the venous circulation.
- The microvascular walls are composed of endothelial cells attached to a basement membrane. These cells lie in a continuous monolayer, and adjacent cells are connected with cell-cell junctions.
- Plasma water and solutes can cross the microvascular membranes by passing through intercellular gaps and pores in the capillary and venular segments. In addition, fluid transport from the plasma to the interstitium occurs through vesicles.
- The microvascular membrane is nearly as permeable to small solutes (e.g., electrolytes, glucose, and urea) as it is water, and the concentration of these solutes in plasma and interstitial fluid are essentially equivalent. In contrast to small molecules, large solutes in plasma—the plasma proteins—are too large to cross the microvascular membrane through the pores that accommodate water and small solutes.

Control of Fluid Movement and Solute Flux Across the Microvascular Membrane

- Starling's hypothesis proposed that an oncotic pressure from plasma proteins exists across the capillary wall that favors the retention of water in the vascular compartment and counterbalances the intraluminal hydrostatic pressure that forces fluid into the interstitium.

- Each organ has different microvascular membrane permeability characteristics, and the influence on total body distribution of ECW between plasma volume and the interstitium is a summation of Starling forces across multiple circulations in parallel.

- The more permeable the microvascular membrane is to plasma proteins, the less effective the difference in colloid osmotic pressure between the plasma and interstitial fluid.

- The term L_pS has two components. L_p represents the permeability of the capillary membrane to water, also designated as hydraulic conductivity. S indicates capillary membrane surface area available for water to move across.

- Ninety percent of hydraulic conductivity in the microcirculation can be attributed to small pores large enough to allow a water molecule to pass but too small to accommodate albumin and other plasma proteins.

- The capillary filtration coefficient (CFC) assumes to measure the combined influence of microvascular hydraulic conductivity (water permeability) and the number of capillaries being perfused at a given point in time per 100 g of tissue. This has been measured in the human forearm with strain-gauge plethysmography, which precisely measures the rate of arm swelling when venous pressure is increased.

- In skin, 50% of interstitial water is ECW, and cell components include primarily fibroblasts, endothelium, and inflammatory cells. Macromolecules constitute a hydrated gel matrix and a major acellular component of the interstitium. The third component is the free-fluid phase of ECW in direct continuity with lymphatics; prenodal lymph and interstitial free fluid are similar in composition. Edema is the pathologic condition of increased interstitial volume.

- The gel matrix of collagen and glycosaminoglycans endows the interstitium with several properties. It provides a structure of fibers that, attached to fibroblasts, resist hydration. Its properties have been speculated to determine the interstitial hydrostatic pressure; experimental evidence indicates that a net pressure to imbibe water and swell exists under normal conditions.

- Lymphatics are endothelial-lined tubes that connect the interstitium to lymph nodes and eventually to major veins in the chest. Lymphatics are thought to be impermeable with the exception of the terminal lymphatics where lymph flow begins.
- Prenodal lymphatics drain into the cortical surface of a lymph node.
- Centripetal flow propels postnodal lymph toward the chest, where it drains into the main thoracic and right thoracic ducts. These vessels have smooth muscle that generates peristaltic contractions.

Pathologic Changes in Interstitial Volume; Dehydration and Edema

- Edema is defined as an excessive increase in interstitial fluid. Several mechanisms that cause edema have been carefully defined. Infusion of a balanced electrolyte solution normally prompts a compensatory renal response and diuresis. In patients with a depleted blood volume following hemorrhage, rapid infusion of isotonic saline expands the blood volume; however, a great proportion of the fluid shifts into the interstitium.
- Congestive heart failure commonly precipitates peripheral edema. Elevated venous pressures shift retrograde into the capillaries, and increased hydrostatic pressure results in higher transmicrovascular fluid shift and edema.
- Resolution of this form of edema depends on reducing the elevated venous pressure; this is often achieved with diuretics to reduce the plasma volume, which is replaced with lymph drainage from the interstitium.
- High permeability edema occurs when the number or size of large pores in the endothelial membrane increases. Two endogenously produced molecules, histamine and the polypeptide bradykinin, cause gaps to develop between venular endothelial cells; other inflammatory agents can also cause these changes.

Control of Blood Pressure in Response to Shock

- The CNS regulates reflexes that sustain a normal blood pressure despite fluctuations in the intravascular volume. Baroreceptors located in the aortic arch and other major vessels respond to perfusion pressure changes that are measures of vessel wall stretch during systole. Increases and decreases in systolic pressure prompt reflex signals to centers in the brainstem that control the catecholamines norepinephrine (NE) and epinephrine (EPI).

- The juxtaglomerular apparatus is located in the nephron at the site where the DCT segment comes close to the glomerulus. The endocrine cells of the apparatus control the renin-angiotensin-aldosterone endocrine reflex.
- The juxtaglomerular apparatus response to hypotension is release of renin, an enzyme that cleaves angiotensinogen in plasma to produce angiotensin I, a peptide of limited physiologic effectiveness. Angiotensin-converting enzyme (ACE) is located on the pulmonary endothelium. ACE converts angiotensin I to angiotensin II, and this second molecule is a potent hormonal vasoconstrictor. Angiotensin II also stimulates secretion of aldosterone by the adrenal glomerulosa.
- Renal function adjusts to restore intravascular volume in the circumstance of hypovolemia.
- Severe hypotension induces a baroreceptor-mediated surge in sympathetic nervous system activity that redistributes blood flow. The increase in vasoconstriction is greatest in the vessels that deliver blood to skin, muscle, and bowel. Available blood flow is diverted to the brain and coronary circulations.

CELLULAR AEROBIC FUNCTION AND DYSFUNCTION

- Shock in patients is ultimately a problem when it comes to the dysfunction of intracellular energy metabolism.
- Successful therapies for patients in shock have focused on restoring organ function.

Cellular Energy Metabolism

- Cellular metabolism depends primarily on hydrolysis of the high-energy bond in ATP.
- Cellular work performed with ATP includes the contraction of actin and myosin, transport of electrolytes across cell membranes, synthesis of constitutive molecules, and generation of heat. ATP is hydrolyzed to ADP, and with cleavage of the terminal phosphate bond, energy is released.

$$ATP^{4-} + H_2O \leftrightarrow ADP^{3-} + P_i^{2-} + H^+ + \textit{energy}$$

- Respiration is a process of biochemical reactions in cells that synthesize ATP from ADP.
- Six-carbon glucose is degraded to a pair of three-carbon pyruvate molecules via a chain of reactions designated the glycolytic pathway. Without consuming oxygen, the glycolytic

pathway can produce two moles of ATP for each mole of glucose that is catabolized.

- Complete oxidation of one mole of glucose generates 38 moles of ATP.

Clinical Syndromes of Cellular Energy Failure

- Several clinical problems demonstrate the consequences for the entire body if the failure of intracellular aerobic metabolism occurs.
- ATP levels fall in the cell while ADP, phosphate, and protons increase.
- As glucose is transported into the cells, aerobic metabolism will rapidly reduce ICW [H^+].
- Pyruvate dehydrogenase requires the cofactor thiamine (vitamin B_1) to convert pyruvate into acetyl-CoA. Patients must ingest thiamine in their diet, which is available in vegetables.
- A specific clinical scenario is that of an alcoholic who has an acute surgical condition and who during treatment develops lactic acidosis and brain damage (resulting from thiamine deficiency) because pyruvate dehydrogenase cannot function and support synthesis of ATP by oxidative phosphorylation.
- In the circumstances of impaired blood flow, the delivery of oxygen to tissues is insufficient to sustain oxidative phosphorylation in the mitochondria at a rate that matches the turnover of ATP to ADP. Patients in shock have an increase in lactate that is coupled with an increase in [H^+].
- However, definitive correction of lactic acidosis caused by hypoxia usually depends on restoring adequate blood flow.

Induced Superoxygen Endpoints of Resuscitation

- A hypothesis regarding treatment of shock that has been debated for decades has asserted that the outcome of seriously ill patients resuscitated from shock was optimal if the resuscitation achieved a supernormal oxygen delivery. The hypothesis's core concept was that during shock cells without sufficient oxygen delivery developed an energy debt.
- Seriously injured patients who require resuscitation from shock should have three sequential interventions in the ICU:
  - First, sufficient blood should be transfused to exceed hemoglobin of 10 g/dL.
  - Second, if cardiac output fails to reach a threshold level after appropriate volume loading, the patient is infused with an inotropic agent such as dopamine or dobutamine.

- Third, adjustments are made in fluid and drug therapy to achieve a goal of a calculated oxygen delivery.
- Randomized clinical trials have been reported that tested the hypothesis that achieving supernormal delivery of oxygen is beneficial. The results have been inconclusive. Boyd et al reported in a randomized control trial of high-risk surgery patients that survival was improved when infusion of inotropes were used to increase oxygen delivery. Gattinoni et al, in large populations of a diverse group of patients requiring resuscitation in an intensive care unit (ICU), were unable to demonstrate a benefit to achieving a supernormal oxygen delivery. Hayes et al reported more deaths in the group pushed to higher oxygen delivery.
- Recent studies suggest that there exists a group of patients who fail to achieve supernormal oxygen delivery and that among these nonresponders death rates are high.

HYPOVOLEMIC SHOCK

- Hypovolemic shock is defined as insufficient delivery of oxygen to tissues caused by a reduced intravascular volume. Surgeons routinely encounter hypovolemic shock, and hemorrhage is the most common specific cause.
- Three forms of hemorrhagic shock have been defined: compensated, uncompensated, and lethal exsanguination.
- Compensated shock occurs with hemorrhage of less than 20% of the blood volume.
- In compensated shock, brain and heart perfusions remain near normal while other less critical organ systems are, in proportion to the blood volume deficit, stressed by ischemia.
- Patients in uncompensated shock are at risk for death because of deficient delivery of oxygen to vital organs and impaired mitochondrial aerobic energy production.
- The third form of hemorrhagic shock is exsanguinating hemorrhage. Patients who lose more than 40% of their blood volume develop profound hypotension; without blood flow to the brain, syncope occurs followed within minutes by cardiopulmonary arrest.
- The patient's intravascular volume often fluctuates during a sequence of therapeutic interventions. Blood loss is treated with first asanguinous fluid and blood product infusions that expand the intravascular volume and restore perfusion.
- Successful treatment of hypovolemic shock is linked to timely and effective interventions that control sites of active hemorrhage.

- Patients survive hemorrhagic shock as a consequence of hemostasis and infusions that replete blood volume and support physiologic mechanisms that restore normal cell and organ function.

- Causes of hypovolemic shock other than hemorrhage exist. Severe dehydration—a substantial reduction in ECW space and total body sodium—can occur over a few hours and result in hypovolemic shock.

- The intravascular volume can also be depleted by shifts of fluid within the ECW space; large body surface area burns or fluid sequestration in the intestinal lumen because of a small bowel obstruction can lead to hypovolemic shock.

- Patients in hypovolemic shock have diaphoresis and pallor of vasoconstricted digits because of increased alpha-adrenergic function.

- Normal volunteers experimentally subjected to hemorrhage of prescribed volumes have enabled investigators to describe the quantitative relationship between blood volume deficit and decline in systolic pressure.

- Tachycardia is not a reliable indication of significant hemorrhage.

PATHOPHYSIOLOGY OF HYPOVOLEMIC SHOCK

- Baroreceptor-mediated vasoconstriction can readily compensate for a sudden hemorrhage of 15% or less of the blood volume. Vasoconstriction of arterial vessels are the consequences of increased sympathetic tone (measurable as elevated plasma NE levels), increased blood levels of angiotensin II generated in response to activation of the renin-angiotensin system, higher levels of circulating EPI released from the adrenal medulla, and a surge in pituitary release of AVP.

- These opposing neuroendocrine influences on heart rate explain why pulse rate is neither a sensitive nor specific indication of the patient's severity of hemorrhagic shock.

- Acidemia has been used as a clinical measure of the severity of shock. The metabolic acidemia of hemorrhagic shock is attributed to impaired delivery of oxygen to cells, resulting in a reduced capacity to conduct aerobic metabolism.

- Patients whose initial base deficit exceeded 6 mmol/L and who did not correct by 24 hours had death rates exceeding 60%. Other investigators have reported the base deficit measurement superior to pH as an indicator of high-risk patients in need of additional resuscitation from hemorrhagic shock.

Treatment of Patients in Hemorrhagic Shock

- The successful resuscitation of patients in hemorrhagic shock depends on two events: restoration of blood volume and therapeutic interventions to stop hemorrhage.

The Three Phases of Hemorrhagic Shock—Events After Resuscitation from Shock

- Three phases have been described in the human response to acute hemorrhagic shock. In *phase I* (beginning with injury and ending with surgery or a procedure to control active hemorrhage), the patient is hypovolemic, is usually vasoconstricted, and has impaired organ perfusion.
- Therapy is infusion of balanced electrolyte solution given in volume ratios of three to four volumes of isotonic saline for every volume of shed blood. Transfusion is essential when patients have sustained a more than 30% blood volume hemorrhage.
- *Phase II* starts at the completion of hemostasis and is a period of fluid sequestration. Both intracellular and interstitial expansions occur during this period of fluid uptake. The duration and magnitude of fluid gain during phase II are proportional to the severity of shock.
- During phase II, patients can develop an abdominal compartment hypertension syndrome, prompting many surgeons to avoid tight closure of the abdomen by inserting a prosthesis.
- *Phase III* involves a diuretic period when the excess fluid gained during phase II is mobilized and excreted by the kidneys. The onset of phase III should occur within 2 to 4 days of phase I.
- In summary, the treatment of hypovolemic shock has two components: repleting blood volume and interventions that terminate the pathologic events that incited the hypovolemia. Patients should follow a sequence of events following an episode of shock, and clinicians should investigate for complications in those patients who deviate from the expected pattern of recovery from hemorrhagic shock.

SHOCK FROM SEPSIS

- Shock associated with the sepsis syndrome is a common cause of death in surgical ICUs.
- Surgeons treating patients with septic shock must consider several issues. First, the patient must be resuscitated from shock. Second, the source of infection and pathogens must

either be identified or predicted pending culture results. Patients in septic shock should receive antibiotics effective against the documented or suspected invading organisms. The surgeon's third problem is to decide whether the sepsis is caused by a condition requiring surgical intervention. To have an optimal probability of survival, patients with an abscess and shock commonly require resuscitation of intravascular volume deficits, antibiotics, and drainage or extirpation of the site of infection.

Systemic Inflammatory Syndrome: A Spectrum of Clinical Disease

- Bone and collaborators convened a consensus conference to define criteria for categorization of sepsis-related inflammatory response.

- These authors defined four categories of clinical disease that represented successive levels of escalating severity of inflammatory response. The core concept of Bone et al was that as the burden of bacterial toxins increases and the extent of endogenous inflammatory response intensifies, the clinical manifestations of the severity of illness become exaggerated and the risk of death increases.

- The consensus conference described the response to infection as beginning with a systemic inflammatory response syndrome (SIRS) characterized by fever, tachycardia, and tachypnea.

- Patients with clinical sepsis meet the SIRS criteria and also have a documented infection.

- Patients with severe sepsis meet the criteria of sepsis and have become hypotensive; these patients exhibit signs of hypoperfusion, including lactic acidemia, oliguria, and depressed level of consciousness. Patients with severe sepsis should be resuscitated by intravenous infusion of balanced electrolyte solution. Many respond with improved perfusion and restored organ function. Patients who remain hypotensive despite adequate intravenous fluid infusion have the most lethal of the four categories: septic shock. Patients in septic shock have organ dysfunction that may progress to organ failure. Although hypotension may respond to resuscitation with inotropic and vasoactive drugs, these patients are at immediate risk for death from shock.

- Patients with an exaggerated inflammatory response to uncontrolled infection risk progression from the mild SIRS to the lethal problem of septic shock.

- Rangel-Frausto et al determined the natural histories of SIRS patients with 1-month follow-up; 61% progressed and met the criteria of sepsis, 18% developed severe sepsis, and 4% developed septic shock.

Clinical Observations; Patterns of Infection or Organisms

- Most SIRS patients have a clinically suspected or culture-positive proven site of infection. Sands et al reported that the four most prevalent sites of infection at university medical centers were—in order of prevalence—pulmonary, blood stream, genitourinary tract, and intra-abdominal wounds.
- Hadley et al, who studied a placebo group of 930 patients in the North American Septic Shock Trial, summarized the bacteria responsible for septic shock. Among 392 patients with positive blood cultures, 44% had gram-positive species, 44% had gram-negative species, and 3% had fungemia (only *Candida species*).
- These findings indicate that clinicians managing patients with a new diagnosis of SIRS should obtain blood cultures, as well as cultures from suspected sites of infection, before instituting empiric antibiotics.

Systemic Inflammatory Response Syndrome as an Exaggerated Inflammatory Response

- The normal response to microbial invasion encompasses a complex immune response that involves circulating immune cells (e.g., neutrophils, macrophages, and lymphocytes), the activation of coagulation and complement cascades, and biochemical alterations within constitutive cells (e.g., endothelial cells and fibroblasts).
- Cytokines are protein molecules produced by activated inflammatory cells that function as messengers and incite production of intermediate metabolites. Pro-inflammatory cytokines include TNF-alpha, IL-1, and IL-8, which induce endothelial cell production of proteases, nitric oxide release, coagulation pathway activation, vasoactive arachidonic acid metabolite production, and increased microvascular membrane permeability, which leads to edema.

Pathogenetic Mechanisms of Shock in Patients with Sepsis

- Patients with severe sepsis or septic shock commonly suffer hypotension because of arteriolar vasodilation. Hyperdynamic patterns in patients with septic shock have been measured with pulmonary artery catheters. Typically, these patients have cardiac outputs twice normal, and their hypotension corresponds to marked reductions in systemic vascular resistance attributed to uncontrolled vasodilation in organs with high capillary densities, such as skeletal muscle.

- Nitric oxide is a potent but effervescent vasodilator synthesized and released into adjacent interstitial fluid by endothelial cells. In response to hypoxia and inflammation caused by invasive infection, an upregulation of enzymes that generate nitric oxide occurs, and nitric oxide release is increased.

- Myocardial dysfunction is a second major factor contributing to hypotension in patients with septic shock. Despite the high cardiac output of patients in septic shock, cardiac function becomes impaired. Parrillo summarized the clinical evidence in support of myocardial dysfunction and proposed that a pathogenetic sequence of events led to shock in infected patients.

- Parrillo et al provided convincing evidence that a substance circulating in the blood accounts for the suppression in myocardial function in patients in septic shock.

Resuscitation of Impaired Hemodynamics in Patients with Septic Shock

- Persistently hypotensive patients who meet the definition of septic shock should be managed with the assistance of invasive hemodynamic monitoring, including pulmonary artery catheters.

- Patients in septic shock may require large volumes of fluid to achieve full resuscitation.

- Patients who remain hypotensive despite increased pulmonary artery wedge pressure should be infused with inotropic agents.

- Patients with restored intravascular volume who remain in septic shock should be given drugs to improve cardiac function, namely dopamine, dobutamine, and EPI. These three inotropic agents have different pharmacologic modes of action.

- In 1994, Marik et al reported that dopamine infusion into patients with septic shock—despite an expanded intravascular volume—effectively increased mean arterial blood pressure.

- These studies support the conclusion that dopamine may have a favorable influence on hemodynamic parameters, but surgeons must remain open to the possibility that drugs that alter one parameter may have unintended consequences on another.

- Dobutamine is a beta-adrenergic agonist that not only increases contractility of the myocardium but also may have a vasodilatory effect at doses of 5 to 15 µg/kg/min.
- Hayes et al also raised the concern that infusion of very large doses of dobutamine can be stressful to cardiac function and detrimental.
- EPI infused in doses of 1 to 20 µg/min acts as a powerful alpha- and beta-adrenergic agonist. EPI was compared with dobutamine-plus-NE infusion in a randomized control trial that studied patients in septic shock. Patients infused with EPI experienced similar improvements in hemodynamic status as the patients infused with the two-drug regime.
- Clinicians treating patients should monitor the individual's hemodynamic response to select the optimal drug and dose.
- Patients in septic shock commonly have profound vasodilatation and often appear flushed and have pink, well-perfused digits with brisk capillary refill despite being hypotensive.
- Improved systolic blood pressure can be accomplished in these patients by infusing a vasoconstrictor agent; the two most commonly used drugs are alpha-adrenergic agents (NE) and vasopressin.
- Alpha-adrenergic agents used effectively in patients with vasodilatory shock include NE and phenylepinephrine.
- Vasopressin infusion has been reported as an effective treatment of vasodilatory shock. This peptide is an antidiuretic hormone synthesized in the hypothalamus and released from the posterior pituitary in response to several stimuli, including increased ECW osmolality, hypoxia, pain, and baroreceptor-detected hypotension.
- Evidence indicates that patients with sustained septic shock (over hours) deplete endogenous vasopressin stores. These observations explain why vasopressin infused into patients with catecholamine-resistant septic shock can reverse vasodilation.
- The surgeon resuscitating a patient must monitor hemodynamic responses and adjust therapies as indicated.
- Rivers et al reported that patients in septic shock who presented to an emergency department benefited from the successful implementation of a protocol intended to rapidly achieve a balance of oxygen delivery and demand.
- Invasive hemodynamic monitoring is essential in complex patients to determine the effectiveness of interventions intended to restore delivery of oxygen to tissues. As a final consideration in the treatment of any patient in septic shock, resuscitation often is futile without amelioration of the source of sepsis.

Antiinflammatory Treatment for Severe Sepsis and Septic Shock

- As sepsis progresses to severe sepsis and septic shock, the risk for organ failure increases in proportion to excessive activation of the inflammatory cascade.
- Bernard et al compared the 28-day survival of patients in severe sepsis who received either placebo or recombinant human activated protein C (APC). This anticoagulant agent inhibits thrombosis and accelerates fibrinolysis. Furthermore, this protein blocks tissue factor monocyte activation and cytokine release. The trial showed a significant reduction in mortality rates from 31% to 25% with APC treatment.
- Severe sepsis has been demonstrated to cause relative adrenal insufficiency, defined as impaired glucocorticoid response to adrenal cortex stimulation. Annane et al reported that treatment of patients in septic shock with low doses of hydrocortisone and fludrocortisone reduced risk of death at 28 days.
- Nonresponders included those patients whose serum cortisol levels increased less than 9 $\mu g/dL$; these patients were considered to have a sepsis-related dysfunction in the hypothalamic-pituitary-adrenal axis.

SHOCK FROM CARDIAC DISEASE

- Surgical patients develop acute hypotension as a consequence of several cardiac diseases that share the general problem that cardiac output from the left ventricle is inadequate. The conditions that cause cardiogenic shock have variable pathophysiologic characteristics, but all are highly lethal. Successful treatment must be directed to correct the specific cause.

Shock from Acute Myocardial Infarction

- Seven to 10% of patients with an acute myocardial infarction develop cardiogenic shock and 70% of patients who develop cardiogenic shock die.
- Patients who develop cardiogenic shock after a myocardial infarction typically have onset of symptoms 6 to 12 hours after initial angina symptoms.
- Other causes of severe cardiac dysfunction associated with myocardial infarction are acute mitral regurgitation, rupture of the interventricular septum, or rarely, right, ventricular dysfunction.
- Cardiogenic shock can be confirmed by echocardiography, which demonstrates poorly contractile left ventricle, or

passing a pulmonary artery catheter, which reveals pulmonary artery wedge pressure greater than 20 mm Hg and cardiac index less than 2.0 L/min m². Initial therapy in patients with myocardial ischemia should include oxygen, nitroglycerin, aspirin, and adequate intravenous morphine to provide pain relief and reduce anxiety.

- Multiple studies have confirmed that fibrinolytic therapy (i.e., tissue plasminogen activator) improves the survival of patients having acute myocardial ischemia. Fibrinolytic therapy is not effective in patients in established cardiogenic shock.

Shock from Cardiac Tamponade and Cardiac Contusion

- A blow to the anterior chest that transmits substantial energy to the myocardium can cause myocardial hemorrhage and tissue edema. Cardiac contusion may be a common cause of immediate death to patients who sustain chest trauma in such high-energy circumstances as a motor vehicle crash. However, cardiac contusion is rarely the cause of shock in a blunt trauma patient who is hypotensive on arrival at a hospital's emergency room. Although several blood tests have been advocated for making the diagnosis of acute cardiac contusion, the cardiac echocardiogram is most specific. Hypotensive patients, who sustained chest trauma and have a dilated ventricular chamber associated with poor contractility of the wall (by echocardiography), either have a cardiac contusion to the ventricle or have sustained a proximal main coronary artery occlusion and an acute myocardial infarction in association with their episode of injury.
- Cardiac tamponade is a readily reversible cause of shock. Tamponade occurs when fluid or blood accumulates between the pericardium and heart. If pericardial fluid develops under significant pressure, filling of the heart cannot occur during diastole; thus, there is little blood within the ventricle available for ejection.
- The physical findings in patients with cardiac tamponade are hypotension, distended neck veins, and pulsus paradoxus, defined as more than 10 mm Hg decline in systolic pressure at the end of the inspiratory phase of respiration.

Shock from Massive Pulmonary Embolism

- A massive pulmonary embolism can cause the acute onset of shock.
- Right-sided heart failure has been identified as the usual cause of death. Echocardiogram shows an enlarged right

ventricle. Clinical examination reveals distended neck veins
and a tricuspid regurgitation murmur.

- Intravenous heparin should be given to most patients in
  whom a diagnosis of acute pulmonary embolism has been
  established.
- For patients with recent wounds or incisions, bleeding complications are a risk following thrombolytic therapy.

SHOCK FROM ADRENAL INSUFFICIENCY

Control of Adrenal Function

- The two adrenal glands release hormones essential for life
  and individuals with sudden stress depend on accelerated
  adrenal hormone release.
- Cortisol is released from the zona fasciculate of the
  adrenal cortex. Cortisol supports accelerated intracellular
  synthesis of proteins in response to stress and is crucial in
  the energy metabolism essential for maintenance of cell
  homeostasis.
- The hypothalamic-pituitary-adrenal axis enables the brain to
  direct the release of cortisol.
- The renin-angiotensin-aldosterone axis starts with cells of the
  juxtaglomerular apparatus of the kidney capable of responding to alterations in perfusion pressure.

Primary and Secondary Adrenal Insufficiency

- Primary adrenal insufficiency is a pathologic process of the
  adrenal gland. The critical nature of adrenal function is dramatically demonstrated by the rapid clinical deterioration of
  patients who have a sudden loss of adrenal function.
- Secondary adrenal insufficiency occurs when there is injury
  or disease of the pituitary or hypothalamus.
- The commonly recommended replacement dose used in
  acute severe stress would be 100 mg intravenously every
  8 hours with a rapid taper over the subsequent days as
  the patient's condition stabilizes. Other glucocorticoids
  used for intravenous replacement therapy include methylprednisolone and dexamethasone, which have been determined to have an anti-inflammatory mg per mg potency
  (relative to hydrocortisone of 1.0) of 5 and 25, respectively.
  Treatment of mineralocorticoid insufficiency in patients
  with primary adrenal failure can be accomplished by
  administration of 0.05 to 0.2 mg day of 9-alpha-fluor-
  hydrocortisone.

Relative Adrenal Glucocorticoid Insufficiency

- Adrenal insufficiency occurs in patients who have received long-term therapy with glucocorticoids. Patients are given these drugs as immunosuppression following transplantation or to treat inflammatory conditions including autoimmune diseases, inflammatory bowel disease, reactive airway disease, and arthritis.

Critical Adrenal Insufficiency in Sepsis

- Annane et al and others have reported evidence that severe sepsis and septic shock are associated with a relative adrenal insufficiency.
- In a randomized, prospective, placebo-controlled trial to evaluate the effectiveness of replacement therapy, these investigators administered low doses of hydrocortisone and fludrocortisone (a synthetic mineralocorticoid) to the treatment group for 7 days. This therapy improved survival of patients, specifically those with occult adrenal insufficiency.

HEMATOLOGIC PRINCIPLES IN SURGERY

CHAPTER 5

HEMOSTASIS AND COAGULATION

- Traditional concepts of coagulation held that two pathways exist by which coagulation could occur: the intrinsic pathway and the extrinsic pathway (Fig. 5–1).
- The clinical relevance of the intrinsic pathway is not associated with clinically significant bleeding *in vivo,* although it does produce aberrations in tests of coagulation.
- The interaction of factor VII with tissue factor (TF), its high-affinity receptor and cofactor, initiates the extrinsic cascade.
- Deficiencies in the cascade model and recent discoveries have prompted a model of cell-based coagulation, with TF-bearing cells and platelets at the center (Fig. 5–2).
- Monroe et al describe three phases of the cell-based coagulation; initiation, priming, and propagation.
- In the second priming phase, platelets release granules containing factor V, which is cleaved to factor Va.
- In the propagation phase, the activated primed platelets are now able to rapidly bind factors Va, VIIIa, and IXa.
- The thrombin-thrombomodulin complex activates protein C in the presence of its cofactor protein S. Activated protein C competitively binds factors Va and VIIIa limiting the production of factor Xa and thrombin. As a clinically important anti-coagulant pathway in humans, either protein C or protein S deficiency is known to cause a significant tendency toward thrombosis. Activated protein C has also been used to treat patients with significant systemic inflammatory response syndrome, who appear to have a procoagulant state with decreased expression of thrombomodulin and decreased levels of protein C.

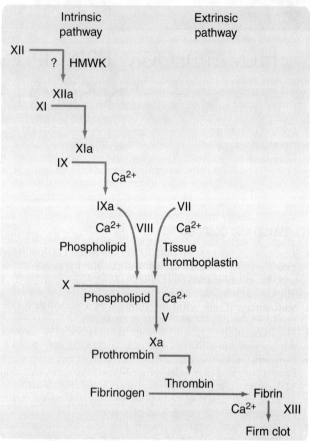

FIGURE 5–1. Traditional schematic version of the coagulation system. HMWK, high-molecular-weight kininogen.

Blood Vessels and Endothelial Cells

- Hemostasis is the physiologic cessation of bleeding.
- Vasoconstriction occurs in response to the release of vasoactive substances from platelets (e.g., thromboxane A_2 and serotonin) and endothelin from endothelial cells. Thromboxane A_2 is produced locally at the site of injury and is a very potent constrictor of smooth muscle, especially in smaller and

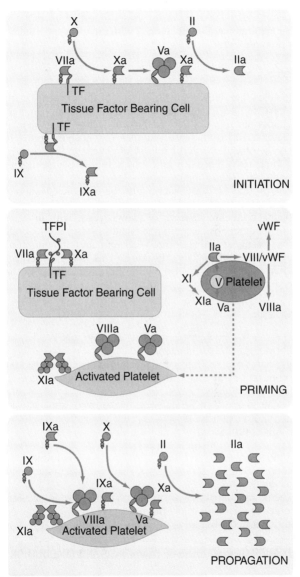

FIGURE 5–2. Cell-based model of coagulation. (From Monroe DM, Hoffman M, Roberts HR: Platelets and thrombin generation. Arterioscler Thromb Vasc Biol 22:1381–1389, 2002.)

medium-sized vessels. Larger vessels constrict in response to innervation and circulating constrictive factors such as norepinephrine.

Platelets

- Platelets are activated with release of the contents of their alpha granules (platelet factor 4, beta-thromboglobulin, thrombospondin, platelet-derived growth factor, fibrinogen, and factor VIIIR) and dense granules (adenosine diphosphate and serotonin). With the release of platelet granule contents, particularly adenosine diphosphate, further platelet aggregation at the site of injury occurs.
- The production of prostacyclin by the endothelial cell serves to counterbalance the local hemostatic process. In particular, prostacyclin elevates levels of adenyl cyclase with an increase in cyclic adenosine monophosphate levels within platelets, decreasing available ionized calcium and limiting further aggregation of platelets. Because of its potent vasodilatory effects, prostacyclin also limits the progress of localized coagulation.

Fibrinolysis

- Plasmin is a powerful proteolytic enzyme that breaks down fibrin into soluble fragments.
- Plasmin acts not only on fibrin but also on fibrinogen and prothrombin, factors V and VIII and, some data suggest, on factors IX and XI.
- The main reaction of the fibrinolytic pathway is the activation of plasminogen to plasmin by the plasminogen activators tPA and urokinase.
- The major inhibitor of plasminogen activation is plasminogen activator inhibitor (PAI-1), which is found in low concentration in plasma but at higher concentration within platelets.
- The major inhibitor of plasmin, alpha$_2$-antiplasmin or plasmin inhibitor, circulates in plasma at relatively high concentrations and can neutralize large amounts of plasmin.

EVALUATION OF DISORDERS OF HEMOSTASIS AND COAGULATION

- An accurate history and physical examination of a patient scheduled to undergo elective operation offers the most valuable source of information regarding the risk of bleeding.

Screening Tests for Bleeding Disorders

- For most patients undergoing either minor operations or procedures that do not involve extensive dissection, laboratory testing is unlikely to provide additional information over a properly performed history and physical examination.
- Prothrombin time (PT) measures the function of factor VII and the *extrinsic pathway* and the *common pathway* factors (factor X, prothrombin/thrombin, fibrinogen, and fibrin).
- The activated partial thromboplastin time (aPTT) detects decreased levels of the intrinsic pathway factors (high-molecular-weight kininogen; prekallikrein; and factors XII, XI, IX, and VIII) and the common pathway factors (fibrinogen, prothrombin, and factors V and X).
- The PT and aPTT can be used together in an attempt to localize coagulation defects. A normal PT with an abnormal aPTT suggests deficiency of the proximal intrinsic pathway factors. A prolonged PT with a normal aPTT suggests abnormalities of the vitamin K–dependent factors such as factor VII. An abnormal PT or aPTT may indicate the presence of an inhibitor (e.g., lupus anticoagulant, heparin, or an inhibitor of a specific factor).
- Patients with Marfan's syndrome, Ehlers-Danlos syndrome, or osteogenesis imperfecta may have abnormal bleeding and poor wound healing despite normal screening tests. Other bleeding disorders often missed by routine coagulation testing include mild von Willebrand's disease, platelet function defect, factor XIII deficiency, hyperglobulinemic states, alpha$_2$-antiplasmin deficiency, and amyloidosis.

CONGENITAL BLEEDING DISORDERS

Hemophilia

- Hemophilia A (classic hemophilia) is a congenital coagulation disorder that results from a deficiency or abnormality of factor VIII. It is transmitted as an X-linked recessive disorder, with males being affected almost exclusively.
- Hemophilia B, also known as Christmas disease, is an inherited X-linked bleeding disorder that reflects a deficiency or defect in factor IX.
- Desmopressin (DDAVP) may temporarily raise factor VIII levels in the patient with mild hemophilia A (basal factor VIII levels of 5% to 10%).

- Two types of concentrates are available for treatment of hemophilia A:
  - Plasma-based factor VIII preparations.
  - Recombinant preparations.
- For treatment of hemophilia B, the traditional therapy is prothrombin complex concentrate, which contains not only factor IX but also all of the vitamin K–dependent factors.
- The transmission of human immunodeficiency virus (HIV) to the hemophiliac population through replacement blood products was a major complication of transfusion therapy, with 55% of hemophiliacs infected with HIV-1 by the mid-1980s. This has been eliminated by viral inactivation procedures, mandatory blood donor screening for HIV, and the use of recombinant products.
- Recombinant factor VIIa (rFVIIa) has been used successfully to stop active bleeding in hemophilia patients and non-hemophilia patients with antibodies to factor VIII.

von Willebrand's Disease

- von Willebrand's disease is the most common congenital bleeding disorder; its frequency is estimated to be as high as 1%.
- Bleeding encountered in patients with von Willebrand's disease is similar to that of patients with bleeding from platelet dysfunction with mucosal bleeding, petechiae, epistaxis, and menorrhagia.
- The administration of DDAVP, 0.3 µg/kg, causes significant shortening in the bleeding time and normalization of factors VIII and VIIIR activities.
- About 48 hours must elapse for new endothelial stores of factor VIIIR to accumulate and so permit a second injection of DDAVP to be as effective as an initial dose. Replacement of factor VIIIR by infusing cryoprecipitate is effective in the control or prevention of bleeding in von Willebrand's disease.

ACQUIRED BLEEDING DISORDERS

Vitamin K Deficiency

- Vitamin K is necessary for the reaction that attaches a carboxy group to glutamic acid, and the proteins containing carboxyglutamic acid residues are, therefore, called *vitamin K–dependent clotting factors* (including prothrombin; factors VII, IX, X; and proteins C and S).

- Vitamin K may be administered parenterally and produces a correction in clotting times within 6 to 12 hours. Up to 5 mg intravenously is given slowly as an initial dose. Older preparations of vitamin K were less purified than those used at present, and anaphylaxis and death were reported with intravenous administration of these older agents. The more purified forms are less likely to cause complications, but intravenous vitamin K should be given cautiously. Intramuscular or subcutaneous vitamin K may be given in doses of 10 to 25 mg/day. Repeated doses of intramuscular or subcutaneous vitamin K allow total body repletion (10 to 25 mg/day for 3 days). Administration of fresh frozen plasma (FFP) rapidly corrects the coagulation deficit and should be given with vitamin K to patients with ongoing bleeding.

Anticoagulant Drugs

- Warfarin acts by blocking the synthesis of vitamin K–dependent factors, prolongs the PT, and causes a slight elevation of the aPTT by reducing the levels of prothrombin and factors VII, IX, and X.
- Unfractionated heparin (UFH) blocks the activation of factor X by binding with antithrombin III (AT-III) and thrombin. All coagulation tests can be affected by UFH, including the PT, but the aPTT is most sensitive. A dose of UFH is cleared from the blood in approximately 6 hours but varies depending on other factors such as hepatic function, body temperature, and shock.
- UFH can cause thrombocytopenia (heparin-induced thrombocytopenia [HIT]) in up to 5% of patients because of the formation of IgG antibodies to heparin-platelet factor 4 complexes.
- In any patient who has a decrease in platelet count, all heparin should be withdrawn immediately, and another anticoagulant such as lepirudin or argatroban initiated if necessary.
- Low-molecular-weight heparins (LMWHs) derived from UFH have more selective anti-Xa activity than UFH. LMWHs have been associated with less bleeding complications and have become the first-line therapy for deep venous thrombosis prophylaxis and treatment and acute coronary syndromes. The PT is not usually affected by LMWH, and

anti-Xa activity should be measured if dose efficacy is questioned.

Hepatic Failure

- The liver is the major site of synthesis of all the coagulation factors except factor VIII.

Renal Failure

- Renal disease and uremia cause a reversible bleeding disorder related to platelet dysfunction.
- The administration of DDAVP helps decrease bleeding problems after procedures in these patients. Intravenous DDAVP, 0.3 µg/kg, decreases bleeding time, increases platelet retention on glass beads, and increases activity of factor VIII. Cryoprecipitate and conjugated estrogens can also shorten the bleeding time.

Thrombocytopathy

- The most common drugs that block platelet function are prostaglandin inhibitors, particularly aspirin, indomethacin, and other nonsteroidal anti-inflammatory drugs (NSAIDs).

Hypothermia

- Hypothermia is one of the most common and least well-recognized causes of altered coagulation in surgical patients, especially those receiving massive transfusion.
- The coagulation system is a series of proteolytic enzymes, the activity of which decreases with decreasing temperature. Hypothermia is characterized by a marked increase in fibrinolytic activity, thrombocytopenia, impaired platelet function, decrease in collagen-induced platelet aggregation, and increased affinity of hemoglobin for oxygen.
- Hemorrhage accounts for 90% of deaths after abdominal injury, and half of these deaths are secondary to a recalcitrant coagulopathy.

DISSEMINATED INTRAVASCULAR COAGULATION (DIC)

- DIC is a systemic thrombohemorrhagic disorder seen in association with many clinical situations with laboratory evidence of coagulant activation, fibrinolytic activation, inhibitor consumption, and end-organ dysfunction.

PREPARATION OF BLOOD COMPONENTS

● Component therapy is the accepted standard for the optimal management of the blood supply.

CLINICAL INDICATIONS AND USE OF BLOOD COMPONENTS

Red Blood Cells

● The use of a hematocrit of 30% (or a hemoglobin of 10 g/dL) as a *transfusion trigger* is no longer acceptable. Oxygen delivery is maintained by a series of complex interactions and compensatory mechanisms when red cell mass (measured by hemoglobin or hematocrit) falls. This includes increased cardiac output, increased extraction ratio, rightward shift of the oxyhemoglobin curve, and expansion of volume.
● The cardiac output does not increase until hemoglobin falls below approximately 7 g/dL. Young healthy patients tolerate acute anemia to hemoglobin levels of 7 g/dL or less, provided they have a normal intravascular volume and high arterial oxygen saturation.
● A University HealthSystem Consortium Expert Panel reviewed the literature and identified four indications for white blood cell (WBC)-reduced blood components:
  ● To decrease the incidence of subsequent refractoriness to platelet transfusion caused by human leukocyte antigen (HLA) alloimmunization in patients requiring long-term platelet support.
  ● To provide blood components with reduced risk for cytomegalovirus (CMV) transmission.
  ● To prevent subsequent febrile nonhemolytic transfusion reaction (FNHTR) in patients who have had one documented FNHTR.
  ● To decrease the incidence of HLA alloimmunization in nonhepatic solid-organ transplant candidates.

Platelets

● Platelets should not be transfused prophylactically in the absence of microvascular bleeding, a low platelet count in a patient undergoing a surgical procedure, or a platelet count that has fallen below 10,000/mm^3 (Box 5–1).

Leukocyte Concentrate

● Leukocyte transfusions are indicated in profound granulocytopenia (<500/mm^3) with evidence of infection (e.g., positive

---

Box 5–1. Suggested Transfusion Guidelines for Platelets

Recent (within 24 hours) platelet count <10,000/cu mm (for prophylaxis)

Recent (within 24 hours) platelet count <50,000/cu mm with demonstrated microvascular bleeding ("oozing") or a planned surgical/invasive procedure

Demonstrated microvascular bleeding and a precipitous fall in platelet count

Adult patients in the operating room who have had complicated procedures or have required more than 10 units of blood **AND** have microvascular bleeding. Giving platelets assumes adequate surgical hemostasis has been achieved.

Documented platelet dysfunction (e.g., prolonged bleeding time greater than 15 minutes, abnormal platelet function tests) with petechiae, purpura, microvascular bleeding ("oozing"), or surgical/invasive procedure

Unwarranted indication:

　Empirical use with massive transfusion when patient is not having clinically evident microvascular bleeding ("oozing")

　Prophylaxis in thrombotic thrombocytopenic purpura/ hemolytic-uremic syndrome or idiopathic thrombocytopenic purpura

　Extrinsic platelet dysfunction (e.g., renal failure, von Willebrand's disease)

---

blood culture, persistent temperature above 38.5°C) unresponsive to antibiotic therapy.

Fresh Frozen Plasma

- FFP is used to replace labile factors in patients with coagulopathy and documented factor deficiency.
- FFP should not be used routinely by preset formula after red blood cell (RBC) transfusion (e.g., two units of FFP for every five units of packed RBCs) or *prophylactically* after cardiac bypass or other procedures.

Cryoprecipitate

- Cryoprecipitate is useful in treating factor deficiency (hemophilia A), von Willebrand's disease, and hypofibrinogenemia and may help treat uremic bleeding.

Perioperative Transfusion

- No specific hematocrit is an indication for preoperative transfusion in a stable patient. A symptomatic patient with anemia who is about to undergo a procedure that involves significant blood loss may benefit from perioperative transfusion.
- The goal of transfusion of a symptomatic patient is the relief of symptoms. Previously a single-unit transfusion was condemned; however, if one unit is sufficient to alleviate symptoms, no additional transfusion should be given because each unit adds to the risk.

Transfusion of the Patient in Shock

- The goal of resuscitation from shock is prompt restoration of adequate perfusion and transport of oxygen.
- Crystalloid is infused at a 3:1 ratio for every unit of RBCs administered, and therapy is monitored by hemodynamic response. Because crystalloid solutions are universally available and some delay is required to prepare blood products, crystalloid is the proper initial resuscitation fluid.

RISKS OF BLOOD TRANSFUSION

- Administrative error leading to ABO incompatibility, bacterial contamination, and transfusion-related lung injury are the three leading causes for fatalities after blood transfusion.

Transfusion Reactions

- Severe acute hemolytic reactions generally involve the transfusion of ABO incompatible blood with fatalities occurring in 1 in 600,000 units.
- Delayed hemolytic reactions tend to present 5 to 10 days after transfusion with approximately 1 in 260,000 patients developing a significant hemolytic reaction.

Bacterial Contamination

- Bacterial contamination of blood is the most frequent cause of transfusion-transmitted infectious disease. After hemolytic reactions, it is the most frequently reported cause of transfusion-related fatalities to the Food and Drug Administration (FDA). A recent Centers for Disease Control and Prevention (CDC) study found the rates of transfusion transmitted bacteremia to be 1 in 100,000 units for single-donor and pooled platelets and 1 in 5 million units for packed red cells.

Transfusion-Related Acute Lung Injury (TRALI)

● The incidence is estimated to be 1 case per 5000 units transfused, but the syndrome is often underdiagnosed. It is believed to be the third most common cause of fatal transfusion reactions.

Hepatitis

● The risk of transfusion-associated hepatitis B virus (HBV) infection is approximately 1:30,000 to 1:250,000 units. With the development of pooled nucleic acid amplification testing (NAT) tests for hepatitis C virus (HCV), the window period has decreased, and the risk of HCV transmission is now as low as 1 in 1 million.

Human Immunodeficiency Virus

● With pooled NAT, the window period for detection of HIV has been reduced by 30% to 50% and the risk of HIV transmission is estimated to be as low as 1 in 2,000,000 units.

Human T-Cell Leukemia Virus

● The risk of human T-lymphotropic virus (HTLV) I and II transmission is estimated to be 1 in 641,000 units.

Immunomodulation

● Allogeneic blood transfusion alters the immune response in individuals and susceptibility to infection, tumor recurrence, and reactivation of latent viruses.

MASSIVE TRANSFUSION

● Massive transfusion is defined as replacement of the patient's blood volume with packed RBCs in 24 hours or transfusion of more than 10 units of blood over a few hours.

Hemostasis

- Prophylactic use of platelet concentrate in the massively transfused patient is not justified without evidence of microvascular bleeding.
- The prophylactic use of FFP along with transfusion of RBCs is no longer acceptable in light of convincing data and the added risk of transfusion.

BLOOD SUBSTITUTES AND ALTERNATIVES TO TRANSFUSION

Autologous Blood

- Because acute normovolemic hemodilution is effective and is less costly than preoperative donation, acute normovolemic hemodilution is more likely to be used in future blood-conserving strategies.

Autologous Cell Salvage

- The procedure is cost effective when at least two shed units are able to be salvaged.

CHAPTER 6

METABOLISM IN SURGICAL PATIENTS

OVERVIEW

Rationale for Provision of Artificial Nutrition

- More than 10% weight loss or 7 to 10 days of inanition are associated with the following:
  - Increased incidence of nosocomial infection.
  - Longer hospital stay.
  - Increased mortality.
  - Impaired wound healing and immune function.
  - Loss of muscle function and strength resulting from muscle wasting.
  - Limitations to all aggressive surgical and medical therapies.

Pitfalls of Artificial Nutrition

- Body tissue is 30% adipose, 30% lean (protein), and 30% extracellular fluid (water). Providing excessive calories during total parenteral nutrition (TPN) administration is associated with the following:
  - Iatrogenic immune and hepatic dysfunction.
  - Further increases in total body water and fat content.
  - No beneficial effect on body protein.

METABOLIC ADAPTATIONS IN CATABOLIC STATES

Amino Acid Metabolism

Roles of Specific Amino Acids

- Essential amino acids include valine, leucine, isoleucine, lysine, methionine, phenylalanine, threonine, and tryptophan. Cysteine and tyrosine are conditionally essential.
- The remaining 10 amino acids alanine, arginine, aspartate, asparagine, glutamate, glutamine, glycine, histidine, proline, and serine are not essential.

- Histidine, proline, glutamine, and arginine may become conditionally essential under catabolic conditions.
- Three major fates of amino acids are (1) protein synthesis, (2) oxidation by the tricarboxylic acid cycle leading to the production of urea and carbon dioxide, and (3) synthesis of nonessential amino acids, purines, and pyrimidines.

Amino Acid Metabolism in Liver

- The liver is the major site for the degradation and synthesis of amino acids and is the most important organ regulating plasma amino acid levels.
- Only 25% of ingested protein reaches the general (nonportal) circulation as free amino acids. Almost 60% is converted to urea, 6% is synthesized to plasma protein, and 14% becomes liver protein.
- In parenteral nutrition, nutrients are supplied to the systemic, rather than the portal, circulation and thus override the liver and the normal postprandial production of gut hormones. As a result, overall nutrient disposal is probably less efficient during TPN administration, and this phenomenon contributes to the difficulty in achieving positive nitrogen balance.

Amino Acid Metabolism in Muscle

- Skeletal and cardiac muscle are the major site in the body for the catabolism of the branched-chain amino acids (BCAAs) leucine, isoleucine, and valine and for the synthesis of alanine and glutamine.
- Leucine is degraded to acetyl-CoA moieties, which are then oxidized in the tricarboxylic acid cycle to provide energy. In many catabolic states, including fasting, diabetes, and trauma, BCAA oxidation increases in muscle and spares glucose.
- Amino groups generated by degradation of BCAAs contribute to the de novo synthesis of alanine and glutamine in muscle, which on release are important gluconeogenic precursors.

Glutamine and Interorgan Relationships

- Most glutamine released from muscle is derived from de novo synthesis, rather than liberated as a result of proteolysis.
- The glutamine released by muscle is an important primary energy source for many cells.
- Glutamine is taken up from the blood primarily by the kidney, where it serves as a precursor for urinary ammonia. Its carbon skeleton is used for gluconeogenesis or energy

production, or some of the carbons are released into the blood as alanine.

- The small intestine metabolizes large amounts of glutamine; it in turn releases appreciable amounts of alanine. The liver then utilizes the released alanine for glucose production. This complex multiorgan process is important for gluconeogenesis from amino acids originating in proteins and converted to glutamine in muscle.
- Glucocorticoids induce glutamine production and release from muscle in starvation and sepsis, when glucocorticoid levels are high.
- The lung has a high capacity for synthesizing glutamine, and this process increases in sepsis.

Regulation of Intracellular Protein Synthesis and Degradation

Biochemical Pathways for Intracellular Protein Breakdown

- Pathways for intracellular proteolysis include the acid-dependent proteases (cathepsins) in lysosomes and proteases active at neutral pH that are found in the cytosol. This latter group includes the calcium-dependent calpains, the caspases, and the ATP-dependent ubiquitin (Ub)-proteasome pathway.
- The Ub-proteasome pathway accounts for the majority of accelerated proteolysis in many different catabolic conditions characterized by muscle wasting, including fasting, diabetes, acidosis, sepsis, and denervation or disuse atrophy.
- Degradation of proteins via the Ub-proteasome pathway is a multistep process that requires the hydrolysis of ATP, in addition to the 8-kDa protein cofactor ubiquitin and the 26S proteasome.

Nutrients and Hormones Regulating Nitrogen Balance

- Insulin inhibits lipolysis and increases nitrogen accrual in muscle, liver, and other tissues. Insulin stimulates amino acid transport into muscle, increases rates of protein synthesis, and inhibits muscle protein breakdown. The rise in insulin after meals promotes net protein accumulation in muscle, while in fasting, when insulin is low, there is a net loss of protein and a release of amino acids from muscle.
- BCAAs stimulate protein synthesis and reduce protein breakdown in muscle.
- The polypeptide insulin-like growth factors (IGF-I and IGF-II) that are synthesized in part under the stimulation of growth

hormone reduce muscle proteolysis and enhance protein synthesis.

- Glucocorticoids retard growth and promote the release of amino acids from muscle by decreasing DNA and protein synthesis and reducing amino acid uptake. In fasting, glucocorticoids promote the breakdown of muscle protein by activation of the Ub-proteasome pathway. Glucocorticoids are also important for the increase in ATP-dependent protein breakdown that occurs in metabolic acidosis, diabetes, and sepsis.
- A lack of tension or disuse is a major signal activating muscle proteolysis, a phenomenon of great relevance clinically.

Physiologic Adaptations in Specific Catabolic States

Short-Term Fasting

- Complete food deprivation leads to a mobilization of body protein to support energy needs. As much as 300 g of protein per day may be lost initially in humans.
  - Amino acid release from skeletal muscle increases markedly.
  - Hepatic glycogenolysis provides a limited store (100 g) for systemic glucose.
  - Lipolysis and fatty acid oxidation for energy increase in response to low insulin.
  - The average adult fat reserve is approximately 10 kg, or 100,000 kcal.
  - BCAA oxidation in muscle rises, sparing glucose.
  - Gluconeogenesis in the liver and kidney is activated, using muscle-derived glutamine and alanine, lactate, and glycerol released from lipid oxidation.
- In muscle, activation of the ATP-Ub-dependent proteolytic pathway is primarily responsible for the increased protein degradation in fasting:
  - Ub mRNA and the mRNAs for several proteasome subunits increase three- to sixfold.
  - Fasted muscles contain higher amounts of proteins conjugated to Ub.
  - A recently identified ubiquitin-ligase named *atrogin-1* is markedly induced.

Inflammation and Sepsis

- Lean tissue losses can approximate 900 g per day in patients with severe sepsis, traumatic injuries, closed head injury, or major burns, with generalized muscle wasting.

- Most of the increased proteolysis results from activation of the Ub-proteasome pathway, although lysosomal cathepsins and the calpains also appear to play a role.
- Sepsis leads to reduced protein synthesis in muscle, whereas hepatic protein synthesis, largely of acute phase reactant proteins found in plasma, is increased.
- Peripheral insulin resistance with impaired skeletal muscle uptake of glucose occurs, and hyperglycemia in response to intravenous feeding during sepsis is common.
- Many of the systemic manifestations of sepsis are mediated by cytokines, for example, interleukin (IL)-1 and IL-6, tumor necrosis factor (TNF), and interferon-γ (IFN-γ).
- Activation of proteolysis by TNF and other cytokines involves activation of a nuclear transcription factor that serves as a common signal for inflammation, termed NF-κB.
- Glucocorticoids are required for activation of the Ub-proteasome pathway in sepsis and are a permissive factor for the response to cytokines.
- Fever also directly increases proteolysis in muscle during systemic infection.

Cancer

- Patients with neoplastic disease may suffer profound weight loss and generalized cachexia resulting from the following:
  - Anorexia with reduced food intake.
  - Altered metabolic rate.
  - Endocrine abnormalities.
  - Direct effects of anticancer treatments.
  - Elevated cytokines, including TNF, IL-1, IL-6, and IFN-γ.
- Marked muscle wasting is a debilitating feature of advanced cancer, although the factors leading to accelerated proteolysis remain unclear.

Regulation of Body Energy Expenditure and Appetite

- Adipose tissue and the gut play an important role in regulating appetite and energy use.
  - Adipose tissue is an important source of endocrine mediators, including leptin, TNF, angiotensinogen, resistin, and adiponectin.
  - Gut-derived mediators include ghrelin, cholecystokinin (CCK), peptideYY (PYY), and insulin.
- These hormones interact at the arcuate nucleus in the brain to control food intake and energy expenditure. In the

arcuate nucleus, two sets of neurons interact with opposing effects:

- Activation of agouti-related peptide (AgRP)/neuropeptide Y (NPY) neurons increases appetite and metabolism.
- Activation of proopiomelanocortin/cocaine and amphet-amine-related transcript (POMC/CART) neurons inhibits eating, in part by causing the release of α-melanocyte-stimulating hormone (α-MSH), a satiety signal.
- Appetite-promoting agents such as ghrelin may improve the inanition accompanying cancer.

FUNDAMENTALS OF ARTIFICIAL NUTRITION

General Indications for Nutrition Support

- Indications for nutritional support include the following:
  - Poor nutritional status (current oral intake meets <50% of total energy needs).
  - Significant weight loss (initial body weight less than the usual body weight by 10% or more or a decrease in inpatient weight by more than 10% of the admission weight).
  - Starvation for more than 7 days.
  - An anticipated duration of artificial nutrition of greater than 7 days.
  - The degree of the anticipated insult, surgical or otherwise.
  - Serum albumin less than 3.0 g per 100 mL in the absence of an inflammatory state.
- There may be a clinical benefit to the initiation of immediate enteral feeding, particularly in the more critically ill patient, regardless of the premorbid nutritional status.

Nutritional Assessment

- Nutritional assessment estimates changes in body composition to predict the risk for surgery or other stressful therapeutic activity and includes clinical history, body composition analysis, and indirect calorimetry.

Clinical History

- The criteria listed previously are most relevant. Burns, sepsis, head injury, or pancreatitis are particularly catabolic and will raise caloric requirements significantly.

Body Composition Analysis

● Lean body mass may be estimated by bioelectrical impedance, the exchange of labeled ions, neutron activation analysis, cross-sectional imaging (magnetic resonance imaging [MRI], computed tomography [CT]), and other experimental methods.

Indirect Calorimetry

● Indirect calorimetry performed using a bedside metabolic cart to measure the following:
  • Oxygen consumption and to estimate caloric requirements.
  • The respiratory quotient (RQ), for an assessment of overfeeding.
RQ = 1 indicates pure carbohydrate utilization.
RQ = 0.8 indicates pure protein oxidation.
RQ = 0.7 is consistent with pure fat utilization.
RQ of greater than 1 is indicative of overfeeding of glucose or fat.

Anthropomorphic Measurements

● The "ideal body weight" (IBW) can be calculated, particularly when the usual body weight (UBW), the patient weight before illness, is unknown. The standardized IBW is as follows:
  • For males: 106 pounds for the first 5 feet and 6 pounds for each inch thereafter.
  • For females: 100 pounds for the first 5 feet and 5 pounds for each inch thereafter.

Biochemical Measurements

● Such methods are often inaccurate but include serum proteins, nitrogen balance, and measurements of protein breakdown and immunologic function.

Serum Proteins

● Albumin less than 3.0 g/dL is the usual indicator.
● Prealbumin or transferrin (<200 mg/dL) may be more sensitive.
● However, the meaning of the lowered serum albumin concentration in patients at risk remains controversial.

Nitrogen Balance

- Nitrogen balance is determined by measuring 24-hour urinary and gastrointestinal (GI) losses, compared with nitrogen intake:
  - = Intake − loss (urine 90%, stool 5%, integument 5%).
  - = [protein intake (g)/6.25] − urinary urea (g) − 2 (for stool and skin) − 2 (for nonurea nitrogen).

Measurement of Protein Breakdown

- Protein turnover can be estimated by the following:
  - Urinary excretion of 3-methylhistidine.
  - *In vitro* measurement in isolated muscle tissue (most accurate).
  - *In vivo* isotopic methods involving infusion of ^{15}N-labeled amino acids.
- All of these methods are subject to a variety of artifacts.

Measurements of Immunologic Function

- These include delayed cutaneous hypersensitivity or anergy and studies of neutrophil function. However, such approaches have little value for measuring specific nutritional or operative risk.

Specific Fuels

Carbohydrate

- Glucose is the preferred carbohydrate source in traditional TPN. Glucose administration decreases urea production, the "protein sparing" effect, by suppressing gluconeogenesis and by sparing amino acids from oxidization for energy.
- Infusion rates of 4 mg/kg/min yield maximal suppression of urea production.
- Infusion rates greater than 9 mg/kg/min lead to net synthesis of lipid.

Toxicity of Hyperglycemia and Excessive Calorie Administration

- Hyperglycemia is a prevalent metabolic disorder and is exacerbated by excessive administration of dextrose. When provided in excess, the following occur:
  - Glucose is converted to fat in the liver, contributing to liver dysfunction.

- The increase in VCO_2 leads to impaired ventilatory function.
- Hyperglycemia causes immunosuppression and nosocomial infections.
- Maintaining blood glucose in the 80 to 110 mg/dL range improves clinical outcomes and mortality. To avoid complications of overfeeding, a short-term option is hypocaloric feeding (20 to 25 kcal/kg body weight/day).

Lipid

- Fat and carbohydrate are similar with respect to their positive effects on nitrogen balance. However, in stress or during sepsis, fat utilization becomes impaired. Many sources of lipid are available for intravenous use.

Long-Chain Triglycerides (LCTs)

- The most commonly used formula is composed of soybean oil and egg lecithin and contains mainly LCT ("Intralipid"). Intralipid is also a source of essential fatty acids. Lipid emulsions are calorically dense (9 kcal/g) and can be safely infused via a peripheral vein.

Medium-Chain Triglycerides (MCTs)

- MCTs contain only 8 to 10 carbons, are cleared more rapidly from plasma than LCTs, are oxidized more rapidly, do not require a carnitine-dependent transport system to enter liver mitochondria, and are more soluble in TPN solutions. Mixed MCT-LCT emulsions are thought to be most desirable. Such mixed emulsions may be of particular benefit in patients with inflammatory disorders, because they may generate fewer potentially deleterious prostaglandins than LCTs alone.

Essential or Unsaturated Fatty Acids

- Unsaturated fatty acids can be classified as monounsaturated fatty acids (MUFAs) or polyunsaturated fatty acids (PUFAs) depending on the location of their double bond.
  - The three families of PUFAs (n-3, n-6, and n-9) start as the "essential" 18-carbon unsaturated fatty acids linoleic acid and α-linolenic acid and as the nonessential oleic acid.

- Via sequential steps of elongation and desaturation, linoleic acid (LA) is converted to arachidonic acid (AA), whereas α-linolenic acid (ALA) is converted to eicosapentaenoic acid (EPA) and docosahexaenoic acid (DHA).
- AA is the precursor of the 2-series of prostaglandins and thromboxanes and the 4-series of the leukotrienes, all proinflammatory mediators.
- EPA and DHA are the precursors of the 3-series of prostaglandins and thromboxanes and the 5-series of leukotrienes.

Omega-3 Fatty Acids in the Clinical Setting

- With the ingestion of fish oil, the primary dietary source of omega-3 fatty acids, EPA and DHA levels rise, and these lipids can displace arachidonic acid in cell membranes. As a result, with omega-3 fatty acid administration there is:
  - Decreased production of prostaglandin E_2.
  - Decreased thromboxane A_2, a platelet aggregator and vasoconstrictor.
  - Reduced leukotriene B_4, an inducer of leukocyte chemotaxis.
  - Increased prostacyclin PGI_3, a vasodilator and inhibitor of platelet aggregation.
- Therefore, omega-3 fatty acids (ALA or its products EPA and DHA) may downregulate an otherwise provasoconstrictive and prothrombotic state.
  - Enteral administration of omega-3 fatty acids in "immune-modulating" feeding formulas appears beneficial and is widely practiced clinically.
  - Intravenous administration of n-3 lipid emulsions requires combination with MCTs and LCTs and remains experimental.

Recognition of Essential Fatty Acid Deficiency

- Fatty acid deficiency is prevented by administering 2% to 5% of daily calories as vegetable oil fat emulsion or 30 to 50 g of lipid emulsion weekly. Plasma alterations include the following:
  - Decreases in linoleic and arachidonic and increased eicosatrienoic acids.
  - An increased "triene-to-tetraene" ratio to greater than 0.2%.
  - Dry, flaky skin with small reddish papules and alopecia may be observed.

Potential Toxicities of Lipid Administration

- LCT lipid administration appears quite safe when infusion rates are less than 0.1 g/kg/hour or 1 kcal/kg/hour. Lipid emulsions are not administered when the following occur:
  - Serum triglyceride levels are greater than 400 mg/dL.
  - Hypertriglyceride-related pancreatitis arises (triglycerides >800 mg/dL).
  - Excessive lipid may also be deleterious in patients with severe acute respiratory distress syndrome (ARDS).
- Impaired plasma clearance of lipids can result in the "fat overload syndrome," manifested by fever, back pain, chills, pulmonary insufficiency, and blocking of the reticulo-endothelial system.

Protein

- A 70-kg man has between 10 and 11 kg of protein or lean body mass. In the fed state, daily protein turnover is between 250 to 300 g, or 3%. Intracellular proteolysis accounts for 50 to 70 g of amino acids daily, but most of these are re-incorporated into protein.

Determining Protein Requirements

- The average normal requirement is 0.8 g of protein per kg or between 56 and 60 g of protein per day. Trauma, infection, and other catabolic conditions will increase this requirement.
  - Protein administration of 1.5 g/kg/day achieves maximal protein sparing.
  - Greater amounts (2 g/day) may be of benefit in severe injury, such as burns.

Alterations for Liver and Renal Failure

- Patients who are intolerant of nitrogen usually manifest renal or hepatic impairment, and patients with advanced hepatic failure may have both hepatic and renal insufficiency, the so-called "hepatorenal syndrome."

Renal Failure

- For patients with acute renal failure who are not yet on dialysis, protein intake may be reduced to 0.8 g/kg. Essential

amino acids and hypertonic dextrose in a restricted volume may also be of benefit:
- Hyperkalemia is improved.
- Dialysis may be averted.
- Survival may be improved, especially if some urine is produced.
- Hyperammonemia may occur in patients receiving only essential amino acids, and sufficient quantities of ornithine should be included and serum ammonia levels monitored.
- For patients on dialysis a more complete amino acid solution is appropriate. Protein intakes of up to 1.2 g/kg are recommended, even if it requires more frequent hemodialysis.

Hepatic Insufficiency

- Most such patients are hypercatabolic, but severe encephalopathy may develop when efforts are made to achieve nitrogen equilibrium (e.g., by giving 1.5 g of amino acids/kg/day).
  - An aromatic amino acid deficient/BCAA enriched solution may be efficacious in this setting.
  - The basis for this approach is the so-called "false neurotransmitter" hypothesis, in which increased aromatic amino acids result in the synthesis of "abnormal" neurotransmitters.

Plasma Electrolytes

- Average daily requirements for patients receiving TPN are as follows: sodium 50 mEq, potassium 20 to 40 mEq, calcium 0.2 to 0.3 mEq/kg, magnesium 0.35 to 0.45 mEq/kg, and phosphate 30 to 40 mmol.
- Extremely cachectic patients during the initiation of TPN may require additional potassium, magnesium, and phosphorus (the so-called phosphate steal or refeeding syndrome).

Vitamins and Micronutrients

- Micronutrient deficiencies in modern parenteral nutrition are rarely seen but result from inadequate provision of essential fatty acids, trace elements, or vitamins.
- Some agents require portal passage for metabolic conversion or activation, which is potentially bypassed during parenteral infusion.

- Following extensive ileal resection, substances that require the enterohepatic circulation for maximal absorption (e.g., zinc, copper, manganese, selenium, and many vitamins [cobalamin; folate; and the fat-soluble vitamins A, D, E, and K]) are particularly vulnerable.

Thiamine

- Severe thiamine deficiency leads to the classic nutritional disease beriberi characterized by a refractory lactic acidosis.

Vitamin D

- Deficiency of vitamin D is primarily an issue during long-term TPN administration. If vitamin D is to be repleted, oral administration is best (50,000 units per week for 6 to 8 weeks).

Vitamin K

- For patients who are entirely dependent on TPN, supplementation weekly with 10 mg intravenous vitamin K is necessary.

Zinc

- Three to 6 mg of elemental zinc per day is required, and up to 20 mg for patients with short bowel syndrome or excessive diarrhea. Signs of zinc deficiency include alopecia, poor wound healing, immunosuppression, night blindness or photophobia, anosmia, neuritis, and a variety of skin disorders.

Copper

- Copper deficiency manifests as microcytic anemia, pancytopenia, depigmentation, and osteopenia. In standard mineral solutions used for TPN, up to 2 mg of copper per day is given.

Chromium

- Chromium is necessary for the adequate utilization of glucose, and deficiency can manifest as a sudden diabetic state, with peripheral neuropathy and encephalopathy. Fifteen to 20 μg per day of chromium is adequate. Molybdenum or selenium deficiency are only very rarely observed.

Iron

- Calcium, iron, and other metals are absorbed in the duodenum, and duodenal bypass or resection may result in long-term deficiencies of these ions. The daily requirement for oral iron is 15 mg/day or 1 to 2 mg/day parenterally. Iron replacement should be avoided in the face of a concurrent inflammatory state or with active infection.

APPROACH TO ARTIFICIAL NUTRITION

- Essential principles are (1) to use the gut if possible and (2) if total nutritional supplementation cannot be provided by the GI tract, to administer at least 20% of the caloric and protein requirements enterally while reaching goal support with TPN until the GI tract returns to full functionality.

Principles of Enteral Feeding

- In addition to mechanical issues related to the feeding tube, the most common complications of enteral feedings result from solute overload:
  - Rapid administration of hyperosmolar solutions may induce diarrhea, dehydration, electrolyte imbalance, and hyperglycemia.
  - Pneumatosis intestinalis with bowel necrosis, perforation, and death may result.

Routes for Administration of Enteral Feeding

- The choice of access route and device must be tailored to the individual, considering their disease process and how long they will likely require nutritional support.

Nasoenteric and Postpyloric Feeding

- This is the least expensive and most widely used modality of enteral nutrition. Nasoenteric feeding tubes can be associated with multiple adverse consequences including tube migration, esophageal and gastric mucosal erosions, pulmonary aspiration, sinusitis, pneumothorax, esophageal stricture, esophageal perforation, and fatal arrhythmias:
  - Aspiration may be minimized by positioning the patient head-up and by monitoring of gastric residuals, which

should generally be less than 150 mL, although tolerance of residuals as great as 300 to 400 mL has been advocated.

- Postpyloric feeding does not appear to improve the incidence of actual aspiration or of clinically definable pneumonia than in patients fed gastrically.

Gastrostomy

- If long-term access to the stomach will be needed, a permanent gastrostomy can be placed either by the open approach or by percutaneous techniques, the latter using endoscopic, radiologic, or laparoscopic methods.

Jejunostomy

- Jejunal or small bowel feeding tube access can be obtained via open jejunostomy, percutaneously via an extension through an existing gastrostomy tube (often termed a G-J tube), or by a laparoscopic approach.

Enteral Formulas and Approach to Feed Advancement

- Almost all enteral products are hyperosmolar. Most formulas provide 1 kcal/mL, although higher calorie formulas (1.5 to 2 kcal/mL) allow smaller volumes of administration.
- Elemental formulations may be more efficiently absorbed in patients suffering from short gut syndrome or in those with chronic diarrhea, although this idea is unproven.
- For gastric feeding, feeds are started at 10 to 20 mL/hour continuously and are advanced in 10 to 20 mL increments until the goal rate is attained.
- For small bowel feeding, volume is increased first, then osmolality. Most patients do not tolerate small bowel administration of tube feeds containing greater than 300 to 400 mOsm, especially when critically ill.

Parenteral Feeding and Calculation of the Ideal Parenteral Formula

- Concentrated TPN (>900 mOsm/L) delivered to a large central vein (termed *central TPN*), with the line tip in the superior vena cava, is the preferred method. In the absence of central access, a less concentrated formula (dextrose not to exceed 5%) may be delivered via a peripheral vein (termed *peripheral TPN*).

Estimation of Energy Needs

- Available methods include indirect calorimetry, use of the IBW, and calculation by standard methods such as the Harris-Benedict equation. Basal metabolic rate (BMR) may be determined by the Harris-Benedict equation:

  Male BMR = 66 + (13.7 × wt in kg) + (5 × ht in cm)
  − (6.8 × age in years)

  Female BMR = 65.5 + (9.6 × wt) + (1.7 × ht in cm)
  − (4.7 × age)

- BMR must be corrected for normal activity (+15%), and for stress. The relevant "stress factor" for an uncomplicated postoperative patient is 10%, for peritonitis 10% to 30%, and for sepsis or trauma 30% to 50%, and in burns caloric requirements may be 50% to 100% greater than normal.
- Caloric requirements can also be estimated using normative values of body weight and the accepted parameter of 25 to 35 kcal/kg/day for the rate of caloric infusion:
  - "Feeding weight" is calculated by determining the IBW, which is then compared to the actual body weight (ABW):
    1. If the patient is underweight, use the ABW as the feeding weight.
    2. If the patient is obese (ABW is >120% of IBW), then add 25% of the difference between the ABW and IBW to the IBW as the feeding weight.
    3. If no reliable weight is available, use the IBW alone.

Formulation of the Total Parental Nutrition Solution

- For the calculation of caloric content in TPN, glucose contains 3.4 kcal/g, protein 4 kcal/g, and fat 9 kcal/g. In general, minimal fluid requirements in the absence of GI or other losses are 25 to 25 mL/kg/day. Using the example of a 70-kg person as the feeding weight, one first calculates the overall caloric goal and the proportion contributed by protein, usually:

  Total kilocalories (25 to 35 kcal/kg/day): 30 × 70 = 2100 kcal
  Protein (1.5 g/kg/day): 1.5 × 70 = 105 g amino acids

- For TPN formulated without lipid (2-in-1 solution):
  - Total kilocalories = 2100 kcal
  - Calories from amino acids = 105 g × 4 kcal/g = 420 kcal
  - Remaining calories = 2100 − 420 = 1680 kcal
  - Then make up the difference with dextrose: 1680 kcal ÷ 3.4 kcal/g = 494 g dextrose
- For TPN formulated with lipid (3-in-1 solution):
  - Total kilocalories = 2100 kcal

- Provide 20% of the total calories as lipid = 2100 × 0.2 = 420 kcal
- Then 420 kcal ÷ 9 kcal/g = 47 g lipid
- Calories from amino acids = 105 g × 4 kcal/g = 420 kcal
- Remaining calories = 2100 − 420 − 420 = 1260 kcal
- Then make up the difference with dextrose: 1260 kcal ÷ 3.4 kcal/g = 370 g dextrose
- Final volume (for 3-in-1, maximally concentrated):
  Amino acids (10% stock solution) 105 g = 1050 mL
  Dextrose (70% stock solution) 370 g = 528 mL
  Lipids (20% stock solution) 47 g = 235 mL
  Total volume = 1813 mL/day
- Final concentrations (wt/vol): amino acids 5.8%, dextrose 20.4%, lipid 2.6%.

Management of Insulin

- All patients who are started on TPN must be provided a subcutaneous sliding scale regimen for regular insulin administration:
  - Never increase the amount of dextrose in the TPN solution until blood sugars are well-controlled (i.e., <150 mg/dL).
  - Determine the amount of sliding scale insulin administered over the previous 24 hours and add ½ to ⅔ of that amount to the new TPN solution for the ensuing 24 hours.
  - Use a constant insulin infusion if it is difficult to gain control.

Mandatory Monitoring During Intravenous Nutrition

Clinical

- Daily fluid balance, body weight, evidence of infection.

Laboratory

- Baseline: electrolytes, blood urea nitrogen (BUN), creatinine, glucose, calcium, magnesium, Pi, liver function, triglyceride, albumin, and prothrombin time.
- Every 6 to 12 hours: glucose, usually for 3 to 5 days or until stable.
- Daily until stable: electrolytes, BUN, creatinine, glucose, calcium, magnesium, and phosphate.
- Weekly: liver function, triglyceride, albumin, and prothrombin time.

Catheter Issues in Parenteral Nutrition

● The avoidance of complications related to catheter placement, avoidance of infection, and preventing late complications (e.g., thrombosis) are paramount.

Catheter Choice and Rationale

● For short duration or inpatient therapy, a percutaneous catheter introduced via the subclavian or internal jugular vein is most common. Peripherally inserted central catheters (PICCs), introduced via the basilic vein, have an increased incidence of complications such as leakage, thrombophlebitis, and malpositioning.
● For long-term TPN administration, appropriate devices are either subcutaneously tunneled central catheters (Hickman, Broviac, Groshong) or self-contained implantable chambers that connect to the central venous system (Portacath).

Catheter Sepsis

● Catheter sepsis is potentially the most lethal complication in patients receiving TPN. Organisms causing infections are generally 80% *Staphylococcus* (50:50 *Staphylococcus aureus* vs. *Staphylococcus epidermidis*), 15% yeast, and 5% gram-negative bacteria. Additional factors include the presence of a percutaneous stoma, hyperglycemia, corticosteroid administration, recent antibiotic therapy, concurrent chemotherapy, or severe neutropenia.
   ● In general, removal of a suspect catheter is safest.
   ● For patients on long-term TPN who may have limited access options remaining because of multiple previous lines, line salvage may be attractive.
   ● For *S. epidermidis* or gram-negative organisms, antibiotic therapy is effective in 60% to 70% of patients.
   ● If *S. aureus* or yeast are cultured, the line should be removed with subsequent intravenous antimicrobial therapy, because these organisms are too virulent to treat in lesser fashion.

Catheter Thrombosis and Other Complications

● Catheter failure resulting from intraluminal thrombus or a fibrin tip sheath, leading to clogging and lack of function, is common:

- This problem can often be corrected by use of tissue plasminogen activator.
- Administering long-term prophylactic low-dose heparin (usually 6000 units/bag) or warfarin (1 to 2 mg/day) is effective.
- Thrombosis of the great veins (subclavian, superior vena cava) occurs less frequently.
- Other complications include pneumothorax, vascular injuries (arterial or venous lacerations, delayed arteriovenous fistulae), brachial plexus injury, chronic pain, thoracic duct injury, air or catheter embolism, erosion of the catheter (into the bronchus, right atrium, or other structures), and hydrothorax.

CONTROVERSIES IN ARTIFICIAL NUTRITION

- Several areas in nutritional practice remain controversial and the subject of ongoing study. These include the following:
  - Whether there is any advantage of enteral compared with parenteral feeding and the optimal timing of such interventions.
  - Whether the immune response can be modulated by diet, termed "immunonutrition."
  - The validity of "nutritional pharmacology" (e.g., the role of conditionally essential and other special metabolites in critical illness). Such agents include glutamine, arginine, BCAAs, and others.

Who Benefits from Artificial Nutrition?

- Indications for parenteral nutrition may be organized into three categories:
  - Primary therapy, in which parenteral nutrition is thought to influence the disease process.
  - Supportive therapy, in which nutritional support does not alter disease processes.
  - Controversial indications or those under study.

Primary Therapy: Efficacy Shown

Gastrointestinal-Cutaneous Fistulas

- GI-cutaneous fistulas represent the classic indication for TPN.
- TPN increases spontaneous closure of fistulas.
- Fistula closure can also be achieved with enteral nutrition, although these rates are slightly lower than with TPN.

Renal Failure

- TPN results in decreased mortality in patients with acute renal failure.
- Essential amino acids and hypertonic dextrose are sometimes used.
- Protein excess may be injurious to patients with renal failure.

Short Bowel Syndrome

- Patients with short bowel syndrome have no alternative to long-term home TPN.
- If a patient is left with 1.5 feet of small bowel anastomosed to the left colon, hypertrophy often enables survival without daily parenteral nutritional support.

Burns

- Early aggressive nutritional support in patients with major burns is associated with improved survival.
- Parenteral nutritional support is reserved for those few patients in whom enteral nutrition cannot meet the patient's caloric needs.
- Well-fed patients have a lower sepsis rate, fewer days of bacteremia, lower mortality, and shorter hospital stay.

Hepatic Failure

- Improved survival is also seen in patients with hepatic failure given aggressive parenteral nutritional support.
- Patients with liver disease are often malnourished secondary to excessive alcohol ingestion, have decreased tolerance to stress, and may be protein intolerant because of hepatic encephalopathy.
- Solutions enriched with BCAAs and deficient in aromatic amino acids result in increased tolerance to administered protein and arousal from hepatic encephalopathy.

Primary Therapy: Efficacy Not Shown

Inflammatory Bowel Disease

- Oral intake often provokes diarrhea, protein-losing enteropathy, bleeding, and abdominal pain.
- TPN and bowel rest are useful in the treatment of Crohn's disease (particularly disease limited to the small bowel); patients with colonic involvement do less well.

Supportive Therapy: Efficacy Shown

Acute Radiation Enteritis or Chemotherapy Toxicity

- TPN administered until the gut mucosa heals and enables the patient to survive.

Prolonged Ileus

- This therapy is only supportive.

Supportive Therapy: Efficacy Probably Present

Weight Loss Preliminary to Major Surgery (Perioperative Parenteral Nutrition)

- Patients who lose more than 15% of their body weight before major operation appear to be at risk for surgical complications; the operant defect is not malnutrition, per se, but immunologic dysfunction.
- A history of greater than 10% or certainly 15% weight loss and an albumin value of less than 3 g/100 mL would place these patients in a high-risk group.
- Delayed cutaneous hypersensitivity testing by injected antigens, hand dynamometry, and serum transferrin are confirmatory.
- In patients who were judged severely malnourished and who had lost more than 15% of their body weight, preoperative nutritional intervention for 7 to 10 days decreased operative septic complications.
- With preoperative repletion, patients begin to feel better at approximately 5 days, a point that generally coincides with an increase in the shortest-turnover proteins, retinol-binding protein, and thyroxin-binding prealbumin.

Cancer

- Initial enthusiasm for nutritional support in patients with cancer waned as evidence suggested that tumor growth is stimulated by such intervention and that nutritional supplementation of patients undergoing chemotherapy and/or radiation therapy might decrease survival and/or the remission-free interval.
- Randomized prospective trials in patients with cancer have shown efficacy for preoperative intravenous nutritional support only in severely malnourished patients with upper GI tumors.

- Several studies in patients with cancer have suggested that postoperative nutritional support using an "immunologically active" tube feeding may improve postoperative outcome.

ADDITIONAL APPROACHES FOR REDUCING CACHEXIA

- In addition to nutritional approaches to promote positive nitrogen balance and improve outcome in critically ill patients, additional strategies are a focus of research. These include inhibition of the stress response, administration of anabolic factors, and inhibition of proteolysis.

Inhibition of the Stress Response

- A variety of approaches have been used to inhibit the actions of inflammatory mediators and catabolic hormones that are released under conditions of stress and are presumably responsible for protein loss and cachexia.
- Included in this category are the omega-3 fatty acids, antagonists of the glucocorticoids, and blocking antibodies for TNF.

Administration of Anabolic Factors

- These include gut-derived hormones such as glucagon-like peptide-2, growth hormone, IGFs, and anabolic steroids such as testosterone.
- Catecholamines may reduce calcium-dependent proteolysis and increase protein synthesis in muscle, as seen with the adrenergic β_2 agonist clenbuterol.

Inhibition of Proteolysis

- An extremely attractive approach to the treatment of muscle wasting is the direct inhibition of intracellular proteolysis.
- Active site inhibitors of the proteasome are now available and have been shown to be fairly safe in humans during initial trials of their use as antineoplastic agents.
- More recently, specific E3s induced in muscle under catabolic conditions have been identified, and these proteins may offer tissue-specific targets for inhibition of ubiquitination and proteolysis.

CHAPTER 7

WOUND HEALING

TISSUE INJURY AND RESPONSE

- Repair by forming scar tissue.
- No return to preinjury status quo.
- All repair is an overlapping series of orchestrated events to limit damage and restore function and integrity.
- All tissues proceed through the same series.
- Phases overlap in both time and activity.
- Wound closure types:
  - *Primary* or first-intention: immediately sealed with simple suturing, skin graft placement, or flap closure.
  - *Secondary* or spontaneous intention: close by reepithelialization and contraction.
  - *Tertiary* intention: also referred to as delayed primary, treated first, ready for closure, surgical intervention (Fig. 7–1).

WOUND HEALING PHASES

- Inflammatory (also called reactive) phase: immediate response, limiting amount of damage, preventing further injury.
- Proliferative (also called regenerative or reparative) phase: reepithelialization, matrix synthesis, and neovascularization.
- Maturational (or remodeling) phase: collagen cross-linking, shrinking, and loss of edema.
- All three phases may occur simultaneously (Fig. 7–2).

Inflammatory Phase

- Hemostasis, inflammation, sealing surface of wound, removing any necrotic tissue, foreign debris, or bacteria.
- Chronic wound is stalled in inflammatory phase; does not proceed to closure.

Hemostasis

- Exposure to Types IV and V collagen promotes platelet aggregation.

Primary healing

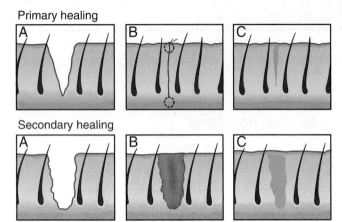

Secondary healing

■ FIGURE 7–1. Wound closure types. Top, Primary or first intention closure: a clean incision is made in the tissue *(A)* and the wound edges are reapproximated *(B)* with sutures, staples, or adhesive strips. *C,* Minimal scarring is the end result. (Adapted from Sabiston D (ed): Sabiston Textbook of Surgery: The Biological Basis of Modern Surgical Practice, 15th ed. Philadelphia, WB Saunders, 1997, p 207.)

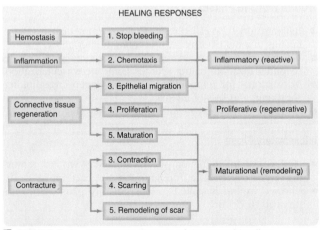

■ FIGURE 7–2. Schematic diagram of the wound healing continuum.

- Activated platelets release biologically active proteins: platelet-derived growth factor (PDGF), transforming growth factor (TGF)-β, insulin-like growth factor (IGF)-1, fibronectin, fibrinogen, thrombospondin, von Willebrand factor, and serotonin.
- Dense bodies contain vasoactive amines that cause vasodilatation and increased vascular permeability.
- Clotting cascade is initiated.
- Thrombin itself activates platelets and serves as catalyst for formation of fibrinogen into fibrin.
- Fibrin strands trap red cells, form a clot, and seal the wound.
- Thromboxane A_2 and prostaglandin $F_{2\alpha}$, formed from degradation of cell membranes, assist with platelet aggregation and vasoconstriction and cause localized ischemia, resulting in further damage to cell membranes.

Polymorphonuclear Cells (PMNs)

- Histamine and serotonin cause vascular permeability.
- Chemoattracted and activated, adhering to the endothelium.
  - C5a and leukotriene B_4 promote neutrophil adherence.
  - Leukotriene C_4 and D_4 further enhance neutrophil adhesion.
- Monocytes and endothelial cells produce interleukin (IL)-1 and tumor necrosis factor (TNF)-α which promote endothelial-neutrophil adherence.
- Neutrophils release contents of their lysosomes and enzymes facilitating migration.
- Complement cascade is activated.
- PMN migration requires sequential adhesive and de-adhesive interactions between β1 and β2 integrins and extracellular matrix (ECM) components.
- Activated neutrophils scavenge necrotic debris, foreign material, and bacteria but are also further destructive to surrounding viable tissue.
  - Oxidative bursts remove bacteria, but more tissue destruction occurs; generate free oxygen radicals.
  - Superoxide anions form hydrogen peroxide and hypochlorous acid.

Macrophages

- Central to wound healing to orchestrate release of cytokines.
- Monocytes are chemoattracted by bacterial debris, C5a, TGF-β, later than leukocytes and at the same time as lymphocytes.

- Monocytes convert to macrophages.
- Some wound macrophages are tissue macrophages that proliferate locally.
- Activated macrophages release free radicals and nitric oxide, which has many functions including antimicrobial properties.
- Activated macrophages also secrete collagenase, which is blocked by nonsteroidal anti-inflammatory drugs.
  - Colchicine and retinoic acid appear to decrease collagenase production.
  - IL-1 secreted by macrophage and further enhances collagenase production.
- Microbial byproducts induce macrophages to release TNF:
  - Induces fever.
  - Increases collagenase.
  - Increases procoagulant activity.
  - Releases PDGF.
  - Produces IL-1.
  - Works synergistically with IL-1.
- IL-6 induces T-cell proliferation and fever and works synergistically with IL-1.
- Macrophages produce PDGF, TGF-α, and TGF-β.
  - These growth factors are important in the proliferative phase.
  - TGF-β is the most potent stimulant of fibroplasia (Table 7–1).

Lymphocytes

- T lymphocytes appear at day 5.
- B lymphocytes are involved in downregulating healing as the wound closes.
- Macrophage-processed foreign debris stimulates lymphocyte proliferation and cytokine release.
- T cells produce interferon-γ (INF-γ).
  - Targets monocyte or macrophage.
  - Releases a cascade of cytokines including TNF-α and IL-1.
  - Results in decreased synthesis of prostaglandins enhancing inflammatory mediators.
  - Inhibits monocyte migration, which probably keeps these cells at site of injury.
  - Causes glycosaminoglycan (GAG) synthesis.
  - Suppresses collagen synthesis.
- T cells synthesize IL-2, which promotes synthesis of IFN-γ; IL-2 potentiates activity of free radicals.

TABLE 7-1. Cytokines that Affect Wound Healing

Cytokine	Abbreviation	Source	Functions
Platelet-derived growth factor	PDGF	Platelets, macrophages, endothelial cells, keratinocytes	Chemotactic for PMNs, macrophages, fibroblasts, and smooth muscle cells; activates PMNs, macrophages, and fibroblasts; mitogenic for fibroblasts, endothelial cells; stimulates production of MMPs, fibronectin, and HA; stimulates angiogenesis and wound contraction; remodeling
Transforming growth factor-beta (including isoforms β_1, β_2, and β_3)	TGF-β	Platelets, T lymphocytes, macrophages, endothelial cells, keratinocytes, fibroblasts	Chemotactic for PMNs, macrophages, lymphocytes, fibroblasts; stimulates TIMP synthesis, keratinocyte migration, angiogenesis, and fibroplasia, inhibits production of MMPs and keratinocyte proliferation; induces TGF β-production
Epidermal growth factor	EGF	Platelets, macrophages	Mitogenic for keratinocytes and fibroblasts; stimulates keratinocyte migration
Transforming growth factor-alpha	TGF-α	Macrophages, T lymphocytes, keratinocytes	Similar to EGF
Fibroblast growth factor-1 and -2 family	FGF	Macrophages, mast cells, T lymphocytes, endothelial cells, fibroblasts	Chemotactic for fibroblasts, mitogenic for fibroblasts and keratinocytes; stimulates keratinocyte migration, angiogenesis, wound contraction, and matrix deposition
Keratinocyte growth factor (also called FGF-7)	KGF	Fibroblasts	Stimulates keratinocyte migration, proliferation, and differentiation
Insulin-like growth factor	IGF-1	Macrophages, fibroblasts	Stimulates synthesis of sulfated proteoglycans, collagen, keratinocyte migration, and fibroblast proliferation; endocrine effects similar to those of growth hormone
Vascular endothelial cell growth factor	VEGF	Keratinocytes	Increases vasopermeability; mitogenic for endothelial cells

HA, hyaluronic acid; MMPs, metalloproteinases; PMNs, polymorphonuclear leukocytes; TIMP, tissue inhibitor of matrix metalloproteinase.
Modified from Schwartz SI (ed): Principles of Surgery, 7th ed. New York, McGraw-Hill, 1999, p 269.

- Presence of incompletely characterized CD4⁻ and CD8⁻ T-lymphocyte population seems to be responsible for promotion of wound healing.

Proliferative Phase

- Scaffolding is made for repair:
  - Angiogenesis.
  - Fibroplasia.
  - Epithelialization.

Angiogenesis

- Basement membrane itself is degraded by activated endothelial cells.
- Cells divide and form a tubule or lumen.
- Upregulation of vascular cell adhesion molecule (VCAM-1), platelet endothelial cell adhesion molecule (PECAM-1), matrix metalloproteinase (MMPs), and plasmin.
- Acidic and basic fibroblast growth factors (FGF) stimulate angiogenesis.
- TGF-α and epidermal growth factor stimulate endothelial cell proliferation.
- TNF-α is chemotactic for endothelial cells and promotes formation of capillary tube.
  - May mediate angiogenesis through induction of hypoxia-inducible factor (HIF-1).
- TGF-β is a chemoattractant for fibroblasts and assists angiogenesis by signaling the fibroblast to produce FGFs.
- Epithelial cells will express vascular endothelial growth factor (VEGF), which is endothelial-cell specific and is both mitogenic and chemotactic.
  - VEGF has potent angiogenic activity.
- Hypoxia and cell disruption induce VEGF.
- Nitric oxide and VEGF appear to enhance one another.
- Fibronectin and hyaluronic acid appear to be angiogenic.
- Collagen appears to interact by causing tubular formation.

Fibroplasia

- Fibroblasts are chemoattracted and divide and produce components of ECM.
- Arrested in the G_0 phase can be made competent to replicate by PDGF or basic FGF.
- Competent fibroblasts must be further stimulated by factors such as IGF-1 and epidermal growth factor.

- Activated monocytes and platelets release PDGF and stimulate fibroblast proliferation.
- Basic FGF, released by fibroblast, is an autocrine stimulant of proliferation.
- TGF-β released with PDGF from platelet granules stimulates PDGF release.

Epithelialization

- Epidermis seals wound to prevent fluid loss and protect against bacterial invasion.
- Tight cell junctions make tissue impermeable and basement membrane zone that gives structural support and attachment.
- Basement membrane zone is several layers in succession including lamina lucida, lamina densa (electron dense), and anchoring fibrils.
    - Basal layer of epidermis attaches to basement membrane zone by hemidesmosomes.
    - Lamina lucida consists of laminin and heparan sulfate.
    - Lamina densa contains Type IV collagen.
    - Anchoring fibrils consist of Type VII collagen.
- When gap occurs in epidermis, wound is first sealed by blood clot.
- Epidermal cells migrate and cellular proliferation occurs.
- Epithelialization involves a sequence of changes in keratinocytes: detachment, migration, proliferation, differentiation, and stratification.
- If basement membrane zone is intact, epithelialization proceeds more rapidly.
- Epidermal cells express integrin receptors, allowing interaction with ECM proteins.
- Basal cells migrate, and leading edge of migration becomes phagocytic.
- Epithelium will migrate under necrotic tissue and foreign material.
- As migration begins, epithelial cells acquire more gap junctions, which are implicated in intercellular communication.
- Epithelial cells move as an intact sheet until edges establish contact.
- If basement membrane zone is not intact, it will be repaired first.
- Wound cleft is coated with fibronectin, laminin, Type IV collagen, and additional fibronectin.
- Migrating epithelial cells release collagenase and plasminogen activator.
- Proteases assist epithelial cells in migration.

- Epithelial adhesion and spreading facilitated by vitronectin; collagen Types I, III, and IV; and laminin.

Extracellular Matrix

- Provisional matrix is a scaffold for cellular migration composed initially of fibrin, fibronectin, and vitronectin.
- GAGs and proteoglycans are synthesized next, supporting further matrix deposition.
- Collagens are the end result.
- Dynamic and reciprocal relationship between fibroblasts and ECM.

Collagen Structure

- Triple helix molecule located extracellularly to provide support.
- 20 types of collagen produced by fibroblasts.
- Synthesis involves transcription from different chromosomes and modifications after translation occurs both intercellularly (preprocollagen) and extracellularly (procollagen).
- Procollagen is released from fibroblasts where extracellular proteases cleave to form collagen monomers that assemble into fibrils.
- Cross-linking occurs forming collagen fiber.
- Ascorbic acid stimulates collagen synthesis.
- TGF-β, IGF-1, and IGF-2 increase collagen synthesis.
- IFN-γ inhibits collagen gene transcription.
- Glucocorticoids inhibit procollagen gene transcription.
- Genetic disorders causing abnormalities in collagen:
  - Osteogenesis imperfecta is caused by deletion of one procollagen α-1 allele.
  - Ehlers-Danlos syndrome caused by abnormal Type III collagen, deletion of part of the Type I collagen gene, abnormal copper utilization, or deficiency in lysyl hydroxylase.

Elastic Fibers

- Present in connective tissue and ECM.
- Provides elastic recoil for skin, blood vessels, ligaments, and lung interstitium.
- Composed of amorphous elastin and elastic fiber microfibrils.
- Elastin is secreted into extracellular space as tropoelastin and form aggregates with cross-linking.
- Amorphous elastin is more prevalent in deeper dermis.
- Microfibrils are more prominent in papillary dermis.

- Very slow turnover rate and typically lasts individual's life.
- Age-related modification is a result of progressive degradation as elastic fibers become tortuous, frayed, and porous.
- IGF-1 and TGF-β stimulate production.
- Glucocorticoids and basic FGF reduce adult skin cell production.
- Mutations resulting in elastin protein deficiency result in internal hyperplasia.
- Fibrillin gene mutations result in Marfan's syndrome; severely affected individuals are prone to aortic rupture.

Glycosaminoglycans and Proteoglycans

- Support cells, provide tissue turgor, facilitate cell-cell inter-action.
- Hyaluronan (HA) is simplest of the GAGs and is especially prevalent in fetal tissues.
- HA facilitates cell migration and is degraded by hyaluronidase.
- Proteoglycans provide hydrated space around and between cells and form gels of different pore size and change density to regulate movement of cells and molecules.
- Proteoglycans function in chemical signaling and bind signal molecules, such as growth factors.
- ECM has other noncollagen proteins, such as fibronectins that can bind to matrix macromolecules and cell surface receptors.
- Fibronectin is important in animal embryogenesis.

Basal Lamina

- Separate cells and epithelia from underlying or surrounding connective tissue.
- Numerous functions: filter, barrier, or scaffold.
- Most mature basal laminae contain Type IV collagen, perlecan, and glycoproteins, laminin and nidogen.

Degradation of the Extracellular Matrix

- Regulated turnover of the ECM is crucial to many biologic processes:
  - For example, metastasis or injury or infection.
- MMPs and serine proteases degrade ECM components.
- Proteolysis is tightly regulated.

Maturation Phase

- Scar contraction is normal; scar contracture is not.

- Contraction caused by cell locomotion, if aborted, appears to cause bunching and contraction of collagen fibers.
- Contracture is a clinical definition that indicates limits of function.
- Normal dermal fibroblasts are trapped by collagen fibers.
- Fibroblasts in a contracting wound change to stimulated cells, referred to as myofibroblasts (function and structure in common between fibroblast and smooth muscle cells).
- Fibroblasts develop a contractile ability related to cytoplasmic actin-myosin contractile activity.
- Tension stimulates actin-myosin structures.
- Colchicine (inhibits microtubules) or cytochalasin D (inhibits microfilaments) inhibit contraction of collagen gels.
- Fibroblasts develop a linear arrangement in the line of tension.
- Overabundance of stimulated fibroblasts or myofibroblasts in diseases of excessive fibrosis that includes the following:
  - Hepatic cirrhosis.
  - Renal and pulmonary fibrosis.
  - Dupuytren's contracture.
  - Desmoplastic reactions.
- Actin microfilaments are arranged linearly and associated with dense bodies that allow attachment to the surrounding ECM.
- Fibronexus is the attachment entity and spans the cell membrane.
- MMPs, which degrade collagen, are also important for wound contraction.
- MMP degrades proteoglycans, laminin, fibronectin, collagen Types IV and IX, procollagen I, and denatured collagens.
- MMPs allow cleavage of attachment between the fibroblast and collagen so that the lattice can be made to contract.
- Stromelysin-1 (also called MMP-3) affects wound contraction.
- Stromelysin-1 allows modification of attachment sites between fibroblast and collagen fibrils involving the β-1 integrins.
- TGF-β1, IGF-1, and PDGF affect contraction by impacting the β-1 integrins.

Remodeling

- Once the wound is healed, it will remodel and mature.
- Fibroblast population decreases, dense capillary network regresses.
- Wound strength increases rapidly within 1 to 6 weeks and then levels off as a sigmoid curve.
- Compared with unwounded skin, tensile strength is only 30% in the scar.

- Cross-linking causes further wound contraction and increase in strength and results in a scar that is more brittle and less elastic.

ABNORMAL WOUND HEALING

- IL-1α is elevated in chronic wounds (Box 7–1).
- Wound collagenase activity is greatly increased.
- Tissue inhibitors of MMPs are increased.
- TNF-α is also apparently increased.
- Stimulants of inflammation increase IL-1α and TNF-α, thus more stimulus to prevent progression to wound healing.
- Proliferative scar: hypertrophic or keloid.
- Pathologic scarring in other areas of the body can cause hepatic cirrhosis, pulmonary fibrosis, scleroderma, retrolental fibroplasia, diabetic retinopathy, or osteoarthritis.
- Keloid more common with darker pigmented skin and tends to occur above the clavicles, in the upper extremities, and on the face.
- Hypertrophic scar can occur anywhere.
- In both cases, collagen deposition far exceeds collagen degradation.
- Hypertrophic scar is in many cases preventable; prolonged inflammation increases risk.
- Insufficient resurfacing leads to hypertrophic scar.
- Tension that signals formation of activated fibroblasts leads to deposition of excessive collagen.
- Hypertrophic scar is limited to area of wound healing.
- Keloid scar tends to occur far beyond the limits of original damage; hypertrophic scar fibroblasts produce more TGF-β1.
- TGF-β1 and TGF-β2 are increased in expression from human keloid cells.

Box 7–1. Factor that Inhibit Wound Healing	
Infection	Vitamin deficiencies
Ischemia	Vitamin C
Circulation	Vitamin A
Respiration	Mineral deficiencies
Local tension	Zinc
Diabetes mellitus	Iron
Ionizing radiation	Exogenous drugs
Advanced age	Doxorubicin (Adriamycin)
Malnutrition	Glucocorticosteroids

- Position of an elective scar can be chosen.
- Scar that is perpendicular to underlying muscle fibers tends to be flatter, more narrow, with less collagen formation.
- Chronically inflamed wounds can develop squamous cell carcinoma.
  - These include unstable burn scars, osteomyelitis, pressure sores, venous stasis ulcers, and hidradenitis; premalignant state is pseudoepitheliomatous hyperplasia.
- Most common cause of healing delays is wound infection.
  - If bacterial count exceeds 10^5 organisms/g tissue or if any β-hemolytic streptococcus is present, the wound will not heal by any means.
  - Bacteria prolong inflammatory phase and interfere with epithelialization, contraction, and collagen deposition.
  - Endotoxins themselves stimulate phagocytosis and release of collagenase.
- Wound hypoxia stimulates angiogenesis; wound will not proceed without tissue oxygen levels of 35 mm Hg or greater.
- Ischemia can be caused by atherosclerosis, cardiac failure, or simple wound tension.
- Diabetes mellitus impairs wound healing at all stages.
  - Basement membrane of capillaries is thickened, causing decreased perfusion.
  - Lymphocyte and leukocyte function is impaired.
  - Increased collagen degradation.
  - Decreased collagen deposition.
  - Collagen that is formed is more brittle.
- Ionizing radiation causes endothelial cell injury with endarteritis resulting in atrophy, fibrosis, and delayed tissue repair.
  - Rapidly dividing cell populations are most sensitive to radiation.
- Elderly patients experience delayed wound healing.
- Aging affects all stages of wound healing, but macrophages are particularly affected.
- Malnutrition, protein catabolism, hypoalbuminemia, and vitamin deficiencies affect wound healing.
- Deficiency of vitamin C decreases rate and quality of collagen production.
- Deficiency of vitamin A will impair monocyte activation, fibronectin deposition, and impairment of TGF-β receptors.
- Vitamin A contributes to lysosomal membrane destabilization and directly counteracts effect of glucocorticoids.
- Vitamin K deficiency limits the synthesis of prothrombin and factors VII, IX, and X.

- Zinc deficiency occurs in large burns, severe multiple trauma, and hepatic cirrhosis.
- Zinc is a cofactor for RNA and DNA polymerase.
- Zinc deficiency decreases bursting strength.
- Some exogenous drugs directly inhibit wound healing:
  - Doxorubicin (Adriamycin).
  - Tamoxifen.
  - Glucocorticosteroid.

FETAL WOUND HEALING

- Fetal wounds heal scarlessly and with regeneration of dermal appendages.
- Fetal wounds differ from adults in inflammatory responses, ECM components, and growth factor expression and responses.
- Fetal repair is both gestational age- and wound size-dependent.
- There are differences in fetal fibroblasts.
  - Higher collagen production.
- There are differences in ECM components of fetal and adult wounds.
  - Higher levels of HA are found in fetal wounds.
  - Larger amounts of fibronectin in fetal wounds stimulate cell attachment, whereas the more rapid deposition of tenascin in the fetus allows cells to migrate and more rapidly reepithelialize the wound.

CHAPTER 8

CRITICAL ASSESSMENT OF SURGICAL OUTCOMES

INTRODUCTION

TWO MAIN APPLICATIONS OF OUTCOMES RESEARCH

- Studies assessing the effectiveness of a clinical intervention
  - By ensuring that patients are as similar as possible between comparison groups, randomized controlled trials (RCTs) minimize the risk that observed differences in outcomes are attributable to other factors (confounding).
- Studies assessing quality of care

DATA SOURCES

- Clinical registries
- Administrative data
  - Most studies using administrative data to examine surgical outcomes rely on hospital discharge abstract files.
  - Because they are generally population-based and often national in scope, administrative databases are often the only way to study surgical outcomes in the real world (i.e., effectiveness rather than efficacy).
  - Such problems in coding and coding accuracy create obvious limitations in the ability to perform risk adjustment, particularly relevant in studies focusing on quality of care.
  - Thus, administrative data are not well suited to assessing nonfatal outcomes of surgical interventions.

IS THE STUDY VALID?

Chance

- Whenever inferences are based on samples, there is always the possibility that results could be inaccurate due to chance alone.
- Type I errors

- The likelihood of a type I error is quantified by statistical testing.
- Type II errors
  - Type II errors cannot be addressed in any way by statistical testing after the study is complete.

Bias

- Bias reflects problems with the design and conduct of the study, not with how the analysis is performed once data are collected.
- Selection bias
- Information bias

Confounding

- Confounding occurs when outcomes differ because of differences in the baseline risks of the comparison groups (often as a result of selection bias).
- Risk adjustment refers to a variety of statistical approaches used to control for patient case mix.
- How reliable are the important risk factors measured?
- Do important risk factors vary between comparison groups?
  - Regardless of the strength of its relationship with the outcome measure or how well it is measured, a variable can only be an important confounder if it varies across comparison groups.
- How large are the observed outcome differences?
  - Finally, in judging the likelihood of confounding, surgeons should consider the magnitude of reported differences in outcomes across comparison groups.

Generalizability

- Clinic trials generally imply careful, standardized protocols for patient selection, operative and perioperative care, and follow-up, often very different than the variable care that patients receive in real-world clinical practice.

IS THE STUDY FOCUSING ON THE RIGHT OUTCOME MEASURE?

- Despite these strengths, however, intermediate outcomes and clinical endpoints may not always correlate with what matters to patients.
- General health status

- Disease-specific symptom scores
- Pain
- Utilities
- Satisfaction

IS THE INTERVENTION COST-EFFECTIVE?

- Cost-effectiveness analysis is only appropriate for assessing interventions that produce benefit at some additional cost.
- A quality-adjusted life years (QALY) is a composite measure reflecting both quality and quantity of life and is obtained by multiplying the length of time spent in a given health state by its associated utility.

CHAPTER 9

PRINCIPLES OF PREOPERATIVE AND OPERATIVE SURGERY

SYSTEMS APPROACH TO PREOPERATIVE EVALUATION

Cardiovascular

- In an attempt to best assess and optimize the cardiac status of patients undergoing noncardiac surgery, the American College of Cardiology/American Heart Association has developed an easily used tool (Fig. 9–1).
- Perioperative risk for cardiovascular morbidity and mortality was decreased by 67% and 55%, respectively in patients receiving beta-blockade in the perioperative period versus those receiving placebo.

Pulmonary

- It is wise to consider assessing pulmonary function for all lung resection cases; thoracic procedures requiring single-lung ventilation; and major abdominal and thoracic cases in patients that are older than 60 years, have significant underlying medical disease, smoke, or have overt pulmonary symptomatology. Necessary tests include the forced expiratory volume at 1 second (FEV_1), the forced vital capacity (FVC), and the diffusing capacity of carbon monoxide (DLCO). Adults with an FEV_1 of less than 0.8 L/second, or 30% of predicted, have a high risk of complications and postoperative pulmonary insufficiency; nonsurgical solutions should be sought. Pulmonary resections should be planned so that the postoperative FEV_1 is greater than 0.8 L/second or 30% of predicted.

Renal

- The patient with end-stage renal disease (ESRD) will often require additional attention in the perioperative period. Pharmacologic manipulation of hypokalemia, replacement

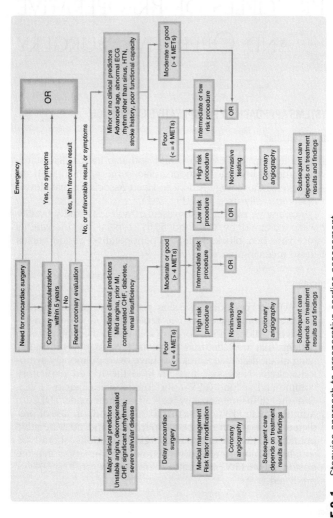

■ **FIGURE 9–1.** Stepwise approach to preoperative cardiac assessment.

TABLE 9–1. Child-Pugh Scoring System

	Points		
	1	**2**	**3**
Encephalopathy	None	Stage I or II	Stage III or IV
Ascites	Absent	Slight (controlled with diuretics)	Moderate despite diuretic treatment
Bilirubin (mg/dL)	<2	2–3	>3
	<4	4–6	>6
Albumin (g/L)	>3.5	2.8–3.5	<2.8
PT (prolonged seconds) INR	<4	4–6	>6
	<1.7	1.7–2.3	>2.3

INR, international normalized ratio; PT, prothrombin time.
Class A = 5–6 points; Class B = 7–9 points; Class C = 10–15 points.

of calcium for symptomatic hypocalcemia, and the use of phosphate-binding antacids for hyperphosphatemia are often required. Sodium bicarbonate is used in the setting of metabolic acidosis when serum bicarbonate levels are below 15. This can be administered in IV fluid as 1–2 amps in D5 solution. Hyponatremia is treated with volume restriction, though dialysis is often required within the perioperative period for control of volume and electrolyte abnormalities.

- The patient with chronic ESRD should undergo dialysis prior to surgery, in order to optimize his or her volume status and control the potassium level. Intraoperative hyperkalemia can result from surgical manipulation of tissue or the transfusion of blood.

Hepatobiliary

- The patient with cirrhosis may be assessed using the Child-Pugh classification, which stratifies operative risk according to a score based on abnormal albumin and bilirubin levels, prolongation of the prothrombin time (PT), and degree of ascites and encephalopathy (Table 9–1).

Endocrine

- The insulin-dependent diabetic should be told to hold long-acting insulin preparations (Ultralente preparations) on the day of surgery; the substitution with lower dosages of intermediate-acting insulin (NPH or Lente) should be made on the morning of operation. These patients should be scheduled for early morning operation, when feasible.

During operation a standard 5% or 10% dextrose infusion is used with short-acting insulin or insulin drip to maintain glycemic control. The patient with diabetes mellitus (DM) that is well controlled by diet or oral medication may not require insulin perioperatively, but those with poorer control or on insulin therapy may require preoperative dosing and both glucose and insulin infusion during surgery. Frequent assessment of glucose levels should be continued through the postoperative period.

Hematologic

- Generally, patients with normovolemic anemia without significant cardiac risk or anticipated blood loss can be managed safely without transfusion; many healthy patients tolerate hemoglobin (Hb) levels of 6 or 7 g/dL (Box 9–1).
- Patients who receive anticoagulation therapy can require preoperative reversal of the anticoagulant effect. In patients taking warfarin the drug can be held for several days preoperatively to allow the international normalized ratio (INR) to fall to the range of 1.5 or less. Patients with a recent history of venous thromboembolism or acute arterial embolism often require perioperative intravenous (IV) heparinization because of increased risk of recurrent events in the perioperative

---

Box 9–1. Guidelines for Red Blood Cell Transfusion for Acute Blood Loss

- Evaluate risk of ischemia.
- Estimate/anticipate degree of blood loss. Less than 30% rapid volume loss probably does not require transfusion in a previously healthy individual.
- Measure hemoglobin concentration: <6 g/dL, transfusion usually required; 6–10 g/dL, transfusion dictated by clinical circumstance; >10 g/dL, transfusion rarely required.
- Measure vital signs/tissue oxygenation when hemoglobin is 6 to 10 g/dL and extent of blood loss is unknown. Tachycardia and hypotension refractory to volume suggest the need for transfusion; O_2 extraction ration >50%, Vo_2 decreased, suggest that transfusion usually is needed.

From Simon TL, Alverson DC, AuBuchon J, et al: Practice parameters for the use of red blood cell transfusions: Developed by the Red Blood Cell Administration Practice Guideline Development Task Force of the College of American Pathologists, Arch Pathol Lab Med 122:130–138, 1998.

period. Systemic heparinization can often be stopped within 6 hours of surgery and restarted within 12 hours postoperatively. When possible, surgery should be postponed in the first month after an episode of venous or arterial thromboembolism. Patients on anticoagulation for less than 2 weeks for pulmonary embolism or proximal deep venous thrombosis (DVT) should be considered for inferior vena cava (IVC) filter placement before operation (Table 9–2).

● Initial prophylactic doses of heparin can be given preoperatively, within 2 hours of operation, and compression devices should be in place before induction of anesthesia.

ADDITIONAL PREOPERATIVE CONSIDERATIONS

Nutritional Status

● Patients with severe malnutrition (as defined by a combination of weight loss, visceral protein indicators, or prognostic indices) appear to benefit most from preoperative parenteral nutrition, as demonstrated in study groups treated with total parenteral nutrition (TPN) for 7 to 10 days before surgery for gastrointestinal (GI) malignancy. Most studies show a reduction in the rate of postoperative complications from approximately 40% to 30%. The use of TPN postoperatively in similar groups of patients is associated with an increase in complication rates of approximately 10%.

TABLE 9–2. Recommendations for Perioperative Anticoagulation in Patients Taking Oral Anticoagulants

Indication	Preoperative	Postoperative
Acute venous thromboembolism		
Month 1	IV heparin	IV heparin
Months 2 and 3	No change	IV heparin
Recurrent venous thromboembolism	No change	SC heparin
Acute arterial embolism		
Month 1	IV heparin	IV heparin
Mechanical heart valve	No change	SC heparin
Nonvalvular atrial fibrillation	No change	SC heparin

IV, intravenous; SC, subcutaneous.
From Kearon C, Hirsh J: Management of anticoagulation before and after elective surgery. N Engl J Med 336:1506, 1997.

Antibiotic Prophylaxis

● Appropriate antibiotics for prophylaxis in surgery depends on the most likely pathogens encountered during the surgical procedure. The type of operative wound encountered (Table 9–3) is helpful in deciding the appropriate antibiotic spectrum, and should be considered prior to ordering or administering any preoperative medication. Prophylactic antibiotics are not generally required for clean (Class I) cases, except in the setting of indwelling prosthesis placement, or in patients who have higher risk; as those with three concomitant diagnoses, or those whose operations are abdominal or longer than two hours in length. Patients who undergo Class II procedures benefit from a single dose of appropriate antibiotic administered prior to skin incision. For abdominal (hepatobiliary, pancreatic, gastroduodenal) cases, cefazolin is generally used. Contaminated (Class III) cases require mechanical preparation or parenteral antibiotics with both aerobic and anaerobic activity. Such an approach should be taken in the setting of emergency abdominal surgery, such as for suspected appendicitis, and

TABLE 9–3. National Research Council Classification of Operative Wounds

Clean (class I)	Nontraumatic
	No inflammation
	No break in technique
	Respiratory, alimentary, or genitourinary tract not entered
Clean-contaminated (class II)	Gastrointestinal or respiratory tract entered without significant spillage
Contaminated (class III)	Major break in technique
	Gross spillage from gastrointestinal tract
	Traumatic wound, fresh
	Entrance of genitourinary or biliary tracts in presence of infected urine or bile
Dirty and infected (class IV)	Acute bacterial inflammation encountered, without pus
	Transection of "clean" tissue for the purpose of surgical access to a collection of pus
	Traumatic wound with retained devitalized tissue, foreign bodies, fecal contamination, or delayed treatment, or all of these; or from dirty source

Adapted from Cruse PJE: Wound infections: Epidemiology and clinical characteristics. *In* Howard RJ, Simmons RL (eds): Surgical Infectious Disease, 2nd ed. Norwalk, CT, Appleton & Lange. 1988.

in trauma cases. Dirty or infected cases often require the same antibiotic spectrum, which can be continued into the postoperative period in the setting of ongoing infection or delayed treatment.

● The appropriate antibiotic should be chosen prior to surgery and administered before the skin incision is made. Repeat dosing should occur at an appropriate interval, generally three hours for abdominal cases or twice the half-life of the antibiotic. Perioperative antibiotic prophylaxis should generally not be continued beyond the day of operation.

PREOPERATIVE CHECKLIST

Review of Medications

● Two notable examples are the additional cardiovascular morbidity associated with the perioperative discontinuation of beta-blockers and rebound hypertension with abrupt cessation of the antihypertensive clonidine.

● Drugs that affect platelet function should be held for variable periods: aspirin and clopidogrel (Plavix) should be held for 7 to 10 days, whereas nonsteroidal anti-inflammatory drugs (NSAIDs) should be held between 1 day (ibuprofen and indomethacin) and 3 days (naproxen and sulindac), depending on the drug's half-life.

PRINCIPLES OF OPERATIVE SURGERY

● There is no substitute for a well-planned and properly conducted operation to provide the best possible surgical outcome.

THE OPERATING ROOM

● The operating room should be an extension of the classroom for surgical trainees and practicing surgeons.

● Alternative procedures should be considered if circumstances require it.

● For more complex and unusual procedures, preoperative communication among surgeons, anesthesiologists, and operating room staff is vitally important.

● The modern operating room for a trauma service, in particular, should have a temperature control panel that allows room temperature to be modified rapidly when dealing with a hypothermic patient.

Hemostasis

- Less blood loss allows for the performance of a technically superior operation. In the presence of adequate hemostasis, one can conduct a more precise dissection and shorten both the operating time and the recovery time of the patient.
- Hemoclip application is acceptable, especially in an operating field with an extremely confined space or when dealing with delicate vessels, such as portal vein branches.
- At times it is necessary to use hemoclips, for example, while performing an oncologic procedure in which outlining of margins provides a radiopaque marker for postoperative radiation.
- Temporary occlusion of the aorta at the esophageal hiatus with a compression device such as a T-bar or vascular clamp or with manual compression should be considered.
- Occasionally, a partial vascular injury may need to be extended or converted to a complete transection to allow for better repair.
- Bleeding that occurs from multiple sites in a trauma patient, such as liver laceration or splenic injury, especially in a hypothermic patient, may best be treated with packing alone or in conjunction with angiographic embolization to achieve temporary control followed by a second look operation.

Wound closure

- In a patient with a condition requiring re-exploration, or one suffering from abdominal compartment syndrome, temporary closure is preferable.
- When proven infection or contamination is a concern, monofilament, nonbraided suture is preferred. For abdominal wall closure in a debilitated, malnourished cancer patient, permanent closure with nondissolvable suture is prudent. In a cirrhotic patient with established ascites or a patient who has the potential to develop postoperative ascites, the abdomen should be closed with running suture, and a multilayer watertight closure must be achieved. In this setting, our practice is to use a tunneled drain that enters the anterior and posterior fascia in different spots. Intermittent drainage helps to reduce the tensile stress on the midline abdominal wound closure in the immediate postoperative period.

CHAPTER 10

ULTRASOUND FOR SURGEONS

PHYSICS AND INSTRUMENTATION

- In diagnostic ultrasonography, the transducer or probe interconverts electrical and acoustic energy (Fig. 10–1).
  - Active element
  - Damping or backing material
  - A matching layer
- There are four main transducer arrays: (1) the rectangular linear array, which yields a rectangular image; (2) the curved array, which yields a trapezoidal image; (3) the phased array, a small transducer in which the sound pulses are generated by activating all of the elements in the array; and (4) the annular array, in which the elements are arranged in a circular fashion.
- Ultrasound beams of different frequencies have different characteristics: higher frequencies penetrate tissue poorly but yield excellent resolution, whereas lower frequencies penetrate well but at the cost of compromised resolution.
- Transmitter
- Receiver or image processor
- Transducer
- Monitor
- Image recorder

CLINICAL USES OF ULTRASOUND

Outpatient Setting

Breast

- Advances in ultrasound technology, including automated biopsy needles, high-resolution transducers, and computer-aided diagnosis programs have prompted a surge of interest

123

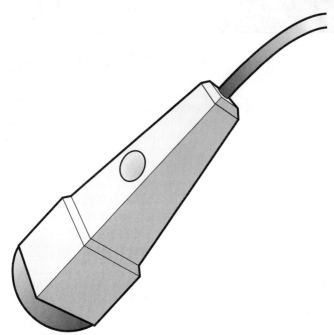

■ FIGURE 10–1. A standard curved array ultrasound probe.

in fine-needle and core biopsy tissue sampling as an alternative to open biopsy.

- Surgeons use ultrasound to evaluate the breast for a solid or cystic lesion and also to identify characteristics of the lesion that suggest whether it is benign or malignant.
- Current indications for breast ultrasonography include (1) evaluation of a nonpalpable, new, or growing mass or microcalcifications detected on mammography; (2) evaluation of duct size in the presence of nipple discharge; (3) assessment of a dense breast or a vaguely palpable mass; (4) differentiation between a solid palpable mass and a cystic one; and (5) guidance of percutaneous drainage of an abscess.

Gastrointestinal Tract

- Endoscopic ultrasonography (EUS) involves the visualization of the gastrointestinal (GI) tract via a high-frequency (12 to 20 MHz) ultrasound transducer placed through an endoscope.

- When done preoperatively, EUS is 80% to 90% accurate at predicting the stage of the upper GI tumor; if an endoscopically directed biopsy attachment is used, the diagnostic potential is even higher.
- Indications for EUS include (1) preoperative staging of esophageal malignancies; (2) preoperative localization of pancreatic endocrine tumors, particularly insulinomas; (3) evaluation of submucosal lesions of the GI tract; and (4) guidance of imaging during interventional procedures (e.g., tissue sampling and drainage of a pancreatic pseudocyst). Recently, endoscopic ultrasound has been used to direct fine-needle aspiration biopsy of submucosal lesions in the GI tract and lesions in the pancreas.
- Endorectal ultrasonography, used in the evaluation of patients with benign and malignant rectal conditions, is commonly performed with an axial 7.0 or 10.0 MHz rotating transducer that produces a 360-degree horizontal cross-sectional view of the rectal wall.
- These layers are important landmarks in ultrasonographic staging, just as they are in postoperative pathologic staging.
- Endoanal ultrasonography is an important part of the evaluation of anal incontinence because it is capable of detecting defects in the internal and external sphincters.
- Ultrasound-detected sphincter disruption correlates well with pressure measurements and operative findings.

Vascular System

- In the office setting, surgeons use ultrasonography to screen for abdominal aortic aneurysm or to follow patients with an aneurysm.
- Ultrasonography is used to examine the patency and size of the portal vein and the hepatic artery in patients who have undergone liver transplantation, to assess the resectability of pancreatic tumors, to detect superior mesenteric artery occlusion, and for diagnosis of pseudoaneurysm or an arteriovenous fistula after percutaneous arterial catheterization.

Intraoperative Use of Ultrasound

Gastrointestinal Tract

- With intraoperative or laparoscopic ultrasonography.
- With this tool, surgeons can detect previously undiagnosed lesions or bile duct stones, avoid unnecessary dissection of

vessels or ducts, clarify tumor margins, and perform biopsy and cryoablation procedures.

- Ultrasonography is much more sensitive in detecting malignant or benign lesions.
- Intraoperative ultrasonography can delineate small lesions (5 mm) and define their relationship to other structures, which facilitates resection, reduces operative time, and frequently alters the surgeon's operative strategy.

Vascular System

- Intraoperative duplex imaging can be used to detect technical errors in vascular anastomoses and abnormalities in flow.

Use of Ultrasound in Acute Settings and Trauma Resuscitation

Trauma Resuscitation: Focused Assessment for Sonography in Trauma (FAST) Examination

- The FAST is designed to assess blood accumulation in dependent areas of the pericardial sac and abdomen while the patient is in the supine position, and the FAST examination is performed in a specific sequence.
- This exam sequentially surveys for the presence or absence of blood in the pericardial sac and dependent abdominal regions, including the right upper quadrant (RUQ), left upper quadrant (LUQ), and pelvis.
- The pericardial area is visualized first so that blood within the heart can be used as a standard to set the gain.
- Blood is most often identified on the RUQ image of the FAST.
- If the subcostal pericardial image cannot be obtained or is suboptimal, a parasternal ultrasound view of the heart should be performed.
- Next, the transducer is placed in the right midaxillary line between the 11th and 12th ribs to identify in the sagittal section the liver, kidney, and diaphragm.
- With the transducer positioned in the left posterior axillary line between the 10th and 11th ribs, the spleen and kidney are visualized and blood is sought in between the two organs and in the subphrenic space.
- Finally, the transducer is directed for a transverse view and placed about 4 cm superior to the symphysis pubis. It is swept inferiorly to obtain a coronal view of the full bladder and the pelvis searching for blood.

Accuracy of the FAST

● Repeating the FAST after the insertion of a tube thoracostomy improves the visualization of the pericardial area,
  thereby decreasing the number of false-positive and negative studies.

● The FAST is accurate when it is used to evaluate hypotensive patients who present with blunt abdominal trauma. In
  this scenario, ultrasound is so accurate that when the FAST
  is positive, an immediate operation is justified.

● Therefore, select patients considered to be at high risk for
  occult intra-abdominal injury should undergo a computed
  tomography (CT) scan of the abdomen regardless of the
  results of the FAST examination. These patients include those
  with fractures of the pelvis or thoracolumbar spine, major
  thoracic trauma (pulmonary contusion, lower rib fractures),
  and hematuria.

Trauma Resuscitation: Hemothorax

● Ultrasound transmission gel is applied to the right and left
  lower thoracic areas in the mid to posterior axillary lines
  between the 9th and 10th intercostal spaces (Fig. 10–2). The
  transducer is slowly advanced cephalad to identify the
  hyperechoic diaphragm and to interrogate the supradiaphragmatic space for the presence or absence of fluid.

Trauma Resuscitation: Pneumothorax

Technique

● A 5.0- to 7.5-MHz linear array transducer is used to evaluate
  a patient for the presence of a pneumothorax.

● Ultrasound transmission gel is applied to the right and left
  upper thoracic areas at about the third to fourth intercostal
  space in the midclavicular line, and the presumed unaffected
  thoracic cavity is examined first.

● The normal examination of the thoracic cavity identifies the
  rib, pleural sliding, and a comet-tail artifact.

● When a pneumothorax is present, visceral pleura is not
  imaged and pleural sliding is not observed.

Trauma Resuscitation: Sternal Fracture

● The ultrasound examination of the sternum is performed
  using a 5.0- or 8.0-MHz linear array transducer that is oriented for sagittal or longitudinal views.

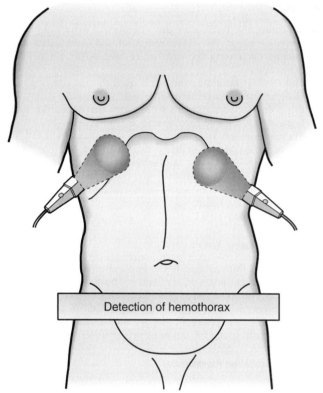

■ FIGURE 10–2.   Transducer positions for hemothorax evaluation.

Intensive Care Unit (ICU)

- Advantages of interventional ultrasound as used by the surgeon in the ICU include the following: (1) visualization in real-time imaging to allow direct placement of a catheter and confirm complete drainage of a fluid collection; (2) performance at the patient's bedside to avoid transport; and (3) safe, minimally invasive, and repeatable, if necessary.
- Education of surgeons in ultrasound.

CHAPTER 11

SURGICAL INFECTIONS AND CHOICE OF ANTIBIOTICS

CAUSES OF SURGICAL SITE INFECTION

- Infections of surgical wounds occur whenever the combination of microbial numbers and virulence in the wound is sufficiently large to overcome the local host defense mechanisms and establish progressive growth.
- All postoperative surgical infections occurring in an operative site are now termed *surgical site infections* (SSI).
- For subclassification, SSIs are defined as *superficial incisional* (involving only the skin and subcutaneous tissues), *deep incisional* (involving fascial and muscle layers of the incision), and *organ space* (involving any part of the anatomy [e.g., organs or spaces], other than the incision, that was opened or manipulated during the operative procedure).
- Organ space SSIs include postoperative intra-abdominal abscesses, empyema, or mediastinitis.

Bacterial Factors

- The deposition and growth of bacteria within wounds are a prerequisite for the development of infections, and the kind and numbers of bacteria contribute significantly to the establishment of overt infection, or the lack of it.
- Exotoxins permit streptococci and clostridia to establish invasive infection after smaller inocula than other pathogens and to evolve much more rapidly.
- Thus, whereas most wound infections do not become evident clinically for 5 days or longer after the operation, infections due to streptococci or clostridia may become severe within 24 hours.
- Wounds classified as clean usually contain skin bacteria such as *Staphylococcus epidermidis* or diphtheroids.
- In traumatic wounds, the most likely organisms are *Staphylococcus aureus* and *Streptococcus pyogenes*.

129

- When a viscus is entered, the resident flora become the expected potential pathogens.
- Normal defense mechanisms are of great importance in preventing infection at its inception, but wound infection is inevitable if the bacterial inoculum is sufficiently large.

Local Wound Factors

- Inhibition of local defense mechanisms for clearing bacteria is perhaps the most important cause of wound infections.
- Foreign bodies including sutures and drains, lack of accurate approximation of tissues, strangulation of tissue with sutures that are too tight, and the presence of any dead tissue, hematomas, or seromas all increase the risk of infection.

Patient Factors

- Wound infections are more common in the very young and the very old, perhaps because of immature or senescent resistance mechanisms.
- Anything that reduces blood flow to the surgical incision—as may be found in vascular occlusive states, hypovolemic shock, or with the use of vasoconstrictors either locally or systemically—increases the incidence of infection.
- Preventing hypothermia during the operative procedure and providing high levels of FIO_2 (80%) in the operating room and recovery room can significantly reduce the rate of surgical site infections.
- Conditions that reduce vascular reactivity as in uremia, old age, or the use of high doses of corticosteroids and other drugs cause an increased susceptibility to infection.
- More complex problems leading to increased infection include cancer and trauma, both of which may be associated with complement activation and the generation of both tissue-derived and complement split product-derived inhibitors of cellular function, which influence both T-cell and phagocytic cell function.

PREVENTION OF WOUND INFECTION

Avoidance of Bacterial Contamination

Environmental Factors

- Two greatest sources of significant microbial contamination of operative wounds are exogenous contact from breaks in technique by the operating team and endogenous contamination from the patient's skin and various bacteria-containing tracts (e.g., gastrointestinal, respiratory, or genitourinary tracts).

- Of the two, endogenous contamination causes a greater number of infections in all types of wounds except those classified as clean (Table 11–1).

Preoperative Preparation of the Patient

- Patients who are in the hospital for prolonged periods of time or who have substantial illness have increased numbers of resident organisms on the skin, especially in the groin and intertriginous areas.
- All cutaneous infections should be controlled or cleared before the time of an elective operation.

TABLE 11–1. Surgical Wound Classification According to Contamination

Wound Class	Definition
Clean	Uninfected operative wound in which no inflammation is encountered and the respiratory, alimentary, genital, or infected urinary tract are not entered. Wounds are primarily closed and, if necessary, drained with closed drainage.Surgical wounds following blunt trauma should be included in this category if they meet the criteria.
Clean-contaminated	Operative wound in which the respiratory, alimentary, genital or urinary tracts are entered under controlled conditions and without unusual contamination.
Contaminated	Open, fresh, accidental wounds. In addition, operations with major breaks in sterile technique or gross spillage from the gastrointestinal tract, and incisions in which acute, nonpurulent inflammation is encountered are included in this category.
Dirty	Old traumatic wounds with retained devitalized tissue and those that involve existing clinical infection or perforated viscera. This definition suggests that the organisms causing postoperative infection were present in the operative field before the operation.

The Importance of Surgical Technique

- Gentle care of the tissues to minimize local damage is one of the most important ways to prevent wound infection.
- All devitalized tissues and foreign bodies should be removed from traumatic wounds.
- Not only must all contaminated foreign bodies be removed from grossly contaminated wounds, but one should try to avoid the introduction of new foreign bodies such as prostheses, grafts, and suture materials.
- Monofilament sutures are preferable to multifilament ones in contaminated wounds.
- The presence of hematomas, seromas, or dead spaces favors bacterial localization and growth and prevents the delivery of phagocytic cells to such foci.
- The best way to prevent fluid collection and infection is to provide a system of closed suction drainage.
- Open drainage of wounds with Penrose-type drains increases rather than decreases the degree of contamination and the incidence of infection.
- In heavily contaminated wounds or in wounds in which all the foreign bodies or devitalized tissues cannot be satisfactorily removed, delayed primary closure minimizes the development of serious infection in most instances.

Systemic Factors

- Host resistance is abnormal in a variety of systemic conditions and diseases, including leukemia, diabetes mellitus, uremia, prematurity, burn or traumatic injury, advanced malignancy, old age, obesity, malnutrition, and several diseases of inherited immunodeficiency.
- Malnutrition, even when subclinical, can significantly impair host defense mechanisms.

Reducing the Bacterial Load by Prophylactic Antibiotic Therapy

- Administration of therapeutic doses of antimicrobial agents can prevent infection in wounds contaminated by bacteria sensitive to the agents.
- Indiscriminate use of antibiotics should be discouraged, because it may lead to emergence of antibiotic-resistant strains of organisms or serious hypersensitivity reactions.
- Prolonged use of prophylactic antibiotics may also mask the signs of established infections, making diagnosis more difficult.
- Prophylactic systemic antibiotics are clearly not indicated for most patients undergoing straightforward clean surgical

operations in which no obvious bacterial contamination or insertion of a foreign body has occurred.

- When the incidence of wound infections is less than 1%, the potential for reducing this low infection rate does not justify the expense and side effects of antibiotic administration.

- Prophylactic antibiotic use is warranted in the following procedures:

  - High-risk gastroduodenal procedures, including operations for gastric cancer, ulcer, obstruction, or bleeding; those operations performed when gastric acid production has been effectively suppressed; and gastric operations for morbid obesity.

  - High-risk biliary procedures, including operations in patients older than 60 years, in patients with acute inflammation, common duct stones, or jaundice, and in patients with prior biliary tract operations or endoscopic biliary manipulation.

  - Resection and anastomosis of the colon or small intestine.

  - Cardiac procedures through a median sternotomy.

  - Vascular surgery of the lower extremities or abdominal aorta.

  - Amputation of an extremity with impaired blood supply, particularly in the presence of a current or recent ischemic ulcer.

  - Vaginal or abdominal hysterectomy.

  - Primary cesarean section.

  - Operations entering the oral pharyngeal cavity in continuity with neck dissections.

  - Craniotomy.

  - The implantation of any permanent prosthetic material.

  - Any wound with known gross bacterial contamination.

  - Accidental wounds with heavy contamination and tissue damage. In such instances, the antibiotic should be given intravenously as soon as possible after injury. The two best-studied situations are penetrating abdominal injures and open fractures.

  - Injuries prone to clostridial infection because of extensive devitalization of muscle, heavy contamination, and/or impairment of blood supply.

  - In the presence of preexisting valvular heart damage, to prevent the development of bacterial endocarditis.

- Prophylactic antibiotic therapy is clearly more effective when begun preoperatively and continued through the intraoperative period, with the aim of achieving therapeutic blood levels throughout the operative period.

- The first dose of prophylactic antibiotics should be given intravenously at the time anesthesia is induced.
- Failure of prophylactic antibiotic agents occurs in part through a neglect of the importance of the timing and dosage of these agents.

NATURE, DIAGNOSIS, AND TREATMENT OF SURGICAL INFECTIONS

- Surgical infections are distinguished from medical infections by the presence of an anatomic or mechanical problem that must be resolved by operation or other invasive procedure to cure the infection.
- The pathogens found in medical infections are usually single and aerobic.
- The pathogens causing surgical infections, in contrast, are frequently mixed, involving aerobes and anaerobes, and usually originate from the patient's own endogenous flora.

Necrotizing Soft Tissue Infections

- Necrotizing soft tissue infections, both clostridial and non-clostridial, are less common than subcutaneous abscesses and cellulitis but are much more serious conditions whose severity initially may be unrecognized.
- These infections are marked by the absence of clear local boundaries or palpable limits.
- A clostridial infection typically involves underlying muscle, and is termed *clostridial myonecrosis* or *gas gangrene.*
- The presence of gas in a soft tissue infection implies anaerobic metabolism.
- Rapid progression of a soft tissue infection, a marked hemo-dynamic response to infection, or the failure to respond to conventional nonoperative therapy may be the earliest signs of a necrotizing soft tissue infection.
- The critical step in diagnosis is to recognize the nonlocal-ized, necrotizing nature of the infection and the need for operative treatment.
- Operative treatment requires excision of involved tissues for clostridial myonecrosis; on an extremity, this may mean amputation.
- All areas of necrotic tissue must be unroofed and débrided.

Intra-Abdominal and Retroperitoneal Infections

- Most serious intra-abdominal infections require surgical intervention for resolution.

- The specific exceptions to the requirement for surgical intervention include pyelonephritis, salpingitis, amebic liver abscess, enteritis (e.g., *Shigella*, *Yersinia*), spontaneous bacterial peritonitis, some cases of diverticulitis, and some cases of cholangitis.
- If the patient is too sick to go without antibiotic therapy, she or he is also too sick to avoid operative intervention and definitive diagnosis and treatment.
- Despite modern antibiotics and intensive care, mortality from serious intra-abdominal or retroperitoneal infection remains high (5–50%) and morbidity is substantial.
- If a corrective operation and effective antibiotics are not employed promptly, the sequence of events termed *multiple-organ dysfunction syndrome* may ensue and cause the death of the patient even after the primary focus of infection has been controlled.
- When a patient is diagnosed with intra-abdominal infection, initial treatment consists of cardiorespiratory support, antibiotic therapy, and operative intervention.
- Specific, targeted antibiotic therapy is not possible at first and the initial choice must be empirical, designed to cover a range of possible organisms.

OPERATIVE INTERVENTION FOR INTRA-ABDOMINAL OR RETROPERITONEAL INFECTION

- The goal of operative intervention in patients with intra-abdominal infection is to correct the underlying anatomic problem that either caused the infection or perpetuates it.
- Computed tomographic scans provide precise localization of intra-abdominal abscesses, permitting selected abscesses to be drained percutaneously under radiologic or ultrasound guidance.
- If percutaneous drainage is not successful, an open operation may be required.
- If a patient has multiple abscesses or abscesses combined with underlying disease that requires operative correction, or if a safe percutaneous route to the abscess is not present, then open, operative drainage may be required.

POSTOPERATIVE FEVER

- Postoperative fever occurs frequently and may be a source of concern to physician and patient.
- The most common nonsurgical causes of postoperative infection and fever—urinary tract infection, respiratory tract

infection, and intravenous catheter-associated infection—are all readily diagnosed.

- The other important causes of postoperative infection and fever—wound infection and intra-abdominal infection—require operative treatment and are not properly managed with antibiotics in the absence of operative treatment.
- The most sensitive test for detecting infection and determining its location continues to be history taking and physical examination conducted by a conscientious physician.
- Fever in the first 3 days after operation most likely has a noninfectious cause.
- However, when the fever starts 5 or more days postoperatively, the incidence of wound infections exceeds the incidence of undiagnosed fevers.
- Only two important infectious causes of fever are likely in the first 36 hours after a laparotomy:

  - The first is an injury to bowel with intraperitoneal leak.
  - The other early cause of fever and infection is an invasive soft tissue infection, beginning in the wound, caused either by beta-hemolytic streptococci or by clostridial species.

- A rare cause of infection in the first 48 hours after operation is wound toxic shock syndrome; this occurs when certain toxin-producing *S. aureus* species grow in a wound.

Nonsurgical Infections in Surgical Patients

- Postoperative patients are at increased risk for a variety of nonsurgical postoperative nosocomial infections; the most common of these is urinary tract infection.
- Lower respiratory tract infections are the third most common cause of nosocomial infection in surgical patients (after urinary tract infection and SSIs) and are the leading cause of death due to nosocomial infection.
- Antibiotic-associated diarrhea is another important problem in hospitalized surgical patients.

PATHOGENS IN SURGICAL INFECTIONS

Gram-Positive Cocci

- Gram-positive cocci of importance to surgeons include staphylococci and streptococci.
- Staphylococci are divided into coagulase-positive and coagulase-negative strains.

- Coagulase-positive staphylococci are *S. aureus* and are the most common pathogen associated with infections in wounds and incisions not subject to endogenous contamination.
- Methicillin-resistant staphylococci do not seem to have intrinsic pathogenicity greater than that of other staphylococci, but they are more difficult to treat because of antibiotic resistance.
- For many years, coagulase-negative staphylococci were considered contaminants and skin flora incapable of causing serious disease; however, in the correct clinical setting, coagulase-negative staphylococci can cause serious disease.

  - Most common in patients who have been compromised by trauma, extensive surgery, or metabolic disease and who have invasive vascular devices in place.
  - Most common organisms recovered in nosocomial bacteremia and are frequently associated with clinically significant infections of intravascular devices.
  - Found in endocarditis, prosthetic joint infections, vascular graft infections, and postsurgical mediastinitis.
  - Most coagulase-negative staphylococci are methicillin resistant.

- The streptococcal species include beta-hemolytic streptococci (especially group A or *S. pyogenes*), *S. pneumoniae*, and other alpha-hemolytic streptococci.
- Other alpha-hemolytic streptococci or viridans streptococci are almost never found as the sole cause of significant surgical infections.
- Enterococci are commonly recovered as part of a mixed flora in intra-abdominal infections; it is rare to recover enterococci alone from a surgical infection.
- Enterococci clearly do cause significant disease in the urinary tract and the biliary tract or as a cause of subacute bacterial endocarditis.
- The most effective antibiotic combination for treating enterococcal infections is gentamicin combined with either ampicillin (or another advanced-generation penicillin) or vancomycin.
- However, vancomycin-resistant enterococci (VRE), resistant to all known antibiotics including gentamicin and vancomycin, have been isolated in increasing numbers.

Aerobic and Facultative Gram-Negative Rods

- A variety of gram-negative rods are associated with surgical infections; most fall into the family Enterobacteriaceae.
- Facultative anaerobic bacteria include *Escherichia, Proteus*, and *Klebsiella*.

- Gram-negative rods recovered from infections originating in the community, such as uncomplicated appendicitis or diverticulitis, are less likely to involve antibiotic-resistant strains.
- Obligate aerobic gram-negative rods that are often found in surgical infections include species of both *Pseudomonas* and *Acinetobacter*; these organisms are most commonly found in hospital associated pneumonias in surgical patients but may also be recovered from the peritoneal cavity or in severe soft tissue infections.

Anaerobes

- Anaerobic bacteria are the most numerous inhabitants of the normal gastrointestinal tract, including the mouth.
- The most common anaerobic isolate from surgical infections is *Bacteroides fragilis*; the other important genus of anaerobic bacteria found in surgical infections is *Clostridium*, which is a gram-positive, spore-forming rod.
- These organisms require an anaerobic environment for growth and invasion and for elaboration of the toxins that account for their dramatic virulence in soft tissue infections.
- The recovery of anaerobes from a soft tissue infection, or even from the blood, implies their growth and multiplication in a focus of dead tissue.
- Anaerobic bacteremia should always prompt a search for an abscess or for an enteric lesion that requires surgical intervention.

Fungi

- Fungi are infrequently the primary pathogens in deep-seated surgical infections, but may be seen frequently as an opportunistic invader in patients with serious surgical infections who have received broad-spectrum antibiotic treatment suppressing normal endogenous flora.
- These infections are best avoided through judicious use of systemic broad-spectrum antibiotics and through prophylaxis with oral nystatin or ketoconazole when broad-spectrum antibacterial therapy is required.

ANTIBIOTICS

Penicillins

- The penicillins are broadly divided into those that are stable against staphylococcal penicillinase and all others.

- Various penicillins have been combined with one of the beta-lactamase inhibitors, clavulanic acid, sulbactam, or tazobactam.
- These combinations provide antibiotic compounds that retain their broad gram-negative activity while also acting against methicillin-sensitive staphylococci and anaerobes, facultative species, and aerobic bacteria that are resistant to the penicillins by virtue of beta-lactamase production.

Cephalosporins

- Cephalosporins are the largest and most frequently used group of antibiotics commonly divided into three generations.
- The first-generation cephalosporins have excellent activity against methicillin-susceptible staphylococci and all streptococcal species, but are not active against enterococci.
- The second-generation cephalosporins have expanded gram-negative activity when compared with the first generation, but still lack activity against many gram-negative rods.
- The third-generation cephalosporins have greatly expanded activity against gram-negative rods, including many resistant strains, and rival the aminoglycosides in their coverage while having much more favorable safety profile.
- In exchange for this gram-negative coverage, most members of this group have significantly less activity against staphylococci and streptococcal species than first- and second-generation cephalosporins.
- Anaerobic coverage is, generally, rather poor as well.

Monobactams

- Aztreonam is the only currently available member of the class of monobactams; it has the safety profile of other beta-lactam antibiotics, but does not cross react in patients who are allergic to penicillins or cephalosporins.

Carbapenems

- Imipenem and meropenem are the first representatives of the class of carbapenems.
- They have a very broad spectrum of antibacterial activity with excellent activity against all gram-positive cocci except for methicillin-resistant staphylococci and only modest activity against enterococci.

- Imipenem is provided only in combination with the enzyme inhibitor cilastatin, which prevents its hydrolysis in the kidneys and resultant nephrotoxicity.

Quinolones

- As a class, the fluoroquinolones are marked by extremely broad activity against gram-negative rods.
- The fluoroquinolones other than norfloxacin are distinguished by excellent tissue penetration and comparable serum and tissue levels with either intravenous or oral administration.

Aminoglycosides

- For many years, the aminoglycoside class of antibiotics was the only reliable class of drugs for the empirical treatment of serious gram-negative infections.
- Aminoglycosides have no activity against anaerobes or against facultative bacteria in an anaerobic environment.
- Clinically, aminoglycosides are difficult to use because the ratio of therapeutic levels to toxic levels is low.
- Primary toxicities are nephrotoxicity and eighth nerve damage, both auditory and vestibular.

Antianaerobes

- The antibiotics with important antianaerobic activity are not logically grouped except by this characteristic.
- Metronidazole currently possesses the most complete activity against all anaerobic pathogens; however, it has no activity against any aerobic or facultative pathogens, either gram negative or gram positive, so it must always be combined with another antibiotic for complete coverage.

Macrolides

- Erythromycin is a macrolide antibiotic with only modest antianaerobic activity in the concentrations that can be achieved systemically.

Tetracyclines

- Tetracyclines previously were an important class of antibiotics with significant antianaerobic activity.

Glycopeptides

- Vancomycin is the only glycopeptide antibiotic available in the United States.

Streptogramins

- The first water-soluble streptogramin antibiotic is actually a combination, quinupristin/dalfopristin.
- It is active against nearly all gram-positive pathogens, including vancomycin-resistant *Enterococcus faecium*, multi-drug resistant *S. aureus*, and penicillin-resistant *S. pneumoniae*.

Oxazolidinones

- The first representative of the class, oxazolidinone, is linezolid; it is available in both parenteral and oral forms.

SUPERINFECTION

- A superinfection is a new infection that develops during antibiotic treatment for the original infection.
- Whenever antibiotics are used, they exert a selective pressure on the endogenous flora of the patient and on exogenous bacteria that colonize sites at risk.
- Bacteria that remain are resistant to the antibiotics being used and become the pathogens in superinfection.
- Careful surveillance of hospitalized patients reveals superinfections in 2 to 10% of antibiotic-treated patients, depending on the underlying risk factors.
- The best preventive action is to limit the dose and duration of antibiotic treatment to what is obviously required and to be alert to the possibility of superinfections.
- The use of increasingly powerful and broad-spectrum antibiotics has also led to an increasing incidence of fungal superinfections.
- Antibiotic-associated colitis is another significant superinfection that can occur in hospitalized patients with mild to serious illness.
- This entity is caused by the enteric pathogen *C. difficile* and has been reported after treatment with every antibiotic except vancomycin.
- *C. difficile* colitis can vary from a mild, self-limited disease to a rapidly progressive septic process culminating in death.

- The most important step in treating this disease is to suspect it; diagnosis is best accomplished by detecting *C. difficile* toxin in the stool.
- Treatment is supportive with fluid and electrolytes, withdrawal of the offending antibiotic if possible, and oral metronidazole to treat the superinfection.
- Vancomycin should be reserved for metronidazole failures.
- In rare instances when an overwhelming colitis does not respond to medical management, emergency colectomy may be required.

CHAPTER 12

SURGICAL PROBLEMS IN THE IMMUNOSUPPRESSED PATIENT

PRIMARY IMMUNOSUPPRESSION

- *Primary immunosuppression* refers to the groups of clinical conditions in which the patient has a genetically predetermined abnormality in host responsiveness (Table 12–1).
- Defects of the primary inflammatory response result in a host that is extraoradinarily susceptible to common bacterial infections.
- Impaired mechanisms of intracellular killing activity are best exemplified in the occasional patients seen with chronic granulomatous disease, myeloperoxidase deficiency, or Chédiak-Higashi syndrome.
- Abnormalities of cellular immunity are identified with increased rates of infection with uncommon pathogens but are also associated with increased rates of specific malignancies; many of these T-cell abnormalities are associated with thymic abnormalities of hypoplasia of the thymus or with thymoma.
- Patients with T-cell abnormalities are at risk for chronic mucocutaneous candidiasis.
- Altered humoral immunity syndrome results from impaired maturation or activation of B cells and results in an increased incidence of pulmonary infections, lymphomas, and gastrointestinal malignancies.

SECONDARY IMMUNOSUPPRESSION

Human Immunodeficiency Virus (HIV) Infection

- Surgical problems in the HIV-infected patient include abnormal presentation of common illnesses and unique problems that are consequences of the acquired immunosuppression.

**TABLE 12–1. General Categories of Primary
Immunodeficiency States***

Host Defense Component	Specific Defect
PRIMARY INFLAMMATION	
Coagulation abnormalities	Congenital decrease in factor XII
Platelets	Congenital amegakaryocytic thrombocytopenia
Complement proteins	Specific protein component deficiencies
Contact activating system (bradykinin production)	Kininogen deficiency state
PHAGOCYTIC PHASE OF INFLAMMATION	
Neutrophils	Defective chemotaxis, mobility, microbicidal activity
Monocytes	Impaired mobility, generalized dysfunction
T-CELL DEFECTS	
Severe combined deficiency states	Reduced T cells and reduced antibody production
Thymoma/hypoplasia of thymus	T-cell deficiency state
B-CELL DEFECTS	
Congenital agammaglobulinemia	Reduction in all immunoglobulin classes
Specific subclass deficiencies	Selective deficiency of IgG, IgA, or IgM

*These abnormalities affect the initiator events of inflammation, inflammatory cell
function, and specific T-cell/B-cell functions.

Pathogenesis

- HIV is a blood-borne infection that is transmitted to the susceptible host after a percutaneous or a mucous membrane exposure to infected blood or body fluids.
- The virus attaches to specific receptors on the host CD4 lymphocytes and is internalized releasing its RNA.
- The unique enzyme, reverse transcriptase, of the virus results in the synthesis of complementary copies of DNA to the RNA template of the virus (cDNA).
- The cDNA then migrates into the nucleus of the infected cell, is incorporated into the chromosomal configuration of the host cell, and initiates the synthesis of new viral particles.
- The viral burden reaches a critical level with lysis of the infected cell and release of viral particles to infect other cells.
- The result of this process over time is the systematic depletion of CD4 T cells, increasing the proportion of CD8 T cells and resulting in immunosuppression of the host.

- The natural history of HIV infection passes through four phases:
  - The first phase is the *acute viral infection,* which includes fever, malaise, and pharyngitis.
  - Second, there is a sustained period of *asymptomatic disease* during which active viral replication is occurring in a slow but progressive reduction in CD4 cells; this indolent second phase is highly variable in different patients.
  - In the third phase, called *acquired immunodeficiency syndrome (AIDS)-related complex,* patients become symptomatic with evidence of regional adenopathy.
  - The fourth phase of the disease, *clinical AIDS,* is considered to exist when the patient has an indicator condition or a CD4 cell count of less than 200 cells/μL (Box 12–1).

Acute Abdomen

- The patient with AIDS has an increased frequency of surgical abdominal conditions.
- Acute appendicitis occurs because of the conventional occlusion of the appendiceal orifice by a fecalith but also can be caused by orifice occlusion by Kaposi's sarcoma lesions or acute CMV infections.
  - Clinical presentation is with characteristic right lower pain, but most HIV patients have a normal white blood cell count.
  - There appears to be an increased rate of perforation, gangrenous appendicitis, and appendiceal abscess among patients with AIDS.
- Perforation of the gastrointestinal tract not related to appendicitis is increased in the patient with AIDS.
  - Cytomegalovirus (CMV) can cause visceral perforation in patients with AIDS.
  - The terminal ilium and colon are the most common sites for CMV-associated perforations.
  - CMV perforation is an indicator of advanced AIDS and carries a grave prognosis.
  - Kaposi's sarcoma, gastrointestinal lymphoma, and severe ileocolitis from *Mycobacterium avium-intracellulare* infection are additional causes of AIDS-related perforations of the gastrointestinal tract and are managed the same as for any other perforation from infectious causes.
- Gastrointestinal obstruction can be caused by AIDS-related diseases.

- Causes of obstruction include lymphoma, mycobacterial disease, intussusception from Kaposi's sarcoma, and a CMV-associated Ogilvie-like syndrome progressing to toxic megacolon.
- Gastrointestinal bleeding is seen with the same array of disease processes that are responsible for perforation and obstruction.

Hepatobiliary Disease

- Hepatobiliary disease is very common in the HIV-infected patient.
- Chronic hepatitis B and C infections share common routes of transmission with HIV infection.
- Infection of the liver parenchyma with *Candida albicans* and *M. avium-intracellulare* can result in small hepatic abscesses that often require liver biopsy for diagnosis.
- AIDS-associated cholangiopathy appears to be the consequence of infection of the bile ducts with opportunistic pathogens, including *Cryptosporidium* species, CMV, and *Microsporidia*.
  - Inflammatory changes from invasion of the ducts result in a sclerosis-like picture with patients having new-onset right upper quadrant pain, fever, and alkaline phosphatase elevations but rarely jaundice.
- Specific antimicrobial therapy is often used for treatment.

Splenomegaly

- Splenomegaly may be the result of multiple causes.
- Patients may have portal hypertension from severe liver disease or portal fibrosis.
- Parenchymal infection of the spleen may be from CMV, mycobacterium, *Pneumocystis carinii*, and other pathogens.
- Splenic enlargement may be from lymphoma or Kaposi's sarcoma.
- Patients will commonly present with left upper quadrant pain and a palpable and tender spleen.

Vascular Disease

- Some infected pseudoaneurysms will be seen among the intravenous drug abuse population with common bacteria.
- *Salmonella* has a particular affinity for atherosclerotic plaque in AIDS patients.

Neoplasms

- B-cell lymphoma, which is medically managed as a lymphoma in a normal patient, is commonly undifferentiated and aggressive among patients with AIDS.
  - Primary management of the lymphoma disease is medical.
- Kaposi's sarcoma in the patient with AIDS occurs at numerous different sites, including skin, gastrointestinal tract, lung, liver, and heart.
  - Surgical involvement is primarily for the diagnosis and management of complications, particularly in the gastrointestinal tract.

Anorectal Disease

- The immunosuppressed patient with AIDS is at increased risk for human papillomavirus infection, which may result in large condylomata acuminata.
- Squamous cell carcinoma of the anus occurs with increased frequency.

Transplant Patients

Infection in Transplant Patients

- Transplant patients may develop all of the infections that might be identified in any patient but are also at risk for an array of infections from minimally virulent pathogens.
- The prevention, diagnosis, and treatment of surgical site infections are the same as would be used for similar infections in nontransplant patients.
- Bacterial nosocomial pneumonia, urinary tract infection, and intravascular device infections will be seen with equal or greater frequency compared with other surgical intensive care patients.
- Because immunosuppression increases the host's vulnerability and preexistent antibiotic therapy may have dramatically changed the host's colonization with resistant microbes, pneumonia is the greatest risk.
- Beginning at approximately 1 month after transplantation, the community-acquired infection with unusual pathogens begins to be a problem.
- Infection with the herpes group of viruses assumes considerable significance, of which CMV infection is most important.
- CMV infection can result in pneumonia, gastrointestinal ulceration, and chorioretinitis.

Box 12–1. Clinical Conditions that Fulfill the Revised Case Definition of Clinical AIDS Diagnosis

Any one of the following combined with a positive HIV serology:
- Candidiasis of the upper aerodigestive tract (e.g., esophagitis lungs)
- Invasive cervical cancer
- Extrapulmonary coccidioidomycosis
- Extrapulmonary cryptococcosis
- Cryptosporidiosis
- Extralymphatic cytomegalovirus infection (e.g., nonlymph nodes, non-spleen or liver)
- Herpes simplex pneumonia or esophagitis
- Extrapulmonary histoplasmosis
- HIV-associated wasting or dementia
- Isoporosis infection
- Kaposi's sarcoma
- Primary central nervous system lymphoma
- Any non-Hodgkin's or B-cell, or undifferentiated type of lymphoma
- Disseminated tuberculosis or atypical *Mycobacterium* infection
- Nocardiosis
- *Pneumocystis carinii* infection
- Progressive multifocal leukoencephalopathy
- *Salmonella* septicemia
- Extraintestinal *Strongyloides* infection
- Toxoplasmosis

AIDS, acquired immunodeficiency syndrome; HIV, human immunodeficiency virus.

- Epstein-Barr virus (EBV) infection begins in the oropharynx epithelial cells and subsequently infects B cells in transit through the area of infection.
- Acute EBV infection may be totally latent, relatively mild, or a florid mononucleosis syndrome before it then lapses into a chronic latent state.
- Sustained EBV infection may lead to the post-transplantation lymphoproliferative disease.
- A decrease in immunosuppression, antilymphoma chemotherapy, and surgery or radiotherapy (or both) to control local disease form the treatment for transplantation-associated lymphoproliferative neoplasms.
- Other opportunistic infections from unusual bacterial, fungi, viruses, and even protozoans can occur (Box 12–2).

**Box 12–2. Unusual Viral, Bacterial, Fungal, and
Protozoan Infections Encountered in
Immunosuppressed Transplant Patients**

VIRAL INFECTIONS
Herpes simplex virus-1 and -2
Human herpesvirus-6
Varicella-zoster
Hepatitis B and C
Human immunodeficiency virus
Papovavirus
Respiratory syncytial virus

UNUSUAL OTHER PATHOGENS
Listeria monocytogenes
Salmonella sp.
Mycobacterium tuberculosis
Mycobacterium avium intracellulare
Cryptococcus neoformans
Coccidioides immitis
Nocardia asteroides
Candida albicans (also non-*albicans* sp.)
Aspergillus fumigatus
Histoplasma capsulatum
Pneumocystis carinii

Neoplasia in Transplant Patients

- Sustained immunosuppression in the transplant patient is associated with increased rates of malignancies, although the types of malignancies differ among the patient groups receiving each type of transplant.
- Viral infection, such as with CMV, EBV, herpesvirus, and human papillomavirus, results in increased malignancies.
- Some immunosuppressive agents may potentiate the effects of other carcinogens or may be carcinogens themselves (e.g., azathioprine, cyclosporine).
- Skin cancers are most common in the kidney transplant patient, whereas lymphomas are most common among liver transplant recipients.
- Other cancers with increased frequencies include Kaposi's sarcoma, lip cancer, carcinoma of the kidney, vulvar and perineal cancers, and hepatobiliary cancers.

Malnutrition

- Malnutrition is an issue for patients with cancer, intestinal fistula, chronic pancreatitis and other malabsorption states, sustained catabolic illnesses, and many others with surgical illnesses.
- Virtually all components of the inflammatory and immune response are affected by malnutrition.
- Neutrophil function, cell-mediated immunity, and humoral immunity are adversely affected by malnutrition.
- Measurement of absolute lymphocyte counts, serum albumin or prealbumin, serum retinol proteins, and creatinine-height indices will give potentially objective measures of malnutrition.
- In general, patients with clinical weight loss or those with acute catabolic illnesses are presumptively considered to be either malnourished or in a state of rapidly diminishing nutritional reserve and must be considered for nutritional support.

Burn and Trauma Injury

- Immunosuppression is an obligatory response of the host to thermal burns and to virtually any form of mechanical trauma.
- Reduced complement protein concentrations, reduced neutrophil chemotaxis/phagocytosis/intracellular killing, reduced B-cell function, and decreased cell-mediated immunity have all been demonstrated in trauma patients.
- The loss of major histocompatibility class II expression on monocytes has been demonstrated as yet another acquired deficiency from trauma that appears to correlate with infectious morbidity and patient outcome.
- The nadir of immunosuppression occurs at 1 to 2 days after injury and lasts for 7 or more days in the absence of intercurrent events.

Shock

- Shock as a clinical event has been proposed to have immunosuppressive consequences.
- Reduced complement protein concentrations, depressed neutrophil function studies, and altered B- and T-cell functions are consistently identified.

Transfusion

- Blood transfusion has been recognized for many decades as having immunosuppressive effects.
- Multiple units of transfusion with homologous blood have been used in the past for transplant kidney immunosuppression.
- Transfusion was a negative independent variable in the outcomes of cancer patients receiving surgical management of their primary disease.
- Blood transfusion was identified as an independent variable for infection morbidity in patients with penetrating abdominal trauma, independent from both shock or injury severity.
- Suppression has been theorized to occur from the release of prostaglandin E derivatives or from other suppressor cell products that are released in response to the transfusion.

Diabetes

- Clinical studies have noted increased rates of infection that occur in diabetic patients with uncontrolled glucose.
- A reduction in neutrophil chemotaxis and phagocytosis in diabetics have been demonstrated but only when blood glucose is poorly controlled.
- Reduced CD4 cell counts have also been reported in diabetics, but as is the case with neutrophil function, this abnormality was not seen when normal glucose control was present.
- Better blood sugar control will likely reduce rates of infection in diabetic patients.

Aging

- Infections are more common and have greater consequences to the elderly patient.
- Several immune changes with aging have been reported that may address increased infection rates:
  - Reduced T-cell stimulation.
  - Reduced immunoglobulin G antibody response to vaccination.
  - Reduced delayed type hypersensitivity (DTH) response.
  - Increased sensitivity of the host to prostaglandin E.

Hypothermia

- Patients undergoing major abdominal procedures who become hypothermic have higher rates of infection than patients who are maintained at normal core body temperature.

Postsplenectomy

- A number of studies have shown that patients, particularly in the pediatric and adolescent age groups, are at increased risk to develop overwhelming postsplenectomy sepsis.
- This septic event is not common in the postsplenectomy trauma patient (<1%) but is somewhat higher in those undergoing splenectomy for medical indications.
- Overwhelmingly, postsplenectomy sepsis is associated with a fulminant course that results in death rates of 70% or higher.
- Splenectomized patients have decreased immunoglobulin M antibodies.
- Splenectomy patients are at risk for infection from encapsulated bacteria of *Streptococcus pneumoniae, Neisseria meningitidis,* and *Haemophilus influenzae.*
- Patients requiring splenectomy should receive the pneumococcal, meningococcal, and *H. influenzae* vaccine.

CHAPTER 13

SURGICAL COMPLICATIONS

INTRODUCTION

- Surgeons can do much to avoid complications by a careful preoperative screening process.
- Once the operation is completed, compulsive postoperative surveillance is mandatory.
- In summary, the wise surgeon will deal with complications quickly, thoroughly, and appropriately.

WOUND COMPLICATIONS

Seroma

- Etiology—a seroma is the collection of liquified fat, serum, and lymphatic fluid under the incision.

Presentation and Management

- Seromas usually present as a localized and well-circumscribed swelling, pressure discomfort, and occasional drainage of clear liquid from the immature wound.
- Seromas that develop in abdominal incisions and extremity incisions can usually be evacuated and packed with saline moist gauze to allow healing by secondary intention.
- Despite repeated aspirations, some seromas persist or becomes secondarily infected; in those cases, the wound must be opened.

Hematoma

Etiology

- A hematoma is an abnormal collection of blood, usually in the subcutaneous layer of a recent incision.
- Bleeding in the involved layer after the skin is closed causes a hematoma.
- Rough handling of the tissues.
- Inadequate hemostasis.
- Coagulopathy.

- Myeloproliferative disorders, liver disease, clotting factor deficiencies, and platelet disorders.
- Presents with physical findings of purplish blue discoloration of the overlying skin and localized wound swelling.
- Management of hematomas depends on the size and age of the wound.
- Hematomas developing under skin flaps usually have to be evacuated in the operating room.
- A small hematoma that occurs 2 weeks after an operation will often resorb with conservative management only.

Prevention

- The most important principle in prevention of hematoma is careful hemostasis of the subcutaneous layer during closure.
- Discontinuing medications that can prolong bleeding times (e.g., warfarin and nonsteroidal anti-inflammatory agents).

Wound Dehiscence

Etiology

- Dehiscence is the separation of fascial layers early in the postoperative course, an event that usually leads to emergency action.
- Evisceration is protrusion of the small intestines through the fascial layers and out onto the abdominal skin surface.
- Dehiscence that occurs soon after operation will usually require a return trip to the operating room.
- However, a small partial dehiscence 10 days postoperation can often be watched and the wound packed without danger of evisceration.
- The etiology of dehiscence is often related to technical errors in placing sutures too close to the edge, too far apart, or under too much tension.

Presentation and Management

- Wound dehiscence usually presents with a sudden, dramatic drainage of relatively large volumes of a clear, salmon-colored fluid.
- Probing with the applicator reveals a large segment of the wound that is open all the way to the omentum and intestines; plans to take the patient back to the operating room immediately should be made.

- Evisceration is a surgical emergency; the eviscerated intestines should be covered with a sterile, saline-moist towel and preparations should be made to return to the operating room emergently.
- Management of the dehisced wound once in the operating room is a function of the condition of the fascia.
- If significant amounts of fascia need to be débrided because of infection or poor tissue integrity, it is poor judgment to attempt to close the fascia under significant tension.
- If the fascial layers cannot be closed without tension, an absorbable mesh may be placed in the wound and sewn to both fascial layers.
- If the dehiscence is small and fairly late postoperatively, the wound can be managed by conservative treatment including débridement of the wound, saline-moist gauze packing of the wound, and keeping an abdominal binder on the patient.
- Certainly, a permanent mesh, such as Marlex, should not be placed in the field under conditions in which there has been significant contamination.

Prevention

- Preventing wound dehiscence is largely a function of careful attention to technical detail during the fascial closure.
- Reduction of massively distended bowel by milking air and fluid back up into the stomach also may facilitate a tension-free closure.

Wound Infection

Etiology

- Wound infections continue to be a significant problem for surgeons in the modern era.
- Although some may view the problem as a merely cosmetic one, that view represents a very shallow understanding of this problem, which causes significant morbidity and expense.
- Wounds are, thus, categorized into three general categories: (1) superficial, which includes skin and subcutaneous tissue; (2) deep, which includes fascia and muscle; and (3) organ space, which includes the internal organs of the body if the operation includes that area.
- Substantial patient suffering and even occasional mortality.
- A host of factors may contribute to the development of postoperative wound infection.

- *Staphylococcus aureus* and coagulase-negative *Staphylococcus* remain the most common bacteria colonized from wounds (Table 13–1).
- Surgical wounds are classified according to the relative risk of postoperative wound infection occurring. The four categories are (1) clean, (2) clean contamination, (3) contaminated, and (4) dirty (Table 13–2).

Presentation and Management

- Postoperative wound infections present with erythema, tenderness, edema, and occasionally drainage.
- Wound infections most commonly occur 5 to 6 days postoperatively.
- A surgical wound is considered infected if (1) there is drainage of grossly purulent material from the wound, (2) the wound spontaneously opens and drains purulent fluid, (3) the wound drains fluid that is culture positive or gram stain positive for bacteria, and (4) the surgeon notes erythema or drainage and opens the wound after deeming it to be infected.
- Management of a postoperative wound infection depends on the depth of the infection.
- Débridement of any nonviable tissue is also an important element of wound management after an infection.

TABLE 13–1. Pathogens Isolated from Postoperative Surgical Site Infections at a University Hospital

Pathogen	% of Isolates
Staphylococcus (coagulase negative)	25.6
Enterococcus (group D)	11.5
Staphylococcus aureus	8.7
Candida albicans	6.5
Escherichia coli	6.3
Pseudomonas aeruginosa	6.0
Corynebacterium	4.0
Candida (non-*albicans*)	3.4
Alpha-hemolytic *Streptococcus*	3.0
Klebsiella pneumoniae	2.8
Vancomycin-resistant *Enterococcus*	2.4
Enterobacter cloacae	2.2
Citrobacter species	2.0

From Weiss CA, Statz CL, Dahms RA, et al: Six years of surgical wound surveillance at a tertiary care center. Arch Surg 134:1041, 1999.

TABLE 13–2. Classification of Surgical Wounds

Category	Criteria	Infection Rate
Clean	No hollow viscus entered Primary wound closure No inflammation No breaks in septic technique Elective procedure	1%–3%
Clean contaminated	Hollow viscus entered but controlled No inflammation Primary wound closure Minor break in aseptic technique Mechanical drain used Bowel preparation preop	5%–8%
Contaminated	Uncontrolled spillage from viscus Inflammation apparent Open, traumatic wound Major break in aseptic technique	20%–25%
Dirty	Untreated, uncontrolled spillage from viscus Pus in operative wound Open suppurative wound Severe inflammation	30%–40%

- Careful evaluation of a wound infection that involves the fascia and muscle layer would include evaluating for the possibility of a fascitis.
- Presence of crepitus in any surgical wound is a surgical emergency.
- Rapid and expeditious surgical débridement is indicated in this setting. After the wound has been adequately cleaned, the wound should be packed to its base with saline-moist gauze to allow healing of the wound from the base anteriorly to prevent premature skin closure.
- Premature closure of the skin should rarely be considered in a wound infection, because it virtually always results in recurrent infection in the deeper spaces.

Prevention

- The operating surgeon plays a major role in reducing or minimizing the presence of postoperative wound infections.
- For patients who are undergoing intra-abdominal surgery, a bowel preparation should be strongly considered.
- The surgeon should make certain that the patient undergoes a thorough skin preparation with appropriate antiseptic solutions.

- The surgeon can make certain that there is careful handling of the tissues. Meticulous hemostasis and débridement of devitalized tissue will be helpful. Similarly, compulsive control of all intraluminal contents is imperative.
- Eliminating a foreign body from the wound is another factor that the surgeon can control.
- Keeping the patient euthermic during the operation plays a major role in avoiding postoperative infections.
- The surgeon's judgment at the end of the case with regards to closing skin or packing the wound plays a major role in lowering infection rates.
- Most surgeons do not believe that preoperative antibiotics are indicated for clean operations.
- For clean-contaminated procedures, the administration of preoperative antibiotics is indicated.
- There is convincing evidence that the timing of the prophylactic antibiotic administration is critical.
- A good time to administer the preoperative dose is as the patient arrives in the operating room.
- The use of drains remains somewhat controversial in preventing postoperative wound infections.

Chronic Wounds

Etiology

- Chronic wounds are wounds that by definition have not healed completely within 30 to 90 days of the operative procedure.

Presentation and Management

- Patients with large chronic wounds require a great deal of patience and willingness to work with them.
- Meticulous wound care in the way of frequent dressing changes or the use of a wound suction system may accelerate healing of these chronic wounds. Recent development of a negative pressure wound treatment device has shown promise in the treatment of these difficult, chronic wounds.

COMPLICATIONS OF THERMAL REGULATION

Hypothermia

Etiology

- Optimal function of physiologic systems in the body occurs within a narrow range of body temperatures. A drop in body temperature of 2°C or an increase of 3°C signifies a health emergency that requires immediate intervention and is life threatening. Hypothermia can result from a number of mechanisms preoperatively, intraoperatively, or postoperatively.

- Trauma patient involved in injuries in a cold environment.
- Paralysis leads to hypothermia.
- Rapid resuscitation with cool intravenous (IV) fluids leads to hypothermia.
- A large, exposed area from the operation can have significant evaporative cooling.
- The body's response to hypothermia includes a decrease in cardiac output, reduction in heart rate, and, at lower temperatures, cardiac arrhythmias.

Presentation and Management

- Meticulous temperature monitoring is an important part of every operation. Most commonly, the monitoring is done with an esophageal thermometer.
- There is significant recent literature suggesting that careful control of body temperature intraoperatively significantly lowers infection rates postoperatively.
- A wide variety of modalities are currently available to assist in maintaining the euthermic patient during surgery or improving the hypothermic patient who arrives in the operating suite.
- Special attention should be paid to cardiac monitoring during the rewarming process, because cardiac irritability may be a significant problem.

Malignant Hyperthermia

Etiology and Presentation

- Malignant hyperthermia is a rare autosomal dominant inherited disorder of skeletal muscle.
- Hypermetabolic state triggered by exposure to certain inhalation agents or succinylcholine.
- The condition is created when uncontrolled amounts of intracellular calcium accumulate in skeletal muscle.
- The disorder may present within 30 minutes after administration of the anesthetic agents, and the clinical presentation is variable both in onset and severity. The most severe cases are associated with high fever, tachycardia, muscular rigidity, and cyanosis.

- Treatment—most cases of malignant hyperthermia will be diagnosed by the anesthesiologist while monitoring during the procedure.
- Immediately discontinue the use of the inhalation agent and administer dantrolene 2.5 mg/kg to treat this life-threatening condition. Correction of any electrolyte disturbances should be done.
- The patient should be hyperventilated with oxygen and the cardiac function monitored carefully.
- A cooling blanket should be used to lower the patient's core body temperature.

Postoperative Fever

Etiology

- A host of infectious and noninfectious agents may cause a postoperative fever, and although most of them do not represent serious threats to the patient, those that do must be sought out and managed.

Presentation and Management

- Postoperative fevers are less concerning for the first 48 to 72 hours postoperatively. During this interval, most fevers are caused by atelectasis.
- Temperatures that are elevated 5 to 8 days postoperatively are a concern and are usually associated with something that must be evaluated or treated by the surgical team.
- Evaluation of the patient 5 to 8 days postoperatively usually involves studying the five Ws associated with postoperative fever. They include wind (lungs), wound, water (urinary tract), waste (lower gastrointestinal [GI] tract), and wonder drug.
- Patients who continue to have a fever and slow clinical progress may require a computed tomography (CT) scan of the abdomen to look for occult, intra-abdominal infection accounting for the fever.

RESPIRATORY COMPLICATIONS

General Considerations

- A host of factors contribute to the abnormal pulmonary physiology present after an operative procedure.
- A loss of functional residual capacity. This loss may be due to a host of problems including abdominal distension, a

painful upper abdominal incision, obesity, a strong smoking history with associated chronic obstructive pulmonary disease (COPD), prolonged supine positioning, and fluid overload leading to pulmonary edema.

- Virtually all patients who undergo an abdominal incision or a thoracic incision have a significant alteration of their breathing pattern.
- Most patients who have respiratory problems postoperatively have mild to moderate respiratory problems that can be managed with aggressive pulmonary toilet.
- Two types of respiratory failure are commonly described. Type I, or hypoxic failure, results from abnormal gas exchange at the alveolar level.
- Type II respiratory failure is associated with hypercapnia and is characterized by a low PaO_2 and a high $PaCO_2$.
- The overall incidence of pulmonary complications exceeds 25% of surgical patients.
- One of the most important elements of this prophylaxis is careful preoperative screening of patients.
- A room arterial blood gas should be obtained on high-risk patients. Any patient with a PaO_2 less than 60 mm Hg is at increased risk.
- The most important parameter in spirometry is the forced expiratory volume in 1 second (FEV_1).
- Consultation with the patient should include a discussion about cessation of cigarette smoking 48 hours before the operative procedure.

Atelectasis and Pneumonia

- The most common postoperative respiratory complication is atelectasis.
- Careful postoperative surveillance will detect the early signs and symptoms of atelectasis, and the prudent surgeon will immediately instigate aggressive pulmonary toilet to obviate the development of a frank pneumonia.

Presentation and Management

- Atelectasis is so common postoperatively that a formal workup is usually not required. With the use of incentive spirometry, deep breathing, and coughing, most cases of atelectasis will resolve without any difficulty. However, if aggressive toilet is not instituted or the patient refuses to participate, frank development of a pneumonia is likely.

- Induced sputum for culture and sensitivity should be sent immediately to the laboratory.
- Broad-spectrum IV antibiotics should be instituted.
- A patient-controlled analgesia device seems to be associated with better pulmonary toilet, as does the use of an epidural infusion catheter.
- The patient should be instructed in use of the incentive spirometer and be held accountable by nurses and physicians during rounds. Encouraging the patient to deep breathe and cough is the single most valuable management approach in resolving atelectasis and pneumonia.

Aspiration Pneumonitis

Etiology

- A host of iatrogenic maneuvers place the patient at increased risk for aspiration pneumonitis in a hospital setting.
- Full stomach.
- Lose control of the ability to clear the airway.
- Patient with a nasogastric (NG) tube and the patient with a recent stroke or debility.
- The patient who is on extremely high doses of narcotics and patients who become obtunded.
- The pathophysiology of aspiration pneumonitis is associated with pulmonary intake of gastric contents at a low pH associated with particulate matter.
- Aspiration pneumonitis often progresses very rapidly and may require intubation soon after the injury occurs.

Presentation and Management

- The patient with aspiration often has associated vomiting at the time the aspiration occurs.
- Often rapidly progresses to frank respiratory failure associated with low oxygen saturation and a low PO_2.
- Close surveillance of the patient immediately after aspiration is absolutely essential.
- After intubation, aggressive suctioning of the bronchopulmonary tree will usually confirm the diagnosis.
- Prevention—identification of the high-risk patient for aspiration pneumonitis is important.
- In the postoperative period, identification of the elderly, overly sedated, or deteriorating patient mandates maneuvers to protect the patient's airway.

Pulmonary Edema, Acute Lung Injury, and Acute Respiratory Distress Syndrome

Etiology

- Three of the commonest manifestations of such injury are pulmonary edema, acute lung injury (ALI), and acute respiratory distress syndrome (ARDS).
- Pulmonary edema is a condition associated with accumulation of fluid in the alveoli.
- ALI and ARDS are associated with hypo-oxygenation resulting from a pathophysiologic inflammatory response that leads to the accumulation of fluid in the alveoli and thickening in the space between the capillaries and the alveoli.

Presentation and Management

- Patients with pulmonary edema often have a corresponding cardiac history of and/or recent history of massive fluid administration.
- The patient with an elevated wedge pressure should be managed with the administration of fluid restriction and aggressive diuresis.
- Administration of oxygen via face mask in mild cases, and intubation in more severe cases, is also clinically indicated.
- The patients presenting with ALI and ARDS usually have tachypnea, dyspnea, and increased work of breathing as manifested by exaggerated use of the muscles of breathing.
- Management of ALI and ARDS should be initiated by immediate intubation associated with careful administration of fluids and invasive monitoring with a Swan Ganz catheter to assess wedge pressures and right heart pressures. The strategy should be one of maintaining the patient on the ventilator with assisted breathing while healing of the injured lung takes place.
- Criteria for extubation are listed in Table 13–3.

Pulmonary Embolism

Etiology

- Risk factors for the development of pulmonary embolus are listed in Box 13–1.
- The ileofemoral venous system represents the site from which most clinically significant pulmonary emboli arise.

TABLE 13–3. Criteria for Weaning from the Ventilator

Parameter	Weaning Criteria
Respiratory rate	<25 breaths/min
Pao$_2$	>70 mm Hg (Fio$_2$ <40%)
Paco$_2$	<45 mm Hg
Minute ventilation	8–9 L/min
Tidal volume	5–6 mL/kg
Negative inspiratory force	−25 cm H$_2$O

Presentation and Management

- Dyspnea, pleuritic chest pain, apprehension, and a cough. Massive pulmonary embolus may be associated with syncope and hemoptysis.
- One third of patients with pulmonary embolus will also demonstrate lower extremity findings consistent with deep vein thrombosis.
- When a patient presents with chest pain and shortness of breath on the wards, an immediate battery of nonspecific tests should be obtained including room air arterial blood gas, electrocardiogram (ECG), and chest x-ray film.
- Any patient who has a room air arterial blood gas with a PaO$_2$ of less than 70 mm Hg should be considered a candidate for pulmonary embolus.
- The patient should be immediately placed on high flow oxygen by face mask.

Box 13–1. Risk Factors for Pulmonary Embolus

Prior pulmonary embolus
Lengthy operative procedures
Oral contraceptives
Traumatic injuries
Malignancy
Immobilization
Paralysis
Inflammatory bowel disease
Chronic heart disease
Coagulation abnormalities
Obesity
Age
Inherited coagulation abnormalities

- For years, pulmonary angiography has been considered the gold standard for making a diagnosis of pulmonary embolus. However, it is an invasive procedure with associated morbidity. For this reason, the ventilation perfusion scan was developed. The development of CT angiography represents a major step forward in diagnosis of pulmonary embolus in a noninvasive fashion and is a very promising new diagnostic modality.
- It is rapidly becoming the diagnostic modality of choice for larger pulmonary emboli.
- Patients who have a diagnosis of pulmonary embolus should be immediately anticoagulated with 10,000 units of heparin followed by approximately 1000 units per hour thereafter.
- Patients should be observed in a surgical intensive care unit.
- The patient should be kept on therapeutic doses of constant IV heparin until the clinician is able to institute warfarin therapy.

Prevention

- The best way to manage patients with potential for pulmonary embolus is to prevent them from occurring.
- Elastic compression stockings, sequential pneumatic compression devices, low-molecular-weight heparin, and platelet inhibitors.

CARDIAC COMPLICATIONS

Postoperative Hypertension

Etiology

- Hypertension is a serious problem that can cause devastating complications in the preoperative, intraoperative, and postoperative periods.
- Twenty-five percent of patients with a prior history of hypertension will develop postoperative hypertension in the postanesthesia periods.

Presentation and Management

- Most cases of perioperative hypertension are detected during the routine preoperative workup.
- The development of new onset postoperative hypertension is an urgent medical matter because of the concerns of stroke and bleeding from the operative wound.

- Any patient who has a diastolic blood pressure greater than 110 mm Hg should be assessed and consideration given to medical management of the hypertension.
- Medications most commonly used in this setting include beta-blockers and alpha II agonists. A number of prospective studies have demonstrated reduced perioperative myocardial complications with beta-blockade.
- There is some evidence that alpha II agonists (clonidine) can reduce perioperative heart complications in some patients.
- Calcium channel blockers, angiotensin-converting enzyme (ACE) inhibitors, and IV vasodilators such as nitroglycerin and nitroprusside might be protective. The latter two should be reserved for the severe, intractable hypertensive who has not responded to other medications.

Prevention

- Tight control of the hypertensive patient who requires emergency surgery is usually not possible.
- Taking antihypertensive medications on the day of surgery with a sip of water.
- In most cases, within 24 to 48 hours postoperative hypertension becomes less labile and more predictable.

Perioperative Ischemia and Infarction

Etiology

- Approximately 30% of all patients taken to the operating room have some degree of coronary artery disease.
- The mortality of a perioperative myocardial infarction remains approximately 30%. Perioperative myocardial complications result in at least 10% of all perioperative deaths.
- Individuals undergoing an operation within 3 months of a myocardial infarction have an 8% to 15% reinfarction rate and between 3 and 6 months only a 3.5% reinfarction rate.

Presentation and Management

- The classic presentation of acute myocardial infarction is chest pain often radiating into the jaw and left arm region.
- Shortness of breath and chest pain remain two postoperative symptoms that should always be carefully evaluated and never written off as postoperative discomfort.
- Immediate ECG assessment and serum troponin levels.
- Echocardiography may be considered.

- Nuclear imaging studies and angiography should be considered.
- Medical management of the infarction once ischemia has been documented includes immediate administration of high flow oxygen and transfer to the intensive care unit.
- Administration of beta-blockers and aspirin should be instituted.
- In most cases thrombolytic therapy is contraindicated in the postoperative period.
- Use of diuretic agents and antiarrhythmic agents should be considered.
- The goal of management of myocardial ischemia is to preserve the maximal amount of myocardial muscle possible.

Prevention

- Preventing the complications of coronary ischemia is a function of prospectively identifying the patient at risk for a perioperative cardiac complication.
- The cardiac risk index system (CRIS) is a commonly used and accepted system of assessing preoperatively the relative risk of a patient undergoing noncardiac surgery.
- The detection of a significant coronary artery disease history or ongoing symptoms from coronary artery disease mandate a preoperative cardiac workup with either thallium scanning or angiography.
- Patients identified as having high risk for myocardial events in the perioperative period should be management with beta-blockers, careful monitoring intraoperatively, and continued pharmacologic management postoperatively.

Cardiogenic Shock

Etiology

- Cardiogenic shock is one of the most serious sequelae of an acute myocardial infarction. Fifty percent or more of the left ventricular muscle mass is irreversibly damaged.
- Other possible causes of cardiogenic shock include ruptured papillary muscle, ruptured ventricular wall, aortic valvular insufficiency, mitral regurgitation, or ventricular septal defect.
- Highly lethal condition.

Presentation and Management

- Aggressive management is required to save the life.

- Mechanical ventilation with high fraction of inspired oxygen (FIO_2) and monitoring with a Swan-Ganz catheter is important.

Arrhythmias and Congestive Heart Failure

Etiology

- Coronary artery disease is the most common cause of arrhythmias and congestive heart failure.
- There are 500,000 new cases of congestive heart failure that develop each year with a 2-year mortality of almost 50%.
- The standard definition of a cardiac arrhythmia is 30 seconds of abnormal cardiac activity; intraoperative occurrence is 60% to 80%.

Presentation and Management

- Patients with well-managed congestive heart failure generally do well during an operation.
- Poorly controlled congestive heart failure is a serious clinical scenario.
- Present with shortness of breath, edema, wheezing, jugular venous distension, and a cardiac gallop.
- In patients with congestive heart failure, management is directed at optimizing preload, afterload, and myocardial contractility.
- Preload is lowered with diuretics and venodilators.
- Afterload reduction is accomplished by lowering vascular resistance against which the heart must contract.
- Afterload reduction can usually be accomplished using vasodilators.
- The initial approach to management of arrhythmias is correction of any underlying medical condition.
- A host of pharmacologic agents are available to treat both atrial and ventricular rhythms once a diagnosis has been made.
- With more serious ventricular arrhythmias, movement from telemetry into an intensive care unit is appropriate.

RENAL AND URINARY TRACT COMPLICATIONS

Urinary Retention

Etiology

- Inability to evacuate a urine-filled bladder is referred to as urinary retention. Urinary retention is a common postoperative complication in perianal operations and hernia repairs.

- Operations for low rectal cancer.
- Reversible abnormality resulting from a discoordination of the trigone and detrusor muscles.
- Spinal or epidermal procedures.

Presentation and Management

- Patients with postoperative urinary retention will complain of a dull, constant discomfort in the hypogastrium.
- Routine straight catheterization if a patient has not been able to void within 6 to 7 hours of the operation.

Prevention

- The most important principle in preventing postoperative urinary retention is awareness of the time from last void to the present time.

Acute Renal Failure (ARF)

Etiology

- ARF is characterized by a sudden reduction in renal output.
- Two types of renal failure have been identified: oliguric and non-oliguric.
- Oliguric renal failure refers to urine in which volumes of less than 480 mL are seen in a day.
- Non-oliguric renal failure involves outputs exceeding 2 L/day.
- Renal failure is divided into three general categories: prerenal, renal, or postrenal.
- Prerenal ARF is usually caused by <u>impaired renal perfusion</u>.
- Hypovolemia, hemorrhage, dehydration, cardiac malfunction, and insufficient fluid administration.
- Renal failure usually involves <u>actual injury to the nephrons</u>, glomerulus, or tubules of the kidney.
- Prolonged prerenal azotemia.
- Hypotension, toxins.
- Radiographic contrast, medications.
- Postrenal causes of ARF involve <u>obstruction</u> of either the urinary excretory pathway or an injury to the bladder.
- Ten percent of patients who undergo operations will have associated ARF during the perioperative course. Some operations appear to be particularly predisposed to associated ARF including major vascular procedures.

- Diabetic patients with vascular disease are at risk for major renal injury when contrast agents are administered.
- Patients with elevated creatinine should be carefully managed in the perioperative period.
- A final special category that can lead to ARF if not quickly diagnosed and treated is the abdominal compartment syndrome.
- This syndrome is due to massive edema of intra-abdominal organs causing intra-abdominal hypertension.
- Causes decreased renal perfusion and significantly reduces venous and urinary outflow.
- Treatment includes laparotomy with fascial closure using absorbable mesh.

Presentation and Management

- Patients who had normal renal function preoperatively and have virtually no urine postoperatively almost always have postrenal dysfunction.
- Causes include a kinked or occluded Foley catheter and irrigation of the Foley catheter should be the first maneuver.
- Ligation of the ureter.
- Prerenal and renal azotemia may be more complicated. Both are heralded by postoperative oliguria.
- Patients with large fluid losses via the GI tract (diarrhea, vomiting, fistula, high ileostomy output) often have associated profound dehydration. In such cases, the rise in blood urea nitrogen (BUN) is usually greater than the rise in creatinine.
- In prerenal causes, the concentrating ability of the nephrons.
- With acute tubular necrosis, the concentrating ability of the kidney is lost and the patient produces urine with a concentration equal to serum.
- The best laboratory test for discriminating prerenal from renal azotemia is probably fractional excretion of sodium (FE_{na}).
- Postrenal problems are usually managed by clearing the Foley catheter or, in rare cases, reoperating to remove ureter or urethral obstructions.
- If the prerenal patient has no history of cardiac disease, administration of isosmotic fluid (normal saline, lactated Ringer's solutions, or blood in patients who have hemorrhaged) is indicated. The IV fluid can be given rapidly (1 L in 20 to 30 minutes).
- If fluid administration does not result in improvement of the oliguria, placement of a central venous pressure (CVP) or Swan-Ganz catheter is indicated.

- If renal azotemia is diagnosed, the treatment must be supportive.
- Most urgent in management of ARF is treating hyperkalemia and fluid overload.
- Administration of a 10% calcium gluconate solution over 15 minutes and simultaneous administrations of IV glucose and insulin (30 units regular insulin in 1 L of 10% dextrose) will rapidly lower serum K^+ levels.
- Indications for hemodialysis.
  - Dialysis may be continued on an intermittent basis until renal function has returned.

Prevention

- Close attention in the preoperative period will reveal the patient with elevated creatinine and pre-existing renal dysfunction.
- Monitoring postoperative renal function closely in all surgery patients is a sound clinical practice.

METABOLIC COMPLICATIONS

Adrenal Insufficiency

Etiology

- Adrenal insufficiency is an uncommon but potentially lethal condition associated with failure of the adrenal glands to produce adequate glucocorticoids.
- The most common cause of adrenal insufficiency is administration of pharmacologic doses of glucocorticoids, which suppresses adrenocorticotropic hormone (ACTH) secretion and, thus, suppresses the adrenal glands.
- All patients on chronic glucocorticoids need to be thoroughly instructed in the dangers of an abrupt termination of their glucocorticoid medication.

Prevention

- Patients present with sudden cardiovascular collapse including hypotension, fever, mental confusion, and abdominal pain.
- Reveals hyponatremia, hyperkalemia, hypoglycemia, and azotemia.
- Treatment involves immediate, rapid administration of hydrocortisone or methylprednisolone with appropriate monitoring until clinical improvement is seen.

Hyperthyroidism

Etiology

- Hyperthyroidism is caused by excess amounts of thyroid hormone in the systemic circulation.
- Graves' disease, thyroid adenoma, toxic multinodular goiter, and self-administration of excessive amounts of thyroid hormone.
- Symptoms associated with the hyperthyroidism include cardiac (tachycardia, atrial fibrillation, dyspnea, congestive heart failure), GI (diarrhea, nausea, vomiting), nervous (anxiety, delirium, restlessness, and irritability), eye (exophthalmos), musculoskeletal (weakness), and cutaneous (warm, moist skin with heat intolerance) manifestations.
- Diagnostic workup includes thyroid function tests, thyroid scan using I^{123}, and occasionally ultrasound.
- Thyroid scan is useful in helping diagnose thyroid disease having abnormal thyroid function.
- Initial treatment involves trying to establish a euthyroid state using one of the two medications: propylthiouracil (PTU) or methimazole.
- For Graves' disease, definitive therapy is accomplished with either radioactive iodine (RAI) or surgery.
- Surgery usually includes one of two operations: total thyroidectomy or a lobectomy on one side with subtotal on the other side.
- Thyroid storm still occurs, and rapid, expeditious management is critical.
- IV placement with hydration and immediate cardiac monitoring. Beta-adrenergic blockade is central to the management strategy along with Lugol iodine solution and PTU administration.

Hypothyroidism

Etiology

- Low systemic levels of thyroid hormone and is associated with cold intolerance, constipation, brittle hair, dry skin, sluggishness, weight gain, and fatigue.
- The hypothyroidism may be primary (surgical removal, ablation, disease); with primary hypothyroidism, serum total thyroxine (T_4), free T_4, and free triiodothyronine (T_3) levels are low and thyroid-stimulating hormone (TSH) is elevated. In secondary disease, TSH, free T_4 index, and free T_3 are low.

- Immediate treatment with thyroid hormone is indicated concomitant with administration of IV hydrocortisone to avoid an Addisonian crisis.

Syndrome of Inappropriate Antidiuretic Hormone Secretion (SIADH)

Etiology

- SIADH occurs when antidiuretic hormone (ADH) continues to be secreted by the pituitary despite sustained hyponatremia.
- The diagnosis should be considered in any patient who remains hyponatremic despite all attempts to correct the imbalance.
- Trauma, stroke, ADH-producing tumors, drugs.
- Anorexia, nausea, vomiting, obtundation, and lethargy.
- Immediate treatment includes fluid restriction (mild disease) and administration of IV normal saline (moderate).
- Correction must be done in a constant, sustained fashion as overly rapid correction can result in seizure activity.

GASTROINTESTINAL COMPLICATIONS

Ileus and Obstruction

Etiology

- Ileus is a general term used to describe intestine that ceases contracting for a brief period of time. Most patients develop a transient ileus after a major abdominal operation. Within 3 to 5 days, however, the patient begins passing flatus, signaling the resolution of the temporary ileus.
- Those who do not resolve their ileus in that time period are felt to have either a prolonged ileus or a mechanical small bowel obstruction (SBO). Distinguishing between these two entities is imperative because their treatment is completely different.

Presentation and Management

- Abdominal distention, nausea, vomiting, obstipation, and varying amounts of abdominal pain depending on the cause.
- Patients with postoperative ileus can be very difficult to distinguish from patients with postoperative SBO.

- Ileus patients have a distended abdomen with diffuse discomfort but no sharp colicky pain.
- Diffusely dilated bowel throughout the intestinal tract with air in the colon and rectum.
- A standard battery of laboratory tests to ascertain the possible cause of the ileus includes complete blood count (CBC) with differential, amylase and lipase, electrolytes including magnesium and calcium, and urinalysis.
- Among all patients who develop SBO (preoperatively and postoperatively), the etiology is most commonly adhesions (70%), malignancy (10%), and hernias (5% to 10%).
- These patients present with abdominal distention, nausea, vomiting, obstipation, and often (but not always) have intermittent, colicky pain.
- The most important task for the involved surgeon is to decide which SBO requires operative management.
- Generally, partial SBO that fails to resolve after 3 to 5 days, those associated with increasing pain, and those associated with tachycardia should be taken to the operating room.
- The diagnostic evaluation of SBO virtually always begins with a flat plate and upright abdominal x-ray films.
- Air-fluid levels, distended small bowel, and a cut-off resulting in no colonic or rectal air.
- High-pitched, tinkling sounds in early obstruction, no improvement—further diagnostic workup is indicated via either enteroclysis or CT scan with contrast.
- Recent studies have revealed that CT scan of the abdomen is highly accurate in diagnosing SBO.
- Management of all SBO patients includes aggressive IV hydration to reverse the hypovolemia secondary to nausea, vomiting, and fluid sequestration into the bowel.
- Nothing by mouth (NPO).
- NG tube placed.
- Operative therapy consists of laparotomy, decompression of the bowel, lysis of the offending adhesions, and closure.

Prevention

- Recent attempts have been made to develop antiadhesion barriers that can be placed in the abdomen after surgery.
- Prospective, randomized studies have demonstrated that these agents effectively inhibit adhesions wherever they are placed.
- No prospective studies have demonstrated a decrease in SBO in patients receiving the agents.

Abdominal Compartment Syndrome

Etiology

- Because of significant bowel edema, fascial closure is extremely difficult and results in high intra-abdominal pressures exceeding 25 cm H_2O. The elevated intra-abdominal pressure causes pulmonary compromise because of pressure on both diaphragms and severely compromises venous return from the kidneys and renal arterial perfusion.

Presentation and Management

- Distended, tense abdomen; hypoxia; inability to adequately ventilate; elevated peak airway pressures; and profound oliguria.
- The diagnosis is made by obtaining intra-abdominal pressure readings through the Foley catheter.
- At pressures of 25 cm H_2O or higher, the patient becomes anuric and begins the cycle of exacerbation of pulmonary failure, cardiac decompensation, and death.

Prevention

- Early diagnosis in the postoperative period by the discerning surgeon can be a life-saving decision.

Postoperative Gastrointestinal Bleeding

Etiology

- Possible sources in the stomach include peptic ulcer disease, stress erosion, Mallory-Weiss tear, and gastric varices.
- In the small intestine, arteriovenous (AV) malformations or bleeding from an anastomosis have to be considered.
- In the large intestine, anastomotic bleed, divesticulosis, AV malformation, or varices should be considered.

Presentation and Management

- Postoperative bleeding can present with slow oozing or rapid hemorrhage that can lead to hypotension. Patients who appear to have lost a unit of blood, have associated tachycardia or hypotension, or have a significant drop in hematocrit should immediately be transferred to the intensive care unit for assessment. Resuscitation begins before any consideration of the diagnosis. Large-bore IVs are placed, the patient is resuscitated with iso-osmotic crystalloids, and laboratory values should be immediately sent to assess hematocrit, platelet count, prothrombin time (PT), and partial thromboplastin time (PTT).

- Serial hematocrits are critical for assessing the patients with ongoing bleeding.
- Placed on histamine-2 (H_2) blockers to keep the pH of gastric contents above 4.
- Those patients with a prolonged PT and PTT or low platelet count should immediately be corrected to normal; upper GI endoscopy should immediately be considered to look for a possible Mallory-Weiss tear, stress erosions, varices, and so forth.
- Local therapy via the endoscope has been successful in a moderately large number of patients.
- For the patient who appears to have lower GI bleeding, emergency colonoscopy may be considered although it is often difficult to clear the colon enough to see adequately.
- Surgery for stress erosions in the stomach occurs very uncommonly.

Prevention

- Maintaining the gastric pH above 4 with the medications mentioned previously seems to protect the patient against stress erosions.

Stomal Complications

Etiology

- Range from a bothersome problem with fit of the stomal appliance to major skin erosion and bleeding around a stoma to a large fistula.
- Complications occur including prolapse of the stoma because of inadequate length obtained during the surgery, prolapse, stomal necrosis, stenosis of the stoma, peristomal hernia formation, placement of the stoma in a crease, and high stoma output.
- Careful, thoughtful stoma placement and taking the required amount of time to get enough length to bring the stoma through the abdominal wall will prevent most complications. The stoma should be below the anterior superior iliac crest, which is usually the belt line, and should be brought through the rectus abdominal muscle.

- Stomal complications are most common in the first couple of weeks postsurgery, but complications may occur 5 or 10 years later including peristomal hernias, fistulae from Crohn's disease, prolapse, or stricture.
- Stoma prolapse is frightening to the patient but uncommonly becomes incarcerated or a surgical problem.
- Cyanotic stoma will usually become better perfused as the postoperative edema resolves. The most severe form of this problem is frank stomal ischemia in which the mucosa turns a grayish-white color and begins to slough. Use of a small penlight to look down into the stoma will indicate whether the mucosa is necrotic just at the skin level or if it extends down into the abdominal wall.
- In most cases, a pulsating artery within 3 cm of the end of the bowel will be compatible with survival of the stoma.
- Approximately 15% of patients will develop a peristomal hernia.
- If the peristomal hernia causes partial obstruction, incarceration, or severe pain, repair of the hernia should be considered.
- Options in the repair of a peristomal hernia include local repair, use of a prosthesis, and movement of the stoma to another location in the abdomen.
- Recurrence of a peristomal hernia is associated with a surprisingly high rate of recurrence on further repairs.

Pseudomembranous Colitis

Etiology

- Use of antibiotics in the preoperative or postoperative period can lead to pseudomembranous colitis in up to 1% of inpatients.
- Etiology appears to be related to alteration of the intestinal flora by the antibiotic, resulting in emergence of *Clostridia difficile.*
- The inflammatory reaction is characterized by the development of the pseudomembrane, which is a whitish membrane consisting of fibrin, white blood cells, necrotic mucosal cells, and mucus.
- Virtually all antibiotics have the potential of causing pseudomembranous colitis.

Presentation and Management

- The clinician should be suspicious of pseudomembranous colitis in the postoperative patient when an individual continues to have copious diarrhea, cramping, and dehydration.

- The diagnosis is made when a stool sample is sent for detection of the exotoxin.
- Two antibiotics have commonly been used for the treatment of pseudomembranous colitis: vancomycin and metronidazole.
- With the emergence of vancomycin-resistant *C. difficile,* metronidazole has become the agent of choice. In both cases, oral administration is always preferable to IV administration.
- In rare cases, if the disease progresses despite antibiotic use, emergency colectomy is indicated and is associated with a mortality of 20% to 30%.

Anastomotic Leak

Etiology

- Leak of an anastomosis between two hollow organs is one of the most serious complications a surgeon will ever encounter.
- Performing an intra-abdominal anastomosis must be done with optimization of the patient preoperatively.
- An anastomotic leak usually suggests that there has been a technical misadventure.
- A pancreaticojejunostomy after Whipple procedure has a leak rate of 15% to 20%.
- Because the esophagus has no serosa, esophagoenterostomies are much higher risk.

Presentation and Management

- Patients presenting with anastomotic leak usually develop fever, abdominal pain, malaise, and general failure to thrive.
- Paralytic ileus develops and the patient refuses to eat or vomits when attempting to eat.
- Wound dehiscence, development of a fistula, or extensive erythema raises the question of anastomotic leak.
- Immediate CT scan is indicated to assess the patient for the possibility of an anastomotic leak.
- If there is a large amount of fluid in the peritoneal cavity, or a large amount of free air in the peritoneal cavity, the diagnosis of an anastomotic leak must be considered.
- When the anastomotic leak is small and a controlled fistula forms, conservative management may be used.
- A bile duct leak or a pancreaticojejunostomy leak, if adequately drained and a controlled fistula forms, may respond to conservative management.

- If infection is uncontrolled, reoperative therapy is indicated.
- If the anastomotic leak occurs at a colon anastomosis, a colostomy should be brought up.
- A pancreaticojejunostomy leak, if small, can probably be drained and a drain placed next to the leak.
- If an anastomosis has virtually fallen apart, the patient will probably require completion pancreatectomy.

Fistulas

Etiology

- A fistula represents an abnormal communication between one hollow epithelialized organ and another epithelialized surface.
- Postoperative fistula is a serious problem that carries a mortality of 15% to 20% if not aggressively managed.
- Most fistulas occur after an abdominal operation involving either an anastomosis under difficult circumstances, a technical mistake, or inadvertent enterotomy during a lysis of adhesions.

Presentation and Management

- A small bowel or colonic fistula to the skin usually presents with initial erythema, abscess, and the subsequent efflux of GI contents.
- A fistula from bowel to bladder is associated with fecaluria and pneumaturia.
- If the fistula is a controlled fistula and is not leaking into the peritoneal cavity, the patient may have a low-grade fever but will usually not be overtly septic.
- A fistula associated with significant sepsis may require urgent surgical intervention.
- Diagnostic modalities used in patients with intestinal fistulae include CT scanning.
- A simple diagnostic maneuver is placement of a catheter into the fistula with placement of contrast material to identify the exact site of the fistula.
- Initial treatment of enterocutaneous fistulas includes fluid resuscitation in the presence of high output, institution of antibiotics to treat any underlying infection, and protection of the skin.
- The patient should be placed NPO, and immediate nutritional supplement with total parenteral nutrition (TPN) should be started in virtually all patients.

- In patients with extremely high outputs exceeding 1 to 2 L/day, careful management of electrolytes is imperative. Use of H_2 blockers and octreotide may decrease the volume of flow through the fistula.
- Fistulas with an output less than 200 mL/day will heal with conservative management.
- Fistulas that are high in the GI tract and have more than 500 mL/day are less likely to heal with conservative management.
- Pancreatic fistulas represent a special problem usually occurring after trauma to the pancreas or after an operative procedure associated with a bowel anastomosis.
- Diagnosis of a fistula is confirmed by amylase measurement of the fluid, which is usually in the tens of thousands.
- Stopping oral intake, placing the patient on TPN, and administering subcutaneous octreotide are indicated initially.
- If the fistula is a low-volume fistula (75 mL/day or less), oral intake may often be instituted as long as the output does not increase significantly. Using conservative management, approximately 60% of pancreatic fistulae will close spontaneously.
- Intestinal fistulae that fail to close are usually associated with an underlying risk factor that includes the presence of a foreign body, radiation injury to the fistula site, an abscess or infection of the fistula site, epithelialization of the fistula tract, a surrounding neoplasm, and obstruction of the bowel distal to the fistula.
- Reoperating on a patient with a controlled fistula early on is fraught with danger because of poor tissue planes, bleeding, and risk of creating additional injury to the bowel.
- Circular excision of the fistula site and mobilization of the intestine until it is freed from the fistula site.
- The fistula should never be closed locally because the incidence of suture line failure is virtually 100%.
- Reoperation may be required to take a Roux-Y limb up to the site of the fistula and suture it to the dense tissue surrounding the fistula site.

HEPATOBILIARY COMPLICATIONS

Bile Duct Injuries

Etiology

- The advent of laparoscopic cholecystectomy has resulted in a significant increase in the number of bile duct injuries treated.

- The incidence of significant bile duct injury is approximately 0.5% today.

Presentation and Management

- Patients with a bile duct injury present with right upper quadrant pain, fever, malaise, and occasionally have associated jaundice.
- Should immediately undergo CT scanning of the abdomen.
- Management of the problem begins with immediate percutaneous drainage of the bile collection with the drain left in place.
- Proceed to endoscopic retrograde cholangiopancreatography (ERCP); the study will indicate the size of the leak, the location of the leak and whether an obstructive component is present.
- Placement of a stent past the area of injury.
- If there is evidence of adequate control of the leak, the surgeon may wait up to 5 to 7 days for inflammation in the area to subside before undertaking operative repair.
- A Roux-Y limb can be brought up to do a hand-sewn anastomosis to the common bile duct.

Prevention and Management

- The surgeon should approach each operation on the biliary tree with caution and respect because of the frequent anomalies and anatomic variations.

NEUROLOGIC COMPLICATIONS

Delirium, Dementia, and Psychosis

Etiology

- Loss of the patient's routine schedule, stresses of the disease process, fear of the operation, loss of personal control, placement in an unfamiliar environment, the addition of mind-altering pain medications, and pain all can lead to dramatic alterations in behavior in postoperative patients. Patients who have particularly high risk for behavioral disorders in the postoperative period include the elderly, patients with a prior history of substance abuse, patients with a prior history of psychiatric disorders, and children.

- Results in disorientation, inappropriate response, depression, agitation, and catatonia.
- The most immediately threatening disorder encountered by physicians is delirium tremens associated with acute alcohol withdrawal.

Presentation and Management

- Patients may present on a spectrum from mild confusion and memory loss to full-blown delirium with confusion, irrational behavior, disorientation, and frank hallucinations.
- In the elderly, these symptoms may become cyclically worse at night-time with dramatic improvements during the daytime.
- Patients who present with a sudden change in behavior should be immediately evaluated for the etiology of the problem.
- Patients who have an abrupt change in their behavior patterns should be considered for CT scan or magnetic resonance imaging (MRI) study after the physical examination and history are taken.
- The patient should be assessed to ascertain whether he or she might be a physical threat to himself or herself or others. On occasion, physical restraints may be required.
- Medical management of the patient with delirium or psychosis involves administration of appropriate sedatives, treatment of underlying disorders, and careful observation.
- Initial restraints may be required while administering sedatives intravenously until the patient is quieted.

Prevention

- Awareness of the high-risk patient for postoperative delirium is the single most important principle in prevention.

Seizure Disorders

Etiology

- Seizures are caused by paroxysmal electrical discharges from the cerebral cortex associated with convulsions, rhythmic myoclonic activity, loss of consciousness, and a change in mental status. Seizures may be primary or secondary.
- Primary causes intracranial tumors, bleeds, trauma, or idiopathic seizure activity.

- Secondary causes metabolic derangements, sepsis, systemic disease processes, and pharmacologic agents.

Presentation and Management

- Patient should be carefully restrained so as not to sustain injury during the course of the seizure. Administration of IV benzodiazepines is the standard for immediate care of the patient undergoing seizure activity. Dilantin is the most commonly used anticonvulsant for a new presentation of generalized or focal seizures.
- The two most commonly used agents for maintenance after seizure or for someone with status ellipticus are carbamazepine (Tegretol) and valproic acid.
- After managing the seizure, a diagnostic workup for etiology of the seizure should be initiated.
- A CT scan or MRI should be ordered in a patient with new onset of seizure activity.

Stroke and Transient Ischemic Attacks

Etiology

- A high percentage of neurologic events are either transient (occurring for seconds to minutes) or reversible (occurring for minutes to hours). Most common causes of stroke include advanced atherosclerotic disease of the internal carotid artery, atrial fibrillation, a ventricular septal defect, acute hepatic failure, or excessive anticoagulation.

Presentation and Management

- Present with focal alteration in motor function, which is unilateral; alteration in mental status; aphagia; and occasionally unresponsiveness.
- Management beyond that point rests on distinguishing between hemorrhagic and nonhemorrhagic.
- Hemorrhagic strokes are commonly associated with poorly controlled hypertension or anticoagulation.
- Management includes pharmacologic reduction of blood pressure, mannitol IV to reduce cerebral swelling, and administration of dexamethasone.
- Nonhemorrhagic: the management principles are similar to those with hemorrhagic stroke, but in addition, anticoagulation is instituted.

EAR, NOSE, AND THROAT COMPLICATIONS

Epistaxis

Etiology

- Epistaxis may be associated with primary disease conditions such as leukemia, hemophilia, excessive anticoagulation, and hypertension.
- The most frequent postoperative cause of epistaxis is injury during placement of an NG tube.
- Epistaxis is divided into two general categories: anterior and posterior. Anterior trauma is often associated with the manipulations mentioned.
- Firm pressure applied between the thumb and index finger to the nasal ala and held for 3 to 5 minutes is generally successful.
- A more serious scenario is posterior nasal septal bleeding that on occasions can even be life threatening. If all attempts to stop anterior nasal septal bleeding are unsuccessful, one may infer the probability of a posterior nasal bleed, which may necessitate placement of a posterior pack of strip gauze covered in petroleum ointment.

Acute Hearing Loss

Etiology

- Abrupt loss of hearing in the postoperative period is an uncommon event. Unilateral hearing loss is usually associated with obstruction or edema associated with an NG or feeding tube.
- Bilateral hearing loss is more often neural in nature and is usually associated with pharmacologic agents such as aminoglycosides and diuretics.
- Examination with an otoscope will often reveal the presence of cerumen impaction. If the otologic examination is completely normal, one should suspect neural injury.

Sinusitis

Etiology

- Present with malaise, a dull aching pain in the maxillary or frontal sinus area, and oftentimes a low-grade fever.

- Because of edema associated with NG tube use, sinusitis is often exacerbated or delayed in healing.
- Unexplained fever in a patient with an NG tube postoperatively should suggest the possibility of sinusitis.
- A CT scan of the head will demonstrate sinusitis, which may be treated with broad-spectrum antibiotics.

Parotitis

Etiology

- Commonly occurs in an elderly male with poor oral hygiene and poor oral intake with associated decrease in saliva production and significant edema and focal tenderness surrounding the parotid gland; the parotitis can cause life-threatening sepsis.
- The patient should be placed on IV, high-dose, broad-spectrum antibiotics with good staphylococcus coverage.
- In the presence of a fluctuant area, incision and drainage is indicated.

SPECIAL CONSIDERATIONS

Complications at the Extremes of Age

Etiology

- The elderly patient frequently will mount very little white blood cell increase with serious infections. They often have less intra-abdominal pain and peritoneal tenderness with serious infections, they often present much later in the course of the disease, and they frequently have comorbid factors.
- Young children and elderly patients process medications in a different fashion than mature adults and, because of a lower lean body mass, may have an exaggerated response to any medications.
- The preoperative period is an important time in not only developing your relationship with your patient but also for sitting down and talking with him or her in great depth regarding the operation, the potential risks, complications, alternatives, and possible benefits.
- Operations that may result in distasteful complications or irreversible alterations in lifestyle should be explained in great detail.
- The surgeon who takes great pains to explain in detail the expected outcome of the operation before the procedure

will have many fewer calls postoperatively and a much more understanding patient in the long run.

- Should the surgeon make an egregious error, the best way to deal with the patient is to be completely honest, frank, and open with regard to any questions that are asked.
- In general, it is unwise to denigrate another surgeon unless it is a clearcut and obvious violation of medical standards.
- Ethics and ethical choices are a part of the practice of every busy surgeon's life.

Public and Regulatory Concerns

- It is likely that in the near future, only those physicians who have low morbidity and mortality rates will be permitted to do more complex operations.
- Those who consistently fall below that norm may even be denied operating room privileges in the future.
- Although reporting of surgical complications and errors had been primarily a local event for the past 50 years, in the future, national data may be available on every surgeon.

CHAPTER 14

SURGERY IN THE ELDERLY

- The population of the United States has increased significantly over the past generation, mostly because of medical and public health interventions.
- The most rapidly growing portion of the population is made up of persons older than 85 years.
- Although reports exist of people living to 120 to 130 years, the calculated life span of humans (without other complications) is estimated at 85 to 115 years.

THEORIES OF AGING

- The aging process is reproducible among species.
- Several characteristics in the aging process have been identified in mammals.
  - Mortality increases with age following maturation.
  - This is the result of progressive changes in biochemical composition of cells and tissues with aging, which lead to a broad spectrum of progressive, deteriorative, and physiologic changes.
  - A decreased ability of the whole organism to respond adaptively to environmental changes develops, as does an increased vulnerability to disease.
- From 1980 to 1996, the percentage of operations in which the patient was older than 65 years increased from 19% to 36%; when obstetric procedures are excluded, this percentage increases to 43%.
- Discharge data in 1996 showed that 36% of the cholecystectomies, 52% of hernia repairs, 56% of coronary artery bypass grafts, and 61% of bowel resections were performed on patients older than 65 years.
- It is currently estimated that at least 50% of patients in most general surgical practices are older than 65 years.
- The increase in the percentage of operations in which the patient is older than 65 years is not entirely due to the increase in the number of older patients; it is also a reflection of a greater willingness to offer surgical treatment to the elderly.
- Emergency surgery in the elderly is poorly tolerated because of the overall decline in physiologic reserve; the operative

mortality rate in the emergency setting is 3 to 10 times higher than in comparable elective cases.
- Chronologic age alone has little effect on surgical outcome; it is rather the age-related decline in physiologic reserves and increase in concomitant illness (comorbidity) that is responsible for this observation.

PYSIOLOGIC DECLINE

- With aging, physiologic function declines in all organ systems, although the magnitude of this decline varies among organs and among individuals.

Cardiovascular

- Morphologic changes are found in the myocardium, conducting pathways, valves, and vasculature of the heart and great vessels with increasing age.
  - The number of myocytes declines as the collagen and elastin content increase, resulting in fibrotic areas throughout the myocardium and an overall decline in ventricular compliance.
  - Nearly 90% of the autonomic tissue in the sinus node is replaced by fat and connective tissue, and fibrosis interferes with conduction in the intranodal tracts and bundle of His.
  - Progressive dilation of all four valvular annuli is responsible for the multivalvular regurgitation demonstrated in healthy older persons.
  - Finally, there is a progressive increase in rigidity and decrease in distensibility of both the coronary arteries and the greater vessels.
- However, it has become generally accepted that systolic function does not change with age.
- Cardiac output and ejection fraction are maintained despite the increase in afterload imposed by the stiffening of the outflow tract.
- The aging heart maintains cardiac output not by increasing the rate but by increasing the ventricular filling (preload).
- Because of the dependence on preload, even minor hypovolemia can result in significant compromise in cardiac function.
- Diastolic function, which depends on relaxation rather than contraction, is affected by aging.
- Diastolic abnormalities are treated with agents that improve preload and ventricular relaxation; digitalis and diuretics

used for systolic failure may in fact worsen diastolic dysfunction.

Respiratory

- With aging, respiratory function diminishes, which is attributable to changes in both the chest wall and the lung.
  - Chest wall compliance decreases as a result of changes in the structure caused by kyphosis and exaggerated by vertebral collapse.
  - Maximum inspiratory and expiratory force decreases by as much as 50% as a result of progressive decrease in the strength of the respiratory muscles.
  - The lung loses elasticity, which leads to increased alveolar compliance, collapse of the small airways, and subsequent uneven alveolar ventilation with air trapping.
  - Forced vital capacity decreases by 14 to 30 mL per year and 1-second forced expiratory volume decreases by 23 to 32 mL per year (in males).
  - Total lung capacity remains unchanged and there is only a mild increase in resting lung volume or functional residual capacity.

Renal

- Between the ages of 25 and 85, there is a progressive decrease in function of the renal cortex in which approximately 40% of the nephrons become sclerotic.
- Sclerosis of the glomeruli is accompanied by atrophy of the afferent and efferent arterioles and by a decrease in renal tubular cell number.
- Renal blood flow also diminishes by approximately 50%.
- Functionally, there is a decline in glomerular filtration rate of approximately 45% by age 80 years.
- Estimates of creatinine clearance in the healthy aged can be made from the serum creatinine by using the following formula derived by Cockcroft and Gault:

$$\frac{(140 - \text{age in years}) \times (\text{weight in kg})}{72 \times (\text{serum creatinine in mg/dL})}$$

- Caution must be exercised when applying this formula to critically ill patients or those on medications that directly affect renal function.
- The ability to conserve sodium and excrete hydrogen ion decreases.

- Dehydration becomes a particular problem because losses of sodium and water from nonrenal causes are not compensated for by the usual mechanisms:
  - Increased renal sodium retention.
  - Increased urinary concentration.
  - Increased thirst.
- The inability to retain sodium is thought to be due to a decline in the activity of the renin-angiotensin system.
- In the bladder, increased collagen content leads to limited distensibility and impaired emptying.
- In women, decreased circulating levels of estrogen and decreased tissue responsiveness to this hormone cause changes in the urethral sphincter that predispose them to urinary incontinence.
- In men, prostatic hypertrophy impairs bladder emptying.

Hepatobiliary

- Morphologic changes in the liver with aging include a decrease in the number of hepatocytes and a decrease in the overall weight and size of the organ.
- There is a compensatory increase in cell size and proliferation of bile ducts.
- Functionally, hepatic blood flow decreases by approximately 1% per year to 40% of earlier values after age 60 years.
- The synthetic capacity of the liver, as measured by the standard test of liver function, remains unchanged.
- Drugs requiring microsomal oxidation before conjugation may be metabolized more slowly, whereas those requiring only conjugation may be cleared at a normal rate.
- The most significant correlate to altered hepatobiliary function in the aged is the increased incidence of gallstones and gallstone-related complications.

Immune Function

- Immunosenescence is characterized by an increased susceptibility to infections, an increase in autoantibodies and monoclonal immunoglobulins, and an increase in tumorigenesis.
- There is
  - A decline in the number of reactive T cells.
  - An increase in the number of memory T cells.
  - A change in the pattern of interleukin-2 production.
- Some B-cell defects have recently been identified, although it is thought that the functional deficits in antibody production

are related to altered T-cell regulation rather than to intrinsic B-cell changes.

- IgM levels decrease; IgG and IgA levels increase slightly.

COMORBID DISEASE

- With age, there is a clear increase in diseases of organ systems other than that for which the older patient seeks surgical care.
- There are numerous studies that document the impact of comorbidity on outcome.
- Studies show that there was a clear increase in mortality from 1.5% in patients with no concomitant diseases to 6.1% in patients with more than three additional conditions.

PREOPERATIVE ASSESSMENT

- The goal of the preoperative assessment of the elderly patient is to define the extent of decline and to identify coexisting diseases or comorbidities.
- Extensive testing for disease in every organ system is not cost effective, practical, or necessary for most patients; a thorough history and physical examination provides information to direct further workup if necessary.
- Of all comorbid conditions, cardiovascular disease is the most prevalent, and cardiovascular events are a leading cause of severe perioperative complications and death.
- Pulmonary complications are at least as common as cardiac complications.
- Poor exercise capacity and poor general health predict pulmonary and cardiac complications.

Functional Status

- The American Society of Anesthesiologists (ASA) functional classification is the most predictive factor of postoperative morbidity and the second most predictive factor for mortality.
- Of all the methods of assessing overall functional capacity, exercise tolerance is the most sensitive predictor of postoperative cardiac and pulmonary complications in the elderly.

Cognitive Status

- Postoperative delirium, defined as an acute confusional state, is associated with a significant increase in mortality rate, major morbidity rate, length of stay, and discharge to a long-term care or rehabilitation facility.

- Delirium must be distinguished from dementia, the more chronic type of baseline cognitive impairment.
- The most frequently cited factors associated with delirium are as follows:
  - Age.
  - Preoperative cognitive impairment.
  - Poor functional status.
  - Alcohol consumption.
  - Multiple drug regimens.
- Intraoperative and postoperative factors have also been studied.
  - No association has been found with the route of anesthesia epidural versus general or the occurrence of intraoperative hemodynamic complications.
  - Intraoperative blood loss, the need for blood transfusion, and postoperative hematocrit less than 30% are associated with a significant increased risk of postoperative delirium.
  - Alterations in the wake-sleep cycle following surgery have also been associated with delirium.
- Mental status changes in the elderly surgical patient are often the earliest signs of postoperative complication.

Nutritional Status

- Malnutrition is estimated to occur in approximately 0% to 15% of community-dwelling elderly persons, 25% to 65% of older patients in acute care hospitals, and 25% to 60% of institutionalized elderly.
- The measurement of nutritional status in the elderly is difficult; standard anthropomorphic measures do not take into account the change in body composition and structure that accompanies aging.
- Serum albumin is probably the strongest nutritional predictor of surgical outcome.

SPECIFIC CONSIDERATIONS

Endocrine Surgery

Breast

- In Western countries, the incidence of breast cancer increases with age.
- Forty-three percent of new cases occur in patients older than 65 years.

- As many as 60% of elderly patients undergoing lumpectomy fail to follow through with radiation.
- The utility of axillary node dissection following lumpectomy is also controversial in the elderly patient; for most patients older than 70 years, tamoxifen is frequently given regardless of node or receptor status, and node dissection may not be necessary.
- Tamoxifen therapy alone has been used for these frail patients; multiple trials have shown that response rates range from 10% to 50%; failure rates range between 23% and 58%.

Thyroid

- The incidence of thyroid nodules increases throughout life.
- Sporadic papillary thyroid cancer has almost a bell-shaped distribution of age at presentation, with a decreasing trend in patients older than 60 years.
- Chronologic age alone appears to be a true independent predictor of survival from well-differentiated thyroid cancer.

Esophagus

- There is a progressive decrease in amplitude of the primary peristaltic waves in the esophagus following deglutition; octogenarians exhibit only 50% of the amplitude of younger control subjects; nonagenarians exhibit only 20%.
- Even though lower esophageal sphincter resting pressure is normal and relaxes appropriately after deglutition, the sphincter fails to rapidly contract back to baseline, resulting in prolonged decreased tone.
- These conditions, in addition to delayed gastric emptying in elderly patients, predispose the elderly patient to gastro-esophageal reflux disease.
- Dysmotility of the cricopharyngeus can result in Zenker s diverticulum.
- Overall 5-year survival rates for curative resection for esophageal cancer in the elderly are 14% to 25%, similar to that observed in younger patients.

Stomach

- Studies have shown that between 25% and 80% of elderly persons have fasting achlorhydria, resulting from progressive loss of parietal cells and decreased antral and serum concentrations of gastrin.

- Achlorhydria results in derangements in folate, iron, and vitamin B_{12} absorption.
- Chronic atrophic gastritis, previous gastric surgery, and chronic *Helicobacter pylori* infection, more frequently found in older patients, are associated with increased risk of gastric cancer.
- In elderly patients, the disease presents with a predominance of intestinal-type tumors rather than the more aggressive diffuse type.
- There is also a progression of the location of the tumor to more proximal areas of the stomach.

Liver

- Persons older than 70 years can undergo liver resection with a morbidity rate of 31% and a mortality rate of 0%.
- Resection for metastatic colorectal cancer is safe, even in elderly patients.
- Multivariate analysis of risk for postoperative complication has shown that only male sex, extent of resection (lobectomy vs resection) operative time, and ASA 3 were statistically significant indicators for morbidity and mortality.
- No difference in survival rate after resection was noted between young and older patients (35% over 5 years).

Biliary Tract Disease

- Biliary tract disease is the most common cause of acute abdominal complaints and accounts for approximately one third of all abdominal operations in the elderly.
- The increased development of gallstones in the elderly is thought to result from changes in the composition of bile and impaired biliary motility.
- Alterations in gallbladder motility and bile duct motility are thought to be central to the development of cholesterol stones and brown pigment stones, respectively.
- The sensitivity of the gallbladder wall to cholecystokinin (CCK) decreases with increasing age in animal models.
- Gallstones are associated with complications in 40% to 60% of older patients requiring treatment for the disease, compared with less than 20% of younger patients.
- Nearly two thirds of the more than 21,000 open cholecystectomies in elderly patients were performed under urgent or emergent conditions.

Small Bowel Obstruction

- Small bowel obstruction (SBO) is the most common and surgically relevant disorder of small intestinal function encountered in the aged.
- Lysis of adhesions is the third most common gastrointestinal procedure after cholecystectomy and partial excision of the large bowel.
- Fifty percent of deaths associated with SBO occur in patients older than 70 years.
- Adhesions are responsible for more than 50% of SBOs, hernias for 15% to 20% of cases, and neoplasms for another 15% to 20%.
- Certain kinds of hernias, such as those that occur through the obturator foramen, are found almost exclusively in the elderly and are particularly difficult to diagnose.
- There are three important management issues, which are even further exaggerated in elderly patients:
  - Distinguishing functional (ileus) from mechanical obstruction.
  - Distinguishing simple from strangulated obstruction.
  - Determining the optimal timing of operation for partial obstruction.
- Many of the factors associated with ileus systemic infections, intra-abdominal infections, metabolic abnormalities, and drug therapy are more common in older persons.

Colorectal

Appendicitis

- Although appendicitis typically occurs in the second and third decades of life, approximately 5% to 10% of cases present in old age.
- Appendicitis in the elderly has increased in recent decades, whereas the incidence in younger patients is declining.
- The overall mortality rate from appendicitis is only 0.8%, but most deaths occur in the very young and the very old.
- For those older than 65 years, the overall mortality rate is 4.6%.
- The indolent nature of the initial symptoms of appendicitis in the elderly usually lead to delays of 48 to 72 hours before medical attention is sought.
- Perforated appendicitis is far more common in elderly patients; rates of perforation increase directly with age.

- The possibility of perforated cancer in this age group requires a thorough evaluation of the colon when the acute process is controlled.

Carcinoma of the Colon and Rectum

- Accounts for two thirds of all gastrointestinal malignancies in patients older than 70 years.
- Some studies report more right-sided lesions and fewer rectal tumors in older compared with younger patients.
- In most studies, the presenting signs and symptoms of colorectal cancer do not vary substantially with age.
- Approximately one third of operations for colorectal cancer in patients of all ages are performed emergently, whereas more than 50% of operations in patients older than 70 years are performed on an urgent or emergent basis.
- Operative mortality rate for colorectal cancer is determined by the same two factors that influence operative mortality rate in the elderly in general:
  - The need for emergency surgery.
  - The presence of coexisting disease.
- The long-term outcome of surgery for colorectal cancer in the elderly is good.
- Most studies show no age difference in 3- or 4-year survival rates, even in patients older than 80 years.

Hernia

- The estimated incidence of abdominal wall hernia in persons older than the age of 65 is 13 per 1000, with a fourfold to eightfold increase in incidence in men.
- The elderly are at risk for the more occult types of hernias that do not become apparent until a complication has occurred.
- Typically, paraesophageal hernias may reach enormous size without symptoms and are only discovered when gastric volvulus or strangulation occurs.
- Similarly, herniation through the obturator canal is rarely diagnosed until SBO occurs.

Vascular Surgery

- The most frequent vascular diseases seen in elderly patients are abdominal aortic aneurysms, carotid artery disease, and peripheral arterial occlusive disease.

- Under elective conditions and in patients with well-managed concomitant disease, vascular surgery is safe and effective.
- Quality of life and preservation and/or restoration of functional independence are most important considerations in older persons.

Cardiothoracic Surgery

Coronary Artery Bypass Grafting

- As the mortality and morbidity rates of cardiac surgical procedures have decreased, there has been a growing willingness to offer surgical therapy to elderly patents with reconstructible coronary artery disease.
- The literature in the late 1980s and early 1990s described series of patients older than 70 years.
- Even in patients older than 80 years, coronary artery bypass surgery is associated with an overall mortality rate of 7% to 12% with elective mortality rates as low as 2.8%; however, morbidity following coronary surgery in the elderly is quite high.
- Pulmonary failure, neurologic events, delirium, and sternal wound infections increase with age and are associated with postoperative death.

Valve Replacement

- The growing willingness to offer aortic valve replacement (AVR) to older patents comes from a better understanding of the natural history of aortic valvular disease; once symptoms such as angina or syncope develop, average life expectancy is only 3 to 4 years.
- Average life expectancy for a 70-year-old is approximately 12 years; for an 80-year-old, life expectancy in approximately 8 years; if AVR could be accomplished with acceptable operative mortality outcome, the benefit would justify the procedure.
- The choice of valve prosthesis is also an important consideration in older patients.
- In patients older than 75 years, the mortality rate from long-term anticoagulation alone is nearly 10% per year.
- Bioprosthetic valves do not require anticoagulation but are somewhat less durable.

Trauma

- Trauma is currently the fifth leading cause of death in the elderly.

- Cerebral atrophy and decreased viscoelastic properties within the cranial vault make the brain more susceptible to blunt trauma.
- Increased body fragility results in increased tendency to fracture.
- The incidence of fracture or serious injury from a simple fall is as high as 40% in the older person.
- A recent study demonstrated the mortality rate for persons older than 60 years with a Glasgow coma score of 5 was 79%, compared with 36% for similarly matched patients aged 20 to 40 years.
- Injury from burns makes up 8% of elderly trauma.
- In general, burns covering more than 40% of total body surface area in older persons have very poor prognosis.

Transplantation

- The rate of both acute and chronic rejection is clearly lower in older patients, attributed to the overall decline in immunocompetence with age.
- The high incidence of lymphoproliferative disorders in older transplant patients in general and the high rate of recurrent hepatitis C in older liver transplant patients in particular may be the result of excessive immunosuppression in the already compromised population.
- It has been suggested that decreasing immunosuppression in older patients may improve both long- and short-term survival.

ETHICAL ISSUES

Do Not Resuscitate Orders

- The Patient Self-Determination Act requires the hospitals and other health care facilities to inform patients of their rights to appoint a proxy (or surrogate) decision maker to act on their wishes regarding life-sustaining care if they become incompetent.
- Only 3% to 15% of the population actually use such documents.

Medical Futility

- In patients in whom medical care is believed futile, studies have shown that withholding care does not decrease health care expenditures significantly.

- The problem really is in predicting futility of medical care.
- Statistical analysis has shown that objective estimates for survival based on Acute Physiology and Chronic Health Evaluation (APACHE) III scores correlate better with actual survival than estimates of experienced clinicians.

Interacting with the Elderly Patient

- Most elderly patients have some degree of hearing loss, so important conversations should occur in a quiet room, with the surgeon speaking in a strong voice, describing the plan slowly and deliberately.
- Even though elderly patients are often frightened by their illness, they usually do not like being told what to do.
- Elderly patients realize that they are old and, therefore, probably have a different outlook of their disease and longevity than we might think.
- Elderly patients tolerate major surgery differently than younger ones; even vigorous persons should be warned preoperatively that easy fatigability is expected after surgery and it may last for weeks after discharge.

CHAPTER 15

Morbid Obesity

OBESITY: THE MAGNITUDE OF THE PROBLEM

- *Morbid obesity* is defined as being either 100 pounds above ideal body weight, twice ideal body weight, or having a body mass index (BMI) (measured as weight in kilograms divided by height in meters squared) of 40 kg/m^2.
- It is estimated that between 3% and 5% of the adult population of the United States is morbidly obese, or clinically severely obese, the highest percentage of population of any country.
- Studies of adolescent obesity have estimated the incidence of obesity (being 40% above ideal body weight) as being in the 35% range for adolescents in the United States but more than 20% in most European countries.
- Obesity is estimated to cause 280,000 deaths annually in the United States.
- After tobacco use, obesity is the second leading cause of preventable death in the United States and is second to smoking on the list of preventable factors responsible for increased health care costs.

PATHOPHYSIOLOGY AND ASSOCIATED MEDICAL PROBLEMS

- There is a clear familial predisposition for severe obesity; it is rare for a single family member to have this problem.
- The rapid increase in obesity from 1980 to 2003 emphasizes the considerable environmental component that contributes to the problem.
- The severely obese individual has, in general, persistent hunger that is not satiated by amounts of food that satisfy the nonobese; this lack of satiety or maintenance of satiety may be the single most important factor in the process.
- Cholecystokinin (CCK) and ghrelin, produced largely in the proximal stomach by food, are involved in satiety.
  - Increased levels of ghrelin seem to produce increased food intake.
  - Individuals who are on low-calorie diets develop increased levels of ghrelin.

- Patients with gastric inflow that is restricted but allows food to pass through the stomach have normal to elevated ghrelin levels postoperatively.
- In contrast, patients undergoing gastric bypass have suppressed postoperative levels of ghrelin.
- Morbid obesity is a metabolic disease associated with numerous medical problems:
  - The most frequent problem is the combination of arthritis and/or degenerative joint disease.
  - The incidence of sleep apnea is high.
  - Asthma is present in more than 25%, hypertension in more than 30%, diabetes in more than 20%, and gastro-esophageal reflux in 20% to 30% of patients.
  - The incidence of these conditions increases with the duration of severe obesity and age.
- The metabolic syndrome includes type II diabetes mellitus, impaired glucose tolerance, dyslipidemia, and hypertension; the syndrome is thought to result in impaired hepatic uptake of insulin, systemic hyperinsulinemia, and subsequent tissue resistance to insulin.

MEDICAL VERSUS SURGICAL THERAPY

- Medical therapy for severe obesity has limited short-term success and almost nonexistent long-term success.
- Once a person is severely obese, the likelihood that he or she will lose enough weight by dietary means alone and remain at a BMI below 35 kg/m^2 is estimated as 3% or less.
- The severely obese patient should be given the chance to comply with a medically supervised diet program to see if any success can be achieved.
- Pharmacologic therapy has focused on two medications: sibutramine and orlistat.
  - Sibutramine blocks presynaptic receptor uptake of both norepinephrine and serotonin, potentiating their anorexic effect in the central nervous system.
  - Orlistat inhibits pancreatic lipase and thereby reduces absorption of up to 30% of ingested dietary fat.
- For the severely obese individual, neither sibutramine nor orlistat has proven effective therapy alone; their efficacy after weight reduction surgery is unknown.

PREOPERATIVE EVALUATION AND SELECTION

Eligibility

- Patients must have a BMI greater than 40 kg/m^2 without associated comorbid medical conditions or a BMI greater than 35 kg/m^2 with an associated comorbid medical problem.
- Patients must have also failed dietary therapy.
- Several practical criteria must also be used as guidelines, including psychiatric stability, motivated attitude, and ability to comprehend the nature of the operation and its resultant changes in eating behavior and lifestyle.
- Medical contraindications are not clear.
- Patients who cannot walk have greater risk than those who can ambulate, even for short distances.
- Patients who weigh more than 600 pounds have even more complications; many options for testing, such as computed tomography (CT) scan, are exceeded by this weight limit.
- The Prader-Willi syndrome is an absolute contraindication; no surgical therapy affects the constant need to eat.
- Age is a controversial contraindication to bariatric surgery.
- For adolescents, most pediatric and bariatric surgeons recommend that the operation be performed after the major growth spurt (mid to late teens), thus allowing for increased maturity on the part of the patient; simple restrictive operations are thought to be most appropriate for patients in this age group.

General Bariatric Preoperative Evaluation and Preparation

- A team approach is required for optimal care of the morbidly obese patient.
- Proper preoperative patient education is essential and attendance at educational sessions is mandatory.
- A first-generation cephalosporin, in a dose appropriate for weight, is given preoperatively, and antibiotics are continued for only 24 hours.
- Three major measures are used for prophylaxis against deep venous thrombosis (DVT) and pulmonary embolism:
  - Ambulation within 4 to 6 hours of surgery.
  - Sequential compression device stockings or shoe sleeves.
  - Low-molecular-weight heparin subcutaneously on call to the operating room and then twice daily until discharge.

- High-risk patients are given subcutaneous injections of heparin at home for a full 2-week course.

Evaluation of Specific Comorbidities

- Patients with a history of recent chest pain or change in exercise tolerance should have a formal cardiology assessment, including stress testing as indicated.
- Central venous and pulmonary hypertension are normal for these patients and should not be interpreted as volume overload.
- The use of transesophageal echocardiography intraoperatively is occasionally helpful for patients with cardiomyopathy.
- Pulmonary assessment includes a search for obstructive sleep apnea.
- Reactive asthma is another common problem of the severely obese.
- Hypoventilation syndrome of obesity (Pickwickian syndrome) is a diagnosis that is often suspected by the patient's clinical appearance and is usually limited to the superobese patient population with a BMI greater than 60 kg/m^2; arterial blood gas analysis in Pickwickian patients reveals $PaCO_2$ higher than PaO_2 and elevated hematocrit.
- Pickwickian patients have an extremely high cardiopulmonary morbidity and mortality and are among the few subsets of patients who require planned intensive care admission postoperatively.
- Because there is a considerable incidence of hypertension or diabetes in those patients with concomitant renal disease, the serum creatinine value is an excellent preoperative screening test for baseline renal function.
- Musculoskeletal conditions, especially arthritis and degenerative joint disease, are the most common group of comorbidities found in the severely obese patient.
- Metabolic problems are common in severely obese patients, particularly hyperlipidemia, hypercholesterolemia, and type II diabetes mellitus.
- Venous stasis disease is associated with a greatly increased incidence of postoperative DVT.
- Cholelithiasis is the most prevalent of the several gastrointestinal conditions and must be sought before bariatric surgery.
- For patients undergoing malabsorptive operations, gallstone formation is so frequent that prophylactic cholecystectomy is a standard part of those procedures; for patients undergoing restrictive operations, a screening ultrasound is recommended; this is particularly true of patients undergoing Roux-en-Y

gastric bypass (RYGB) because endoscopic retrograde cholangiopancreatography (ERCP) is not possible.

- Current recommendations for patients undergoing laparoscopic bariatric surgery are for simultaneous cholecystectomy if gallstones are present and ursodiol therapy for 6 months after surgery if the gallbladder is normal.

- Gastroesophageal reflux disease (GERD) is common in severely obese patients because of the increased abdominal pressure and its shortened lower esophageal sphincter.

- Preoperative upper endoscopy is indicated for all patients who have GERD to detect Barrett's esophagus and to evaluate the lower stomach and duodenum in patients undergoing RYGB.

- The patient with nonalcoholic steatotic hepatitis (NASH) presents a potential problem. Ultrasound screening to determine the size of the left lobe of the liver is done because the enlarged liver may interfere with access or visualization of the stomach at operation. Bariatric surgery is beneficial for NASH; weight loss improves the prognosis. NASH is not a contraindication for bariatric surgery if there is no cirrhosis and portal hypertension or hepatocellular decompensation.

OPERATIVE PROCEDURES

- Bariatric operations are performed using either an open or laparoscopic approach.
- Bariatric operations produce weight loss because of two factors:
  - Restriction of oral intake.
  - Malabsorption of ingested food (Box 15–1).

Box 15–1. Bariatric Operations: Mechanism of Action

Restrictive
Vertical banded gastroplasty (VBG) (historic purposes only)
Adjustable gastric banding (AGB)

Largely Restrictive/Mildly Malabsorptive
Roux-en-Y gastric bypass (RYGB)

Largely Malabsorptive/Mildly Restrictive
Biliopancreatic diversion (BPD)
Duodenal switch (DS)

Vertical-Banded Gastroplasty

- Vertical-banded gastroplasty has now largely been abandoned in favor of other operations, because of the poor long-term weight loss, high rate of late stenosis of the gastric outlet, and tendency of patients to adopt a high-calorie liquid diet, leading to regain of weight.

Adjustable Gastric Banding

- The adjustable gastric banding (AGB) procedure may be performed with any one of three types of adjustable bands.
- All of the bands work on the principle of restriction of oral intake by limiting the volume of the proximal stomach.
- The advantage over the traditional vertical banded gastroplasty is the adjustability.
- Excess weight loss may lead to actual removal of a small amount of saline, whereas inadequate weight loss is an indication for the addition of more saline to the system, increasing the restriction of the band.
- The incidence of metabolic problems is low after AGB because there is no disruption of the normal gastrointestinal tract.
- The pattern of weight loss is such that weight loss continues after the first year, up to a maximal amount usually by the third year.
- The decrease in BMI in series with more than 5-year follow-up shows a decrease from a baseline BMI average of 42 to 46 kg/m^2 to a BMI of 30 to 36 kg/m^2 at 5 years.
- The success of AGB in treating existing medical comorbidities for severely obese patients has been equally good.
  - Improved blood glucose control resulted for all patients, with resolution of type II diabetes in two thirds of patients.
  - Hypertension was resolved in 55% of one cohort of patients after AGB.
  - Patients also experienced a decrease in fasting triglyceride levels and elevation of high-density lipoprotein levels.
  - Obstructive sleep apnea was reduced from an incidence of 33% preoperatively to 2% postoperatively.
  - Asthma symptom scores fell from 44.5 before operation to 14.3 at 1 year, with all patients showing improvement.
  - Gastroesophageal reflux was resolved or improved in 90% of patients with this problem.

Roux-en-Y Gastric Bypass

- The gastric bypass described by Itoh in 1969 incorporated a loop of jejunum anastomosed to a proximal gastric pouch; this proved unacceptable, because of bile reflux.
- Griffen and colleagues popularized the use of the Roux limb as drainage for the proximal gastric pouch.
- The RYGB has become the most commonly performed bariatric operation in the United States (Box 15–2).
- Patients with a BMI in the 40 to 50 kg/m^2 range will be well served with a Roux limb of 80 to 120 cm, whereas those patients with a BMI significantly in excess of 50 kg/m^2 are usually given a Roux limb of approximately 150 cm.
- The incidence of small bowel obstruction after laparoscopic RYGB has actually been greater than open RYGB for the first postoperative year.
- Long-term follow-up studies show that there is a tendency for patients to regain some weight after the first year.
- An 85% incidence of resolution of type II diabetes after RYGB has been reported.
- Hypertension was resolved in 54% to 69% of patients undergoing RYGB and improved in 15% of patients.
- Resolution of sleep apnea occurred in 67% of patients, and resolution of obesity hypoventilation syndrome symptoms occurred in 76% of patients undergoing RYGB.
- RYGB resulted in a mean decrease of more than 15% in cholesterol and more than 50% in triglycerides, changes that remained stable for 5 years even if patients regained 15% of the 55% excess weight lost after 2 years.
- Excellent efficacy of RYGB in resolving the symptoms of pseudotumor cerebri, as well as curing the difficult problem of venous stasis ulcers, was demonstrated.

Box 15–2. Essential Components of the Roux-en-Y Gastric Bypass

Small proximal gastric pouch
Gastric pouch constructed of cardia of stomach to prevent dilation and minimize acid production
Gastric pouch divided from distal stomach
Roux limb at least 75 cm in length
Enteroenterostomy constructed to avoid stenosis or obstruction
Closure of all potential spaces for internal hernias

- Immediate resolution of symptoms of patients with GERD occurs in more than 90% of cases.
- The extremely small gastric pouch has a limited reservoir for holding gastric juice, and the cardia is a low acid-producing area of the stomach.

Biliopancreatic Diversion

- Biliopancreatic diversion (BPD) is based on largely malabsorption to produce weight loss but does have a mild restrictive component.
- The operation serves to promote malabsorption, particularly of fat and protein.
- The intestinal tract is reconstructed to allow only a short "common channel" of the distal 50 cm terminal ileum for absorption of fat and protein; the alimentary tract beyond the proximal stomach is rearranged to include only the distal 200 cm of ileum, including the common channel.
- The proximal end of this ileum is anastomosed to the proximal stomach, after performing a distal hemigastrectomy.
- The ileum proximal to the end that is anastomosed to the stomach is, in turn, anastomosed to the terminal ileum within the 50 to 100 cm distance from the ileocecal valve.
- Appendectomy is optional.
- The alimentary tract limb can be lengthened beyond 200 cm in total length if there is concern the patient may not eat a protein-rich diet.
- A maximum length of 300 cm has been used without significantly compromising weight loss.
- Gastric volume may be tailored to the patient's degree of obesity, with larger volumes of 250 mL being created for patients with a BMI less than 50 kg/m^2 and smaller size pouches to a lower limit of 150 cm for patients with a BMI greater than 50 kg/m^2.
- Weight loss after BPD has been reported up to 78% at 12 years of follow-up.
- Patients who undergo malabsorptive procedures such as BPD typically experience the highest weight loss of any of the standard bariatric procedures; this is particularly true of patients with higher BMI.
- Relatively selective malabsorption of starch and fat provide the major mechanism of weight loss, but the partial gastric resection does contribute a restrictive component to the operation.
- In most patients, a "postcibal" syndrome is present immediately after surgery and resolves during the first year, which

causes early satiety and is often associated with vomiting and epigastric pain; these symptoms are not true dumping, because the vasomotor response of dumping is absent.

- Most patients can absorb adequate protein; however, protein malnutrition may occur, and patients must achieve adequate protein intake to prevent this.
- Patients must also be aware that their ability to absorb simple sugars, alcohol, and short-chain triglycerides is good and that overindulgence of sweets, milk products, soft drinks, alcohol, and fruit may produce excess weight gain.
- The BPD has also been highly effective in treating comorbidities, including hypertension, diabetes, lipid disorders, and obstructive sleep apnea.
- Lipid disorders and type II diabetes are almost uniformly resolved after BPD.
- Supplemental fat-soluble vitamins, including D, K, and A, are indicated monthly.

Duodenal Switch

- The duodenal switch (DS) was conceived using the concept for the treatment of bile reflux gastritis and combining it with the BPD concept.
- This modification was developed to help lessen the high incidence of marginal ulcers after BPD.
- The mechanism of weight loss is similar to that of a BPD.
- An appendectomy is followed by measurement of the terminal ileum.
- In the DS, however, the common channel is 100 cm and the entire alimentary tract is 250 cm.
- The major difference between the DS and the BPD is the gastrectomy and the proximal anatomy; instead of a distal hemigastrectomy, a sleeve gastrectomy of the greater curvature of the stomach is performed.
- Cholecystectomy is a routine part of the DS operation.
- A relative indication for selecting either a BPD (or possibly a DS) operation for patients includes those patients who are morbidly obese and who have undergone a previous fundoplication for the treatment of GERD.
- Such patients, because of the potential heavy scarring present in the gastroesophageal junction area, are more amenable to a BPD or DS, which can be performed with little (BPD) or less (DS) disturbance of the proximal gastric area than can either a banding type procedure or a gastric bypass.

- Patients undergoing DS achieved a mean excess weight loss at 8 years of 70%; this was true if patients had a BMI either greater or less than 50 kg/m^2.
- DS patients also had less stool frequency than the BPD patients.
- DS patients had improved food variety tolerance, less vomiting, and improved appetite compared with BPD patients.

POSTOPERATIVE CARE AND FOLLOW-UP

- A potential complication after bariatric surgery is a gastrointestinal tract leak.
- Tachycardia, at times accompanied by tachypnea or agitation, is often the only manifestation of this severe intra-abdominal problem.
- The severely obese patient may not develop a fever or signs of peritonitis, as would the patient with normal body habitus.
- Higher than expected fluid requirements, oliguria, and tachycardia are a constellation of postoperative findings, suggesting intra-abdominal problems.
- DVT prophylaxis is important; pulmonary embolism is the leading cause of death after bariatric surgery.

COMPLICATIONS

Adjustable Gastric Banding

- Mortality for the AGB has been significantly lower than that for RYGB or either of the malabsorptive operations.
- The overall complication rate of AGB is 11.3% and of LAP-BAND is 11.3%.
- The rate of perioperative complications for laparoscopic AGB is 1.5%.
- The rate of band slippage or prolapse is 13.9%, of erosion is 3%, and of port access problems is 5.4%.
- Slippage is by far the most common cause of obstruction, but on occasion erosion and fibrosis can also cause similar symptoms; erosion of the band into the lumen of the stomach is a far less frequent complication but requires reoperation.
- Reoperation is the appropriate treatment for band slippage.

Roux-en-Y Gastric Bypass

- Mortality rates after RYGB have generally been 0.3% to 1.0%.

- Causes of mortality have varied, but include pulmonary embolism, anastomotic leak, cardiac events, intra-abdominal abscess, and multiorgan failure.
- The incidence of complications is not different for patients older than age 50 undergoing RYGB, but these patients are much more likely to have a fatal outcome.
- Male gender is also associated with an increased risk of morbidity and mortality.
- The wound infection rate, of all severity, is about 7%.
- Pulmonary embolism is the most feared complication after any form of bariatric surgery, and its incidence in large reported series of RYGB is about 1%.
- Postoperative atelectasis is relatively common after open RYGB but less frequently seen after laparoscopic RYGB.
- The incidence of pneumonia after either approach is about 1% to 3%.
- Major cardiovascular complications have less than a 1% incidence.
- Complications specific to the RYGB include anastomotic leaks from the proximal or distal anastomosis.
- Leaks from the gastrojejunostomy are more common and are generally the cause of a significant percentage of the life-threatening complications and deaths.
- Another specific life-threatening complication that may result after RYGB is that of bowel obstruction or internal hernias.
- Stenosis of the gastrojejunostomy may occur after RYGB and has been reported in 2% to 14% of patients.
- Postoperative anastomotic stenosis usually presents at 4 to 6 weeks postoperatively as progressive intolerance to solids then liquids in a setting where these were previously tolerated; the problem is quite successfully treated with endoscopic or fluoroscopic balloon dilation.
- Marginal ulcer occurs in 2% to 10% of RYGB; the incidence can be decreased by preoperative treatment of patients with *Helicobacter pylori* colonization of the stomach.
- Another problem, both short- and long-term, may be severe dumping; this should be initially addressed by diet modification.
- Long-term metabolic complications of RYGB are limited to iron and vitamin B_{12} deficiencies.
- The major differences between open and laparoscopic RYGB have been in the lower incidence of wound and hernia complications and splenectomy.

- The incidence of bowel obstruction, especially early bowel obstruction, appears higher in patients undergoing laparoscopic RYGB.

Biliopancreatic Diversion

- Mortality rates after BPD have been reported as being 0.66% in large series.
- Surgical complications occur in 1.2% to 2.8% of patients.
- The most significant and specific complication seen after BPD is protein malnutrition in 11.9% of patients; treatment is hospitalization with 2 to 3 weeks of parenteral nutrition.
- Other complications that are unique to BPD include those associated with excess amounts of diarrhea.
- Marginal ulcers are a distinct problem of BPD and occur in 3.2% of patients; most marginal ulcers appeared within 1 year of surgery, and 75% are successfully treated with medical therapy.
- There was a reported 20% incidence of stenosis with healing, requiring subsequent endoscopic dilatation or surgical revision.
- Malabsorption of fat-soluble vitamins is one of the major problems associated with BPD and may result in low levels of vitamins D and A.
- The incidence of bone resorption was very high, and the incidence of bone pain resulting from such problems was believed to be in the 6% range for patients after BPD.

Duodenal Switch

- Mortality and complications after DS are similar to those seen after BPD but have a few distinct differences.
- A 1.4% mortality with pulmonary embolus being the leading cause of death has been reported.
- Revisional surgery to increase the length of the common channel was performed in 5.7% of patients; in 4.8% it was for protein-calorie malnutrition.
- Major perioperative complications including gastrointestinal leaks, bleeding, gluteal rhabdomyolysis, bowel obstruction, and wound dehiscence represented a 2.9% complication rate.
- Half the patients at 3-year follow-up were anemic, and 30% were hypocalcemic.

CHAPTER 16

ANESTHESIOLOGY PRINCIPLES, PAIN MANAGEMENT, AND CONSCIOUS SEDATION

PHARMACOLOGIC PRINCIPLES

- Intravenous induction agents most commonly initiate the anesthetic state, which then is maintained using inhalation agents, supplemented with intravenous opioids, benzodiazepines, and muscle relaxants.

Inhalational Agents

Nitrous Oxide

- Nitrous oxide provides only partial anesthesia at atmospheric pressure.
- Because nitrous oxide diffuses into closed gas spaces faster than nitrogen diffuses out, it is contraindicated in patients with pneumothorax, small bowel obstruction, or middle ear surgery.

Halothane

- Halothane is a potent anesthetic agent with potent bronchodilator effects.
- Halothane has numerous shortcomings:
  - Is a powerful cardiac depressant that substantially reduces cardiac output.
  - Sensitizes the myocardium to catecholamines.
  - Is associated with a rare form of fulminant hepatitis.
  - Like other potent inhalational agents, occasionally triggers malignant hyperthermia (MH).

Enflurane

- Enflurane is metabolized to fluoride (F^-) and, after prolonged administration, especially in obese patients, is associated with mild renal dysfunction.
- Enflurane is relatively contraindicated in patients with seizure disorders.

Isoflurane

- Isoflurane is now the most commonly used potent inhalational agent.
- Advantages include less reduction of cardiac output, less sensitization to the arrhythmogenic effects of catecholamines, and minimal metabolism.
- Isoflurane-induced tachycardia is an occasional clinical problem.
- Isoflurane causes little increase in intracranial pressure (ICP) and depresses cerebral metabolic activity more than halothane or enflurane.

Sevoflurane

- Low solubility in blood facilitates rapid induction and emergence.
- Sevoflurane is well suited for outpatient surgery, mask induction, and maintenance of patients with bronchospastic disease.
- Although sevoflurane also is metabolized to F^-, renal damage is quite rare.

Desflurane

- Desflurane is very rapidly taken up and eliminated.
- Desflurane is associated with tachycardia and hypertension if the concentration is increased too rapidly.

Intravenous Agents

- Intravenous agents can be used alone (total intravenous anesthesia) or more commonly for induction of anesthesia.

Induction Agents

- The five most commonly used intravenous agents are sodium thiopental, ketamine, propofol, etomidate, and midazolam.

- Sodium thiopental is associated with rapid emergence.
- Ketamine produces a dissociative state; increases blood pressure, heart rate, and ICP; decreases bronchomotor tone; and is associated with emergence delirium and bad dreams.
- Propofol, popular as an induction agent for ambulatory surgery, is a short-acting induction agent that is associated with smooth, nausea-free emergence; propofol also produces excellent bronchodilation.
- Etomidate produces minimal hemodynamic changes but may cause adrenal suppression when given as a prolonged infusion for sedation.
- Midazolam causes minimal cardiovascular side effects and has a much shorter duration of action than diazepam.

Opioids

- Synthetic opioids, such as fentanyl, sufentanil, and remifentanil, produce profound analgesia and minimal cardiac depression but also produce ventilatory depression and inconsistent hypnosis and amnesia.
- Opioids provide analgesia that extends through the early postemergence interval and facilitates a smoother awakening from anesthesia.
- In doses 10 to 20 times the analgesic dose, opioids can be used as complete anesthetics in selected patients.

Neuromuscular Blockers

- The use of muscle relaxants permits reduction of the doses of inhalational and intravenous agents, while still providing satisfactory operating conditions.
- Two categories of neuromuscular blockers in clinical use are depolarizing (noncompetitive) agents and nondepolarizing (competitive) agents.
- The depolarizing agents initially cause muscle fasciculations, followed by an interval of profound relaxation.
  - Succinylcholine is the only depolarizing agent still in use.
  - Because the duration of action is only 5 minutes, a patient who cannot be successfully intubated can be ventilated by mask for a short time until spontaneous respiration resumes. However, if mask ventilation is difficult, severe desaturation will occur before succinylcholine is metabolized.
  - Side effects of succinylcholine include bradycardia, especially in children, and severe, life-threatening hyperkalemia

in patients with burns, paraplegia, quadriplegia, and massive trauma.
  - Succinylcholine, when combined with a volatile agent, is implicated in triggering malignant hyperpyrexia in susceptible patients.
- Nondepolarizing neuromuscular blockers compete for receptor sites with acetylcholine.
- At the conclusion of anesthesia, nondepolarizing relaxants are usually pharmacologically reversed using an anticholinesterase (neostigmine or edrophonium), accompanied by atropine or glycopyrrolate to counteract the muscarinic effects of the anticholinesterase.
- Specific nondepolarizing agents are chosen based on duration of action and metabolism. Pancuronium and vecuronium have prolonged half-lives in patients with renal disease.

Local Anesthetics

- Two classes of local anesthetic drugs are the *esters* and *amides*.
- Local anesthetics dose-dependently block sodium currents in nerve fibers.
- Local anesthetic toxicity involves the central nervous system (CNS) and cardiovascular system.
  - The earliest signs of an overdose or inadvertent intravascular injection are numbness or tingling of the tongue or lips, a metallic taste, light-headedness, tinnitus, or visual disturbances.
  - The signs of toxicity can progress to slurred speech, disorientation, and seizures.
  - With higher doses of local anesthetics, cardiovascular collapse ensues.
  - The best defenses against local anesthetic toxicity are aspiration to detect unplanned vascular entry before injecting large doses of local anesthetics and knowledge of the maximal safe dose of the drug being injected.

PREOPERATIVE EVALUATION

Airway Examination

- Assessing the patient's airway is a crucial step in developing any anesthetic plan.

TABLE 16–1.   Patient-Related Risk Factors Associated with Postoperative Pulmonary Complications

Potential Risk Factor	Type of Surgery	Relative Risk Associated with Factor
Smoking	Coronary bypass	3.4
	Abdominal	1.4–4.3
ASA class >II	Unselected surgery	1.7
	Thoracic or abdominal	1.5–3.2
Age >70 yr	Unselected surgery	1.9–2.4
	Thoracic or abdominal	0.9–1.9
Obesity	Unselected surgery	1.3
	Thoracic or abdominal	0.8–1.7
COPD	Unselected surgery	2.7–3.6
	Thoracic or abdominal	4.7

ASA, American Society of Anesthesiologists; COPD, chronic obstructive pulmonary disease.
Modified from Smetana GW: Preoperative pulmonary evaluation. N Engl J Med 340:937–944, 1999.

Cardiovascular Disease

- Five major predictors of postoperative myocardial ischemia are: electrocardiogram (ECG) evidence of left ventricular hypertrophy, history of hypertension, diabetes mellitus, definite coronary artery disease (CAD), and use of digoxin.
- Clinical predictors of increased cardiac risk have been proposed and are listed in Table 16–1.
- Cardiac risk also varies among specific surgical procedures.
- Perioperative beta-blockade has been shown to decrease long-term mortality in patients with or at risk for CAD undergoing high-risk noncardiac surgery.
- In general, antihypertensive medications should be continued throughout the perioperative period.

Pulmonary Disease

- Important preoperative considerations include functional status, exercise tolerance, severity of disease, current medications, and recent worsening of symptoms.
- Preoperative preparation should treat reversible pulmonary pathology, optimize medical management, and plan postoperative ventilatory management.

Neurologic Disease

- Important preoperative neurologic conditions include seizure disorders and upper motor neuron lesions.
- Careful documentation of deficits is required to facilitate evaluation of apparent postoperative neurologic complications.

Renal and Hepatic Disease

- Chronic renal insufficiency presents many perioperative management challenges, including acid-base abnormalities, electrolyte disturbances, and coagulation disorders.
- Dialysis should be performed 18 to 24 hours before surgery to avoid fluid and electrolyte shifts that occur immediately after dialysis.
- Chronic liver disease alters anesthetic drug metabolism, predisposes to coagulopathy, encephalopathy, ascites and malnutrition, and hypoalbuminemia increases the free (active) fraction of many drugs.

Diabetes

- Diabetic evaluation includes duration and type of diabetes and current medical regimen.
- Potential end-organ dysfunction includes autonomic dysfunction, delayed gastric emptying, gastroesophageal reflux, cardiovascular disease, renal insufficiency, retinopathy, and neurologic complications.
- In diabetic patients undergoing surgery, both severe hyperglycemia and hypoglycemia must be prevented.
  - Substitute shorter-acting for longer-acting insulin.
  - Provide a reduced dose in insulin on the morning of surgery.
  - After giving insulin, provide glucose in intravenous fluids.
  - In Type 2 diabetic patients, long-acting sulfonylurea drugs should be stopped, and shorter-acting agents should be substituted.
  - Metformin should be stopped because of the slight risk for perioperative drug-induced lactic acidosis.
  - Tight control of blood glucose has been associated with improved outcome in critically ill surgical patients, including nondiabetic patients.

Chronic Glucocorticoid Administration

- Because of the remote risk for adrenal insufficiency during anesthesia, patients who receive chronic glucocorticoids generally receive perioperative steroid coverage.

Assessment of Physical Status

- The American Society of Anesthesiologists (ASA) has developed a graded, descriptive scale as a means of categorizing preoperative comorbidity:
  - *ASA I*—No organic, physiologic, biochemical, or psychiatric disturbance.
  - *ASA II*—A patient with mild systemic disease that results in no functional limitation. Example: uncomplicated diabetes mellitus.
  - *ASA III*—A patient with severe systemic disease that results in functional impairments. Example: diabetes mellitus with vascular complications.
  - *ASA IV*—Severe systemic disease that is a constant threat to life. Examples: congestive heart failure, unstable angina pectoris.
  - *ASA V*—Moribund condition in a patient who is not expected to survive with or without the operation. Example: ruptured aortic aneurysm.
  - *ASA VI*—Declared brain dead patient for organ harvest.
  - *E*—Emergency operation is required.

SELECTION OF ANESTHETIC TECHNIQUES AND DRUGS

- The selection of anesthetic techniques and drugs is influenced by preexisting conditions, chronic medications, operative site, positioning during surgery, duration of surgery, need for postoperative hospital admission, and relative costs of various techniques.

Risk of Anesthesia

- The risk of cardiac arrest attributable to anesthesia appears to be less than 1 in 10,000 cases.

Selection of Specific Technique

- There are four general ways in which to provide sedation or analgesia for surgical procedures: moderate sedation (previously termed conscious sedation), monitored anesthesia care, regional anesthesia, and general anesthesia.
- Moderate sedation, usually provided by a specially trained nurse, implies that the patient can respond purposefully to verbal or tactile stimulation, has a patent airway requiring no intervention, has adequate spontaneous ventilation, and has maintained cardiovascular function. In contrast, deep sedation

may result in airway compromise and cardiovascular and ventilatory depression and requires greater expertise to manage.

- Monitored anesthesia care supplements local anesthesia performed by surgeons. Anesthesiologists usually participate because an individual patient or procedure requires sedation or analgesia exceeding moderate sedation or because an acutely or chronically ill patient requires close monitoring and hemodynamic or respiratory support.

- Regional anesthesia is useful for operations on the upper and lower extremities, pelvis, and lower abdomen. Certain other procedures, such as carotid endarterectomy and "awake" craniotomy can also be successfully performed under regional or field block.

- General anesthesia achieves the four components of general anesthesia (amnesia, analgesia, inhibition of noxious reflexes, and skeletal muscle relaxation) by a combination of agents.

- Rapid-sequence induction is indicated for patients who are at high risk for acid aspiration.

COMMON INTRAOPERATIVE PROBLEMS

- Several important problems that can arise after induction of anesthesia include difficulty establishing an airway, hypotension, hypoxemia, myocardial ischemia, increased peak inspiratory pressure, and increased body temperature.

- Difficult direct laryngoscopy occurs in 1.5% to 8.5% and failed intubation occurs in 0.13% to 0.3% of general anesthetics (for management guidelines, see Fig. 16–1).

- The laryngeal mask airway (LMA), the Combitube, the lighted stylet, the Bullard laryngoscope, and the fiberoptic bronchoscope facilitate intubation in many patients who have failed intubation using a conventional laryngoscope.

- Hypotension, which is operationally defined as a decrease in blood pressure by more than 25%, usually is easily treated with fluid boluses or short-acting pressors; however, hypotension arising during anesthesia may also indicate more serious complications.

- Hypoxemia can result from multiple causes, including right mainstem intubation, pneumothorax, bronchospasm, and aspiration of gastric contents.

- Myocardial ischemia is a particular risk in patients with known CAD or who have major risk factors for CAD.

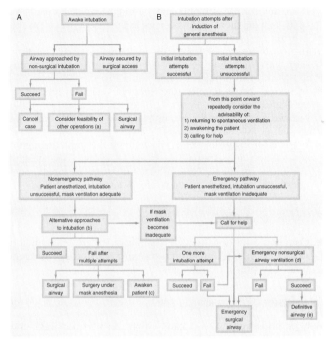

FIGURE 16–1. The American Society of Anesthesiologists (ASA) difficult airway algorithm. The likelihood and clinical impact of basic management problems such as difficult intubation, difficult mask ventilation, and difficulty with patient cooperation or consent should be assessed in all patients in which airway management is contemplated. The clinician should consider the relative merits and feasibility of basic management choices including the use of awake intubation techniques, preservation of spontaneous ventilation, and the use of surgical approaches to establish a secure airway. Primary and alternative strategies should be established: (a) other options include, but are not limited to, surgery under mask anesthesia, surgery under local infiltration or nerve block, and intubation attempts after induction of general anesthesia; (b) alternative approaches include use of different laryngoscope blades, awake intubation, blind oral or nasal intubation, fiberoptic intubation, use of intubating stylet or tube changer, light wand, retrograde intubation, and surgical airway access; (c) see awake intubation; (d) options for emergency nonsurgical airway include transtracheal jet ventilation, laryngeal mask airway, and Combitube. *(Reproduced from American Society of Anesthesiologists: Practice guidelines for management of the difficult airway: A report by the American Society of Anesthesiologists task force on management of the difficult airway. Anesthesiology 78:597–602, 1993.)*

Most myocardial ischemia can be diagnosed from leads V_5 or II. Management of myocardial ischemia depends on the precipitating cause.

- Increased peak inspiratory pressure gauge may have multiple etiologies, including light anesthesia, bronchospasm, pneumothorax, and aspiration pneumonia.
- Increased body temperature may be due to release of cytokines from an area of infection as it is surgically drained, to overzealous attempts to prevent hypothermia, or to MH.
- If MH is strongly suspected, discontinue the triggering agent (usually an inhalational anesthetic), replace the existing anesthesia machine with a machine free of inhalational anesthetic, and intravenously infuse dantrolene.

POSTANESTHESIA CARE

- Common anesthesia-related complications are encountered in the recovery room and must be promptly recognized and treated to prevent serious injury.

Postoperative Agitation and Delirium

- This nonspecific complication may result from pain and anxiety but also from hypoxemia, hypercarbia, acidosis, hypotension, hypoglycemia, surgical complications, and adverse drug reactions. More serious conditions must be excluded before empirical treatment with pain medications, sedatives, or physical restraints.

Respiratory Complications

- Respiratory problems are the most frequent major complications.
- Airway obstruction is most commonly a result of obstruction of the oropharynx by the tongue or oropharyngeal soft tissues caused by the residual effects of general anesthetics, pain medications, or muscle relaxants.
- Other causes include laryngospasm; blood; vomitus or debris in the airway; glottic edema; vocal cord paralysis; and external compression of the airway by a hematoma, dressing, or cervical collar.
- Characteristics physical signs of airway obstruction are sonorous respiratory sounds and paradoxical chest movement.

- Many obstructions can be relieved by applying a head-tilt and jaw-thrust maneuver, placement of an oral or nasopharyngeal airway, or suctioning.
- In children, glottic edema or postextubation croup are treated with humidified oxygen and, if severe, systemic steroids and racemic epinephrine by nebulization.
- Hypoxemia can result from hypoventilation, ventilation-perfusion mismatching, or right-to-left intrapulmonary shunting; reluctance to inspire deeply after abdominal or thoracic surgery may also result in hypoxemia.
- Hypoxemia must be excluded as an underlying problem in patients exhibiting restlessness, tachycardia, or cardiac irritability.
- Treatment of hypoxemia requires administration of oxygen, assurance of adequate ventilation, and treatment of underlying causes.
- Hypoventilation (hypercarbia) can result from airway obstruction or central respiratory depression and may present as prolonged somnolence, bradypnea, airway obstruction, shallow breathing, tachycardia, and arrhythmias.
- If severe, hypoventilation can result in hypoxemia.
- Treatment is aimed at identification and treatment of the underlying problem.

Circulatory Complications

- Hypotension in the recovery room is most commonly a result of hypovolemia, left ventricular dysfunction, or arrhythmias but may also indicate anaphylaxis, transfusion reactions, cardiac tamponade, pulmonary emboli, adverse drug reactions, adrenal insufficiency, and hypoxemia.
- Treatment involves circulatory support with fluids, inotropic agents, Trendelenburg position, and oxygen until the underlying cause is diagnosed and treated.
- Common causes of hypertension in the Post Anesthesia Care Unit (PACU) include pain, anxiety, and inadequately managed essential hypertension, but hypoxemia and hypercarbia must be excluded.
- Less common causes include hypoglycemia; drug reactions, hyperthyroidism, pheochromocytoma, or MH; and bladder distention.
- Treatment is to identify and correct the underlying cause.

ACUTE PAIN MANAGEMENT

- *Acute* pain is of relatively short duration and should stop, usually within minutes, hours, or days, as tissue heals and noxious stimuli resolve.

Mechanisms of Acute Pain

- Pain has both sensory and affective components.
- Tissue injury produces pain through a process called nociception, which has four steps: transduction, transmission, modulation, and perception. The fourth step, perception, is integral to the subjective and emotional experience.

Methods of Analgesia

- Agents include opioids, nonsteroidal anti-inflammatory drugs (NSAIDs), and local anesthetics. Routes of administration include oral, parenteral, epidural, and intrathecal.
- The oral route is the preferred route for analgesic delivery. Patients experiencing mild to moderate acute pain and who can receive agents orally can obtain effective analgesia.
- Parenteral administration is preferred for moderate to severe pain, rapid control of pain, and patients who cannot receive oral agents.
- Strong opioids (e.g., morphine sulfate) are ideal for moderate to severe pain and for pain that is constant in frequency. Meperidine now is rarely used because it is metabolized to normeperidine, a unique toxic metabolite that can accumulate and cause seizures.
- Weak opioid agents, such as hydrocodone and codeine, are commonly combined with aspirin or acetaminophen and are suitable for mild to moderate pain that is intermittent.
- Common opioid-related side effects include nausea, pruritus, sedation, mental clouding, decreased gastric motility, urinary retention, and respiratory depression.
- Addiction (psychological dependence) is extremely rare as a consequence of postoperative analgesia. Postoperative opioid use may result in tolerance (when a previously effective opioid dose fails to provide adequate analgesia) and rarely in physical dependence (resulting in a withdrawal syndrome when a drug is stopped suddenly or when an antagonist is given).
- NSAIDs reduce pain and can decrease opioid consumption.
- Traditional NSAIDs are nonselective inhibitors of cyclooxygenase (COX). Selective COX-2 inhibitors appear to offer similar analgesia with a somewhat reduced risk of causing gastrointestinal bleeding, bleeding diathesis, and renal compromise.
- Local anesthetics are used to provide regional anesthesia for surgery, but their effects persist into the perioperative period and contribute to preemptive analgesia. Postoperative

analgesia requires lower doses of local anesthetics than are required for surgical anesthesia.

● Combining agents from different analgesic classes permits reduced dosage of each individual agent and fewer, less severe side effects from each agent.

● Pre-emptive analgesia, which aims to interrupt processing of painful stimuli before surgical incision, may decrease post-operative pain, postoperative analgesic requirement, side effects from analgesics, and the incidence of chronic post-surgical pain syndromes and may improve compliance with postoperative rehabilitation.

Neuraxial Analgesia

● Neuraxial routes of administration include the epidural and intrathecal (subarachnoid) routes. An important relative con-traindication to neuraxial analgesia is the presence of abnor-mal coagulation, including concurrent use of antiplatelet and anticoagulant agents.

● Small doses of agents such as opioids and local anesthetics are given neuraxially to achieve analgesia.

● Local anesthetics are delivered in smaller doses and weaker concentrations than are required to achieve surgical anes-thesia. Neuraxial analgesia for acute pain commonly com-bines opioids and local anesthetics. Many clinicians believe that epidural analgesia provides superior analgesia in com-parison to parenteral opioids.

Intravenous Patient-Controlled Analgesia

● For alert, cooperative patients, intravenous patient-controlled analgesia (IV PCA) minimizes the steps involved in the deliv-ery of analgesia and increases patient autonomy and control. IV PCA provides prompt analgesia, uses smaller doses of opioids at more frequent intervals, can maintain drug con-centrations within the analgesic range, and has a lower incidence of drug-related side effects.

● The use of structured protocols and guidelines is encour-aged for facilities using IV PCA.

Selection of Methods of Postoperative Analgesia

● The choice of postoperative pain management strategies is a function of patient factors, surgeons' preferences, anesthesi-ologists' skills, and availability of resources for postoperative care and monitoring.

Specific Types of Acute Pain Patients

- Patients who have a history of chronic pain may manifest tolerance to opioid therapy and a decreased pain threshold.
- In patients with a history of substance abuse, effective analgesia can be obtained with strict guidelines, patient education, and modalities such as regional analgesia.
- Effective analgesia for the pediatric patient experiencing acute pain can be achieved with pain assessment tools that are tailored for this population and the use of modalities and agents similar to those used for adults.
- Elderly patients require pain assessment and evaluation tailored to their mental status, cognitive abilities, underlying disease states, and decreased organ function.

CHAPTER 17

MINIMALLY INVASIVE SURGERY

LAPARASCOPIC SURGERY

Introduction and Indications

Physiology

- Insufflation of gas into the peritoneum, preperitoneal space, or retroperitoneal space increases intra-abdominal pressure impairing ventilation, decreasing venous return, depressing circulation, reducing renal perfusion, and increasing intracranial pressure. The process is analogous to, although less marked than, abdominal compartment syndrome.

Pulmonary Effects

- Peak airway pressures rises, whereas pulmonary compliance and vital capacity fall in proportion to intra-abdominal pressure, but patient positioning does not significantly alter the effects of insufflation on pulmonary function.
- Patients at risk for acidosis include those with high metabolic and cellular respiratory rates (i.e., septic patients), impaired regional blood flow, a large ventilatory "dead space" (i.e., patients with chronic obstructive pulmonary disease), or poor cardiac output.
- Pneumoperitoneum also induces locoregional acidosis, in the absence of systemic acidosis, by impairing microcirculation and decreasing organ blood flow.
- Laparoscopic surgery results in less pain and subsequently less pulmonary embarrassment postoperatively compared with the corresponding open procedure.

Circulatory Effects

- Capillary wedge pressure (preload), mean arterial pressure, and systemic vascular resistance (afterload). These changes have a dual effect; increased preload tends to augment cardiac

227

output, whereas increased afterload decreases it and increases cardiac work.

- The net result of the cardiovascular changes on cardiac output, therefore, depends on the patient's volume status, autonomic response, and cardiac reserve (Fig. 17–1).
- Reverse-Trendelenburg position leads to reductions in cardiac output by decreasing preload and may cause hypotension. Hypercarbia, resulting from CO_2 absorption, causes arteriolar dilation and myocardial depression, which tend to lower blood pressure. These effects are counteracted by an autonomic response, mostly resulting from the sympathetic nervous system, that elevates heart rate, systolic blood pressure, central venous pressure, left ventricular stroke, and volume cardiac output.
- Patients with cardiac disease tolerate the effects of laparoscopy poorly.

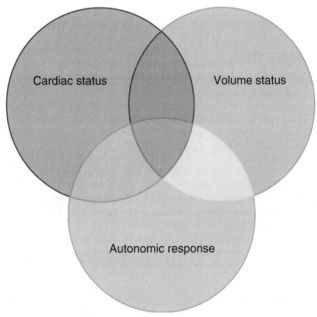

■ **FIGURE 17–1.** Factors influencing tolerance of laparoscopic surgery.

Renal Effects

- Randomized studies demonstrate that urine output is lower with a pneumoperitoneum versus either open techniques or gasless laparoscopy.
- The actual effect of pneumoperitoneum on renal blood flow is highly dependent on volume status of the patient. The effects on both renal blood flow and urine output can be overcome by optimizing the patient's volume status.

Immune Function and Inflammatory Response

- Peritoneal macrophages play a primary role in this inflammatory response.
- High CO_2 results in less interleukin (IL)-1 and tissue necrosis factor (TNF)-α production by peritoneal macrophages challenged with lipopolysaccharide and less peritoneal macrophage TNF-α production in a tumor model.
- Recent large series now show that port site recurrence rates approximate wound recurrence rates from open surgery.

Miscellaneous Effects

Intracranial Pressure

- Hypercarbia with pneumoperitoneum is, therefore, undesirable in patients with head injuries.

Intestinal Function

- Multiple randomized studies demonstrate that bowel function returns quicker after laparoscopic procedures.

Technical Considerations

- Skills training taught outside the operating room improves operative task performance.

Laparoscopy during Pregnancy

- An open approach is recommended for placement of the first trocar and establishment of pneumoperitoneum, because of the risk of injury to the gravid uterus by misplacement of a Veress needle.

Complications

- Although usually resulting from "blind" placement of the device, major vascular injury has been reported with the open approach.
- Bowel injury is the second most common cause of death from laparoscopic surgery. About one third of these injuries occur during abdominal access by mechanisms similar to those described previously for vascular injuries.
- Potential complications of specimen removal are infection, recurrence (port site and regional intra-abdominal recurrence), splenosis, and endometriosis. The pathophysiology is similar in all during the dissection or specimen extraction; viable bacteria or cells are released within the abdomen or at the port site.
- Clinically, gas embolus presents as bradycardia, hypotension, arrhythmia, or a "mill wheel" heart murmur, during or shortly after insufflation. Transesophageal echocardiography definitively establishes the diagnosis. Treatment includes immediate desufflation of the abdomen and placing the patient in the head-down, left lateral decubitus position.
- Using the lowest insufflation pressure that allows adequate working space minimizes both pneumothorax and pneumomediastinum.

Specific Procedures

Diagnostic Laparoscopy

- Laparoscopy diagnoses 81% to 96% of patient problems accurately. Most importantly, the information obtained changes the planned operation to a more limited approach in at least two thirds of cases.
- Laparoscopy is ideally suited to evaluation and repair of diaphragmatic and isolated visceral injuries.
- The greatest gains are derived in patients with isolated abdominal stab wounds, especially if ultrasound or local exploration indicates that the posterior fascia of the abdomen is violated.

Biliary Disease

- Recent meta-analysis suggest that routine intraoperative cholangiography lowers the incidence of duct injury by approximately 50%.
- Preoperative endoscopic retrograde cholangiopancreatography (ERCP) is commonly performed for transient episodes

of pancreatitis or jaundice, persistently elevated liver function tests, or a dilated bile duct. However, it identifies pathology in 20% or less of patients with such presentations.

Laparoscopic Common Bile Duct Exploration

- Choledochotomy is used for large stones when the bile duct is dilated.
- Recently, primary duct closure without T-tube placement has gained popularity.

Gastroesophageal Reflux Disease

- Today, more than 90% of antireflux operations are performed laparoscopically, and surgical treatment competes effectively with medical therapies for patients.
- Several trials show comparable relief of symptoms by laparoscopic and open antireflux surgery. Although data are still evolving, laparoscopic operations afford equivalent durability when compared with open surgery.
- It also improves asthma in children and adults.
- A "shoeshine" maneuver ensures that there is sufficient laxity of the plication and that the esophagus is invaginated into the stomach rather than the stomach being twisted around the esophagus.

Achalasia

- Most surgeons use intraoperative endoscopy to gauge the length of the myotomy and to test the integrity of the esophageal mucosa at the conclusion of the procedure.
- Myotomy effectively alleviates symptoms in 90% of patients, but 10% to 15% of patients develop significant reflux.
- Laparoscopic approaches are also used for patients who have a perforation during balloon dilatation. Results are best if the perforation is recognized promptly and addressed quickly.

Appendicitis

Colorectal Procedures

- Randomized, prospective studies by Milsom et al and Stage et al show that laparoscopic patients have less pain, earlier return of bowel function, earlier discharge from the hospital, and no increase in the rate of wound or port site recurrences, although follow-up was short.

Bariatric Surgery

● Randomized prospective studies demonstrate that laparoscopic gastric bypass results in less blood loss, less pain, shorter hospital stays, faster convalescence, and lower rates of incisional hernia than open surgery.

Laparoscopic Splenectomy

● Several retrospective and nonrandomized prospective studies show that there is less pain and blood loss, quicker return of bowel function, and shorter hospital stay, but a longer operative time with laparoscopic splenectomy performed for nontraumatic splenic diseases.
● There has been no difference in the detection of accessory spleens.
● As with open operation, it is important to examine the abdomen for accessory spleens that are located, in descending order of frequency, in the splenic hilum and vascular pedicle, gastrocolic ligament, pancreatic tail, greater omentum, greater curve of the stomach, splenocolic ligament, small and large bowel mesentery, left broad ligament in women, and left spermatic cord in men.

Adrenalectomy

● Laparoscopic adrenalectomy is particularly well suited for the resection of nonmalignant adrenal lesions such as aldosteronomas, pheochromocytomas, Cushing's disease with adrenal hyperplasia, nonfunctional adenoma, and rare entities such as cyst or myelolipoma.
● On both sides, dissection can be performed on the anterior, posterior, and inferolateral aspects with ultrasonic shears, or with electrocautery, because these areas are relatively avascular.

Inguinal Hernia

● The preperitoneal space does not expand properly during totally extraperitoneal approach (TEP) when the patient has had lower abdominal surgery, particularly prostatectomy. Complications such as bladder injury are also more common. Transabdominal preperitoneal (TAPP) or open repair may be preferable in this situation or with incarcerated hernias, because the bowel can be reduced and inspected for viability.

Incisional Hernia

- Successful laparoscopic incisional hernia requires placement of a prosthetic material, which should overlap the edges of the fascial defect by at least 3 cm. The introduction of composite ("double-sided") mesh, which is coated/covered by polytetrafluoroethylene on one side, allowing ingrowth of abdominal wall tissues into the mesh, but minimal adhesions to bowel, has facilitated this procedure.

Miscellaneous Procedures

- Patients who are the best candidates for primary laparoscopic treatment of bowel obstruction are those with a history of only one or two previous operations, early (less than 24 hours) obstruction, and minimal to moderate distension of the bowel. Bowel obstruction after recent laparoscopic surgery, early bowel obstruction associated with incarcerated inguinal hernias, and obstruction after localized operations such as appendectomy may be particularly good candidates for laparoscopic exploration.

VIDEO-ASSISTED THORASCOPIC SURGERY (VATS)

Introduction and Indications

- The benefits of VATS include less postoperative pain, less pulmonary trauma, shorter hospitalizations, and improved patient satisfaction.
- The greatest controversy surrounds the suitability of VATS for definitive resection of pulmonary malignant lesions.

Physiology

- Physiologic changes during VATS largely result from one-lung ventilation and patient positioning.
- One-lung ventilation decreases the surface area available for gas exchange and results in loss of normal pulmonary autoregulation in which hypoxic pulmonary vasoconstriction results in redistribution of blood flow to better-ventilated segments improving arterial oxygenation. These compensatory mechanisms are obliterated when 70% of the lung is atelectatic and further suppressed by volatile anesthetics.

Technical Considerations

- Complete collapse of the operative lung is mandatory for locating deep lesions.

- Alternately, wire-guided needle localization, subpleural dye injection, and intraoperative ultrasound have been used as adjuncts.

Complications

- The most common problems are atelectasis, prolonged air leak, hemorrhage, and infection (Box 17–1).
- Air leaks lasting greater than 7 days occur in 2% to 6% of cases and are a common reason for reoperation, often requiring a formal thoracotomy.
- Port site recurrence has been reported in several series of VATS procedures and tends to be more common when specimens are not placed within a protective bag prior to removal from the chest. They are more common with mesothelioma, metastatic sarcoma, melanoma, or malignant effusion.

Specific Procedures

Pulmonary Resection for Cancer

- Thorascopic wedge resection may not be possible or prudent if there is dense pleural symphysis, inability to tolerate one-lung ventilation, lesion size greater than 3 cm, or known

---

Box 17–1. Complications of Video-Assisted Thoracoscopic Surgery

Air leak with persistent/recurrent pneumothorax
Atelectasis
Pneumonia
Barotrauma
Re-expansion pulmonary edema
Dissemination of malignant disease
Infection
    Pulmonary abscess
    Empyema
    Wound infection
Hemorrhage
Myocardial infarct
Arrhythmias
Hypotension/hypertension
Intercostal neuritis

cancer. A patient requiring anticoagulation is also a relative contraindication to the procedure.

- Anatomic resections are performed less commonly because of concern about adequate tumor margins with minimally invasive approaches and chest wall (port-site) recurrence. However, disease-free survival appears to be equivalent in nonrandomized studies.

- Biopsy may be required in up to one third of patients with diffuse interstitial disease of the lung, to establish a diagnosis.

- VATS has a diagnostic accuracy (94% or greater) and operating time comparable to open biopsy but has less morbidity. If both lungs are affected equally, the right chest presents more free edges for biopsy, whereas the left lung tends to collapse more completely during one-lung ventilation.

Lung Volume Reduction

- Ideal candidates for lung reduction surgery have a localized pattern of parenchymal destruction with hypoperfusion in the diseased segments by pulmonary perfusion scanning.

- One study of 42 patients showed that lung volume reduction by VATS takes longer to perform but resulted in fewer days on the ventilator, in the intensive care unit, and with an air leak. Patients also experienced shorter hospital stays and lower hospital costs.

Pneumothorax

- Stapled bullectomy yields a 95% to 100% success rate compared with 78% to 91% success with chemical pleurodesis alone.

Pleural Effusion

- Thoracoscopy is also indicated for selected cases of empyema and hemothorax. In acute empyema, VATS allows evacuation and lavage of the pleural space, thus removing the fibrin that prevents lung re-expansion.

Mediastinal Disease

- VATS allows the surgeon to widely inspect the entire mediastinum and hemithorax and to obtain generous biopsies. This improves diagnostic accuracy and staging of

mediastinal masses by detecting tumor invasion or metastatic spread not apparent on preoperative imaging.
- Total thymectomy for myasthenia gravis is very effective compared with medical treatment alone.
- Invasiveness represents an absolute contraindication to VATS resection.

CHAPTER 18

EMERGING TECHNOLOGY IN SURGERY: INFORMATICS, ELECTRONICS, ROBOTICS

- Informatics, electronics, and robotics are changing the way that we practice medicine.
- Despite decades of technologic developments, the performance of surgical operations (the open cutting and suturing) remained unchanged.
- Minimally invasive surgery (MIS), however, brought about a major deviation from traditional surgery. Large surgical problems do not require large incisions for adequate treatment any longer.
- Robotic surgery is aimed at improving surgical outcomes through increased precision in a setting of minimal invasiveness.
- Robotics is facilitating the development of new fields: telementoring and telepresence.

MINIMALLY INVASIVE SURGERY AND ROBOTICS

- The principle *first do not harm* is central to the practice of medicine.
- In surgery, however, significant pain and morbidity derive at large from the surgical access (e.g., laparotomy, thoracotomy) alone.
- Development of MIS (or minimally access surgery) has been a logical and ethically justified process.
- Many MIS operations (e.g., appendectomy, antireflux procedures, hernia repairs, adrenalectomy) yielded better outcomes than their open counterparts: less pain, decreased blood loss, less systemic response, less wound complications, shorter hospital stay, faster recovery, and better cosmetics.
- Reduced surgical stress, less impairment of physiologic functions, and improved immune responses expanded the indications for MIS to include the elderly and the high-risk patient.

- More complex operations (e.g., colectomy, pancreatectomy, coronary bypass), however, have not found an easy transition to MIS. The problem has been the technical limitations inherent to traditional videoscopic platforms.
- Videoscopic surgery is hindered by (1) replacement of the normal open three-dimensional (3-D) sight by a two-dimensional (2-D) vision of the field displayed on a monitor, (2) unstable video camera positioning, (3) inferior operative ergonomics, and (4) loss of the normal degrees of freedom for manipulation of surgical instruments.
- Robotic technology has been envisioned as one way to overcome physical obstacles of MIS and improve on the surgeon s natural limitations.

THE CONCEPT AND FUNCTIONS OF SURGICAL ROBOTS

- The term *robot* (Czechoslovakian word *robata*) means forced labor or worker.
- Replacement of the surgeon is not the intent of a surgical robot.
- A surgical robot is as a powered, computer-controlled device that can be programmed to aid in the positioning and manipulation of surgical instruments; the central requirement is to be self-powered.
- The terms *computer-enhanced* and *computer-assisted* surgery (CAS) have been coined also for surgical systems that operate without autonomy.
- Tasks assigned to surgical robots include percutaneous biopsy of solid organs (e.g., brain, prostate, kidney), high-precision drilling or cutting of bone, automated resection of prostate, image processing (e.g., magnification and reproduction of 3-D vision), motion scaling (e.g., microsurgery), suturing, endoscope holding, and biohazardous procedures (e.g., radiosurgery, brachytherapy).
- Surgical robots are becoming integral components of a more comprehensive network of clinical information.
- A surgical robot linked to another robotic system such as a computed tomography (CT) or magnetic resonance imaging (MRI) scanner can have access to imaging studies to be imported into the operative theater. Robots can assist with the preoperative planning and with the rehearsal of individualized operations. For example, Robodoc (see later) functions by using the actual patient s anatomy obtained by preoperative imaging examinations.
- Robotic technologies offer solutions for updating our methods of surgical training.

- *Telementoring,* a class of telemedicine, has been carried out successfully in surgery using standard means of transmission and over various distances.
- Short-distance telementoring has shown to be a safe method for the assessment of competency during training of laparoscopic cholecystectomy.
- Long-distance telementoring (e.g., over thousands of miles apart) has been accomplished successfully using standard telephone, cellular, and satellite systems. Telementoring represents a feasible method of conveying proctorship and expert consultation in MIS.
- In *telepresence* surgery, the surgeon does not operate in direct contact with, but rather at a distance from, the patient. The robots used for telepresence surgery are called telerobots.
- A transatlantic telerobotic cholecystectomy was performed in July 2001: the operating surgeon was in New York City and the patient was in Strasbourg, France.
- Telepresence surgery may help to outreach underserved areas.
- Telerobots enable the surgeon to (1) take personal control of the optical system (e.g., camera positioning, zooming, magnification), (2) operate with 3-D vision, (3) increase precision (e.g., dumping of tremor and scaling of motion, and (4) improve dexterity (e.g., increased degrees of freedom).

CLASSIFICATION OF SURGICAL ROBOTS

Passive Robots

- In passive robots, the energy to propel the system is provided by the surgeon; in turn, the system provides information about the tracking and relative position of the device with regard to the target.
- Prerobotic devices are passive retractors adapted to assist with the holding of the camera and other laparoscopic instruments. These devices, however, are considered prerobotic devices.

Semiactive and Synergistic Robots

- Semiactive robots are devices that combine the capability of some autonomous function with other actions carried out by the surgeon.

- One example is Laparoscopic Assistant Robotic System (LARS) (Johns Hopkins University and IBM). LARS is a robotic arm that has four degrees of freedom for positioning of video camera or retracting instruments and is fitted with sensors that monitor forces and torque.
- Synergistic robots are devices simultaneously powered by both the robot s engine and the surgeon. Active Constraint Robot (ACROBOT) (Imperial College, London) is an example of a synergistic robot. ACROBOT was designed to cut bone with maximum precision and safety in preparation for knee replacement.

Active Robots

- Active surgical robots are powered devices that can function with significant independence from the surgeon. These robots carry the greatest safety concerns and have been developed for specific purposes.

Camera Holder Robots

- Robots for camera holding were the first active robots to be developed for commercial use. Automated Endoscopic System for Optimal Positioning (AESOP) (Computer Motion Inc.) and EndoAssist (Armstrong Healthcare Ltd.) are the better known robotic camera holder systems. They have successfully replaced the camera assistant and have allowed for the performance of *solo-surgery*.
- AESOP is composed of a control computer, a power system, and an articulated, electromechanical arm for holding and maneuvering the telescope. The arm attaches to the operating table and its action can be controlled via foot pedals, hand controls, or a voice activation/recognition system. AESOP has been used extensively to assist in urologic, gynecologic, gastrointestinal, and thoracic videoscopic operations. The use of AESOP significantly reduces smudging, fogging, need for cleaning, inadvertent movements of the telescope, and sometimes reduces the operative time.
- EndoAssist is a head-mounted navigation system that allows the laparoscopic camera to follow the surgeon s head movements by tracking a headband sensor. The robot is in active mode only when a foot switch is pressed by the surgeon. In active mode, any glance of the operator in one direction on the video monitor causes the camera to pan in the same direction (left/right, up/down, zoom in/out).

Orthopedic Robots

- Orthopedic operations are especially suited for automated tasks because the target site can be effectively stabilized. Goals for using robots in orthopedic surgery include decreased frequency of iatrogenic fractures, more precise bone drilling, better alignment of fragments and prosthesis, improved contact areas, better bone ingrowth, and, hopefully, improved long-term performance.

- Robodoc (Integrated Surgical Systems) has been developed for bone drilling in total hip replacement, revision hip replacement, and total knee replacement. The contact area achieved with Robodoc is 98% (or better). Robodoc is a computer-controlled mechanical arm capable of five degrees of freedom and force sensing in all axes.

- Robodoc functions in coordination with a preoperative planning station, Orthodoc (Integrated Surgical Systems). Orthodoc is a computer workstation that converts actual CT scan images of the patient to create a 3-D reconstruction of the joint to be replaced. Using computer modeling, the surgeon can choose the prosthesis (from a software library) with the best fit and can simulate the joint replacement (virtual surgery).

- CASPAR, CRIGOS, and the Loughborough manipulator are other computer-assisted robotic systems under development for different orthopedic applications that integrate image reconstruction and guidance.

Neurosurgery Robots

- The rigid structure of the skull and the delicateness of access to specific regions in the cranial cavity are suitable for the use of robots in neurosurgery to assist with image-guided, frameless neuronavigation.

- Minerva is a powered neurosurgery robot that functions under the guidance of a dedicated CT imaging system. Minerva, using specifically designed instruments loaded onto a rotary carrousel, can carry out an entire operation without assistance from the surgeon.

- NeuroMate (Integrated Surgical Systems) is a computer-assisted, image-guided device for stereotactic procedures in neurosurgery. Neuromate consists of a mechanical arm, an image-planning computer station, and a head stabilizer. Preoperatively, CT scan, MRI, or other images are correlated to the individual characteristics of the patient. During the operation, the robot moves and positions the instruments as programed preoperatively. The surgeon can manually drive instruments to preselected areas of the central nervous system using the fixture provided by the robot.

- PathFinder (Armstrong-Healthcare Ltd.) is a powered, image-guided robot for accurate positioning of stereotactic instruments. PathFinder consists of a planning workstation and a gyratory mechanical arm mounted on a wheeled trolley. The workstation accepts standard output formats from CT and MRI scanners and enables the surgeon to view and mark images to plan the path to a designated target within the brain; the preoperative planning also includes a demarcation of no-go zones for safety purposes.

- CyberKnife (Accuray) is a system for stereotactic radiosurgery composed of a computer-controlled robotic arm, a compact 6-MV linear accelerator, and an image guidance system. The linear accelerator is mounted on the robot arm, and the arm has six degrees of freedom. The maneuverability of the system enables for nonisocentric delivery of radiotherapy, thus limiting unwanted radiation of normal tissue. The imaging system (built into the treatment room) uses the body s skeletal structure and small implanted fiducial markers as a reference frame. The image guidance system uses preoperative CT or MR scans, along with intraoperative x-rays and video cameras, to register the target and monitor any movements of the patient; any displacement of the target is compensated by repositioning of the robot arm.

Urology Robots

- The prostate and the kidney are relatively fixed solid organs amenable for MIS.

- Transurethral resection of the prostate (TURP) is a good candidate procedure for automation to improve precision.

- Probot (Mechatronics in Medicine, Imperial College, London) is a powered, image-guided, computer-controlled robot for TURP. Probot moves in four axes to carry out TURP within the constraints of the prostate s size exclusively. The surgeon docks Probot to the patient and measures the length of the prostate under direct endoscopic visual cues. The prostate is then imaged using transurethral, thin-cut ultrasound scanning. In a computer station, the ultrasound images create a 3-D reconstruction of the prostate and the surgeon can specify the cavity to be cut. Probot carries out TURP by cutting tissue cones in a sequence of concentric rings, starting at the bladder neck and moving toward the verumontanum. The operation is completely performed by Probot under the supervision of the surgeon.

- The Remote Center of Motion (RCM) robot (Brady Urological Institute, Johns Hopkins University) was developed for percutaneous, radiologic access of the kidney, for MIS interventions and delivery of therapy. The device also has been referred to as the PAKY-RCM robot. The RCM robot is a three-module system consisting of the RCM unit, the PAKY unit, and a passive mechanical arm. The mechanical arm mounts on the operating table, confers seven degrees of freedom for positioning, and accommodates both the RCM and the PAKY units. The RCM unit has two degrees of freedom for motorized rotation in two planes (x and y directions) about the RCM point. The PAKY unit is a motorized needle driver that holds and inserts the trocar needle.

Master-Slave Robots

- Master-slave robots are powered, computer-controlled devices that do not perform autonomous tasks but are completely governed by the surgeon; thus, the surgeon is the master and the robot is the slave. The master surgeon is seated at a control console and the slave robotic arm is located at the surgical field over the patient.

- Master-slave robots are also called telemanipulators, implying that the master and the slave are separated from each other by a distance but communicated through data cables.

- At the console, the surgeon observes the surgical field on a video display and actuates his hands on mechanical transducers (masters or joysticks). The surgeon s motions are telecasted from the console to the robotic arms that, in turn, manipulate instruments (needle drivers, forceps, scissors) and the telescope. The surgeon s console also holds commands for special functions (e.g., focusing, motion scaling) and accessory equipment (e.g., electrosurgical and ultrasonic units).

- The separation between master and slave components may vary, from a few meters (e.g., inside the operating room) to several kilometers apart (e.g., transatlantic operation).

- Advantages of these systems include (1) the surgeon holds control of a stable camera-telescope platform, eliminating the dependence from a camera assistant; (2) the surgical field is presented to the surgeon in a 3-D display; (3) the robotic instruments have articulations near the tip that increase the degrees of freedom to function more like a human hand; (4) the computer eliminates hand tremor and the scale of motion is programmable; and (5) the console provides a more ergonomic operating position for the surgeon.

- Master-slave robots of today, however, have significant limitations: (1) the major drawback is the lack of tactile feedback and, therefore, the force applied in tissue dissection and suturing must rely on visual cues exclusively; (2) there is a scant number of instruments available; and (3) the hardware is extremely bulky and heavy and clutters the operating room easily.

- da Vinci robotic surgical system (Intuitive Surgical). da Vinci gives a true 3-D view of the surgical field by using a dual-lens, three-chip digital camera system. The dual-lens system is bundled into one large telescope. Each camera transmits to separate cathode ray tube (CRT) screens located inside the console, and each screen projects separately to an individual eye (i.e., binocular system). At the surgeon s console, the binocular viewer is anatomically aligned with the position of the masters (i.e., the hands). Such an arrangement creates the feeling of being immersed into the surgical field, much like in open surgery. Both the instruments and the telescope are driven via the masters, switching control from one to the other with the press of a clutch. The robotic arms of the da Vinci system are floor mounted; therefore, the patient cannot be moved after the robotic arms become attached to the cannulas. Both thoracic and abdominal operations have been performed with da Vinci.

- Zeus robotic surgical system (Computer Motion). Zeus produces 3-D views of the field by merging right and left video frames (from right and left cameras) over a single video monitor fitted with an active matrix and polarizing filters. The broadcast alternates between right and left frames that synchronize with clockwise or counterclockwise polarization filters, respectively. The surgeon wears glasses fitted with different polarizing filters, a clockwise filter for the right eye and a counterclockwise filter for the left eye. This causes the right eye to see right video frames only and the left eye to see left video frames only. The telescope is driven by a voice-activation system. The robotic arms are mounted on the operating table; therefore, it is possible to change the patient s position without undocking the robot. Thoracic and abdominal operations have been performed with Zeus.

- Advanced Robotics and Telemanipulator System for Minimally Invasive Surgery (ARTEMIS) (Karlsruhe Research Center). ARTEMIS consists of two master-slave units for manipulation of surgical instruments and a guiding system for a 3-D endoscope. ARTEMIS is still a project under development for both abdominal and thoracic MIS.

Robotic Abdominal Surgery

- Both da Vinci and Zeus have been successfully used for interventions in general surgery, gynecology, and urology.
- Operations described in general surgery include cholecystectomy, antireflux procedures, Heller s cardiomyotomy, distal pancreatectomy, gastrojejunostomy, esophagectomy, gastric bypass, gastric banding, pyloroplasty, colectomy, adrenalectomy, and splenectomy.
- Pediatric operations include Thal fundoplication, Nissen fundoplication, cholecystectomy, and salpingo-oophorectomy.
- Operations in gynecologic include hysterectomy and tubal reanastomosis.
- Urologic procedures include donor nephrectomy, nephrectomy for pathology, radical prostatectomy, and pelvic lymph node dissection.

Robotic Cardiothoracic Surgery

- Significant morbidity results from the median sternotomy used for access (e.g., thoracic cage deformation and fractures, pain, prolonged rehabilitation time, large amount of blood loss, ventilatory problems, sternitis, and mediastinitis) and from the cardiopulmonary bypass (CPB) needed to obtain a stable and dry operative field (e.g., hemolysis; complement activation; immunosuppression; and impairments of visual, memory, and intellectual functions, among others).
- Cardiothoracic MIS (CT-MIS) techniques have been developed to improve on both the access and the dependence of CPB.
- A high-resolution videoscope introduced into the chest can reach targets and replace or even improve over the classical open exposures; for instance, the 10× to 20× optic magnification capable by the digital videocamera is more powerful than the typical 2.5× to 3× magnification provided by conventional surgical glasses.
- 3-D video displays have been refined that eliminate the lack of depth perception given by the conventional 2-D videoscopic systems.
- Current digital technology has made totally endoscopic and closed-chest cardiothoracic operations a reality. Robot-assisted CT-MIS has been performed since 1998; the procedures include repair of atrial septal defect, repair or replacement of mitral valve, and coronary artery bypass.

- The complexity of CT-MIS has been divided into four levels. In Level I CT-MIS or direct-vision/mini-incision approach, the procedure is performed under direct vision through small incisions by conventional means (e.g., Limited Anterior Small Thoracotomy [LAST] and Minimally Invasive Direct Coronary Artery Bypass [MIDCAB]). In Level II CT-MIS or video-assisted/microincision approach, a videoscope is passed through the incision to function as secondary visual aid for portions of the operation (e.g., mitral valve surgery and internal mammary artery [IMA] harvest). An intracardiac minicamera can be used to aid with lighting and to close-up on anatomic details. In Level III CT-MIS or video-directed/port-incision approach, most of the operation is conducted videoscopically and instruments are passed through operative ports. A helmet-mounted 3-D videoscopic system (Vista Medical Technologies, Becton, MA) driven by an assistant or docked to an AESOP mechanic arm has been used successfully to improve on visualization and dexterity. This video-directed/port-incision technique has been used in mitral valve surgery with outcomes that challenge the conventional open approach but achieving faster recovery times and significant cost savings. Level IV or video-directed—robot-assisted approach represents the current cutting-edge of CT-MIS; at this level of technologic sophistication and skill, complex procedures are performed through port incisions only using 3-D video-displays and robotic articulated micro-instruments (e.g., de Bakey forceps, Potts scissors, micro clips).
- Surgical robots have been used for heart valve surgery, dissection of the IMA, anastomosis of coronary bypass grafting, and correction of atrial septal defect; both the da Vinci and Zeus systems have been used in various phases of development of these procedures.
- The culprit of CT-MIS is the totally endoscopic coronary artery bypass or TECAB where both conduit preparation (IMA) and anastomosis for a single- or two-vessel disease are completed through a three-port operation.
- Alternatives to conventional CPB that have been developed to permit closed chest CT surgery.
- The Port-Access (Heartport, Redwood City, CA) is a device for femoro-femoral CPB and endovascular balloon clamping of the aorta. The Heartport system allows for antegrade and retrograde perfusion for systemic and coronary circulation. The Heartport technology has been used for videoscopic valve surgery and coronary bypass.

- Off-pump or beating-heart technique has been used in coronary artery bypass. For this purpose a myocardial stabilizer (e.g., Genzyme, Intuitive Surgical) is deployed over the target coronary artery to be anastomosed. Off-pump TECAB with bilateral IMA harvest for single- and double-vessel coronary disease has been performed.
- In summary, robotic technology has the great promise to expand the spectrum of MIS not only on the technical aspects of surgery but also in areas such as training and telesurgery. To this point, however, all the studies have documented and proven the feasibility and safety of these emerging technologies as used under ideal conditions. Although early results are encouraging, the cost-effectiveness of robotic technology has not yet been established.

CHAPTER 19

MANAGEMENT OF ACUTE TRAUMA

INTRODUCTION

● Trauma is a major worldwide public health problem. It is one of the leading causes of death and disability in both industrialized and developing countries.

Mortality Following Traumatic Injury

● Trauma deaths occur at traditionally recognized time points after injury (Fig. 19–1).

Access and Emergency Medical System (EMS) Response

● The vital components of prehospital care include committed medical control, established lines of communication,

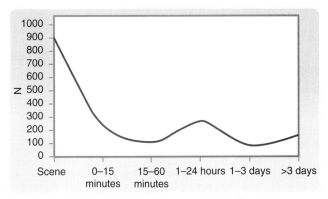

■ **FIGURE 19–1.** Trimodal distribution of death. The time to mortality for a population of trauma patients admitted to a single trauma center from a unified geographic area over a 10-year period is shown above. All deaths at the scene and hospital deaths are included. *(From Resources for Optimal Care of the Injured Patient: 1999. Chicago, Committee on Trauma, American College of Surgeons, 1999.)*

tested triage criteria, effective transportation, and a cadre of prehospital providers well trained in specific field intervention.

Triage

- The goal of civilian prehospital triage is to identify high-risk injured patients who would benefit from the resources available in a trauma center.
- Perhaps the most useful currently available system is that advocated by the Committee on Trauma of the American College of Surgeons, which assesses four components simultaneously: physiologic response, injury anatomy, injury biomechanics, and comorbid factors (Fig. 19–2).

Prehospital Care

- The principles of prehospital care of the trauma victim are (1) securing the area, (2) determining the need for emergency treatment, (3) initiating treatment according to protocols for medical direction, (4) communicating with medical control, and (5) rapid transfer of the patient to a trauma center.

Transportation

- The best method for transportation depends on the patient's condition, distance to the regional trauma center, accessibility of the scene, and weather conditions.

Hospital Care

- Trauma center care consists of care provided in the emergency department, the operating room (OR), the intensive care unit, and the floor and may extend even to rehabilitation in some hospitals.
- The importance of predesignated "trauma team" members with assigned duties cannot be overemphasized. Equally important is the team leader who accepts the responsibility of leadership and is responsible for making overall assessment and management decisions.

The Surgeon's Role in a Trauma System

- It is essential for the surgeon to maintain active involvement in the initial resuscitation and to prioritize and orchestrate

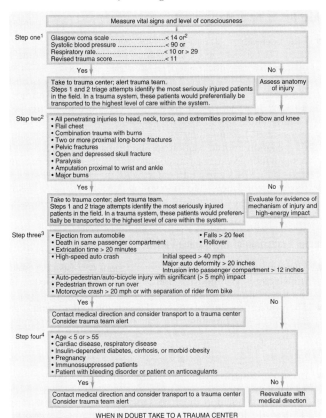

| Measure vital signs and level of consciousness |

Step one[1]

| Glasgow coma scale ....< 14 or[2]
Systolic blood pressure ....< 90 or
Respiratory rate.....................................< 10 or > 29
Revised trauma score.............................< 11 |

Yes ↓   No ↓

| Take to trauma center; alert trauma team.
Steps 1 and 2 triage attempts identify the most seriously injured patients
in the field. In a trauma system, these patients would preferentially be
transported to the highest level of care within the system. | Assess anatomy
of injury |

Step two[2]

| • All penetrating injuries to head, neck, torso, and extremities proximal to elbow and knee
• Flail chest
• Combination trauma with burns
• Two or more proximal long-bone fractures
• Pelvic fractures
• Open and depressed skull fracture
• Paralysis
• Amputation proximal to wrist and ankle
• Major burns |

Yes ↓   No ↓

| Take to trauma center; alert trauma team.
Steps 1 and 2 triage attempts identify the most seriously injured
patients in the field. In a trauma system, these patients would preferen-
tially be transported to the highest level of care within the system. | Evaluate for evidence of
mechanism of injury and
high-energy impact |

Step three[3]

| • Ejection from automobile   • Falls > 20 feet
• Death in same passenger compartment   • Rollover
• Extrication time > 20 minutes
• High-speed auto crash   Initial speed > 40 mph
                  Major auto deformity > 20 inches
                  Intrusion into passenger compartment > 12 inches
• Auto-pedestrian/auto-bicycle injury with significant (> 5 mph) impact
• Pedestrian thrown or run over
• Motorcycle crash > 20 mph or with separation of rider from bike |

Yes ↓   No ↓

| Contact medical direction and consider transport to a trauma center
Consider trauma team alert |

Step four[4]

| • Age < 5 or > 55
• Cardiac disease, respiratory disease
• Insulin-dependent diabetes, cirrhosis, or morbid obesity
• Pregnancy
• Immunossuppressed patients
• Patient with bleeding disorder or patient on anticoagulants |

Yes ↓   No ↓

| Contact medical direction and consider transport to a trauma center
Consider trauma team alert | Reevaluate with
medical direction |

WHEN IN DOUBT TAKE TO A TRAUMA CENTER

■ FIGURE 19–2. American College of Surgeons (ACS) field triage algorithm.

the sequence of evaluation and management of complex injuries.

INITIAL MANAGEMENT

● The thoughtful and accurate ordering of diagnostic and therapeutic interventions is critical to provide the optimal outcome and is perhaps the most important task of the trauma surgeon.

Priorities in Initial Management

- The necessity to balance various conflicting priorities and accurately direct the initial diagnosis and treatment requires an approach to the patient as a whole not as an isolated organ system. The overall management of the patient is best directed by one person, who has the experience and authority to make difficult immediate decisions under stressful circumstances.
- In general, establishing a patent airway with adequate oxygenation and ventilation are the primary concerns during resuscitation. Next, the physiologic stabilization of the patient and control of significant hemorrhage must be addressed.
- Once immediately life-threatening problems have been controlled, management of possible brain injury is the next priority.

Initial Evaluation of the Trauma Patient

- The initial evaluation of the trauma patient consists of a rapid primary survey, aimed at identifying and treating immediately life-threatening problems.
- The primary survey is conducted according to the mnemonic ABCDE: airway, breathing, circulation, disability, and exposure.

Airway

- In most patients, this is accomplished by endotracheal intubation.
- Excessive ventilation must be avoided following intubation particularly in the hypovolemic patient because excessive ventilation will increase mean intra-thoracic pressures and compromise cardiac filling.
- Indications for a surgical airway include massive maxillofacial trauma, anatomic distortion resulting from neck injury, and inability to visualize the vocal cords because of the presence of blood, secretions, or airway edema.

Breathing

- Inspection, palpation, and auscultation of the chest will demonstrate the presence of normal, symmetric ventilatory effort and adequate bilateral tidal exchange. A supine antero-posterior (AP) chest radiograph is the primary diagnostic adjunct, demonstrating chest wall, pulmonary parenchymal, and pleural abnormalities.

- Serial measurement of arterial blood gases should be used to monitor patients who are at risk and to assist in appropriate adjustment of the ventilator.
- There is also a body of evidence that suggests that hyperventilation may be detrimental to cerebral perfusion, accentuating the need for accuracy in ventilator management and vigilance in monitoring pH and $Paco_2$.

Circulation

- The primary goal is the identification and control of the hemorrhage. External hemorrhage is controlled by direct pressure on the wound, while the possibility of hemorrhage into the chest, abdomen, or pelvis is rapidly assessed.
- While steps are being taken to control hemorrhage, at least two large-bore intravenous lines should be placed to allow fluid resuscitation.
- Fluid resuscitation begins with a 1000-mL bolus of lactated Ringer's solution for an adult or 20 mL/kg for a child.
- If there is no response or only transient response to the initial bolus, a second bolus should be given. If ongoing resuscitation is required after two boluses, it is likely that transfusion will be required, and blood should be initiated early.
- The clinician must be vigilant for possible causes of hypotension that require immediate intervention during the primary survey, such as pericardial tamponade or tension pneumothorax.
- Needle catheter decompression can be done with relative impunity, even bilaterally, in patients who are intubated and on positive pressure ventilation.

Disability

- Level of consciousness measured by the Glasgow Coma Scale (GCS) score (Table 19–1), pupillary response, and movement of extremities are evaluated and recorded.

Exposure

- The final step in the primary survey is to completely undress the patient and do a rapid head-to-toe examination to identify any injuries to the back, perineum, or other areas that are not easily seen in the supine, clothed position.
- This secondary survey is often done in a head-to-toe manner, and includes ordering and collecting data from appropriate laboratory and radiologic tests.

TABLE 19–1. The Glasgow Coma Scale

Eye Opening

No response	1
To painful stimulus	2
To verbal stimulus	3
Spontaneous	4

Best Verbal Response

No response	1
Incomprehensible sounds	2
Inappropriate words	3
Disoriented, inappropriate content	4
Oriented and appropriate	5

Best Motor Response

No response	1
Abnormal extension (decerebrate posturing)	2
Abnormal flexion (decorticate posturing)	3
Withdrawal	4
Purposeful movement	5
Obeys commands	6
Total	**3–15**

● It is very important for the physician to return and perform a tertiary survey, which is another complete head-to-toe physical examination aimed at identifying injuries that may have escaped notice in the first several hours.

MANAGEMENT OF SPECIFIC INJURIES

Head Injury

● Traumatic brain injury (TBI) is the leading cause of death in trauma patients and is responsible for more than 50% of all traumatic deaths.

Resuscitative Priorities

● Secondary TBI is primarily due to cerebral ischemia. Hypotension and hypoxemia have proven to be the most significant factors leading to a poor neurologic outcome or death. Hypotension appears to be the more deleterious than hypoxemia and in one study resulted in a twofold increase in the mortality from closed head injuries.
● In patients with severe brain injury the airway should be secured immediately, taking care to remember that spinal

cord injury is present in as many as 10% of head injury patients.

Assessment of Injury Severity

- The severity of brain injury can be rapidly estimated by determining the level of consciousness and presence or absence of lateralizing signs of central nervous system dysfunction, including pupillary changes and motor findings.
- The GCS is based on an evaluation of eye opening, best motor response, and verbal response (Table 19–1).
- Signs of central nervous system dysfunction that are unilateral or asymmetric, so-called lateralizing signs, are highly suggestive of focal intracranial lesions that may require surgical intervention.
- It is essential to obtain a computed tomography (CT) scan of the head as rapidly as possible to ensure accurate localization of the lesion.

Definitive Management Strategy

- Evidence-based guidelines for the management of severe head injury were published in 1995 and revised in 2000. Institutions that adhere to these guidelines and are aggressive in their management principles may have better outcomes than those institutions with a more empiric approach.
- Patients with focal intracranial pathology that is causing significant mass effect require urgent surgical evacuation of the mass lesion. The outcome in these patients is improved by rapid decompression; therefore, time is of the essence.
- Therapy is directed at two major goals. First is general supportive care of the patient, maintenance of pulmonary and cardiovascular function to provide adequate oxygen delivery, treatment of infection, and early use of enteral nutrition. The second goal of treatment is to optimize cerebral perfusion, which is primarily achieved through control of intracranial pressure (ICP).

Vertebrae and Spinal Cord

- Despite this low incidence, spinal cord injuries are often devastating in both socioeconomic and psychological impact.

Resuscitative Priorities

- High cervical spinal injuries can result in acute ventilatory decompensation resulting from loss of phrenic nerve function (roots C3 to C5) and intercostal muscle function (primarily thoracic roots).

- High spinal cord injuries also can result in systemic hypotension because of loss of sympathetic tone.
- The essential priority in initial care of patients with potential spinal cord injury is to maintain strict immobilization of the entire spine.
- The lower portion of the cervical spine is often difficult to visualize well on lateral views, especially in large patients. If the region of C7 to T1 is not visualized, there is potential for dramatic missed injury.

Assessment of Injury Severity

- If the injury appears to be complete, the presence of spinal cord reflexes, especially the sacral reflexes, yields important prognostic information. After acute spinal cord injury, a transient phenomenon known as "spinal shock" is seen, in which all cord function is absent below the level of injury. The affected muscle groups are flaccid and are flexic.
- The second pattern of spinal cord injury is the incomplete injury. Under these circumstances, the patient will exhibit some sensory and motor function below the level of injury.
- Most common is the central cord syndrome. A patient with central cord syndrome will present with motor weakness and sensory loss primarily involving the distal muscles of the upper extremity.
- A second clinical syndrome is the Brown-Sequard syndrome, anatomically interesting but uncommon in clinical practice.
- The assessment of the severity of injury to the spinal column itself is independent of the nature and type of spinal cord injury. The primary question that must be answered is one of stability.
- CT of the spine, and more recently magnetic resonance imaging (MRI), provide much better detail of bony and ligamentous structures, respectively. These more detailed studies should be used whenever there is a suspicion of injury on plain radiographs.

Definitive Care

- General support of the patient's cardiovascular function is important to optimize spinal cord perfusion and prevent ischemic secondary injury.
- Therefore, decompressive surgery is unlikely to be of benefit in complete lesions and is rarely done.

- The need for surgical intervention for the injury to the spinal column itself is dictated by the degree of deformity and the perceived stability of the injury. Displaced fractures of the cervical spine are usually treated with careful application of traction, using a halo or Gardner-Wells.
- Unstable injuries usually require surgical stabilization. Stabilization can be achieved by placement of hardware posteriorly, by use of hardware and bone grafting anteriorly or in some cases using both techniques simultaneously.

Neck Injuries

- Because of the high likelihood of injury to the airway or major blood vessels, accurate and aggressive initial evaluation and treatment are required to optimize outcome.
- The major vascular and aerodigestive structures in the neck are located in the anterior triangle, and all are deep to the platysma.
- Injuries that do not penetrate the platysma can be considered superficial, and no further investigation is needed. Wounds that penetrate the platysma must be further evaluated. Injuries that are anterior to the sternocleidomastoid present a high likelihood of significant injury, whereas those that track posterior to the sternocleidomastoid are unlikely to involve major vascular or aerodigestive injury.
- In analyzing wounds based on cranio-caudad location, the neck is commonly divided into three horizontal zones (Fig. 19–3). Zone I is the thoracic inlet.
- Zone II is the mid portion of the neck.
- Zone III extends from the angle of the mandible to the base of the skull.

Resuscitative Priorities

Assessment of Injury Severity

- Patients with overt clinical signs of vascular or aerodigestive tract injury require surgical exploration of the neck.
- Significant controversy exists regarding the optimal approach to patients with injuries that penetrate the platysma but who exhibit no suspicious clinical findings. One school of thought favors mandatory surgical exploration for all penetrating injuries, citing a low rate of complications and the potentially devastating effect of delay in diagnosis of aerodigestive tract injuries. The second school of thought favors selective exploration based either on the results of extensive

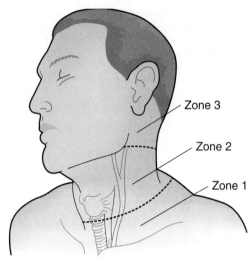

■ FIGURE 19–3. Zones of the neck. The border between Zone 1 and Zone 2 is at the level of the cricoid cartilage. The border between Zone 2 and Zone 3 is at the angle of the mandible. These zones are primarily useful in management of injuries in the anterior triangles of the neck.

evaluation including angiography, esophagoscopy, and esophagography or on progression of clinical symptoms.
- Current data show similar outcome for both approaches and do not favor one approach over the other.

Definitive Therapy

Technique of Neck Exploration

- Whether one adopts a policy of mandatory or selective exploration for penetrating injuries of the neck, once a decision to operate has been made, the approach is the same. From a strategic point of view it is important to remember that the goal is to explore the structures of the neck to identify injuries, not to explore the wound per se.

Vascular Injuries

Airway Injuries

- Penetrating injuries to the airway are either clinically overt, with bubbling and air movement through the wound, or they are found at the time of neck exploration done for other indications.

Pharynx and Esophagus

● Injuries of the esophagus present a difficult problem. If early diagnosis is made, primary surgical repair is usually possible. If the diagnosis is delayed for more than 12 hours, primary repair may be impractical, leaving diversion and drainage as the only alternative.

Nerve Injury

● There are many important nerves that run through the neck and are at risk, both from the primary injury and from operative attempts to repair the primary injury. It is important to document a full neurologic examination before operative intervention, including cranial nerve function, vocal cord function, and peripheral nerve function, whenever possible.

Maxillofacial Injuries

● Most maxillofacial injuries do not present with initial threat to life, and definitive evaluation and care are often deferred in patients with multiple injuries.

Resuscitative Priorities

● Severe maxillofacial injuries have the potential to lead to airway obstruction, either as a direct result of anatomic derangement or secondarily resulting from the presence of blood and debris in the upper airway.

Evaluation of Injury Severity

● The diagnosis of facial fractures is now largely done through the use of CT. CT scan of the face is far more accurate than plain radiographs in determining the presence and significance of fractures of the facial bones.
● Fractures of the maxilla are classified according to a system proposed by Le Forte in 1901. There are three types, Le Fort I, II, or III, determined by the type and location of fractures.
● Fractures of the mandible are also classified by anatomic location. The need for surgical intervention and its nature are determined by the type and location of the fracture; thus, complete radiographic evaluation is important.

Definitive Care

Facial Fractures

- Operative repair of facial fractures is usually undertaken for one of two indications, either to restore function or to improve cosmetic outcome. Fractures that can cause significant functional impairment are listed in Box 19–1.

Facial Lacerations

- It is important to determine if deeper structures are at risk and to identify any such injuries before closure of the laceration.

Ocular Injuries

- The presence of ocular trauma mandates a thorough examination of the structural and functional components of the eye.
- A functional eye examination includes visual acuity, papillary response, and assessment of extraocular eye movements.
- Simple lacerations to the corneal, lens, or anterior chamber may be repaired using microsurgical techniques. Rupture of the globe requires débridement and suture repair.

Thoracic Trauma

- Thoracic injuries account for 20% to 25% of all trauma-related deaths, and complications of chest trauma contribute to another 25% of all deaths.
- Most thoracic injuries are managed with simple procedures such as clinical observation, thoracentesis, respiratory support, and adequate analgesia. The remaining 15% to 20% of

---

Box 19–1. Facial Fractures of Functional Significance	
Fracture Type	**Functional Impairment**
Blowout fracture of muscles inferior orbital floor	Entrapment of extra-ocular muscles
Maxilla, alveolar ridge	Malocclusion
Mandible	Malocclusion
Depressed zygomatic arch fracture	Entrapment of temporalis muscle

patients sustaining chest trauma will require a thoracotomy for definitive repair of major intrathoracic injuries.

Pathophysiology

Initial Evaluation

- The initial evaluation of a patient sustaining chest trauma follows the same principles and guidelines outlined by the advanced trauma life support (ATLS) course.
- The chest x-ray film is of the utmost importance in thoracic trauma.
- With the development of the helical scanners, CT has been used more liberally in the evaluation of chest trauma and some authors have recommended its routine use despite the results of plain chest x-ray films.

Tube Thoracostomy

- Tube thoracostomy is the most common procedure performed in the management of thoracic trauma. In fact, 85% of the patients sustaining chest injuries will require only clinical observation or tube thoracostomy.

Thoracotomy

Specific Injuries

Rib Fractures

- One or two rib fractures without pleural or lung involvement are usually treated on an outpatient basis. However, in the elderly, because of decreased bone density, reduced chest wall compliance, and increased incidence of underlying parenchymal disease, rib fractures may lead to decreased ability to cough, reduced vital capacity, and infectious complications.

Flail Chest

- Flail chest occurs in 10% to 15% of patients sustaining major chest trauma, and the chance of having an intrathoracic injury in this situation increases several fold.
- It is now understood that underlying pulmonary contusion and pain during inspiration are the most important components in the pathophysiology of respiratory failure (Fig. 19–4).

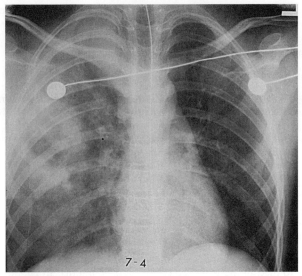

7 - 4

■ FIGURE 19–4. Chest x-ray film showing a pulmonary contusion.

Sternal Fractures

Pulmonary Contusion

● Management is directed toward maintaining good oxygenation and adequate pulmonary toilet. Judicious crystalloid infusion is important to avoid fluid overload and pulmonary edema; however, intravascular volume depletion also should be avoided to decrease the risk of global ischemia and multiple organ failure.

Pneumothorax

● Clinical findings suggestive of a pneumothorax include decreased breath sounds, hyperresonance to percussion, and decreased expansion of the affected lung during inspiration.
● A tension pneumothorax is characterized by complete lung collapse, tracheal deviation, mediastinal shift leading to decreased venous return to the heart, hypotension, and respiratory distress.

Open Pneumothorax

- Open pneumothorax, also known as sucking chest wound, occurs when there is a significant defect in the chest wall (e.g., large-caliber gunshot wounds, traumatic thoracotomy) large enough to exceed the laryngeal cross-sectional area, allowing the air to enter from the exterior into the pleural cavity and leading to lung collapse because of a rapid equilibration between the intrathoracic (pleural) pressure and the atmospheric pressure.

Hemothorax

- The pleural space can accumulate up to 3 L of blood. Massive hemothorax is usually the result of major pulmonary vascular injury or major arterial wounds, whereas minor lung injuries cause small hemothorax.
- Hemothoraces are initially treated by chest tube placement (36-French tube), and in approximately 85% of the cases, the bleeding will stop as the lung is re-expanded because of the low pressure in the systemic circulation.
- As previously described, indications for emergent thoracotomy are initial chest tube output of 1,500 mL of blood or persistent drainage of 200 to 300 mL/hour.

Pulmonary Parenchyma Injury

- Massive hemorrhage from extensive lung injuries can be treated by oversewing or stapling the wound or, more rarely, by performing wedging or lobar resections.

Tracheobronchial Injuries

- Patients may present with pneumothorax, massive air leak, subcutaneous emphysema, hemoptysis, pneumomediastinum, and respiratory distress. Bronchoscopy is always required if one of the previously listed signs is present and should be performed, ideally, before intubation.

Blunt Cardiac Injuries

- Myocardial contusion may occur in less severe chest trauma. Its definition, diagnosis, clinical significance, and management are still subject to debate.
- The combination of electrocardiogram (ECG) and troponin (TnI) at admission and 8 hours after injury rules out the

diagnosis of significant blunt cardiac injury. Patients with normal tests at both time points can be safely discharged from the hospital.

Penetrating Cardiac Injuries

- All patients with penetrating injuries within an area determined by the midclavicular line bilaterally, a line at the level of the clavicles superiorly, and a line at the level of the costal margins inferiorly potentially have a cardiac injury until proven otherwise.
- Diagnosis usually is made by echocardiography, identifying abnormal amounts of pericardial fluid, or more accurately by performing a subxiphoid pericardia window.
- Pericardial tamponade must be suspected in all patients sustaining penetrating injuries to the anterior chest. Classic signs of pericardial tamponade include muffled heart tones, distended neck veins, and hypotension, also known as the Beck's triad.

Diaphragmatic Injuries

- Patients sustaining penetrating injuries below the nipples and above the costal margins should be investigated to rule out diaphragmatic injury.
- Following blunt trauma, injury to the diaphragm involves both sides equally, as reported in autopsy and CT scan studies, although in clinical practice, left-sided injuries are more frequent.
- Acute diaphragmatic rupture is usually repaired through a midline abdominal incision because of the increased incidence of associated intra-abdominal injuries.

Esophageal Injuries

- The diagnosis is confirmed with esophagography and esophagoscopy. These tests have a reported sensitivity varying from 50% to 90%.
- Delay in diagnosis of traumatic esophageal injuries is accompanied by high morbidity and mortality rates.
- Treatment consists of early débridement, primary repair, and drainage if identified within 24 hours after injury. Injuries diagnosed after 24 hours with mediastinal contamination are treated by cervical esophagostomy and distal feeding access.

Transmediastinal Gunshot Wounds

- Hemodynamically unstable patients are treated with exploratory thoracotomy and the diagnosis of specific injuries will be made during the operation. Hemodynamically stable patients can be evaluated by multiple diagnostic modalities and significant controversy remains regarding the best methods and the most appropriate sequence of tests used.
- More recently, contrast-enhanced CT scan has been used as a screening modality to determine the trajectory of the projectile, to identify specific injuries, and to determine the need of further evaluation by other diagnostic modalities.

Abdominal Trauma

Introduction

- Several diagnostic modalities evolved during the last three decades including diagnostic peritoneal lavage (DPL), ultrasound (US), CT, and laparoscopy, all of them with advantages, disadvantages, and limitations.

Mechanism of Injury

Diagnosis

- We consider that an objective abdominal evaluation is necessary and should be obtained by using any of the available diagnostic modalities in addition to the physical examination. The test of choice will depend on the hemodynamic stability of the patient and the severity of associated injuries.
- Hemodynamically stable patients sustaining blunt trauma are adequately evaluated by an abdominal US or CT scan, unless other severe injuries take priority and the patient must go to the OR before the objective abdominal evaluation. In such instances, a DPL is usually performed in the OR to rule out intra-abdominal injury requiring an immediate surgical exploration.
- Blunt trauma patients with hemodynamic instability should be evaluated by US in the resuscitation room, if available, or by DPL to rule out intra-abdominal injuries as the source of blood loss and hypotension.
- Patients with isolated penetrating abdominal trauma who are admitted hypotensive, in shock, or with peritoneal signs should go to the OR despite the mechanism of injury. Stab wound (SW) victims without peritoneal signs, evisceration,

or hypotension benefit from wound exploration and DPL. Gunshot wound (GSW) victims generally should be explored.

Plain Radiographs

Diagnostic Peritoneal Lavage

- Standard criteria for a positive DPL include aspiration of at least 10 mL of gross blood; a bloody lavage effluent; a red blood cell count greater than 100,000/mm³; a white blood cell count greater than 500/mm³; an amylase greater than 175 IU/dL; or the detection of bile, bacteria, or food fibers.
- DPL results can be misleading in the presence of a pelvic fracture. False-positive results are expected because of bleeding from the retroperitoneum into the peritoneal cavity. Anterior abdominal and flank wounds can be accurately evaluated by DPL. False-positive results are frequent following DPL resulting from bleeding of the abdominal wall, increasing the number of negative explorations. Another potential disadvantage of DPL is the low accuracy in the diagnosis of hollow viscus injuries.

Ultrasound

- The advantages and disadvantages of abdominal US are listed in Box 19–2. The sensitivity ranges from 85% to 99% and the specificity from 97% to 100%.

Box 19–2.　Advantages and Disadvantages of Ultrasound

Advantages
Noninvasive
Does not require radiation
Useful in the resuscitation room or emergency department
Can be repeated
Used during initial evaluation
Low cost

Disadvantages
Examiner dependent
Obesity
Gas interposition
Lower sensitivity for free fluid <500 mL
False-negatives: retroperitoneal and hollow viscus injuries

Box 19–3. Indications and Contraindications for Abdominal Computed Tomography

Indications
Blunt trauma
Hemodynamic stability
Normal or unreliable physical examination
Mechanism: duodenal and pancreatic trauma

Contraindications
Clear indication for exploratory laparotomy
Hemodynamic instability
Agitation
Allergy to contrast media

Abdominal Computed Tomography Scan

- CT scan is the most frequently used method to evaluate the stable blunt abdominal trauma patient. The retroperitoneum is best evaluated by CT scan. The indications and contraindications of abdominal CT scan are listed in Box 19–3.
- The most important disadvantage of CT scan is its inability to reliably diagnose hollow viscus injury (Box 19–4).
- The accuracy of CT scan ranges from 92% to 98% with low false-positive and false-negative rates.

Box 19–4. Advantages and Disadvantages of Abdominal Computed Tomography

Advantages
Adequate assessment of the retroperitoneum
Nonoperative management of solid organ injuries
Assessment of renal perfusion
Noninvasive
High specificity

Disadvantages
Specialized personnel
Hardware
Duration: helical vs. conventional
Hollow viscus injuries
Cost

Other Diagnostic Modalities

Gastric Injuries

- Gastric injuries often result from penetrating trauma.
- Most penetrating wounds are treated by means of débride-ment of the wound edges and primary closure in layers. Injuries with major tissue loss may be best treated by gastric resection.
- Because of its proximity with the diaphragm, the stomach is frequently injured following thoracoabdominal wounds.

Injuries to the Duodenum

- The incidence of duodenal injuries varies from 3% to 5%. Most of duodenal injuries are accompanied by other intra-abdominal injuries. This occurs because of its close anatomic relationship with other solid organs and major vessels.
- Failure to recognize this injury is associated with the devel-opment of intra-abdominal abscesses, sepsis, and high mortality rates.
- Definitive diagnosis requires a Gastrografin upper gastroin-testinal (GI) series or CT scan of the abdomen with oral and intravenous contrast in the hemodynamically stable patient. Extravasation of contrast material is an absolute indication for laparotomy.
- The appropriate repair of duodenal injuries depends on injury severity (Table 19–2) and elapsed time from injury to treatment.

Pancreatic Injuries

- Major abdominal vascular injuries are present in more than 75% of cases of penetrating pancreatic trauma, and injuries to the solid organs and hollow viscus are common following blunt trauma.
- The diagnosis of a pancreatic injury with the use of newer generation CT scanners has improved significantly; however, some injuries may be identified only during follow-up scans obtained for changes in the clinical status.
- The presence of a pancreatic duct injury appears to be an essential factor in postoperative morbidity.
- Pancreatic injuries are divided into proximal or distal accord-ing to the location on the right or left of the superior mesen-teric vessels. The classification of pancreatic injuries according to injury severity is described in Table 19–3.

TABLE 19-2. Duodenum Injury Scale

Grade*	Type of Injury	Description of Injury
I	Hematoma	Involving single portion of duodenum
	Laceration	Partial thickness, no perforation
II	Hematoma	Involving more than one portion
	Laceration	Disruption <50% of circumference
III	Laceration	Disruption 50%–75% of circumference of D2
		Disruption 50%–100% of circumference of D1, D3, D4
IV	Laceration	Disruption >75% of circumference of D2 involving ampulla or distal common bile duct
V	Laceration	Massive disruption of duodenopancreatic complex
	Vascular	Devascularization of duodenum

*Advance one grade for multiple injuries up to grade III. D1, first position of duodenum; D2, second portion of duodenum; D3, third portion of duodenum; D4, fourth portion of duodenum.
From Moore EE, Cogbill TH, Malangoni MA, et al: Organ injury scaling: II. Pancreas, duodenum, small bowel, colon, and rectum. J Trauma 30:1427–1429, 1990, with permission.

● Penetrating wounds to the right of the superior mesenteric vein should be treated with débridement and direct suture ligation of areas of bleeding.

Small Intestine Injuries

● Several tests may help in the diagnosis of blunt intestinal trauma in patients without a clear indication for surgical exploration.

TABLE 19-3. Pancreas Injury Scale

Grade*	Type of Injury	Description of Injury
I	Hematoma	Minor contusion without duct injury
	Laceration	Superficial laceration without duct injury
II	Hematoma	Major contusion without duct injury or tissue loss
	Laceration	Major laceration without duct injury or tissue loss
III	Laceration	Distal transaction or parenchymal injury with duct injury
IV	Laceration	Proximal transaction or parenchymal injury involving ampulla†
V	Laceration	Massive disruption of pancreatic head

*Advance one grade for multiple injuries up to grade III. II631.51, 863.91—head; 863.99, 862.92—body; 863.83, 863.93—tail.
†Proximal pancreas is to the patient's right of the superior mesenteric vein.
From Moore EE, Cogbill TH, Malangoni MA, et al: Organ injury scaling: II. Pancreas, duodenum, small bowel, colon, and rectum. J Trauma 30:1427–1429, 1990, with permission.

● At laparotomy, a careful examination of the entire small bowel should be performed. Bleeding should be initially controlled and clamps or sutures should be applied to prevent further leakage of intestinal contents into the peritoneal cavity. Penetrating injuries caused by firearms should be débrided, and usually small tears are closed primarily. If two adjacent holes are found, they can be connected across the bridge of normal bowel and closed transversally to avoid narrowing of the intestinal lumen. Extensive lacerations, devascularized segments, or multiple lacerations in a short segment of bowel are better treated by resection and reanastomosis. All mesenteric hematomas should be explored because these can hide small bowel injuries.

Injuries to the Colon

● Colon injuries are usually the result of penetrating trauma. The colon is the second most frequently injured organ following gunshot wounds and the third following stab wounds to the abdomen.
● The operative management of colonic injury is still controversial.
● Primary repair can be selected when known associated complicating factors have been excluded. General criteria for primary repair include early diagnosis (within 4 to 6 hours), absence of prolonged shock or hypotension, absence of gross contamination of the peritoneal cavity, absence of associated colonic vascular injury, less than six units of blood transfusion, and no requirement for the use of mesh to permanently close the abdominal wall.
● A multicenter prospective study comparing the staples with hand-sewn anastomosis following penetrating colon trauma concluded that the method of colonic anastomosis does not affect the incidence of abdominal complications.

Rectum

● Primary closure of extraperitoneal rectal injuries, particularly those located in the inferior third of the rectum, should be attempted, although this is not always possible. A diverting colostomy, washout of the distal rectal stump, and wide presacral drainage are mandatory. Rectal stump irrigation in this setting decreases the incidence of pelvic abscess, rectal fistulas, and sepsis. Intraperitoneal rectal injuries are usually managed by primary closure and by a diverting colostomy.

Liver Injuries

- Because of its size and location in the abdominal cavity, the liver is frequently injured in both blunt and penetrating trauma.
- Spontaneous hemostasis is observed in more than 50% of small hepatic lacerations at the time of laparotomy.
- Some small, nondeep, bleeding lacerations are easily controlled with simple suture or with the use of hemostatic agents.
- The type of injury dictates surgical management. The principles of surgical management of liver injury are the same, regardless of the severity of injury.
- Simple lacerations, which are not bleeding at the time of surgery, do not require drainage unless they are deep into the parenchyma with the possibility of postoperative biliary fistula.
- Bleeding vessels and biliary radicals should be individually ligated.
- If a Pringle maneuver is applied, caution regarding the duration of inflow occlusion is necessary. Hypothermic patients do not tolerate liver ischemia for prolonged periods, and significant damage to the liver parenchyma because of ischemia may occur.
- Packing the liver wound is used when the previously described techniques fail in controlling hemorrhage.

Nonoperative Treatment

- Blunt hepatic injuries in hemodynamic stable patients without other indications for exploration are best served by a conservative, nonoperative approach.
- The overall reported success of nonoperative management of blunt hepatic injuries is greater than 90% in most series.

Porta Hepatis

- The management of common bile duct injury is challenging. Primary repair and placement of a T-tube should be attempted in partial or minor injuries involving less than 50% of the duct's circumference. Major injuries or complete transections of the common bile duct are best managed by means of a choledochoenteric anastomosis. This procedure significantly reduces the incidence of late postoperative complications, in particular the development of strictures.

Postoperative Complications

Splenic Injuries

- The diagnosis is confirmed by abdominal CT scan in the hemodynamically stable patient or during exploratory laparotomy in the unstable patient with a positive DPL.
- The true incidence of overwhelming postsplenectomy sepsis is not well defined, although a commonly used estimation of the incidence of overwhelming postsplenectomy infection (OPSI) is 0.6% in children and 0.3% in adults, which may be a low estimate.
- Because of the severity of the disease process and the high mortality rates, the universal use of polyvalent pneumococcal vaccine (Pneumovax 23, Merck; Pnu-Immune, Lederle) and close follow-up after trauma splenectomy is routine.
- Patients should receive the vaccine before discharge.

Management

- Hemodynamic stable patients now undergo US examination. If US is positive for free fluid and the patient remains stable, an abdominal CT scan is obtained to identify the source of bleeding, to evaluate for contrast extravasation and other intra-abdominal injuries that would require an operation, and to grade the severity of the splenic injury. The finding of contrast extravasation or "contrast blush" observed during the arterial phase of the intravenous contrast on abdominal CT scanning is indicative of persistent bleeding.
- Some institutions advocate for routine use of angiography, but overall splenic salvage rates are similar to institutions following more selective use of angiography. Prospective studies should clarify this issue in the future.
- More than 70% of all stable patients are currently being treated by means of a nonoperative approach.
- Patients are usually admitted to the intensive care unit and kept on bed rest, with a nasogastric (NG) tube in place. Serial abdominal examinations and hematocrit are obtained during the initial 48 to 72 hours.
- A repeat CT scan before discharge does not seem to be necessary.
- The surgical treatment of a splenic injury will vary depending on its severity (Table 19–4), the presence of shock, and associated injuries.
- Major lacerations involving less than 50% of the splenic parenchyma and not extending into the hilum can be treated with segmental or partial splenic resection.

TABLE 19–4. Spleen Injury Scale (1994 Revision)

Grade*	Type of Injury	Description of Injury
I	Hematoma	Subcapsular, <10% surface area
	Laceration	Capsular tear, <1-cm parenchymal depth
II	Hematoma	Subcapsular, 10%–50% surface area: intraparenchymal, <5 cm in diameter
	Laceration	Capsular tear, 1- to 3-cm parenchymal depth that does not involve a trabecular vessel
III	Hematoma	Subcapsular, >50% surface area or expanding; ruptured subcapsular or parenchymal hematoma; intraparenchymal hematoma >5 cm or expanding
	Laceration	>3-cm parenchymal depth or involving trabecular vessels
IV	Laceration	Laceration involving segmental or hilar vessels producing major devascularization (>25% of spleen)
V	Laceration	Completely shattered spleen
	Vascular	Hilar vascular injury that devascularizes spleen

*Advance one grade for multiple injuries up to grade III.
From Moore EE, Cogbill TH, Jurkovich GJ, et al: Organ injury scaling: Spleen and liver (1994 revision). J Trauma 38:323–324, 1995, with permission.

Complications

Urinary Tract Injuries

- Injuries to the genitourinary tract are often clinically unsuspected and frequently overlooked. Gross hematuria is the most frequent sign associated with urinary tract injuries.
- The workup of patients with suspected urinary tract injuries depends on the hemodynamic status.
- Victims of blunt trauma with blood at the urethral meatus should undergo a urethrocystogram to rule out the presence of a urethral injury before bladder catheterization. Once urethral injury has been ruled out, a cystogram is performed by injecting 250 to 300 mL of contrast medium through the Foley catheter to maximally distend the bladder.

Renal Injuries

- Blunt renal injuries are generally divided into minor and major injuries. Minor injuries compose approximately 85% of cases.
- It is our opinion that all perinephric hematomas caused by penetrating mechanisms, not previously evaluated by intravenous pyelogram (IVP), should be explored. If a preoperative IVP shows renal pedicle injury, extensive parenchymal laceration, or urinary extravasation, surgical exploration remains the best option.

Ureteral Injuries

- Injury to the ureter is uncommon and occurs mostly following penetrating trauma.
- In hemodynamically unstable patients, the diagnosis of ureteral injury may be made at the time of laparotomy by intravenously injecting 5 mL of methylene blue or indigo carmine dye. Extravasation of the blue-stained urine confirms the presence of a ureteral injury. The principles of ureteral repair are adequate débridement, tension-free repair, spatulated anastomosis, watertight closure, ureteral stenting, and drainage.

Bladder Injuries

- Approximately 70% of patients with bladder rupture have associated pelvic fractures.

Injuries to the Urethra

- It is found mostly in men, frequently following either pelvic fractures or straddle injuries.

Pelvic Fractures

- Mortality rates vary depending on the amount of bleeding and number of associated injuries.
- Pelvic fractures can be classified according to the resultant vector force (AP compression, lateral compression, and vertical shear), anatomy of the fracture lines, and pelvic stability.
- The objectives of the initial management of pelvic fractures are directed to control hemorrhage. This can be accomplished in unstable fractures, and particularly in those known as the open book type, with external fixation in the acute setting. Posterior fractures with involvement of the sacroiliac joint are frequently associated with arterial bleeding, which can be controlled with embolization of the bleeding vessel, usually branches of the internal iliac artery.

Damage Control

- Recently, a new approach has been proposed in these circumstances. Damage control includes an abbreviated laparotomy and temporary packing and closure of the abdomen used as an effort to blunt the physiologic response to prolonged shock and massive hemorrhage.
- When the patient is stable and organ function is maintained, usually 48 to 72 hours after the initial operation, the patient is taken back to the OR for packing removal, débridement of nonviable tissue, and definitive repair.

Abdominal Compartment Syndrome

- This syndrome is characterized by a sudden increase in intra-abdominal pressure, increased peak inspiratory pressure, decreased urinary output, hypoxia, hypercarbia, and hypotension resulting from decreased venous return to the heart.
- The physiologic consequences of persistent elevated intra-abdominal pressure are listed in Box 19–5.

Box 19–5.   Physiologic Consequences of Increased Intra-abdominal Pressure

Decreased
Cardiac output
Central venous return
Visceral blood flow
Renal blood flow
Glomerular filtration

Increased
Cardiac rate
Pulmonary capillary wedge pressure
Peak inspiratory pressure
Central venous pressure
Intrapleural pressure
Systemic vascular resistance

CHAPTER 20

EMERGENT CARE OF MUSCULOSKELETAL INJURIES

EPIDEMIOLOGY OF ORTHOPAEDIC INJURIES

TERMINOLOGY

- A fracture is considered *open* when an overlying wound produces communication between the fracture site and the outside environment.
- Although the skin laceration is the most obvious component, the energy of the fracture, the degree of contamination, and the soft tissue injury must all be taken into account when grading the severity of the injury.
- Displaced intra-articular fractures require urgent, anatomic reduction and rigid fixation to avoid post-traumatic arthritis.
- Epiphysis.
- Metaphysis.
- Diaphysis.
- Comminution.
- Translation.
- Angulation.
- Rotation.
- Sprain.
- Strain.

FIXATION PRINICIPLES

- The primary uses of external fixation are in the treatment of open fractures, of fractures in unstable patients who cannot tolerate significant anesthesia times or blood loss, of complex fractures in which open reduction and internal fixation (ORIF) is not warranted, of fractures with associated vascular injuries requiring stabilization and urgent vascular repair, and of those in specialized limb reconstruction surgery.
- ORIF implies that an incision is made at or near the site of injury with reduction of the fracture under direct vision (open reduction) and rigid stabilization with plates, screws, wires, or combinations thereof (internal fixation).

- This technique uses a variety of implants to convert tension forces on one side of a fracture into a compressive force across the entire contact area.
- In contrast to wires, plates, and screws, intramedullary (IM) nails are placed in the medullary canal of long bones. They are used to splint or bridge a fracture while still controlling axial, bending, and rotational forces. IM nailing also permits the fixation of a fracture through an incision distant from the fracture site.
- Reaming.

PATIENT EVALUATION

- *Sterile dressings* placed at the scene or in the trauma room should be left in place until the patient reaches the operating room.
- Urgent stabilization of fractures, vascular repair, débridement, and fasciotomy in severely injured extremities has reduced the incidence of acute respiratory distress syndrome (ARDS) and multisystem organ failure.
- Severe pelvic fractures are addressed in the primary survey because of the possibility of exsanguination. Cervical spine injuries, with associated neurologic compromise, also deserve immediate attention.
- At all times, the trauma team must take steps to protect the patient from self-inflicted or iatrogenic spinal cord injury.
- The presence of sacral sparing (intact perianal sensation, rectal tone, or great toe flexion) represents at least partial continuity of the white matter long tracts. In one large series, sacral sparing was predictive of the completeness of injury in 97% of patients with spinal cord injury.
- Burst fracture.
- Compression fractures.
- All joints should be put through a passive range of motion at minimum.
- Gross alignment and interim immobilization of long bone fractures are achieved before the transportation of the patient from the trauma room. This will facilitate transfer, decrease pain, decrease soft tissue trauma and hemorrhage, reduce the chance of turning a closed fracture into an open one, improve the quality of radiographic studies, and prevent potential neurovascular injury.
- When filming long bone injuries, it is important to verify the integrity of the adjacent limb segments. Therefore, the joints above and below the level of injury are always included in the films.

- Cervical spine ligamentous injuries are often diagnosed this way, using *active* flexion-extension radiographs. *Passive* flexion-extension should not be attempted.
- Knee dislocations are a common cause of arterial injury secondary to the proximity of the popliteal vessels. Prompt reduction of these injuries is mandatory followed by reevaluation of the vascular status. In cases in which pulses return after reduction, arteriography is still indicated because of the probability of intimal damage to the artery and late thrombosis.

INITIAL MANAGEMENT

- Careless wound management in the emergency room has been shown to increase the ultimate infection rate by 300% to 400%.
- All displaced fractures and dislocations are gently reduced to regain gross limb alignment.
- Difficulty of reduction increases as does edema and muscle spasm. Therefore, reduction should be attempted as soon as possible and with the patient as relaxed as possible.
- Reduction maneuvers follow the same principles for all fracture and dislocation types. First, inline traction is applied to the limb. If the soft tissue envelop surrounding the fracture fragments is intact, this may be all that is required to obtain satisfactory alignment. The deformity is then re-created and exaggerated to unhook the fragment ends. Finally, the mechanism of injury is reversed and the fracture immobilized. Neurovascular status is again checked after any reduction maneuver or splint application. Once satisfactory reduction or alignment is achieved, it must be maintained by immobilization through casting, splinting, or continuous traction. The joints above and below the fracture must be included to provide the greatest control against displacement. Postreduction radiographs are required to confirm alignment and rotation.
- The rationale of immobilization is threefold. First, splinting, particularly with traction or compression devices, reduces bleeding. Second, additional soft tissue injury may be averted. The chance of converting a closed to an open fracture is reduced. Third, immobilization of the fracture leads to reduced pain.
- Pin care is performed every nursing shift and includes cleaning of the pin sites with 0.5% hydrogen peroxide and placing of sterile dressings.

- In addition to hemorrhage, immediate surgery is also indicated for the prevention of the pulmonary failure septic state; the prevention of local and systemic infections from open, devitalized wounds; and limb salvage. Stabilization of severe open and femoral shaft fractures may be performed simultaneously or after hemodynamic stabilization of the surgical patient. Limb-threatening vascular injuries are managed emergently because warm ischemia time is limited to 6 hours for optimal limb salvage.

ORTHOPAEDIC EMERGENCIES

- Mortality rates in the patient with high-energy pelvic ring injuries are approximately 15% to 25%.
- Early recognition of unstable pelvic ring disruptions is essential because they are more likely to be associated with fatal hemorrhage.
- Lateral compression and vertical shear-type fractures are associated with intra-abdominal and head injuries. The most common cause of death in a lateral compression injury to the pelvis is associated closed head trauma. The anteroposterior compression-type injuries have the greatest risk for retroperitoneal hemorrhage. Intrapelvic visceral injuries are also more common in the anteroposterior patterns. Mortality in anteroposterior compression-type injuries relates to a combination of retroperitoneal bleeding and visceral injuries.
- Recently, devices called pelvic C-clamps have been developed that can be rapidly applied to reduce and provisionally stabilize the pelvis in the emergency room.
- Orthopaedic injuries most frequently associated with vascular insults include posterior knee dislocations, supracondylar humerus fractures, and elbow dislocations. Vascular injuries associated with posterior knee dislocations occur 40% of the time, and delay in diagnosis or repair has led to amputation rates as high as 85%. Fractures such as supracondylar femoral, tibial plateau, or combined tibial-fibular fractures are rarely associated with vascular injury.
- Early recognition and treatment of compartment syndrome is critical in the trauma patient to avoid death, early amputation, and limb dysfunction.
- Compartment syndrome occurs secondary to increased pressure in the enclosed osteofascial space. The most common cause of compartment syndrome in the orthopaedic patient is muscle edema, resulting from direct trauma to the extremity

or from reperfusion after vascular injury. This edema causes an increase in compartment pressure, which prevents venous outflow from the affected extremity, causing backflow congestion and furthering the cycle of increasing pressure and muscle ischemia.

- Investigators have established that peripheral nerve and muscle can survive for as long as 4 hours under ischemic conditions without irreversible damage. However, total ischemic time for longer than 8 hours resulted in irreversible nerve and muscle injury. Ischemic time of 6 hours resulted in a variable return to function in both muscle and nerve tissue.

- The presence of distal pulses and the absence of pallor cannot exclude the diagnosis of compartment syndrome because tissue perfusion in a compartment is dependent on both arterial and capillary perfusion gradients.

- Ischemia of muscles, however, causes pain. Patients are typically said to have "pain out of proportion to that expected for the injury."

- Passive stretching of the ischemic muscle of the compartment in question causes exquisite pain and is the most sensitive clinical finding in developing compartment syndrome.

- The two-incision approach to fasciotomy (Fig. 20–1) of the lower leg is a reliable and straightforward procedure, given that the anatomy is well understood.

- Open fractures are surgical emergencies. The long-term complications are limb threatening and, in cases of systemic sepsis, life threatening.

- Early irrigation and débridement are the mainstays of treatment.

- If skin grafting or muscle flap coverage is necessary, it should be performed within the first week before secondary colonization and wound fibrosis develop.

- Patients with poor nutrition, multisystem injuries, or psychoses and those not able to cooperate with a lengthy reconstructive process may not be candidates for limb salvage.

- Severely injured upper extremities have a far greater impact on the overall functioning status of the patient. Likewise, the indications for upper extremity amputation are significantly more limited.

- Lange and colleagues described indications for primary below-knee amputation in 1985. Absolute indications were defined as anatomically complete disruption of the tibial nerve in an adult and warm ischemia time longer than 6 hours in a crush injury.

- A score of 7 or higher consistently predicted the need for amputation, whereas all limbs with initial scores of 6 or less remained viable in the long term.
- Many investigators have reported a high incidence of infection when reamed intramedullary nailing was attempted after a substantial period of external fixation. Osteomyelitis after intramedullary nailing was associated with long periods of external fixation and history of pin tract infection. If this technique is to be used, the external fixator should be left on no longer than 2 weeks.
- Until further evidence is available, some form of external fixation should be applied initially and then converted to a reamed, locked nail within 2 weeks in these difficult fractures. Coverage for all wounds is accomplished within 1 week, whenever possible. Using these guidelines, the amputation rate has fallen dramatically.
- Dislocations of major joints (e.g., shoulder, elbow, hip, knee, ankle) are considered orthopaedic emergencies. Prolonged

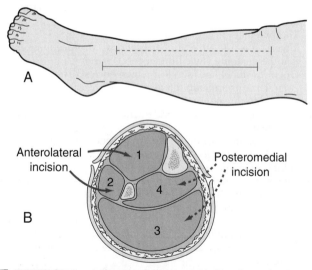

FIGURE 20–1.   *A,* The double-incision technique for performing fasciotomies of all four compartments of the lower extremity. *B,* Cross section of the lower extremity shows a position of anterolateral and posteromedial incisions that allows access to the anterior and lateral compartments (1 and 2) and the superficial and deep posterior compartments (3 and 4).   *Continued*

dislocation can lead to the development of cartilage cell death, post-traumatic arthritis, neurovascular injury, ankylosis, and avascular necrosis.

- Dislocations of the hip require special discussion because of the extreme consequences of failing to recognize and address them in a timely fashion. Sciatic nerve injury, cartilage cell death, and avascular necrosis can result from delay in treatment of these injuries. Of these, avascular necrosis is the most devastating because of its propensity to cause collapse of the femoral head and subsequent development of degenerative joint disease. This problem can lead to total-hip replacement or hip fusion at a young age. After these procedures, multiple major reconstructive operations are common during the patient's lifetime.

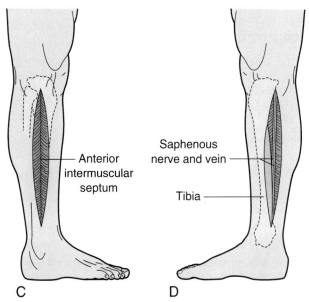

■ FIGURE 20–1, cont'd. *C,* A vertical anterior incision is centered midway between the tibia and the fibula. The anterior intermuscular septum is identified, and two fasciotomy incisions are made, one anterior and one posterior to the septum. *D,* A vertical posteromedial incision is centered 2 cm to the rear of the tibia. Care is taken to avoid injury to the saphenous vein and nerve. *(A to D, Modified with permission from AAOS Instructional Course Lectures, Vol 32. St. Louis, Mosby, 1983, pp 519–520.)*

COMMON LONG BONE FRACTURES

- Except for the rare pathologic or insufficiency fracture in the elderly, these fractures are always the result of a high-energy injury and in the trauma setting are predictive of small bowel injury.
- Leaving a displaced fracture unsplinted leads to increased edema and bleeding and risks further damage to the surrounding soft tissues and neurovascular structures. Continued motion at the fracture site will also lead to increased fat embolization and contribute to the development of ARDS.
- In patients with severe trauma (injury severity score [ISS] >40), delayed fixation of femoral shaft fractures leads to a fivefold increase in the incidence of ARDS.
- In the trauma setting, right-sided humerus shaft fractures are significantly predictive of concomitant liver injury.

COMPLICATIONS

- The incidence of pulmonary embolism in major trauma patients ranges from 2% to 22% and is the third leading cause of death among these patients.
- In particular, long bone fractures, pelvic fractures, advanced age, spinal cord injuries, and surgical procedures are associated with an increased risk of deep venous thrombosis in trauma patients.
- Marrow fat from the fracture site after musculoskeletal trauma can enter into the pulmonary vasculature. This causes activation of the coagulation cascade and platelet dysfunction with the subsequent release of vasoactive substances.

POSTOPERATIVE MOBILIZATION

- Early joint mobilization will decrease the likelihood of fibrosis and, therefore, increase early mobility. Furthermore, joint motion is necessary for good health of articular cartilage. Cartilage is nourished from synovial fluid most efficiently when the joint is moving. Early joint mobilization has become a basic tenet of orthopaedic care and has led to decreased stiffness and improved cartilage health.

CHAPTER 21

BURNS

PATHOPHYSIOLOGY OF BURNS

Local Changes

- Burns cause coagulative necrosis of the epidermis and underlying tissues, with the depth depending on the temperature to which the skin is exposed and the duration of exposure.
- Burns are classified into five different causal categories. The causes include injury from flame, hot liquids (scald), contact with hot or cold objects, chemical exposure, and conduction of electricity. The first three induce cellular damage primarily by the transfer of energy, inducing coagulative necrosis. Chemicals and electricity cause direct injury to cellular membranes in addition to the transfer of heat.
- The area of cutaneous injury has been divided into three zones: zone of coagulation, zone of stasis, and zone of hyperthermia.
- The necrotic area of burn, where cells have been disrupted, is termed the *zone of coagulation;* this tissue is irreversibly damaged at the time of injury.
- *The zone of stasis* is the area immediately surrounding the necrotic zone that has a moderate degree of insult with decreased tissue perfusion and, depending on the wound environment, can either survive or go on to coagulative necrosis.
- The last area is termed the *zone of hyperemia,* which is characterized by vasodilation from inflammation surrounding the burn wound and contains the clearly visible tissue from which the healing process begins; it is generally not at risk for further necrosis.

Burn Depth

- First-degree burns
  - Injury confined to the epidermis.
  - Painful, erythematous, and blanch to the touch with an intact epidermal barrier.
  - Do not result in scarring, and treatment is aimed at comfort.

- Second-degree burns
  - Divided into two types, superficial and deep.
  - Superficial second-degree burns are erythematous, painful, blanch to touch, and often blister.
  - Spontaneously re-epithelialize from retained epidermal structures in the rete ridges, hair follicles, and sweat glands in 7 to 14 days.
  - Deep second-degree burns into the reticular dermis appear more pale and mottled, do not blanch to touch, but remain painful to pinprick.
  - Heal in 14 to 35 days by re-epithelialization from hair follicles and sweat gland keratinocytes, often with severe scarring as a result of the loss of dermis.
- Third-degree burns
  - Full thickness through the epidermis and dermis and are characterized by a hard leathery eschar that is painless and black, white, or cherry red in color.
  - No epidermal or dermal appendages remain; thus, these wounds must heal by re-epithelialization from the wound edges.
  - Deep second-degree and full-thickness burns require excision with skin grafting from the patient to heal the wounds in a timely fashion.
- Fourth-degree burns
  - Involve other organs beneath the skin, such as muscle, bone, and brain.

Burn Size

- Burn size is generally assessed by the "rule of nines" (Fig. 21–1).
- Children have a relatively larger portion of the body surface area in the head and neck, which is compensated for by a relatively smaller surface area in the lower extremities.

Systemic Changes

- Significant burns are associated with massive release of inflammatory mediators, both in the wound and in other tissues.
- These mediators produce vasoconstriction and vasodilation, increased capillary permeability, and edema locally and in distant organs.
- T helper cell function is depressed after a severe burn that is associated with polarization from T helper 1 (TH1) response toward the T helper 2 (TH2) response.

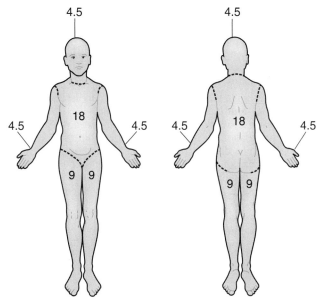

■ **FIGURE 21–1.** Laser Doppler flowmeter. The sensor is placed on the skin in question, which returns a value of perfusion units. A value of 0 is obviously necrotic, whereas values about 80 indicate viable skin that will heal.

- Burns also impair cytotoxic T-lymphocyte activity as a function of burn size, thus increasing the risk of infection, particularly from fungi and viruses.
- After severe burn and resuscitation, *hypermetabolism* develops, which is characterized by tachycardia, increased cardiac output, elevated energy expenditure, increased oxygen consumption, massive proteolysis and lipolysis, and severe nitrogen losses.
- Hypermetabolism is seen in its most dramatic form in severe burn injuries in which it may be sustained for months leading to massive weight loss and decreased strength (particularly when strength is needed to recover from the complications associated with the injury).
- These alterations in metabolism are due in part to the release of catabolic hormones, which include catecholamines, glucocorticoids, and glucagon.

INITIAL TREATMENT OF BURNS

Initial Assessment

- Airway injury must be suspected with facial burns, singed nasal hairs, carbonaceous sputum, and tachypnea.
- Upper airway obstruction may develop rapidly, and respiratory status must be continually monitored to assess the need for airway control and ventilatory support.
- Progressive hoarseness is a sign of impending airway obstruction, and endotracheal intubation should be instituted early before edema distorts the upper airway anatomy.
- The presence of pulses in the distal extremities may be adequate to determine adequate circulation of blood until better monitors, such as arterial pressure measurements and urine output, can be established.
- Other traumatic injuries are possible with severe burns, and if life threatening should be addressed first.
- Pain is a common component of burns and may be addressed with small doses of intravenous morphine after the initial assessment is made.

Resuscitation

- Venous access is best attained through short peripheral catheters in unburned skin; however, veins in burned skin can be used.
- Saphenous vein cutdowns are useful in cases of difficult access and are used in preference to central vein cannulation because of lower complication rates.
- In children younger than 6 years, intramedullary access in the proximal tibia can be used.
- Lactated Ringer's solution without dextrose is the fluid of choice except in children younger than 2 years, who should receive 5% dextrose Ringer's lactate.
- The initial rate can be rapidly estimated by multiplying the total body surface area (TBSA) burned by the patient's weight in kilograms and then dividing by 8.
- The amount of fluid necessary to maintain adequate perfusion is easily monitored in burned patients with normal renal function by following the volume of urine output, which should be at 0.5 mL/hour in adults and 1.0 mL/kg/hour in children.
- Changes in intravenous fluid infusion rates should be made on an hourly basis determined by the response of the patient to the particular fluid volume administered.

- For burned children, formulas are commonly used that are modified to account for changes in surface area to mass ratios.
- All of the formulas listed calculate the amount of crystalloid volume given in the first 24 hours, one half of which is given in the first 8 hours (Table 21–1).
- A nasogastric tube should be inserted in all patients with major burns to decompress the stomach.
- All patients with burns of greater than 10% TBSA should receive 0.5 mL tetanus toxoid. If prior immunization is absent or unclear, or the last booster dose was more than 10 years ago, 250 units of tetanus immunoglobulin is also given.

Escharotomies

- When deep second- and third-degree burn wounds encompass the circumference of an extremity, peripheral circulation to the limb can be compromised.
- Development of generalized edema beneath a nonyielding eschar impedes venous outflow and eventually affects arterial inflow to the distal beds.
- This can be recognized by numbness and tingling in the limb, increased pain in the digits, and decreased capillary refill.
- Arterial flow can be assessed by determination of Doppler signals.
- Compromised extremities require escharotomies, which are releases of the burn eschar performed at the bedside by incising the lateral and medial aspects of the extremity with a scalpel or electrocautery unit.

TABLE 21–1. Resuscitation Formulas

Formula	Crystalloid Volume	Colloid Volume	Free Water
Parkland	4 mL/kg per % TBSA burn	None	None
Brooke	1.5 mL/kg per % TBSA burn	0.5 mL/kg per % TBSA burn	2.0 L
Galveston (pediatric)	5000 mL/m² burned + 1500 mL/m² total	None	None

These are used as guidelines for the initial fluid management after burn. The response to fluid resuscitation should be continuously monitored, and adjustments in the rate of fluid administration should be made accordingly.
TBSA, total body surface area.

- The entire constricting eschar must be incised longitudinally to completely relieve the impediment to blood flow.
- Increased muscle compartment pressures may necessitate fasciotomies.
- Any decrease in ventilation of a burn patient should produce inspection of chest excursion with appropriate truncal escharotomies to relieve the constriction and allow adequate tidal volumes.

INHALATION INJURY

- In inhalation injury, damage is caused primarily by inhaled toxins and not by heat. Heat is dispersed in the upper airways, whereas the cooled particles of smoke and toxins are carried distally into the bronchi and alveoli to cause chemical injury.
- The response to smoke inhalation includes edema formation and increases in lung lymph flow.
- Increasing volume leads to localized increases in pressure that are associated with numerous complications, including pneumothorax and decreased lung compliance.
- Smoke inhalation injury is often seen with a clinical history of closed space smoke exposure, hoarseness, wheezing, and carbonaceous sputum.
- It may also be associated with facial burns and singed nasal hairs.
- The definitive diagnosis must be established by the use of bronchoscopy or less commonly by xenon ventilation scanning.
- The clinical course is divided into three stages:
  - The first stage is acute pulmonary insufficiency in which patients may begin to show signs of pulmonary failure from the time of injury with asphyxia, carbon monoxide poisoning, bronchospasm, and upper airway obstruction.
  - The second stage occurs from 72 to 96 hours after injury and is associated with increased extravascular lung water, hypoxia, and development of diffuse lobar infiltrates.
  - In the third stage, clinical bronchopneumonia dominates and appears in up to 60% of these patients.
- Management of inhalation injury is directed at maintaining open airways and maximizing gas exchange while the lung heals.
- If respiratory failure is imminent, intubation should be instituted, with frequent chest physiotherapy and suctioning performed to maintain pulmonary toilet (Table 21–2).
- Inhalation treatments with heparin and Mucomyst have been effective in improving the clearance of tracheobronchial secretions and decreasing bronchospasm.

TABLE 21–2. Clinical Indications for Intubation

Criteria	Value
Pao$_2$ (mm Hg)	<60
Paco$_2$ (mm Hg)	>50 (acutely)
Pao$_2$/Fio$_2$ ratio	<200
Respiratory/ventilatory failure	Impending
Upper airway edema	Severe

- Steroids have not been shown to be of benefit and should not be given unless the patient is steroid dependent before injury or if the patient is bronchospasm resistant to standard therapy.
- Novel ventilator therapies have been devised to minimize barotrauma, including high-frequency percussive ventilation, which successfully recruits alveoli at lower airway pressures.
- In the presence of significant inhalation injury, resuscitation needs may be up to 2 mL/kg per percent TBSA burn more than would be required for an equal size burn without an inhalation injury.

WOUND CARE

- Current therapy directed specifically toward burn wounds can be divided into three stages: assessment, management, and rehabilitation.
- Once the extent and depth of the wounds have been assessed and once the wounds have been thoroughly cleaned and débrided, the management phase begins.
- First-degree wounds are minor with minimal loss of barrier function; these wounds require no dressing and are treated with topical salves to decrease pain and keep the skin moist.
- Second-degree wounds can be treated with daily dressing changes with topical antibiotics, cotton gauze, and elastic wraps, or alternatively with skin substitutes such as Biobrane.
- Deep second-degree and third-degree wounds require excision and grafting for sizable burns.

Antimicrobials

- The timely and effective use of antimicrobials decreases invasive wound infections.

- As the untreated burn wound organisms proliferate to high wound counts ($>10^5$ organisms per gram of tissue), they may penetrate into viable tissue and then invade blood vessels, causing a systemic infection.
- Silver sulfadiazine.
  - Most commonly used topical antibiotic salve.
  - A broad spectrum of activity to gram-positive, most gram-negative, and some fungal forms.
  - Is painless on application and is easy to use.
  - A transient leukopenia develops 3 to 5 days following its continued use.
- Mafenide acetate.
  - A broad-spectrum topical agent and is particularly useful against resistant *Pseudomonas* and *Enterococcus* species.
  - Can also penetrate eschar, which silver sulfadiazine cannot.
  - Disadvantages include painful application, and it has carbonic anhydrase inhibitory characteristics that can result in a metabolic acidosis.
- Polymyxin B, neomycin, and bacitracin.
  - Clear on application, painless, and allow for easy wound observation.
  - Commonly used for treatment of facial burns, graft sites, healing donor sites, and small partial-thickness burns.
- Mupirocin has improved activity against gram-positive bacteria, particularly methicillin-resistant *Staphylococcus aureus* and selected gram-negative bacteria.
- Nystatin can be applied to wounds to control fungal growth.
- Silver nitrate soaks.
  - Painless on application and have complete antimicrobial effectiveness.
  - Disadvantages include staining of surfaces to a dull gray or black; the solution is hypotonic and continuous use can cause electrolyte leaching.
- Dakin's solution.
  - A dilute solution of sodium hypochlorite.
  - Has effectiveness against most microbes.
  - Has cytotoxic effects of the healing cells of patients' wounds.

Synthetic and Biologic Dressings

- These types of dressings provide for stable coverage without painful dressing changes, provide a barrier to evaporative losses, and decrease pain in the wounds.

- They do not inhibit epithelialization.
- They should generally be applied within 48 hours of the burn, before high bacterial colonization.
- Synthetic and biologic dressings are used to cover second-degree wounds while the underlying epithelium heals or are used to cover full-thickness wounds for which autograft is not yet available.
- Xenografts from swine and allografts from cadaver donors engraft and perform the immunologic and barrier functions of normal skin.
- These biologic dressings are the optimal wound coverage in the absence of normal skin.
- Eventually, these biologic dressings will be rejected by usual immune mechanisms.
- They can be used to cover any wound as a temporary dressing.
- Disadvantages include the possible transmission of viral diseases and the possibility of a residual mesh pattern.

Excision and Grafting

- Deep second- and third-degree burns usually require early excision and grafting.
- There are benefits over serial débridement in terms of survival, blood loss, and length of hospitalization.
- Attempts are made to excise tangentially to optimize cosmetic outcome.
- Rarely, excision to the level of fascia is necessary to remove all nonviable tissue, or it may become necessary at subsequent operations for infectious complications.
- To maximize cosmetic outcome, the skin grafts are not meshed, or they are meshed with a narrow ratio (2:1 or less).
- In major burns, a typical method of treatment is to use widely expanded autografts (4:1 or greater) covered with cadaver allograft to completely close the wounds for which autograft is available.
- The portions of the wound that cannot be covered with even widely meshed autograft are covered with allograft skin in preparation for autografting when donor sites are healed.
- Ideally, areas with less cosmetic importance are covered with the widely meshed skin to close most of the wound before using nonmeshed grafts at later operations for the cosmetically important areas, such as the hands and face.

- Infection is controlled by the appropriate use of perioperative antibiotics and covering the grafts with topical antimicrobials at the time of surgery.
- Cultured epithelial autografts are of use in truly massive burns (>80% TBSA) because of their limited donor sites.
- Disadvantages of cultured epithelial autografts are the length of time required to grow the autografts (2 to 3 weeks), a 50% to 70% take rate of the grafts, the low resistance to mechanical trauma, an increase in scarring potential, and expense to produce.
- The use of anabolic agents to accelerate wound healing has been investigated and the most effective agent to date has been systemic administration of recombinant human growth hormone and insulin.
- Full-thickness skin grafts that include the entire dermal and epidermal layers provide the best outcomes in wound coverage, with diminished contracture and superior skin appearance compared with split-thickness skin grafts.

MINIMIZING COMPLICATIONS

- Sepsis and subsequent multiple organ failure is the leading cause of death associated with burns.
- Multiple organ failure is often associated with infectious sepsis, but infection is by no means required to develop multiple organ failure; what is required is an inflammatory focus.
- The progression to multiple organ failure exists in a continuum with the systemic inflammatory response syndrome.
- Nearly all burn patients meet the criteria for systemic inflammatory response syndrome.

Etiology and Pathophysiology

- Most responsible mechanisms are found in patients with inflammation from infectious sources that most likely emanate from invasive wound infection or from lung infections (pneumonia).
- Occasionally, endotoxins can cause failure of the gut barrier and result in organ damage and progression toward organ failure.
- Arachidonic acid metabolites, cytokines, neutrophils and their adherence molecules, nitric oxide, complement components, and oxygen-free radicals are among other potentially harmful circulating mediators.

Prevention

- Early excision and early removal of devitalized tissue prevents wound infections and decreases inflammation associated with the wound.
- Oxidative damage from reperfusion after low-flow states makes early aggressive fluid resuscitation imperative.
- Topical and systemic antimicrobial therapy has significantly diminished the incidence of invasive burn wound sepsis.
- Perioperative antibiotics clearly benefit patients with injuries of greater than 30% TBSA burns.
- Vigilant and scheduled replacement of intravascular devices minimizes the incidence of catheter-related sepsis.
- Every attempt should be made to wean patients as early as possible from the ventilator.
- Early ambulation is an effective means of preventing respiratory complications.
- Early enteral feeding reduces septic morbidity and prevents failure of the gut barrier.

Organ Failure

- The presence of the systemic inflammatory syndrome that is ubiquitous in burn patients may progress to organ failure, particularly of the lungs, kidneys, and coagulation systems.

NUTRITION

- Hypermetabolism occurs dramatically after severe burn, and increases in oxygen consumption, metabolic rate, urinary nitrogen excretion, lipolysis, and weight loss are directly proportional to the size of the burn.
- The response can be as high as 200% of the normal metabolic rate and this can persist for months after complete closure of the wound.
- Energy requirements are immense and are met by mobilization of carbohydrate, fat, and protein stores.
- Energy stores are quickly depleted, leading to loss of active muscle tissue and malnutrition.
- This malnutrition is associated with functional impairment of many organs, delayed and abnormal wound healing, decreased immunocompetence, and altered cellular membrane active transport functions.
- The goals of nutrition support are to maintain and improve organ function and prevent protein-calorie malnutrition.

- The Curreri formula used commonly in adult burned patients calls for 25 kcal/kg/day plus 40 kcal per percent TBSA burned per day, but may lead to overfeeding.
- Another formula that can be used gives 1500 kcal/m^2 + 1500 kcal/m^2 burned.
- The optimal dietary composition contains 1 to 2 g/kg/day of protein, which with the previously mentioned caloric requirements provides a calorie-to-nitrogen ratio around 100:1.
- Carbohydrates over fats have the advantage of stimulating endogenous insulin production.
- Total parenteral nutrition delivered centrally in burned patients has been associated with increased complications and mortality rate compared with enteral feedings; total parenteral nutrition is reserved only for those patients who cannot tolerate enteral feedings.

ELECTRICAL BURNS

Initial Treatment

- Visible areas of tissue necrosis represent only a small portion of the destroyed tissue.
- Electrical current enters a part of the body and proceeds through tissues with the lowest resistance to current, generally the nerves, blood vessels, and muscles; it then leaves the body at a "grounded" area.
- Heat generated by the transfer of electrical current then injures the tissues.
- Muscle is the predominantly damaged tissue, which generally resides deep and close to bones.
- Blood vessels initially remain patent, but they may proceed to progressive thrombosis and thus further damage from ischemia.
- Injuries are divided into high- and low-voltage injuries.
- In low-voltage injury, zones of injury from the surface extend into the tissue.
- High-voltage injury consists of varying degrees of cutaneous burn at the entry and exit sites, combined with hidden destruction of deep tissue.
- Initial evaluation consists of cardiopulmonary resuscitation if ventricular fibrillation is induced.
- Thereafter, if the initial electrocardiogram findings are abnormal or there is a history of cardiac arrest associated with the injury, continued cardiac monitoring is necessary along with pharmacologic treatment for any dysrhythmias.
- The most serious cardiac derangements occur in the first 24 hours after injury.

- If patients with electrical injuries have no cardiac dysrhythmias on initial electrocardiogram or recent history of cardiac arrest, no further monitoring is necessary.
- Assessment should include circulation to distal vascular beds, because immediate escharotomy and fasciotomy may be required.
- Early exploration of affected muscle beds and débridement of devitalized tissues should be done.
- Muscle damage results in release of hemochromogens (myoglobin), which are filtered in the glomeruli and may result in obstructive nephropathy.
- Thereafter, vigorous hydration and infusion of intravenous sodium bicarbonate (5% continuous infusion) and mannitol are indicated to solubilize the hemochromogens and maintain urine output.
- These patients require additional intravenous volumes over predicted amounts based on the wound area.
- Urine output should be maintained at 2 mL/kg/hr in the setting of myoglobinuria.

Delayed Effects

- Central nervous system effects have been reported up to 9 months after injury.
- Others report delayed peripheral nerve lesions characterized by demyelination and reactive gliosis.
- Another devastating long-term effect is the development of cataracts.

CHEMICAL BURNS

- Chemical injury persists while the agent is in contact with the skin.
- Initial treatment is complete removal of the causative agent and lavage with copious quantities of clean water.
- Dry powders should be brushed from the affected areas before irrigation.
- Spent lavage solution pH gives a good indication of lavage effectiveness and completion.
- Patients may have metabolic disturbances and respiratory difficulty.
- Total fluid needs may be dramatically different from the calculated volumes.
- Patients should be observed closely for signs of adequate perfusion, such as urine output.

- Operative débridement, if indicated, should take place as soon as a patient is stable and resuscitated.
- Wounds are covered with antimicrobial agents or skin substitutes.
- Once the wounds have stabilized with the indicated treatment, they are taken care of as with any loss of soft tissue.

Alkali

- Alkalis, such as lime, potassium hydroxide, bleach, and sodium hydroxide, are among the most common agents involved in chemical injury.
- Accidental injury frequently occurs in infants and toddlers.
- There are three factors involved in the mechanism of alkali burns: (1) saponification of fat causes the loss of insulation of heat formed in the chemical reaction with tissue; (2) massive extraction of water from cells causes damage because of the hygroscopic nature of alkali; and (3) alkalis dissolve and unite with the proteins of the tissues to form alkaline proteinates, which are soluble and contain hydroxide ions.
- Attempts to neutralize alkali agents with weak acids are not recommended.
- Particularly strong bases should be treated with lavage and consideration for the addition of wound débridement in the operating room.
- Tangential removal of affected areas is performed until the tissues removed are at a normal pH.

Acids

- Acids induce protein breakdown by hydrolysis, which results in a hard eschar that does not penetrate as deeply as the alkalis.
- Metabolic acidosis, renal failure, intravascular hemolysis, and pulmonary complications (adult respiratory distress syndrome) are common.
- Acidemia should be corrected with intravenous sodium bicarbonate.
- Hemodialysis may be required.
- Mannitol diuresis is required if severe hemolysis occurs after deep injury.
- A formic acid wound is best treated by surgical excision.
- Hydrofluoric acid produces dehydration and corrosion of tissue with free hydrogen loss.

- Systemic absorption of the fluoride ion induces intravascular calcium chelation and hypocalcemia, which causes life-threatening arrhythmias. Beyond initial copious irrigation with clean water, the burned area should be treated immediately with copious 2.5% calcium gluconate gel.
- These wounds in general are very painful because of the calcium chelation and associated potassium release.
- If pain relief is incomplete after several applications or symptoms recur, intradermal injections of 10% calcium gluconate ($0.5 \ mL/cm^2$ affected) or intra-arterial calcium gluconate into the affected extremity may be required to alleviate symptoms.
- Serum electrolytes must be closely monitored.
- Any electrocardiographic changes require a rapid response with intravenous calcium chloride to maintain heart function.

CHAPTER 22

BITES AND STINGS

SNAKEBITES

Epidemiology

- In the United States, approximately 8000 bites by venomous snakes occur with approximately six deaths each year.

Species

- In the United States, bites by snakes of the subfamily Crotalinae (pit vipers), which include the rattlesnakes, copperheads, and cottonmouths, account for 99% of medically significant bites.

Toxicology

- Snake venoms are complex, possessing many peptides and enzymes.

Clinical Manifestations

Local

- Actual venom poisoning produces burning pain within minutes, followed by edema and erythema. Swelling progresses over the next few hours, and ecchymoses and hemorrhagic bullae may appear.

Systemic

- Patients may complain of weakness, nausea, vomiting, perioral paresthesias, metallic taste, and muscle twitching. Diffuse capillary leakage leads to pulmonary edema, hypotension, and eventually shock. In victims of severe bites, a consumptive coagulopathy can develop within an hour.
- Laboratory abnormalities may include hypofibrinogenemia, thrombocytopenia, prolonged prothrombin and partial thromboplastin times, increased fibrin split products, elevated creatinine and creatine phosphokinase, proteinuria, hematuria, and anemia or hemoconcentration.

Management

Field Treatment

- Most pit viper bites in the United States pose more of a threat to local tissues than to the life of the victim, and the use of any method to limit venom to the bite site may be ill advised.
- Field measures must not delay transport to the nearest hospital appropriately equipped to handle a venomous snakebite.

Hospital Management

- Physical assessment should emphasize vital signs, cardio-pulmonary status, neurologic examination, and wound appearance and size. The bitten extremity should be marked in two or three locations so that circumferences can be measured every 15 minutes to judge progression of local findings.
- Necessary laboratory analyses include a complete blood count, coagulation studies (prothrombin time, partial thromboplastin time, fibrin degradation products, fibrinogen level), electrolytes, blood urea nitrogen, creatinine, creatine phosphokinase, and urinalysis.
- All envenomed patients are best observed for at least 24 hours in the hospital.

Antivenom Therapy

- Currently, antivenom should be administered to any patient with evidence of venom poisoning and clear progression in severity after arrival at the hospital or without delay in any patient with clearly serious poisoning (severe swelling, hypotension, respiratory distress, etc.).
- CroFab is given intravenously as 4 to 6 vials in 250 mL of diluent over approximately an hour. If, after the initial dose, there is progression of venom poisoning severity over the next hour, the loading dose should be repeated. This sequence should be repeated as needed until the victim has stabilized. Following stabilization, to prevent recurrence of venom effects, repeat dosing of CroFab should occur at a dose of 2 vials intravenously every 6 hours for three additional doses.
- Epinephrine should always be immediately available when such products are being administered, and patients should

be warned of the symptoms of serum sickness before discharge from the hospital.

Wound Care and Blood Products

- Antibiotics should be reserved for the rare wound that develops secondary infection.
- However, antivenom must be started before these second-line agents are infused.

Fasciotomy

- Fasciotomies should be considered only if pressures are documented to exceed 30 to 40 mm Hg despite antivenom treatment and elevation.
- There is no role for routine or prophylactic fasciotomy in venomous snakebite.

MAMMALIAN BITES

Epidemiology

Treatment

Evaluation

- Radiographs should be obtained to diagnose potential fractures, joint penetration, severe infections, and presence of foreign bodies, such as teeth. The patient s tetanus status should be updated as necessary.

Wound Care

- Early wound cleansing is the most important therapy for preventing infection and contracting rabies.
- Copious irrigation of the wound with normal saline or tap water using a 19-gauge needle and syringe significantly decreases the likelihood of infection.
- Contrary to past beliefs, primary closure of selected bites produces the best outcome for patients without increasing the risk of infection. This is especially true for head and neck wounds, for which aesthetic results are more important and infection rates are low.
- Bites involving the hands or feet have a much greater chance of becoming infected and should be left open initially.

- A common human bite wound associated with a high morbidity rate is the clenched fist injury. Regardless of the history obtained, injuries over the dorsum of the metacarpophalangeal joints should be treated as clenched fist injuries resulting from striking another person s mouth.
- Potentially deeper injuries and infected bites that are seen after 24 hours require exploration and d bridement in the operating room and administration of intravenous antibiotics.
- Delayed primary repair or healing by secondary intention should be considered for high-risk bites, whereas early primary closure can be performed safely in low-risk bites. Primary closure can be used for low-risk wounds to the arms and legs presenting within 6 to 12 hours and for the face presenting in 12 to 24 hours or possibly days. Puncture wounds have an increased incidence of infection and should not be sutured.

Microbiology

- Infections are usually polymicrobial, with both aerobic and anaerobic bacteria.
- *Pasteurella multocida* is the primary microorganism responsible for infections in cat bites (including large, wild cats) and is isolated in 25% of infected dog bites.

Antibiotics

- Prophylactic antibiotics are recommended for patients with high-risk bites.
- Initial antibiotic selection should cover *Staphylococcus* and *Streptococcus* species and anaerobes for all bites, in addition to *Pasteurella* species for dog and cat bites, and *Eikenella corrodens* for human bites.
- Rabies virus from bats accounts for greater than 80% of the rabies cases reported in this country during the last 20 years with most patients unaware of contact with a bat.
- Rabies is caused by a rhabdovirus found in the saliva of animals and is transmitted through bites or scratches. Patients with rabies develop acute encephalitis and almost invariably die.
- Adequate wound care and postexposure prophylaxis can prevent the development of rabies.
- Guidelines for administering rabies prophylaxis can be obtained from local public health agencies or from a recent publication by the Advisory Committee on Immunization Practices.

- All wild carnivores should be considered rabid, but birds and reptiles do not contract rabies. In cases of bites by domestic animals, rodents, or lagomorphs, the local health department should be consulted before beginning rabies prophylaxis.
- Passive immunization consists of administering 20 IU per kg of rabies immunoglobulin (Ig). As much of the dose as possible should be infiltrated into and around the wounds. The rest can be given intramuscularly at an anatomic site remote from the site of vaccine administration. Active immunization consists of administering 1 mL of human diploid cell vaccine, purified chick embryo cell vaccine, or rabies vaccine absorbed intramuscularly into the deltoid in adults and into the anterolateral thigh in children on days 0, 3, 7, 14, and 28.

ARTHROPOD BITES AND STINGS

Black Widow Spiders

Toxicology

- The black widow spider produces a neurotoxic venom with minimal local effects.

Clinical Manifestations

- Neuromuscular symptoms may occur as early as 30 minutes after the bite and include severe pain and spasms of large muscle groups. Abdominal cramps and rigidity could mimic a surgical abdomen, but rebound is absent. Dyspnea can result from chest wall tightness. Autonomic stimulation produces hypertension, diaphoresis, and tachycardia. Other symptoms include muscle twitching, nausea and vomiting, headache, paresthesias, fatigue, and salivation.

Treatment

- Narcotics and benzodiazepines are more effective agents to relieve muscular pain.
- In the United States, antivenom derived from horse serum is available (Black Widow Spider Antivenin, Merck & Co., Inc., West Point, PA). Because it can cause anaphylaxis and serum sickness, however, it should be reserved for serious cases.
- The initial recommended dose is one vial intravenously (IV) or intramuscularly (IM), repeated as necessary.

Brown Recluse Spiders

Toxicology

- Although several enzymes have been isolated from the venom, sphingomyelinase D is the major deleterious factor, causing both dermonecrosis and hemolysis.
- Local findings at the bite site range from mild irritation to severe necrosis with ulceration.
- Systemic features can include headache, nausea and vomiting, fever, malaise, arthralgias, and maculopapular rash. Additional findings may include thrombocytopenia, disseminated intravascular coagulation, hemolytic anemia, coma, and, possibly, death. Renal failure can result from intravascular hemolysis.
- Appropriate laboratory tests include a complete blood count (with platelet count) and a bedside urine test for blood. If any of these are abnormal, electrolytes, liver function studies, and coagulation studies are in order, but there are no truly diagnostic studies available.

Treatment

- The bite site should be splinted, elevated, and treated with cold compresses.
- Early surgical intervention, other than simple, conservative d bridement of obviously necrotic tissue should be avoided.
- Steroid administration, by any route, has never been shown to be beneficial in limiting dermonecrosis. A short course (few days) of oral steroids can help stabilize red cell membranes and reduce hemolysis in the setting of viscerocutaneous loxoscelism.
- Patients with rapidly expanding, necrotic lesions or a clinical picture suggesting systemic loxoscelism should be admitted for close observation and management.

Scorpions

- In this group, the bark scorpion *(Centruroides exilicauda)* is the only potentially dangerous species in the United States.

Clinical Manifestations

- The bark scorpion, whose sting can, in very rare cases, be lethal, produces a neurotoxin that prevents sodium channel closure. When stung, a patient typically experiences local paresthesias and burning pain. Systemic manifestations may include cranial nerve and neuromuscular hyperactivity, and respiratory distress.

Treatment

- Victims of bark scorpion sting with signs of systemic envenomation require supportive care, with close monitoring of cardiovascular and respiratory status in an intensive care setting.

Ticks

- Proper removal involves grasping the tick by the body as close to the skin surface as possible with an instrument and applying gradual, gentle axial traction, without twisting.
- If the tick was embedded for less than 24 hours, the risk of infection transmission is very low.
- Patients in whom a local rash or systemic symptoms develop within 4 weeks of exposure to tick-infested areas (even in the absence of a known bite) should be evaluated for infectious complications such as Lyme disease (LD), the most common vector-borne disease in the United States.
- LD is caused by the spirochete *Borrelia burgdorferi* and may present at any of three stages early localized (stage 1), early disseminated (stage 2), or late/persistent (stage 3). Stage 1 findings of limited infection include a skin rash in at least 80% of patients that develops after an incubation period of approximately 3 to 30 days. The rash, termed erythema migrans (EM), is typically a round or oval erythematous lesion that begins at the bite site and expands at a relatively rapid rate (up to a centimeter each day) to a median size of 15 cm in diameter. As the rash expands, there may be evidence of central clearing, and less commonly, a central vesicle or necrotic eschar. The rash may be accompanied by fatigue, myalgias, headache, fever, nausea, vomiting, regional lymphadenopathy, sore throat, photophobia, anorexia, and arthralgias.
- Neuroborreliosis occurs in approximately 15% of untreated patients and presents with central or peripheral findings such as lymphocytic meningitis, subtle encephalitis, cranial neuritis (especially facial nerve palsy which may be unilateral or bilateral), cerebellar ataxia, and motor neuropathies. Cardiac findings occur in approximately 5% of untreated patients and usually presents with atrioventricular nodal block (AVB) or myocarditis. Oligoarticular arthritis is a

common presentation of early, disseminated LD and occurs in approximately 60% of untreated victims.

- Over time, as much as a year following the initial tick bite, LD can progress to its chronic form manifested by chronic arthritis, chronic synovitis, neurocognitive disorders, and/or chronic fatigue.

- Diagnosis of LD is largely based on the presence of a classic EM rash in a patient with a history of possible tick exposure in an endemic area or the presence of one or more findings of disseminated infection (nervous system, cardiovascular system, and/or joint involvement) and positive serology on acute and convalescent plasma samples (enzyme-linked immunosorbent assay [ELISA] and Western blot testing for IgM and IgG antibodies to *B. burgdorferi*).

- First-line treatment of early or disseminated LD, in the absence of neurologic involvement, is oral doxycycline for 14 to 21 days.

- If the patient has any evidence of neuroborreliosis, treatment should be with daily intravenous ceftriaxone for 14 to 28 days. Likewise patients with cardiac manifestations should be treated via the intravenous route for at least part of their course, and should receive cardiac monitoring if AVB is significant (i.e., PR interval greater than 0.3 second). Oral antibiotics for 30 to 60 days or intravenous therapy for 30 days are usually effective for Lyme arthritis, although approximately 10% of patients will have persistent joint complaints following treatment.

- A vaccine is available for use in patients at significant risk for LD adults living or traveling regularly to endemic regions.

Hymenoptera

Envenomation

Clinical Reactions

- Bee-sting anaphylaxis develops in 0.3% to 3% of the general population and causes approximately 40 reported deaths annually in the United States.

Treatment

- Mild anaphylaxis can be treated with 0.3 mL of 1:1000 subcutaneous or intramuscular epinephrine (0.01 mL per kg in children, up to 0.3 mL) and an oral or parenteral antihistamine. More severe cases should also be treated with steroids and may require oxygen, endotracheal intubation, intravenous epinephrine infusion, bronchodilators, intravenous fluids, or vasopressors. These patients should be observed for approximately 24 hours in a monitored environment for any recurrence of severe symptoms.

- Venom immunotherapy effectively prevents recurrent anaphylaxis from subsequent stings in certain patients with positive skin tests.
- Patients with a history of anaphylaxis resulting from Hymenoptera stings should carry injectable epinephrine with them at all times; they should also wear an identification medallion identifying their medical condition.

MARINE BITES AND STINGS

Initial Assessment

- Injuries from marine organisms can range from mild local skin reactions to systemic collapse from major trauma or severe envenomation.

Microbiology

- Most marine isolates are gram-negative rods. *Vibrio* species are of primary concern, particularly in the immunocompromised host. In fresh water, *Aeromonas* species can be particularly aggressive pathogens. *Staphylococcus* and *Streptococcus* species are also frequently cultured from infections.

General Management

- Initial management is focused on airway, breathing, and circulation.
- Antivenom can be administered if available.
- Third-generation cephalosporins provide adequate coverage for the gram-positive and gram-negative microorganisms found in ocean water, including *Vibrio* species.
- Outpatient regimens include ciprofloxacin, trimethoprim-sulfamethoxazole, or doxycycline. Patients with large abrasions, lacerations, puncture wounds, or hand injuries and immunocompromised patients should receive prophylactic antibiotics. Infected wounds should be cultured.

Wound Care

- Meticulous wound care is necessary to prevent infection and to optimize aesthetic and functional outcome.

- The decision to close a wound primarily must balance the cosmetic result against the risk of infection. Wounds should be loosely closed and drainage allowed. Primary closure should be avoided in distal extremity wounds, punctures, and crush injuries.

Antivenom

- Antivenom is available for several envenomations, including those from the box jellyfish, sea snake, and stonefish.
- Regional poison control centers or major marine aquariums can sometimes assist in locating antivenoms.

Injuries from Nonvenomous Aquatic Animals

Sharks

- Approximately 50 to 100 shark attacks are reported annually. However, these attacks cause fewer than 10 deaths each year.
- Powerful jaws and sharp teeth produce crushing, tearing injuries. Hypovolemic shock and near drowning are life-threatening consequences of an attack.
- Most wounds require exploration and repair in the operating room.

Moray Eels

- Puncture wounds and bites to the hand from all animals, including eels, are at high risk for infection and should not be closed primarily if the capability exists for delayed primary closure.

Alligators and Crocodiles

- Injuries from alligator and crocodile attacks should be treated like shark bites.

Miscellaneous

Envenomation by Invertebrates

Coelenterates

- Coelenterates carry stinging cells called nematocytes, which in turn carry the nematocysts.

- Mild envenomations, typically inflicted by fire coral, hydroids, and anemones, produce skin irritation.
- Severe envenomations are caused by anemones, sea nettles, and jellyfish. Patients have systemic symptoms in addition to the local manifestations.
- Fever, nausea, vomiting, and malaise can develop. Any organ system can be involved, and death is attributed to hypotension and cardiorespiratory arrest.
- Therapy consists of detoxification of nematocysts and systemic support. The wound should be rinsed in seawater and gently dried.
- Dilute (5%) acetic acid (vinegar) can inactivate the toxin and should be applied for 30 minutes or until the pain is relieved. This is critical with the box jellyfish. For a sting from this creature, Australian authorities also recommend the pressure-immobilization technique.
- To decontaminate other jellyfish stings, isopropyl alcohol should be used only if vinegar is ineffective. Baking soda may be more effective than acetic acid for inactivating the toxin of U.S. eastern coastal Chesapeake Bay sea nettles. Do not apply baking soda after vinegar without a brisk saline or water rinse in between the two substances to avoid an exothermic reaction. Powdered or solubilized papain (meat tenderizer) may be more effective than other remedies for seabather s eruption (often misnomered sea lice), caused by thimble jellyfishes or larval forms of certain sea anemones.
- After the skin surface has been treated, remaining nematocysts must be removed. One method is to apply shaving cream or a flour paste and shave the area with a razor. The affected area should again be irrigated, dressed, and elevated.

Sponges

- Two syndromes occur after contact with sponges. The first is an allergic plantlike contact dermatitis characterized by itching and burning within hours of contact. This can progress to soft tissue edema, vesicle development, and joint swelling.
- The second syndrome is an irritant dermatitis after penetration of the skin with small spicules.
- Treatment consists of washing the affected area and drying gently. Dilute (5%) acetic acid (vinegar) should be applied for 30 minutes three times daily. Remaining spicules can be removed with adhesive tape. A steroid cream can be applied to the skin after decontamination. Occasionally, a systemic glucocorticoid and an antihistamine are required.

Echinodermata

● Starfish and sea cucumbers produce venoms that can cause contact dermatitis. Sea cucumbers occasionally feed on coelenterates and secrete nematocysts; therefore, local therapy for coelenterates should also be considered. Sea urchins are covered with venomous spines capable of producing local and systemic reactions similar to those from coelenterates. First aid consists of soaking the wound in hot, but tolerable, water. Residual spines can be located with soft tissue x-rays or magnetic resonance imaging. Purple skin discoloration at the site of entrance wounds may be indicative of dye leached from the surface of an extracted urchin spine. This temporary tattoo disappears in 48 hours, which generally signifies the absence of a retained foreign body. A spine should be removed only if it is easily accessible or if it is closely aligned to a joint or critical neurovascular structure. Reactive fusiform digit swelling attributed to a spine near a metacarpal bone or flexor tendon sheath may be alleviated by a high-dose glucocorticoid administered in an oral 14-day taper.

Mollusks

● Octopuses and cone snails are the primary envenoming species in the phylum Mollusca.
● Both species can produce local symptoms such as burning and paresthesias. Systemic manifestations are primarily neurologic. Management of the bite site is controversial. Options include pressure and immobilization to contain the venom. Treatment of systemic complications is supportive.

Envenomation by Vertebrates

Stingrays

● Local damage can be severe, with occasional penetration of body cavities. This is worsened by vasoconstrictive properties of the venom, producing cyanotic-appearing wounds. The venom is often myonecrotic. Systemic complaints include weakness, nausea, diarrhea, headache, and muscle cramps. The venom can cause vasoconstriction, cardiac dysrhythmias, respiratory arrest, and seizures.
● The wound should be irrigated and then soaked in nonscalding hot water (up to 45° C) for an hour. D bridement, exploration, and removal of spines should occur during or after hot water soaking. Immersion cryotherapy is detrimental.

The wound should not be closed primarily. Lacerations should heal by secondary intention or be repaired by delayed closure. The wound should be dressed and elevated. Pain should be relieved locally or systemically. Radiographic studies should be obtained to locate remaining spines. Acute infection with aggressive pathogens should be anticipated. In the event of a nonhealing, draining wound, suspect foreign body retention.

Miscellaneous

- An equine-derived antivenom exists for administration in the event of a significant stonefish envenomation.

Sea Snakes

- Venom produces neurologic signs and symptoms, with possible death from paralysis and respiratory arrest. Local manifestations can be minimal or absent. Therapy is similar to that for coral snake (Elapidae) bites. The pressure-immobilization technique is recommended in the field. Antivenom should be administered if any signs of envenomation develop. The initial dose is 1 ampule, repeated as needed.

CHAPTER 23

SURGICAL CRITICAL CARE

CENTRAL NERVOUS SYSTEM

- Intensive care unit (ICU) psychosis should be considered strictly a diagnosis of exclusion.
- There are specific criteria for the diagnosis of death: absence of cerebral function, pupillary light reflex, corneal reflex, vestibulo-ocular reflex, and oropharyngeal reflex and apnea in the face of "adequate stimulation" ($PaCO_2$ >60 mm Hg for 30 seconds).
- It is important that there be a reason sufficient to cause death and no complicating conditions.
- Drug intoxication is one of the most common causes of coma of unknown etiology.
- A computed tomography (CT) scan is indicated in any patient with coma or focal neurologic findings and many patients with depressed level of consciousness.
- A dose of 50 mL of 50% dextrose should be given immediately to any patient with coma of unknown etiology.
- Naloxone (0.2 to 0.4 mg) should be given to patients with coma of unknown etiology.
- Patient self-reporting is the "gold standard" for the assessment of pain and the adequacy of analgesia.
- In noncommunicative patients, assessment of behavioral (movements, facial expressions, posturing) and physiologic (heart rate, blood pressure, respiratory rate) indicators is necessary.
- Opioids are the mainstay of pain management in the ICU.
- Preventing pain is more effective than treating established pain.
- Epidural opioid analgesia provides better postoperative pain relief compared with parenteral opioids.
- A patient who is calm, easily arousable, and follows commands is appropriately sedated.
- In paralyzed patients, assessment of adequate analgesia and sedation is extremely difficult, and patients must be presumptively medicated.

CARDIOVASCULAR SYSTEM

- An Allen's test should be performed before placement of a radial artery catheter to document adequate collateral flow from the ulnar artery.
- Mean arterial pressure (MAP) = diastolic blood pressure (DBP) + 1/3 (systolic blood pressure [SBP] − DBP).
- Measurement should be made at end expiration, because it is relatively independent of the ventilatory status.
- Insertion of a PAC is warranted in any patient with severe cardiopulmonary derangement.
- Shock is defined as perfusion that is inadequate to meet metabolic needs.
- Shock commonly presents with hypotension, but it is important to recognize that it can exist in the face of normal blood pressure.
- Shock may be classified into five categories: hypovolemic, cardiac compressive, neurogenic, septic, and cardiogenic.
- Septic shock represents cardiovascular collapse associated with an infectious process.
- Cardiogenic shock refers to pump failure.
- The factors that determine perfusion are the O_2 content of the blood (CaO_2), the pumping function of the heart, and the tone of the vasculature.
- $DO_2 = CaO_2 \times CI \times 10$.
- $CaO_2 = [Hb \times SaO_2 \times 1.39] + [.003 \times PaO_2]$.
- Dysrhythmias are common in the ICU, and correct interpretation of the rhythm is the key to proper treatment.
- Cardioversion should be performed for hemodynamic instability.
- The principal determinants of cardiac output (CO) are preload, afterload, and contractility.
- Hypotensive patients may require medication to augment cardiac contractility, increase systemic arterial vasoconstriction, or both.
- In patients who have an adequate MAP but who need help with myocardial contractility, inotropic drugs are useful.
- Prospective randomized clinical trials (PRCTs) have demonstrated that survival is no better and possibly worse when albumin is given instead of crystalloid.
- There should be an objective measure of the success of resuscitation in meeting tissue metabolic needs. In the early 1990s, Bishop, Shoemaker, and colleagues identified values for CI (4.5 L/min/m^2), DO_2 (600 mL O_2/min/m^2), and VO_2 (170 mL O_2/min/m^2) above which survival could be predicted in critically ill patients.

- With few exceptions, every prospective, goal-directed clinical trial that has shown a survival advantage has espoused the principles of the "supranormal DO_2" strategy.
- In the face of an acute surgical emergency, the preoperative risk assessment is limited to vital signs, volume status, and electrocardiogram (ECG).
- Three or more risk factors mandate noninvasive testing.
- Exercise ECG is generally advocated as the first test.
- An abnormal noninvasive test mandates cardiac catheterization with coronary arteriography.
- An abnormal noninvasive test mandates cardiac catheterization with coronary arteriography.
- Echocardiography may be a more useful tool in patients with acute heart failure.
- Diuretics and vasodilators are the mainstays of treatment for heart failure.

RESPIRATORY SYSTEM

- Indications for intubation and mechanical ventilation include "SOAP": excessive Secretions requiring pulmonary toilet; impaired Oxygenation requiring positive pressure ventilation; Airway obstruction or inability to protect the airway; compromised Pulmonary function (i.e., inability to generate adequate respiratory effort or to meet minute ventilatory needs).
- The goal in acute respiratory failure is to achieve a PaO_2 that lies on the upper plateau of the curve.
- Hypoxemia is affected by inspired O_2, ventilation, and V/Q matching.
- Defects can be quantified as the alveolar – arterial O_2 gradient ($AaDO_2$):
  - $AaDO_2 = PAO_2 - PaO_2$
  - where $PAO_2 = [FiO_2 \times (PATM - PH_2O)] - PACO_2$
- In healthy individuals, ventilation and perfusion are well matched and the $AaDO_2$ is low (10 to 25 mm Hg).
- Treatment of aspiration is to mechanically clear the airways of debris, decompress the stomach to prevent further events, and provide supportive respiratory care (e.g., bronchodilators, bronchoscopy, mechanical ventilation) as needed.
- The clinical presentation involves fever, leukocytosis, hypoxia, a distinct radiographic infiltrate, and purulent sputum with bacterial colonization.
- Criteria for the diagnosis of acute respiratory distress syndrome (ARDS) include acute onset, bilateral pulmonary infiltrates on chest x-ray, the absence of cardiogenic pulmonary edema

(i.e., pulmonary arterial wedge pressure [PAWP] <18 mm Hg), and hypoxemia (PaO_2/FiO_2 ≤200).

- The pathogenesis of ARDS involves three stages.
- The optimal ventilatory strategy for ARDS patients remains elusive.
- Low tidal volume (TV) ventilation has been the focus of a number of PRCTs.
- There may be benefit to increasing positive end-expiratory pressure (PEEP) to improve oxygenation and to protect the lung by preventing repetitive recruitment/derecruitment of alveoli.
- The different modes of volume-cycled ventilation include controlled mandatory ventilation (CMV), assist control ventilation (AC), and intermittent mandatory ventilation (IMV).
- Pressure-controlled ventilation (PCV) is designed to protect the lung from alveolar overdistension and epithelial injury.
- Pressure support ventilation (PSV) is the most comfortable mode of ventilation because the patient is able to control all elements of inspiration and expiration.
- It is important to first ensure that the underlying problem leading to intubation has been rectified and the patient is hemodynamically stable.
- Perhaps the most reliable single test is the f/TV ratio, or rapid shallow breathing index.
- The preferred strategy may be to assess parameters daily and perform a single T-piece trial for at least 30 minutes.

GASTROINTESTINAL SYSTEM

- Risk factors for stress gastritis include mechanical ventilation for more than 48 hours, coagulopathy, significant burns, and head injury.
- Histamine-2 (H_2) receptor antagonists were superior to sucralfate in preventing clinically important bleeding. The rate of ventilator-associated pneumonia (VAP) was similar between the groups.
- The abdominal compartment syndrome (ACS) is fundamentally defined as an increased intra-abdominal pressure (IAP) that is associated with adverse physiologic consequences.
- Secondary ACS refers to ACS in the absence of abdominal or pelvic pathology and is entirely due to edema and ascites following shock and aggressive resuscitation.
- The organ systems that appear most affected are the cardiovascular, pulmonary, and renal systems.
- The diagnosis (and treatment) is, therefore, based on the patient's physiologic responses to increased IAP.

- All patients with IAP greater than 35 mm Hg (grade IV) require immediate decompression.
- BEE = 66 + (13.7 × weight) + (5 × height) − (6.8 × age) (males).
- BEE = 665 + (9.6 × weight) + (1.8 × height) − (4.7 × age) (females).
- MEE = [(3.9 × VO$_2$) + 1.1 + VCO$_2$] × 1.44 − (2.8 × UUN).
- Protein loss = [UUN + (4 g insensible + nonurea nitrogen loss)].
- The optimal route for delivery of nutritional support is debated.
- Immune-enhancing diets provide specific nutrients (glutamine, arginine, nucleotides, and ω-3 fatty acids) that exert favorable immunomodulatory effects.

ACUTE RENAL FAILURE

- It is typically heralded by oliguria (<0.5 mL/kg/hour or <400 mL/24 hours) or rising serum creatinine.
- A U$_{Na}$ less than 20 mEq/L is consistent with a prerenal cause and a U$_{Na}$ greater than 40 mEq/L with a renal parenchymal cause.
- An FE$_{Na}$ less than 1% indicates a prerenal etiology of acute renal failure (ARF), whereas FE$_{Na}$ greater than 3% suggests a renal parenchymal or postrenal problem.
- The creatinine clearance (C$_{Cr}$; mL/minute) can be used for medication dose adjustment.
- C$_{Cr}$ = (U$_{Cr}$ × V)/P$_{Cr}$
- C$_{Cr}$ = [(140 − age) × weight]/(P$_{Cr}$ × 72)

HEPATIC DYSFUNCTION

- Patients with an exacerbation of chronic liver disease usually present with a complication that must be treated.
- The hepatorenal syndrome is a functional renal problem that probably results from a combination of systemic vasodilation, relative hypovolemia, and increased activity of the renin-angiotensin-aldosterone system.

ENDOCRINE SYSTEM

- Steroids should be administered based on the anticipated degree of stress.
- An acute adrenal crisis may present with unexplained hypotension, fever, abdominal pain, or weakness. If adrenal crisis is suspected, administer hydrocortisone 200 mg along with glucose and saline while awaiting confirmatory laboratory values (hyponatremia, hyperkalemia, hypoglycemia, azotemia).

- For cortisol levels between 15 and 34 μg/dL, a cosyntropin stimulation test should be performed.
- Diabetic ketoacidosis (DKA) is typically seen in patients with type 1 diabetes mellitus (DM), because of noncompliance with insulin therapy or as a result of an illness or injury.
- Hyperosmolar nonketotic dehydration syndrome (HONK) is more common in patients who have sufficient insulin to prevent ketoacidosis but not hyperglycemia.
- The free water deficit may be calculated based on the corrected serum sodium level (add 1.6 mmol/L for every 100 mg/dL elevation in glucose):
  - Free Water Deficit = $0.6 \times$ Weight $[1 - (140/\text{Serum Na})]$
- The consequences of protracted hyperglycemia include increased postoperative infectious complications and worse outcomes following myocardial infarction, stroke, and head injury.
- A large prospective, randomized clinical trial in a surgical ICU demonstrated improved survival associated with intensive insulin therapy.

HEMATOLOGIC SYSTEM

- Virchow's triad of stasis, endothelial injury, and hypercoagulability are common among ICU patients; indeed, deep venous thrombosis (DVT) occurs in 30% of these patients.
- Because ICU patients typically have at least one risk factor, and often more, prophylaxis should be considered routine.
- The clinical signs and symptoms (leg pain, swelling, rubor, fever) of DVT are unreliable in the ICU.
- Duplex ultrasonography is noninvasive and portable and has sensitivity and specificity of greater than 95%, making it an excellent screening tool.
- The combination of a normal D-dimer concentration and a low pretest probability is safe to rule out DVT.
- Low-molecular-weight heparin (LMWH) is preferred over low-dose unfractionated heparin (LDUH).
- CT pulmonary angiography is reportedly accurate, in addition to demonstrating additional or alternative pathology.
- The diagnosis should be suspected if a patient develops resistance to anticoagulation, thromboembolic events, a fall in the platelet count of more than 30%, or a platelet count of less than 100,000/mm^3.
- 29% of patients admitted to ICUs had Hb less than 10 g/dL, and 37% were transfused during their stay.
- The in-hospital mortality was lower among the restrictive-strategy group.

- Weekly administration of 40,000 units of recombinant human erythropoietin increase Hb and decreases transfusions.
- There are at least four Hb-based red blood cell (RBC) substitutes that have been investigated in clinical trials.
- Clinical trials have demonstrated the safety and physiologic function of PolyHeme, as well as the ability to avoid transfusions of allogeneic blood. Unlike the other solutions, there is no evidence that PolyHeme increases systemic or pulmonary vascular resistance.

SEPSIS AND MULTIPLE ORGAN FAILURE

- The fundamental strategy in managing septic patients involves resuscitation and treatment of the underlying infection.
- There may be a role for vasopressin administration in patients with septic shock.
- Patients with septic shock who have adrenal insufficiency have significant reductions in 28-day ICU mortality and hospital mortality if they receive a course of steroids.
- There are a number of adjunctive therapies that have shown promise in preclinical studies or small clinical trials but in large multicenter PRCTs have not demonstrated survival benefits.
- One of the only compounds that has been shown to improve survival in patients with severe sepsis is recombinant human activated protein C.

CHAPTER 24

THE SURGEON'S ROLE IN UNCONVENTIONAL CIVILIAN DISASTERS

INTRODUCTION

- Disasters, especially terrorist attacks, have the potential to produce mass casualties and destroy infrastructure needed to sustain the health care system.
- Terrorist attacks differ from most natural disasters in the capacity to rapidly produce very large numbers of dead and injured.
- The emergency medical service (EMS) and trauma system are designed to be an organized response to injury.
- It is imperative that surgeons and their communities understand these differences and become educated and participate in disaster planning and training.

DISASTER RESPONSE PLANNING

- Joint Commission on Accreditation of Healthcare Organizations (JCAHO) standards require hospitals to have a disaster plan and prepare for patients contaminated by hazardous materials.

PREDICTING CASUALTY LOAD AND SEVERITY

- Casualties tend to arrive quickly at the nearest hospital following a mass trauma event. Typically half of the casualties a hospital can expect will arrive within 1 hour of the arrival of the first casualty.

PREDICTING HOSPITAL CAPACITY

- If the number of predicted or actual critical casualties exceeds the number of operating rooms (ORs) that are available, consider diverting further critical casualties to other hospitals.

INITIAL RESPONSE TO TERRORIST ATTACK—METROPOLITAN MEDICAL RESPONSE SYSTEM (MMRS)

- MMRS allows a metropolitan area to manage the event until state or federal response resources are mobilized.

NATIONAL DISASTER MEDICAL SYSTEM

- The National Disaster Medical System provides federal level resources to any incident that exceeds the capability of any local, state, or federal health care system, with a planned capacity of up to 100,000 victims.
- Medical response
- Patient evacuation
- Hospitalization

TRIAGE—START SYSTEM

- Triage, from the French "sorting," can be characterized as doing the greatest good for the greatest number.

INCIDENT COMMAND SYSTEM (ICS)

- More than 6000 emergency services agencies and hospitals have adopted ICS without modification of the basic concepts because it provides a common structure for management of any disaster.

Structure and Function of Incident Command

- First and foremost, the incident commander is responsible for the entire rescue and recovery operation.
- Hospital emergency incident command system (HEICS).
  - Adoption of HEICS into the hospital disaster plan will provide an ICS-based response that reduces the amount of chaos by improving communication within the facility and with outside agencies.
- Role of the surgeon at the scene.
  - Surgeons are more effectively used away from the incident site at a facility where patients are sorted to a level where surgical intervention is required.
- Hospital response.
- Operating room.
  - OR personnel who treat casualties from weapons of mass destruction (WMD) that have been previously decontaminated do not need personal protective equipment (PPE)

beyond usual Standard Precautions surgical garb of gloves, tight-fitting mask, gown, and goggles/face shield.
- Isolation and the intensive care unit (ICU).
  - Excess use of isolation will overwhelm isolation beds and resources.

BACTERIAL AGENTS

- Various microbes and microbial products have been developed specifically for purposes of use in germ warfare.
- Requirements for a biologic agent to be used as a weapon include ease of production and stability of the agent when stored or stockpiled after it is produced.
- For airborne pathogens, weaponized microbes need to be easily dispersed, and particle size after dispersal becomes very important.

Anthrax

- *Bacillus anthracis* is a gram-positive rod that is a naturally occurring pathogen of sheep, cattle, and other quadrupeds.
- Infection with anthrax can occur via three different routes. Cutaneous anthrax, or woolsorter's disease, occurs when open wounds or abrasions become inoculated with anthrax spores. This is the most common naturally occurring form of anthrax infection in humans.
- Oropharyngeal/gastrointestinal anthrax occurs from ingestion of the spore from uncooked or poorly cooked meat products.
- Gastrointestinal anthrax patients have abdominal pain, nausea, vomiting, and fever, which rapidly proceed to systemic toxemia.
- Inhalational anthrax has been the proposed use for the spores as a biologic weapon.
- The disease is fulminate with a picture of rapidly developing systemic sepsis without a readily apparent source. The subsequent pulmonary failure that develops is the result of the septic process and not pulmonary infection.
- The treatment for inhalational anthrax infection is the usual supportive care of the septic patient and specific antibiotic therapy.
- Ciprofloxacin appears effective in animal models and its favorable oral pharmacology has made it a choice for early presumptive therapy or for postexposure prophylaxis.
- A vaccine for anthrax is available.
- Standard infection control practices are satisfactory for handling patients that are infected with anthrax. Infected patients are not infectious to others.

Plague

- *Yersinia pestis* is the plague bacillus. It is a gram-negative bacterium that is responsible for several of the most deadly pandemics in recorded history. It is a naturally occurring infection of rodents. Fleas become the vectors that transmit the disease from rats to humans.
- Primary septicemic plague occurs when the site of cutaneous infection actually bypasses the regional lymph nodes and gains systemic access directly. These fulminate infections are associated with disseminated intravascular coagulation and purpuric skin lesions.
- Primary septicemic plague is nearly a 100% fatal illness.
- It is the airborne pulmonary form of the disease that poses the greatest threat for a civilian biologic attack.
- A pneumonia develops with systemic dissemination of the microbe from the lung tissue.
- The Food and Drug Administration (FDA)-approved treatment for infection secondary to *Y. pestis* has been streptomycin.
- Gentamicin is recommended as the alternative treatment.

Tularemia

- The bacterial pathogen of tularemia is *Francisella tularensis*. It is a gram-negative intracellular pathogen. Like the plague bacillus, this bacterium is a pathogen of rodents that is transmitted to man by insect vectors.
- The *F. tularensis* has been the focus of potential germ warfare applications because a very low number of inhaled bacteria are necessary to cause infection. Engineered plasmids that will promote resistance to many different antibiotics have been used to enhance the virulence of wild strains of this species to make it a more formidable weapon.
- Pulmonary tularemia is the greatest concern for a biologic attack. Very few organisms need be inhaled to result in clinical infection.
- The clinical picture is one of severe pneumonia, and it is not easily differentiated from any of a number of gram-negative pneumonias.

Brucellosis

- Brucellosis is caused by an aerobic, coccobacillus that is gram negative.
- Although airborne *Brucella* sp. would be the most likely route in a biologic attack, the infection is a systemic illness rather than a pneumonia.

- The disease has about a 5% mortality rate, but its value in terrorism is the chronic incapacitation that affects the host.
- The recommended treatment for brucellosis is combination therapy with doxycycline and rifampin.

Other Bacteria

See Table 24–1.

VIRUSES

- Viruses have been sources of concern as potential biologic weapons. Viruses are more difficult to generate in large quantities, and storage of viruses is more problematic than bacteria.

Smallpox

- Of all of the potential biologic weapons, none has generated more debate than smallpox. Variola is the virus of smallpox.
- Smallpox creates grave concern as a biologic weapon for several reasons. The population of the world is unvaccinated or is greater than 20 years from having received vaccination against this virus. The natural transmission of the virus is as an airborne pathogen, so that aerosolization would efficiently infect many individuals. Furthermore, the virus is quite stable for a period of time in aerosol form. Of greatest significance

TABLE 24–1. Other Agents That Have Been Proposed for Acts of Bioterrorism

Disease	Organism	Route of Transmission	Treatment
Cholera	*Vibrio Cholerae*	Oral	Rehydration; Doxycycline; Quinolones
Salmonellosis	*Salmonella typhi*	Oral	Quinolones
Glanders	*Burkholderia mallei*	Airborne	Quinolones, Doxycycline, Rifampin
Q Fever	*Coxielia burnetii*	Airborne	Quinolones
Shigella Dysentery	*Shigella dysenteriae*	Oral	Quinolones
Cryptosporidium	*Cryptosporidium parvum*	Oral	No effective chemotherapy

is that infected smallpox patients are highly infectious to others, thus making a large outbreak in a densely populated urban area an infection control nightmare.

- Mortality rates from smallpox infection are 30%, with the hemorrhagic and malignant forms of the disease having higher mortality rates.
- There is no established antiviral therapy for smallpox infection, although some are being investigated (e.g., cidofovir). Acutely infected individuals require supportive care as the only meaningful treatment at present. Vaccinia immune globulin is thought to be of value in the first week after exposure. Vaccination is also recommended within the first postexposure week.
- The concern about the return of smallpox infection as a biologic weapon against civilian populations has stimulated interest in the renewal of public vaccination.
- Although this vaccination process is safe for the vast majority of the population, it is not without risk.

Other Viruses

- Many other viruses have been the subjects of interest as potential biologic weapons. Particular interest has focused on the hemorrhagic fever viruses.

TOXINS

- Biologic toxins have also been hypothesized as potential agents for biologic attacks on civilian populations. Bacterial and plant toxins have been the principal ones to be sources of concern at present.

Botulinum Toxin

- Botulinum toxin refers to the accumulated seven different neurotoxins that are specifically produced by *Clostridium botulinum*.
- Botulinum toxin prevents the release of acetylcholine from the presynaptic nerve terminal at the neuromuscular junction. The result is paralysis.
- The greatest concern for botulinum toxin is for it to be inhaled as a finely dispersed powder. The toxin has incredible toxicity in small quantities. The lung becomes an efficient absorptive surface to result in systemic paralysis very quickly.
- The initial management of the patient with botulism is the use of the antitoxin.

- The antitoxin will only influence potential effects from botulinum toxin that has not been absorbed systemically.
- Because the illness is due to toxin and not bacterial infection, antibiotics have no role other than to manage nosocomial infections that will attend the care of these patients.

Ricin

- Ricin is a complex toxin that is extracted from the castor bean. The process for extraction is relatively simple, and large quantities of the toxin can be produced and stored, which makes this a source of concern for use as an agent for a biotoxin attack.
- Inhalation would appear to be the most likely scenario for a terrorist incident.
- Ricin can be identified from a nasal swab specimen within 24 hours of the episode.
- Therapy would be supportive care for the patient with a severe pulmonary insult. Intubation and ventilator support would be required.
- Ricin remains at this point as an agent of concern but one with minimal clinical experience to assist in making a diagnosis or providing specific treatment.

Other Toxins

- The potential toxins that could be derived from bacterial cultures or other plants are numerous. Staphylococcal enterotoxin B and the vast array of potential mycotoxins are examples. The presentation of patients with toxic conditions without explanation should create an index of suspicion about malicious use of toxins. Although culturing patients with clinical syndromes that resemble infection is a standard, the presentation of patients with an unexplained toxic condition should stimulate the observant physician to obtain nasal swabs, blood samples, and other body fluids for subsequent analysis.

CHEMICAL AGENTS

- Chemical agents have been used in World War I and other military conflicts. Chemicals are generally more easily produced and stored than are biologic agents. Most are dispersed as gases or vapors and have posed problems of delivery because of environmental conditions at the time they are used.

Cyanide

- Cyanide is an ubiquitous substance that occurs by natural processes.
- Cyanide was used as a military weapon by the French during World War I.
- Cyanide may be present as a sodium or potassium salt, but military applications have focused on the volatile liquids of hydrogen cyanide or cyanogens chloride.
- The cyanide ion binds to the iron of cytochrome oxidase within the mitochondria of the cell. This results in complete inhibition of electron transport and ATP synthesis. Oxygen is available as the electron acceptor of oxidative phosphorylation, but cyanide inhibits the process.
- Acute symptoms of cyanide poisoning include weakness, fatigue, anxiety, dyspnea, nausea and vomiting, headache, and confusion. Large exposures are associated with rapid onset of convulsions, coma, and death.
- Treatment of acute cyanide poisoning requires immediate administration of an antidote.
- The recommended treatment of cyanide poisoning at the present time is the combination of sodium nitrite (10 mL of solution of 30 mg/mL) and sodium thiosulfate (50 mL of 250 mg/mL solution, or 12.5 g). The patients also require the usual elements of vigorous supportive care.

Nerve Agents

- The nerve agents are a group of organophosphate compounds. These agents include sarin, tabun, soman, and VX.
- The proposed dispersal of the agent as a weapon has been as a vapor to be inhaled by the victims.
- These agents are potent and irreversible inhibitors of acetylcholinesterase.
- Blockade of the cholinesterase enzyme results in accumulation of the acetylcholine and continuous postsynaptic stimulation, which results in a cholinergic crisis.
- The effects on human physiology after inhalation of nerve agents are extensive. Profound sweating, rhinorrhea, and excessive salivation begin quickly. Severe miosis and eye pain are experienced. The pulmonary system demonstrates copious secretions, wheezing, rhonchi, dyspnea, and cough. Nausea, vomiting, and cramping abdominal pain followed by diarrhea are the results of increased smooth muscle constriction in the gut.
- Severe exposures result in loss of consciousness and seizures, followed by respiratory arrest and death.

- The treatment of the individual exposed to nerve agents begins by removing him or her from the exposure; quick decontamination of the skin if there is dermal exposure (not necessary for vapor exposure); and adherence to fundamental principals of airway, breathing, and immediate cardiovascular support while the individual is being transported.
- The antidotal treatment of nerve agent exposure is atropine and pralidoxime chloride.

Lung Toxicants

- Phosgene gas is the prototype agent in this category.
- Phosgene gas as a chemical agent for human injury is delivered for inhalation.
- It wounds and kills people by injury to the respiratory epithelium and lung tissue. Severe, noncardiogenic pulmonary edema and suffocation is the result.
- The treatment for phosgene poisoning is supportive care until the injured lung recovers.
- There is no antidote for phosgene.

Vesicants

- The vesicants are a group of military chemicals that were designed to injure and incapacitate the enemy rather than to kill them.
- The most recognized vesicant is sulfur mustard.
- The principal injuries from mustard are the skin, eyes, and lung.
- Severe exposures are associated with partial thickness blistering of large surface areas of the skin.
- The severity of injury can be reduced by rapid decontamination within minutes of the injury.

RADIATION TERRORISM

- The use of radioactive contamination or even a nuclear detonation as an unconventional civilian act of terrorism looms as a perceived threat.

Basics of Radioactivity

Radiation Injury

- Acute radiation exposure will give a variable pattern of illness depending on the exposure dose.

- Long-term effects of radiation exposure are generally identified as oncogenic effects that may occur after a lengthy latent period of many years.

Medical Management of Radiated Patients

- In the "dirty bomb" scenario, management is relatively simple. Surface decontamination is achieved by removal of clothing, surface rinsing of the skin, and washing the hair.
- With a nuclear detonation, patient management requires effective triage of those with significant exposure into groups of those with and those without physical injuries from the kinetic force of the explosion.

SUMMARY

- Surgeons can ensure a successful response to terrorist attack by taking a proactive role in the planning, training, and management of terrorist incidents involving mass trauma and WMD (Box 24–1).

Box 24–1.   Things Surgeons Can Do To Enhance Their Response To Terrorist Attack

- Participate in the development of your MMRS.
  Understand the model of incident command that exists within your community so that in the event of a disaster you will know your role and participate accordingly, Determine if your hospital uses an ICS-based disaster plan. Appropriate people to contact can be identified by linking to your state or local EMS agency at the National Association of Emergency Medical Directors at www.nasemsd.org.
- Participate in hospital, WMD planning.
  Within each hospital, surgeons should participate to define and develop the internal response capabilities of their hospital for injury from biological and chemical agents using the DHHS OEP guide at www.bt.cdc.gov or www.ahapolicy-forum.org.
- Learn WMD effects and treatment.
  Individual surgeons need to expand their own knowledge of biological and chemical agents by learning: (1) agents that are most likely to be used, (2) appropriate initial injury control and risk reduction and barrier precaution procedures, (3) presenting signs and symptoms and the natural history of exposure, and (4) definitive treatment. A primary resource for didactic information is at the CDC web site at www.bt.cdc.gov.
- Surgeons' role in education on WMD—local.
  The surgeon should participate in the education of colleagues, hospital staff, and administration. Surgeons should partner with local public health officials to educate the public regarding the thoroughness of the local disaster response, the need for specific prevention measures, and the comprehensiveness of our national systems for disaster response and management.
- Surgeons' role in response to WWD—national.
  Beyond participating in the local hospital and community plan, surgeons should ask how they might participate at the national or international level in either a homeland disaster or war. They may participate in the NDMS by joining a local DMAT team. Further information is provided at www.ndms.dhhs.gov.

CDC, Center for Disease Control and Prevention; DMAT, Disaster Medical Response Team; EMS, Emergency Medical Service; ICS, Incident Command System; MMRS, Metropolitan Medical Response System; NDMS, National Disaster Medical System; WMD, Weapons of Mass Destruction. From Committee on Trauma, American College of Surgeons: Disasters from Biological and Chemical Terrorism—what should the Individual Surgeon Do? A Report from the Committee on Trauma. Available http://www.facs.org/civiliandisasters/trauma.html. Accessed 7-8-2004.

CHAPTER 25

TRANSPLANTATION, IMMUNOLOGY, AND IMMUNOSUPPRESSION

CONCEPTUAL APPROACHES TO IMMUNOSUPPRESSIVE THERAPY

- Lymphocytes have an essential, central role in the immune response and mediate its specificity.
- Chemical communicators called soluble proteins or glycoproteins that are effective across short distances and that, in turn, amplify the response and activate other cells.

CELLS INVOLVED

- The key components of the immune system: T cells, B cells, and antigen-presenting cells (APCs) are produced by the hematopoietic stem cell.
- Cytokines.
- If they react too strongly to self-antigen major histocompatibility complexes (MHCs), they are deleted from the immune repertoire, a phenomenon termed programmed cell death.
  - Apoptosis is a form of regulated cell death.

CELL-TO-CELL INTERACTIONS

- Critical to this response are the professional APCs: dendritic cells and macrophages, which bind antigen and present it to T and B cells.
- T-lymphocyte activation.
  - Associated with the T-cell receptor (TCR) is the CD3 molecule. Together they comprise the TCR complex.
  - After interleukin (IL)-2R binds IL-2, T-cell proliferation begins.
- Costimulatory pathways.
  - Two signals are required for T-cell activation: an antigen-specific signal and a costimulatory signal. The TCR/CD3

interaction (signal 1) required for cell activation has been well defined. The costimulatory pathways present on APC surface molecules provide the second signal for T-cell activation (signal 2).

- T-cell effector functions.
  - In addition to acquiring the TCR complex during thymic maturation, T cells also acquire differentiation receptors called cluster of differentiation (CD) antigens.
- B lymphocytes.
  - B cells are responsible for the humoral or antibody-mediated immune response against foreign antigen.
- Monocytes.
- Dendritic cells.
  - The most potent APCs are CD11c$^+$ bone marrow-derived dendritic cells, which are distributed ubiquitously throughout the lymphoid and nonlymphoid tissues of the body.
- Natural killer cells.

MAJOR HISTOCOMPATIBILITY LOCUS: TRANSPLANTATION ANTIGENS

- There are two types of cell-surface MHC molecules: class I and class II.
- Human histocompatibility complex.
  - In conventional antigen recognition, the foreign antigen is ingested by the host APC, digested into small peptides, and presented to T cells that recognize the antigen as well as class I or class II of the APC. This is termed *indirect antigen presentation* or the *indirect pathway.*
- HLA typing: prevention and rejection.
  - Occurs within minutes to days after transplantation and is mediated primarily by preformed antibody.
  - *Rejection* is mediated primarily by T lymphocytes and first occurs between 1 and 3 weeks after solid organ transplantation without immunosuppression.
  - Risk factors for development of the lesions of chronic rejection include (1) previous acute rejection episodes, with increased severity and increased number of episodes further increasing risk of chronic rejection; (2) inadequate immunosuppression, including patient noncompliance; (3) initial delayed graft function; (4) donor issues such as age and hypertension; (5) organ recovery-related issues including preservation and reperfusion injury; and (6) recipient diabetes, hypertension, or post-transplant infections.

CLINICAL IMMUNOSUPPRESSION

- Overall risks of immunosuppression.
- Induction agents.
  - Antilymphocyte globulin.
  - Monoclonal antibody.
  - OKT3.
  - IL-2 receptor inhibitors.
  - Anti-CD20 monoclonal antibody (Rituximab).
  - Intravenous immunoglobulin.
- Maintenance agent.
- Hypertension, weight gain, peptic ulcers and gastrointestinal bleeding, euphoric personality changes, cataract formation, hyperglycemia that could progress to steroid diabetes, pancreatitis, muscle wasting, and osteoporosis with avascular necrosis of the femoral head and other bones.
  - Azathioprine.
  - Mycophenolate mofetil.
  Mycophenolate mofetil is another immunosuppressant that functions by the inhibition of purine metabolism.
  Leukopenia and gastrointestinal upset.
  - Leflunomide.
  Pyrimidine synthesis.
- T-cell-directed immunosuppressants.
  - Cyclosporine.
  Medications that increase or decrease cytochrome P-450 function can dramatically increase or decrease cyclosporine or tacrolimus levels.
  Nephrotoxicity, hypertension, hyperkalemia, hirsutism, gingival hyperplasia, tremor and other neurotoxicities, diabetogenicity, and hepatotoxicity.
  - Tacrolimus.
  The drug-immunophilin complex blocks the phosphatase activity of calcineurin that is important in regulation of IL-2 gene transcription.
  The side effects of cyclosporine and tacrolimus are similar.
  - Sirolimus.
  Sirolimus does not block T-cell cytokine gene expression but instead inhibits the transduction of signals from the IL-2R to the nucleus.
  - FTY720.
  Bradycardia.
- Positive crossmatch protocols.
- Possible immunosuppressive regimens.
  - From experimental "tolerizing" protocols using alemtuzumab or rabbit antithymocyte globulin followed by

low-dose monotherapies with tacrolimus, cyclosporine, or sirolimus, to more traditional triple-therapy regimens with or without induction agents, to steroid avoidance—no standard protocols exist today.

- Treatment of acute rejection.
  - Biopsy.

CHAPTER 26

TRANSPLANTATION OF ABDOMINAL ORGANS

RENAL TRANSPLANTATION

Indications

- The three diseases most commonly leading to renal failure and treated by kidney transplantation are insulin-dependent diabetes mellitus, glomerulonephritis, and hypertensive nephrosclerosis, accounting for about 60% of the total. Other important causes include polycystic kidney disease, Alport's disease, immunoglobulin (Ig) A nephropathy, systemic lupus erythematous, nephrosclerosis, interstitial nephritis, pyelonephritis, and obstructive uropathy. In African Americans, hypertensive nephrosclerosis is the most common of all causes of renal failure.
- Although history of a successfully treated cancer is not a contraindication to transplantation, it is a general rule to wait at least 2 years before transplantation is justified.
- Predicted noncompliance is another contraindication because careful adherence to immunosuppression is necessary.
- Indeed, the current results of transplantation mandate serious consideration of this therapy in virtually any patient with terminal renal disease. Not only is the quality of life far better with transplantation than with dialysis but, because the mortality of patients in the first year after transplantation is now less than 5%, survival is also superior.

Recipient Evaluation and Preparation

- The evaluation of all transplant candidates, in addition to a standard medical workup, should include cytomegalovirus (CMV) antibody titer; creatinine clearance; serology for syphilis, human immunodeficiency virus (HIV), and hepatitis B virus (HBV) and hepatitis C virus (HCV); evaluation of parathyroid status; coagulation profile; Papanicolaou smear; ABO and histocompatibility typing; urologic evaluation (including a voiding cystourethrogram in selected patients to assess outlet obstruction and reflux); gastrointestinal evaluation (as warranted by history of ulcer, diverticulitis, or other symptoms); and psychiatric evaluation.

Histocompatibility Typing and Crossmatching

- Although opinions vary regarding the significance of histocompatibility testing for selection of unrelated donors, its importance is unquestionable for selection of the optimal donor within a family. Regardless of the donor source, compatibility for ABO blood groups and a negative leukocyte crossmatch are mandatory.
- ABO blood groups.
- Lymphocytotoxic crossmatching.
- Sensitization to human leukocyte antigen (HLA), as indicated by the presence of lymphocytotoxic antibodies in the recipient's serum, may occur as a result of pregnancy, blood transfusions, or prior transplantation. Presence of donor-reactive antibodies, detected by incubation of recipient serum with donor cells in the presence of complement (a positive crossmatch), is a contraindication to renal transplantation because of its strong association with hyperacute renal allograft rejection.
- There is controversy whether the most sensitive crossmatching methods such as antiglobulin and flow cytometry techniques should be used because they may exclude donors that might have been used successfully. In addition, the clinical relevance of positive crossmatches to B lymphocytes (especially if performed in the cold) and those caused only by IgM antibodies is questionable. Attempts have also been made to define the role of antibodies against minor (non-HLA) specificities. For example, there is evidence that antibodies reactive to determinants on vascular endothelial cells can damage renal allografts.
- To allow transplantation of sensitized patients, several methods have been tried to remove cytotoxic antibody (including thoracic duct drainage, total lymphoid irradiation, and plasmapheresis). Recently several groups have explored the ability of intravenous immunoglobulin (IVIG) to inhibit anti-HLA antibodies by an anti-idiotypic mechanism.

Pretransplant Operations

- Any necessary urinary tract reconstructions must be carried out before transplantation (e.g., lysis of posterior urethral valves, transurethral resection for obstructing prostatic hypertrophy).

The patient's own bladder should be used for ureteroneocystostomy, even if this necessitates bladder reconstruction or augmentation of a small bladder by ileocecocystoplasty. Careful intermittent catheterization of a neurogenic bladder three or four times daily after transplantation is preferable to the use of an intestinal conduit. In the absence of an alternative strategy, ileal conduits should be constructed at least 6 weeks before the transplant operation to avoid risk of infection.

Selection and Management of Living Donors

● For the prospective recipient, there are major advantages to obtaining a living donor that obviates the discomfort, expense, and risks of prolonged dialysis while waiting for a cadaver kidney. Post-transplant morbidity is also minimized by decreasing the chances of acute tubular necrosis (ATN).

Histocompatibility Considerations in Living Donor Selection

● The HLA antigens are gene products of alleles at a number of closely linked loci on the short arm of chromosome 6 in humans. At least six HLAs (A, B, C, DQ, DP, DR) have been defined, and the existence of several others has been deduced from family studies and immunochemical findings. The extreme polymorphism of the HLA system, which is the basis of infinite genetic variability of the human species, plays a pivotal role in regulation of the immune response. The gene products of the HLA-A, B, and C loci are referred to as Class I major histocompatibility complex (MHC) antigens, and the products of the D region are Class II MHC antigens. Class I MHC antigens are expressed on all nucleated cells and can be readily detected serologically using lymphocytotoxicity assays. Class II MHC antigens are important in antigen presentation and are expressed on B lymphocytes, dendritic cells, endothelium, and activated T cells.

● HLA antigens are inherited as codominant alleles, and, because of the relatively low recombinant frequency, the HLA genes are usually inherited en bloc from each parent. In immediate families, inheritance of the HLA, which is of overriding importance in transplant outcome, can be determined serologically and falls into four different combinations of haplotypes. Any two siblings have a 25% chance of being HLA identical, that is, of having inherited the same chromosome 6 (haplotype) from each parent, a 50% chance of sharing one haplotype, and a 25% chance of sharing neither haplotype. Parent-to-child donation always involves a one-haplotype identity.

● The importance of matching HLA antigens in the selection of living related donors for renal transplantation is well established. Excellent graft survival (>95%) can be expected when a related donor and a recipient are HLA identical. There is a progressively lower graft survival associated with one or zero haplotype matches, although even totally mismatched related living donor grafts have a significantly better outcome than cadaveric grafts.

Risks to the Living Donor

● Despite the major advantages of related donors, their use is justified only if the risks to the donor are minimal. Nevertheless, it is important to frankly present these risks to the donor. In addition to discomfort and morbidity associated with any operation, there is an operative mortality of about 0.05%. Concern for even a small mortality rate has led to a traditional policy of accepting as donors only individuals between 18 and 55 years and in virtually perfect health. Because donor age limits are now being extended at most centers, it is important to exercise even greater care to avoid unacceptable risks.

Living Unrelated Donors

● Until recently, unrelated volunteers were excluded from donation because the results were assumed not sufficiently advantageous compared with those of cadaver grafts to warrant the risk. However, the improvement in unrelated kidney allograft survival with cyclosporine and the shortage of cadaver donors provoked reexamination of this issue. Whereas the use of paid donors is unlawful, genetically unrelated but emotionally related donors (especially spouses) are now considered acceptable by most centers and, by 2002, accounted for about 25% of living donor transplants. Surprisingly these transplants have graft survival as good at 5 and 10 years as living related transplants, except for those from HLA identical sibling donors and were significantly better than the survival of cadaveric transplants.

Selection and Management of Cadaveric Donors

● In the absence of a family donor, cadaveric renal transplantation is a satisfactory alternative. In most countries, acceptance of the concept of brain death allows removal of viable organs from heart-beating donors. The donor shortage is perhaps the most important impediment to transplantation. Although in the United States the Uniform Anatomical Gift Act has been adopted in all 50 states, few cadaver kidneys are actually removed because of donor cards alone without permission of the next of kin. Only about half of U.S. citizens currently consent to donation of organs from deceased relatives, and organs are in fact recovered from fewer than half of potentially acceptable donors. In the United States, it has been estimated that only about 20,000 brain-dead patients per year are acceptable donors. However, only the approximately 9000 cadaveric kidney transplants are performed annually, a number that has changed little over the last decade.

- The use of cadaver donors raises the ethical and legal problems of defining brain death. Consideration of transplantation should never be allowed to influence the treatment of patients who have any chance to survive or the definition or declaration of death, which must always be the responsibility of the patient's primary physician or of a neurologic consultant, with the full understanding and permission of the family. To avoid any conflict of interest, the transplant team must never be involved with care of the donor or with decisions regarding prognosis or therapy.

Donor Pretreatment

Human Leukocyte Antigen Considerations in Cadaver Donor Selection

- Although the benefit of matching for HLA-A and B antigens in selection of family donors is well established, its value for cadaveric grafts remains controversial.
- Even in the United States, the benefits of six antigen-matched (or zero antigen-mismatched) kidney transplants are now uncontested, causing United Network for Organ Sharing (UNOS) to mandate their sharing on a national basis. Whether lesser degrees of matching are important is controversial (especially because of the introduction of cyclosporine and other potent new immunosuppressive agents) and is the central issue of an ongoing debate whether to change UNOS's point system for cadaveric kidney allocation, which currently emphasizes HLA matching. Two analyses on the outcomes of over 30,000 renal transplants led to opposite conclusions. Takemoto and coworkers noted that HLA matching and transplant success were correlated, whereas Held and colleagues, who stratified other risk factors, found

little benefit and argued that the ischemic damage inherent in transportation necessary for national sharing would outweigh the advantage of matching. An additional consideration in sharing nationally is the potential negative impact on a second kidney that will subsequently need to be shipped to "pay back" the first shipped kidney.

Post-Transplant Management

● If the transplanted kidney has not suffered ischemic damage, a brisk diuresis is likely to begin within minutes of revascularization. Responsible for the diuresis (which may reach 1000 mL per hour) are (1) osmotic factors secondary to uremia or high glucose concentrations in intravenous fluids, (2) total body fluid and electrolyte overload secondary to chronic uremia, and (3) mild proximal tubular damage resulting from allograft ischemia. Early in the postoperative period, mild diuresis is reassuring and should be encouraged by replacement of urine volumes and, if necessary, by diuretics. Initial under replacement of fluid may lead to oliguria or impaired transplant function interfering with diagnosis of vascular occlusion, urinary obstruction, or early rejection. Severe dehydration can be the outcome of inadequate replacement of losses during a massive diuresis, especially in children.

Immunosuppression

● Thus far, the success of solid organ transplantation has been dependent on lifelong administration of nonspecific pharmacologic immunosuppressants. Since the early 1980s, advances in understanding mechanisms of T-cell activation have facilitated the development of more powerful and somewhat more selective immunosuppressive drugs that target the distinctive cell surface molecules of T cells, which initiate rejection.

Azathioprine

Adrenal Corticosteroids

● The previously known immunosuppressive effects of adrenal corticosteroids, although not sufficient in themselves to prevent rejection, were noted in the early 1960s to be synergistic with those of azathioprine. The combination of azathioprine and steroids then became standard therapy for the next two decades. The complex impact of steroids on the immune system involves blockade of postreceptor events occurring after engagement of the T-cell receptor with antigen and the inhibition of certain cytokine gene activation such as interleukin-1 (IL-1), and IL-6. Steroids also possess potent anti-inflammatory properties, which reduce the migration of monocytes to sites of inflammation. This probably explains why brief intensification of steroid therapy often aborts the "rejection crises" that ensue despite baseline immunosuppression. Because of the adverse impact of chronic steroid therapy attempts are being made at many centers to withdraw these agents or to avoid their use altogether. Although this may be possible in some patients, others appear to suffer either acute or chronic rejection when steroids are withdrawn from immunosuppressive protocols.

Antilymphocytic Antibodies

- The effectiveness of anti-lymphocyte serum (ALS) was the basis for the introduction by Cosimi and coworkers of monoclonal mouse antihuman anti–T-cell antibodies. Monoclonal anti–T-cell antibodies induce rapid depletion of T lymphocytes from peripheral blood while having little detrimental effect on other populations, such as red blood cells, platelets, or granulocytes, all of which are affected by cross-reacting antibodies present in the polyclonal ALG preparations. Because of lower cost and greater availability, specificity, and standardization of the preparation, monoclonal antibodies such as OKT3 have largely replaced ALS and ALG in many centers. The structure recognized by OKT3, the CD3+ antigen, is linked to the T-cell antigen receptor, which is critical for the activation of human T cells. *In vivo* depletion of T cells following exposure to OKT3 is believed to be mediated by mechanisms such as complement mediated lympholysis or opsonization of cells. In the presence of bound OKT3, the CD3+ T-cell receptor complex is internalized by the cell, further rendering the T-cell population inactive. Multi-institutional, randomized prospective trials revealed the efficacy of OKT3 in reversal of acute rejection in 94% of cadaveric renal allograft rejections, a figure significantly better than that obtained with steroid treatment.
- Side effects associated with OKT3 therapy (particularly the initial doses) include fever, shaking chills, headache, nausea, vomiting, diarrhea, wheezing, and pulmonary edema. These phenomena are probably due to release of cytokines, especially tumor necrosis factor, and have been termed the

cytokine release syndrome. Fortunately, such side effects can often be ameliorated by pretreatment with methylprednisolone, acetaminophen, and antihistamines or, more recently, antibodies against tumor necrosis factor or its receptor. As with polyclonal ALG, the use of monoclonal antibody OKT3 may induce rapid sensitization to mouse antibody, which results in the neutralization of OKT3 and reappearance in the peripheral blood of CD3+ cells. Concomitant administration of azathioprine and steroids may delay the production of anti-OKT3 antibody and prolong its immunosuppressive effect. Beyond return of graft function, *in vivo* efficacy of OKT3 may be monitored by sequential analyses of the CD3+ T-cell populations in the peripheral blood and the circulating level of OKT3 and by measurement of human antibodies to the murine immunoglobulin.

- Other monoclonal antibodies that have been developed for the prevention or treatment of rejection are currently under clinical investigation. These include mouse antihuman monoclonal antibodies directed against various T cell surface markers including, the IL-2 receptor, adhesion molecules (e.g., anti-intercellular adhesion molecule [ICAM]-1), and CD52. Also promising is the development of monoclonal antibodies in which the entire protein backbone structure of the antibody molecule is replaced with corresponding human sequences, except for the idiotypic specific region. Such engineered molecules, termed *humanized* antibodies, appear to retain their *in vivo* efficacy for T-cell depletion but may have limited side effects (diminished cytokine release syndrome) and prolonged effectiveness because their elimination through the development of human antimurine immunity is less.

Cyclosporine

- The introduction of cyclosporine (a calcineurin inhibitor) in the early 1980s revolutionized transplantation by facilitating successful extrarenal transplants and improving cadaveric kidney graft survival. Cyclosporine is a fungal derivative that appears to block T-lymphocyte production of the lymphokine IL-2 through inhibition of the production of its messenger RNA. Like azathioprine, cyclosporine is most useful for prophylaxis rather than reversal of rejection.
- Cyclosporine has the major advantage over azathioprine of lacking bone marrow toxicity but the disadvantage of nephrotoxicity, which is its major side effect. Nephrotoxicity may be manifest as a delay in function of a newly transplanted

kidney or impairment of function of a well-established renal allograft.

- Doses are determined by trough levels in whole blood, which are maintained at 100 to 200 µg per liter (as determined by high-performance liquid chromatography). Absorption and bioavailability of cyclosporine were found to be quite variable after oral administration, complicating regulation of blood levels. A microemulsion formulation of cyclosporine (Neoral) allows faster and more consistent absorption and facilitates management.

Tacrolimus (FK-506)

- Tacrolimus has properties similar but perhaps superior to those of cyclosporine. The antilymphocytic effect of tacrolimus results from the formation of active complexes between the drug and the respective intracellular binding protein or immunophilin. The FK-506 immunophilin complex inhibits the phosphatase activity of calcineurin, which is important in the regeneration of IL-1 gene transcription. Tacrolimus was first described by Kino and colleagues in 1987, introduced clinically in the United States at the University of Pittsburgh in 1989. It is about 100 times more potent as an anti–T-cell agent than is cyclosporine (on a per milligram basis). Initially, tacrolimus was used to "rescue" liver transplants observed to be failing on cyclosporine-based immunosuppression.
- The adverse effects of tacrolimus are similar to those of cyclosporine: nephrotoxicity, neurologic problems (tremor, headache), and diabetes.

Mycophenolate Mofetil

- Mycophenolate mofetil (MMF), the morpholino-ethyl ester of mycophenolic acid (MPA), which *in vivo* is hydrolyzed to free MPA (the active immunosuppressive moiety), is a potent and specific inhibitor of de novo purine synthesis. MPA blocks the proliferation of both T and B lymphocytes because these cells lack a significant purine biosynthetic salvage pathway activity. The use of MMF in combination with cyclosporine dramatically reduced both the incidence and the severity of acute rejection. Subsequent trials combining MMF with cyclosporine indicated that the risk of biopsy-proven acute rejection declined to less than 20% and the frequency of resistant rejection was markedly decreased. As a result, MMF has virtually replaced azathioprine at many transplant centers.

Sirolimus (Rapamycin)

- Sirolimus, which is structurally similar to tacrolimus, was discovered in a search for novel antifungal agents. It is a macrocyclic triantibiotic produced by *Streptomyces hygroscopicus,* an actinomyces that was isolated from a soil sample collected from Rapa Nui (Easter Island). Although sirolimus also binds to FKBP25, its effect is distinct from the calcineurin-inhibition activity of tacrolimus or cyclosporine.
- Sirolimus is not nephrotoxic but may cause thrombocytopenia and hypercholesterolemia. It also appears to be associated with delayed wound healing.

Other Immunosuppressive Agents

- Development of new, less toxic immunosuppressive therapies is very important. A new class of biologic agents that target costimulatory molecules necessary for T-cell activation hold great promise for this purpose. Unlike conventional agents such as tacrolimus and cyclosporine that inhibit T-cell activation by blocking the effects of T-cell receptor triggering by antigen (termed *signal I*), these agents target the interaction of T cell CD28 with antigen-presenting cell (APC) B7 molecules, or T cell CD154 with APC CD40 *(signal II).* The theoretical attractiveness of this approach is based on considerable experimental research indicating that T cells receiving signal I in the absence of signal II are rendered anergic. This may allow for the design of immunosuppressive protocols with a greater probability of inducing a state of tolerance to the graft. In large animal studies, Kirk and coworkers reported long-term survival of kidney allografts using simultaneous blockade of CD154 and B7. In subsequent work, even monotherapy with anti-CD154 alone administered for a 5-month course resulted in prolonged function of all grafts without graft loss because of rejection. Interesting in these studies was the finding that combination therapy with conventional agents and anti-CD154 produced inferior results to monotherapy with anti-CD154, perhaps indicating that conventional therapy inhibits anergy induced by costimulatory blockade.

Rejection

- Considerable effort has been made to correlate allograft morphology with the clinical course of rejection. However, histologic study of a kidney biopsy can never provide more than a narrowly focused "snapshot" of the target of a complex systemic process that is in continuous evolution while also being modified by immunosuppression. Rejection is conveniently categorized as hyperacute, acute, or chronic, but there are overlapping features and transitions among these categories. The introduction of newer potent immunosuppressives has also changed the classic histologic changes of rejection. The outcome of an interventional conference in Banff was the proposal of new criteria for the semiquantitative analysis of rejection and the development of standardized nomenclature.

Hyperacute Rejection

- In the 1960s, several instances were noted in which transplanted kidneys that initially seemed viable were rejected within minutes of revascularization, as evidenced by bluish discoloration of the kidney, deterioration of perfusion, and cessation of function. Histologically, extensive intravascular deposits of fibrin and platelets and intraglomerular accumulation of polymorphonuclear leukocytes, fibrin, platelets, and red blood cells along with accumulation of leukocytes in the peritubular and glomerular capillaries were seen. This process proved refractory to immunosuppressive or anticoagulant therapy and inevitably led to rapid destruction of the kidney. It soon became evident that the occurrence of hyperacute rejection was usually correlated with the presence of preformed circulating antibodies against donor antigens and that these could be identified by a pretransplant crossmatch. The classic form of hyperacute rejection has become rare because transplants are no longer performed when the crossmatch is positive.

Acute Cellular Rejection

- Acute cellular rejection most commonly becomes evident during the early days or weeks following transplantation, although it may occasionally occur months or years later. The diagnosis of acute rejection is based on a constellation of findings that include clinical signs and symptoms, laboratory assays of blood and urine, radioisotope studies, and allograft biopsies.
- Because the diagnosis of rejection on clinical grounds alone may be difficult, a biopsy is often performed when rejection is suspected. This procedure may be performed transcutaneously with little risk. Early microscopic signs of acute rejection include the adherence of lymphocytes to the endothelium of peritubular capillaries and venules, which then progresses to disruption of these vessels, tubular necrosis, and interstitial infiltrates. Cellular infiltration, which is the

hallmark of rejection, is composed at first of small lympho-cytes and later consists of a variety of cells such as large lym-phocytes and macrophages. As rejection proceeds toward irreversibility, there is greater involvement of the vascular elements of the graft.

- In the Banff schema, glomerular, interstitial, tubular, and vas-cular lesions are graded 0 to 3+, depending on whether they are absent (0), mild (1), moderate (2), or severe (3). Total reliance cannot be placed on a biopsy as the "gold standard" for diagnosing acute rejection. Not only are biopsies subject to sampling error but also lymphocytic infiltration in itself cannot be taken as conclusive evidence of rejection because, for obscure reasons, even perfectly functioning renal allografts may exhibit some degree of mononuclear infiltration.

Chronic Rejection

- The border between acute and chronic rejection is not always sharply defined, but the typical course of chronic rejection is gradual, progressive loss of renal function. It may begin after years of stable function but is more often seen in patients who have had multiple early and incompletely reversible episodes of acute rejection. Humoral injury (thought to be a more important factor in this condition than in acute cellular rejection) is manifested histologically by intimal fibroproliferative arterial lesions that probably stem from repetitive cycles of immune injury to the endothelium with focal thrombosis and incorporation of thrombus into the arterial wall (also seen in chronic rejection are glomeru-lar changes). Histologically, increased mesangial matrix and mesangial proliferation are seen. The glomerular basement membrane is thickened and focal deposition of IgM, IgG, and complement may be identified along capillary walls and within the mesangium. Clinically, these are manifested by proteinuria, microscopic hematuria, and slowly deteriorating function. As with acute rejection, a semiquantitative analysis of assessing renal progress for chronic rejection has been proposed under the Banff schema.
- In the presence of these morphologic vascular and glomerular changes, antirejection therapy is ineffective.
- It is important to remember that acute cellular rejection is also occasionally encountered after years of stable transplant func-tion, sometimes as the result of discontinuation of immuno-suppression by the careless or noncompliant patient. This must be distinguished from chronic rejection if possible, although a timely diagnosis of late acute rejection is usually fortuitous because symptoms are uncommon. A prompt

biopsy is warranted in cases of unexpected or precipitous deterioration in stable function because late cellular rejection (unlike chronic rejection) can often be reversed if treated before severe damage occurs.

Recurrent Disease in Transplanted Kidneys

- Because transplantation does not modify the underlying etiology of the renal disease, it is not surprising that the transplanted kidney is sometimes regarded by the host as an appropriate new target for destruction by the original disease process, especially in autoimmune or metabolic diseases.

Glomerulonephritis

- In identical twin donor transplants performed in the 1950s, Murray recognized recurrent glomerulonephritic damage, which sometimes became apparent within only a few months.
- Fortunately, recurrent disease is less common in allografts, but in this setting, it is more difficult to diagnose because its clinical manifestations and even histologic changes may be confused with those of chronic rejection.
- It appears to be most likely in twins and next most likely in recipients of closely matched related donor allografts.

Complications of Renal Transplantation

Technical Complications

- Vascular complications.
  - Partial occlusion of the transplant vessels may be caused by kinking from unfortunate positioning of the kidney. Although radioisotopic scanning and arteriography will confirm suspected vascular occlusion, immediate reoperation without delay for diagnostic studies is usually the only chance for salvaging such a graft because only a few minutes of total ischemia can be tolerated before damage becomes irreversible.
- Hemorrhage.
  - Imperfect operative hemostasis in the setting of uremic coagulopathy or anticoagulation during hemodialysis are the usual causes of early postoperative bleeding. Fracture or frank rupture of the transplanted kidney are unusual causes of bleeding, but these may occur from rapid swelling of the transplant during acute rejection. Rupture is more common in kidneys from infant or child donors, in which the small organ is sometimes unable to tolerate adult levels of blood pressure and flow.

- Hypertension and renal transplant artery stenosis.
- Urinary tract complications.
  - The most common cause of sudden cessation of urinary output in the immediate postoperative period is the presence of a blood clot in the bladder or urethral catheter, which can be relieved by irrigation. Other more serious causes of urinary obstruction are unusual and should be investigated simultaneously with consideration of vascular occlusion, acute tubular necrosis (ATN), or rejection.
  - Devascularization of the ureter during donor nephrectomy is a more serious problem that may lead to ureteral necrosis and fistula within the first few days or weeks.
- Acute tubular necrosis.
  - Ischemia occasionally precipitates ATN in a related donor transplant, but in cadaver transplants, the incidence is much higher. Even in transplants from "heart-beating cadavers," some degree of ATN occurs in 5% to 30%. Therefore, in the absence of vascular or ureteral problems, initially nonfunctional cadaver kidneys may be assumed to suffer from ATN, especially if technetium and iodohippurate scans demonstrate good blood flow and poor tubular function.
- Lymphoceles.
  - Extensive mobilization of the iliac vessels during the transplant operation or failure to ligate lymphatics crossing them may predispose to lymphoceles, which have a variable reported incidence (0.6% to 18%). Possible manifestations that can occur weeks or months postoperatively are swelling of the wound; edema of the scrotum, labia, and lower extremity; and urinary obstruction resulting from pressure on the collecting system or ureter. Ultrasound to identify a fluid-filled mass is the most useful diagnostic study.
  - The treatment of choice is fenestration of the cyst into the peritoneal cavity. This can often be accomplished by laparoscopic technique. We have also successfully used a nonoperative treatment of percutaneous drainage followed by repeated instillation of tetracycline or povidone iodine to sclerose and obliterate the cyst.

Nontechnical Complications

Infections

- Factors predisposing to infection of transplant recipients include a major surgical operation involving the urinary tract;

infection carried over from the donor; and indwelling catheters in the bladder, bloodstream, and peritoneal cavity. Because of these and the immunodepression associated with uremia and antirejection therapy, 30% to 60% of patients suffer some type of infection during the first transplant year, and in half of the deaths that occur during the first year, infection is an important contributing feature. More cautious use of immunosuppression in the 1980s and the introduction of cyclosporine have reduced the magnitude of this problem, but infection remains the most common and most lethal complication of renal transplantation.

- Bacterial infections.
  - The incidence of wound infections (reported to be anywhere from 1% to 10%) can probably be reduced by preoperative or intraoperative prophylaxis with a cephalosporin, which should not be continued for more than 24 to 48 hours.
  - Urinary tract infections, which are the most common bacterial infections in transplant recipients, can be decreased by 50% by using trimethoprim-sulfa antibiotics for the first 6 months after transplantation. This is also helpful in decreasing the incidence of *Pneumocystis carinii.*
- Opportunistic infections.
  - The period between 30 and 180 days after transplantation, usually the time of most intense immunosuppression, is the most common time for infection with opportunistic organisms, which in normal individuals rarely cause significant illness.
- Cytomegalovirus (CMV).
  - CMV, a member of the herpes virus family, is the most important viral pathogen. This ubiquitous agent infects most normal people at some point in their lives.
  - Seronegative recipients who receive a kidney from a seropositive donor are subject to a three times greater incidence of symptomatic illness, and of affected patients 25% have severe disease. CMV disease (as distinguished from asymptomatic seroconversion) varies in severity from mild fever and malaise to a debilitating syndrome marked by leukopenia, hepatitis, interstitial pneumonia, arthritis, central nervous system changes including coma, gastrointestinal ulceration and bleeding, renal insufficiency, bacterial or fungal infection, and even death.
  - A rapid diagnosis can be made by using tests for antigenemia or polymerase chain reaction assays using blood samples or the demonstration of virus on biopsy of infected tissues.
- Polyomavirus nephropathy.

- Primary infections with the polyomavirus (type BK) are known to occur in up to 90% of the population typically without specific signs or symptoms. This virus persists in the kidney where reactivation and shedding into the urine may be detected in 0.5% to 20% of healthy individuals depending on the sensitivity of the assay (polymerase chain reaction vs detection of viral inclusion bearing "decoy cells" on urinary cytology).
- It now appears that up to 5% of renal allograft recipients can be affected. The diagnosis can be suspected on the basis of screening urinary cytology but definitive diagnosis requires allograft biopsy to demonstrate nuclear inclusions in tubular epithelial cells and to rule out rejection or drug toxicity. Progression from an inflammatory stage to a fibrotic stage and finally to sclerosis and irreversible allograft failure has been observed in as many as 45% of affected cases. Current management is based on judicious decreases in immunosuppression to allow clearance of viral replication. In a few instances the antiviral agent cidofovir has been used with success.

Tumors

- It has been known for many years that both naturally occurring and iatrogenic states of immunodeficiency are accompanied by an increased risk of neoplasia.
- One hypothesis invoked to explain the more striking prevalence of malignancies in immunosuppressed patients is a breakdown of normal immunologic surveillance mechanisms that allows persistence of mutant malignant cells that would be recognized and destroyed by an intact immune system.
- Transplant recipients in all parts of the world have a disproportionately high incidence of lymphomas (350 times normal) that compose 20% of all tumors in this population.
- There has been considerable disagreement regarding the classification of the more usual lymphomatous lesions of transplant patients. Therefore, the nonspecific term *post-transplant lymphoproliferative disease* (PTLD) is now widely used, covering a spectrum of lesions ranging from benign hyperplasia to frankly malignant lymphomas. According to the UNOS database of 205,114 recipients transplanted between 1988 and 1999, 2365 (1.15%) developed PTLD.
- Hyperplastic PTLDs are polyclonal in origin, whereas neoplastic PTLDs contain a monoclonal component that can be detected by sensitive assays.

- Compelling evidence of this is the finding of Epstein-Barr virus incorporated into the genome of lymphoma cells.

Results of Renal Transplantation

- During the early days of transplantation, the success of HLA identical sibling donor grafts was twice that of cadaveric transplants. Since then, the short-term results of cadaveric grafts have improved greatly and, now at least for a year, approach the success of HLA identical sibling grafts (89% vs 96%) (Fig. 26–1). However, when long-term survival is examined, the importance of histocompatibility remains obvious. At 5 years, 90% of HLA identical sibling grafts survive and at 10 years 65%, but despite striking advances in immunosuppressive therapy, the survival of cadaveric grafts at 5 years is only 65% and at 10 years less than 40% unless they are matched for the recipient's HLA antigens, which improves their 5-year survival to about 73%.
- A disappointing aspect of the results of renal transplantation is evident from examining long-term cadaveric graft survival. Despite the dramatic short-term improvements in both patient and graft survival since about 1980, substantive attrition of

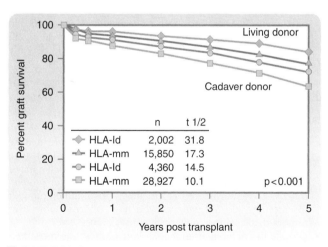

	n	t 1/2
HLA-Id	2,002	31.8
HLA-mm	15,850	17.3
HLA-Id	4,360	14.5
HLA-mm	28,927	10.1

p<0.001

■ FIGURE 26–1. Although the short-term success of kidneys transplanted from cadaveric donors approaches that of related donors, the long-term survival increasingly favors related donor grafts. The half-life of HLA identical living donor grafts is three times longer than that of HLA-mismatched cadaveric donor grafts.

cadaveric grafts continues after 1 year. Until 1988, this attrition remained almost constant at about 7% per year despite the introduction of cyclosporine. Since then, the half-life of cadaveric grafts has improved to 14.5 years if they were HLA-matched with the recipient but to only 10.2 years for other cadaveric grafts.

- Continuing damage of grafts appears to be the result of chronic rejection, and in some patients recurrence of glomerulonephritis, entities for which we still lack effective therapy.
- The excellent results of transplantation relative to dialysis and the donor shortage have resulted in a growing list of patients awaiting transplantation. By 2001 more than 50,000 candidates awaited cadaveric kidneys in the United States, whereas only about 9000 renal transplants were done. For older patients, a 3- to 5-year waiting time represented a significant portion of their remaining life.
- Impatience with long waiting times for cadaveric donor kidneys (during which many dialysis patients die) has led to a considerable increase in the use of in living donors, which now exceed the number of cadaveric donors in the United States compared with less than 20% a decade ago.
- Another impact of the donor shortage has had an adverse effect on overall results: the use of kidneys from suboptimal donors. The percentage of cadaveric kidneys from donors older than 50 years increased from 26% in 1988 to 46% in 2000. Unfortunately age has a profound effect on 5-year graft survival, which was 72% for donors 6 to 18 years old but only 50% for donors older than 60 years.

LIVER TRANSPLANTATION

Indication for Liver Transplantation

- Liver transplantation is the procedure of choice for a wide range of diseases that result in acute or chronic end-stage liver disease (ESLD) and for several diseases in which a major genetic error affects production of an essential liver protein. It may also be considered as a treatment for a limited number of carefully selected patients who have nonresectable liver tumors that have not metastasized outside the liver.
- Despite the differences in the etiology of these diseases, their shared pathophysiology leads to a common set of symptoms and signs typical of end-stage liver failure.
- In 2002, UNOS put into place a new system for allocation.
- A statistical model for end-stage liver disease (MELD) was used for adult patients that had been shown to have a high

predictive capacity in identifying those patients with ESLD at greatest risk of mortality within 3 months. The MELD score was based on three laboratory values; total bilirubin, international normalized ratio (INR), and creatinine and demonstrated a better correlation with 3 month survival than the Child-Turcote-Pugh (CTP) score (Table 26–1). A similar approach was developed for pediatric patients although the relevant variables suffer slightly (pediatric end-stage liver disease [PELD] score).

- Specific exclusion criteria for liver transplantation are not formally established, although it is generally agreed that the presence of active sepsis or the findings of extrahepatic malignancy should be considered absolute contraindications. However, controversial are conditions such as HIV infection in the absence of acquired immunodeficiency syndrome (AIDS), large size hepatocellular cancer (HCC) (>6 cm), or cholangiocarcinoma. Several other entities such as portal vein thrombosis once considered contraindications for transplantation are no longer so categorized.

- It is essential for the general surgeon to recognize the dynamics of chronic liver disease and to be able to assess the residual liver function in the presence of chronic liver disease. It is not uncommon for minor surgical procedures to exhaust the residual reserve and precipitate the development of acute on chronic failure. Management of these complications is extremely difficult. If liver transplantation must be performed during such circumstances it is associated with higher morbidity and mortality.

Disease Treated by Liver Transplantation

- The conditions that result in an end-stage acute or chronic liver failure are different in the pediatric and adult populations. Although the incidence of most liver diseases has

TABLE 26–1. Concordance with 3-Month Mortality: MELD and CTP

Score	Concordance	95% Confidence Interval
Model for End-Stage Liver Disease (MELD)	0.88	0.85, 0.90
Child Turcote-Pugh (CTP)	0.79	0.75, 0.83

remained relatively constant over recent times, the prevalence of liver failure from viral hepatitis is increasing, reflecting the increased rate of infection in the last two decades. It is expected that the relatively recent availability of the hepatitis B vaccine and the ability to detect HCV in donated blood will lower the rate of new infections and the number of individuals who subsequently develop chronic disease.

- Hepatitis B.
  - As with other forms of liver cancer, tumors associated with hepatitis B result from chronic inflammation and repeated cellular regeneration, typically occurring only after 25 to 30 years of infection. Most patients with chronic hepatitis B undergoing liver transplantation will reinfect the hepatic graft, and some undergo rapidly progressive liver failure. Fortunately, prophylaxis consisting of high-titer hepatitis B immune globulin and/or lamivudine is highly effective in the control of viral replication and recurrent disease post transplant.

- Hepatitis C.
  - HCV is an RNA virus of the flavivirus family, which leads to chronic inflammation of the liver in about 85% of infected individuals. It is detected by the persistence of anti-HCV antibodies, serum viral proteins, and HCV RNA. Virtually all patients with chronic HCV infection develop histological features of chronic hepatitis, and as many as 20% of patients develop cirrhosis within 10 to 20 years of HCV infection. They develop the typical complications of chronic liver disease including portal hypertension, hepatocellular failure, and hepatic encephalopathy. Hepatocellular carcinoma may ensue in 1% to 4% per year of chronic active hepatitis C (CAHC) patients with established cirrhosis.
  - For patients with advanced liver disease, liver transplantation is often the only therapeutic option.
  - However, virtually all patients become reinfected with HCV after transplantation and about half of them develop histologic evidence of chronic hepatitis within a few months. There is growing concern regarding the eventual recurrence of liver failure in these patients 5 to 10 years after transplantation, and recent evidence indicates that the long-term survival for patients transplanted for HCV may be significantly inferior in comparison to transplantation for other causes of liver disease.

- Alcoholic liver disease.
  - Alcoholic liver injury results from toxic effects of ethanol to hepatocytes, the accumulation of fatty acids within the

cells, and subsequent degeneration and necrosis. The intensity of the inflammatory process is directly related to the amount of alcohol consumed and is associated with fibrosis and subsequent cirrhosis. The coexistence of hepatitis C infection accelerates liver injury in most cases. Discontinuation of alcohol consumption may arrest hepatocyte destruction and allow regeneration and relatively compensated cirrhosis. Continued deterioration of liver function in the absence of alcohol and an appropriate CTP score are an indication for transplantation just as in other liver diseases. Transplant candidates with alcoholic cirrhosis should undergo careful psychosocial evaluation in an attempt to document their sobriety for at least 6 months and the likelihood of post-transplant recidivism.

- Primary biliary cirrhosis (PBC) and primary sclerosing cholangitis (PSC).
  - PBC and PSC share many clinical, biochemical, and pathologic features. Clinically, both give rise to characteristic symptoms and signs of chronic biliary tract disease (e.g., pruritus and jaundice). In both conditions, the most characteristic biochemical abnormality is an increased serum alkaline phosphatase level. Central to the pathologic changes in both PBC and PSC is damage to bile ducts; in the case of PBC, this involves mainly the smaller intrahepatic ducts, whereas in PSC it also affects large ducts outside the liver and the gallbladder and even pancreatic ducts. Unique to PSC is its association with inflammatory bowel disease, which occurs in 70% of the patients. There is an increased incidence of cholangiocarcinoma in PSC patients. Liver failure in both diseases is manifested by hyperbilirubinemia. Transplantation is highly successful in both groups leading to long-term survival of greater than 90% and an insignificant incidence of recurrence.

- HCC.
  - The rationale for liver transplantation in patients with nonresectable HCC is based on the logical potential of complete removal of disease that is confined to the liver. Unfortunately, it has become evident that in most cases the tumor recurs. However, the procedure can provide significant benefit in a specific subpopulation of patients identified by the following characteristics: histologic grading of G1 to G2, tumor size less than 5 cm, and limited multifocally.
  - The results of transplantation for this selected group are variable but have been reported to have a disease-free survival of 60% to 85% at 3 years. It is yet to be determined

whether the addition of adjuvant chemotherapy following transplantation could be an important factor in the control of recurrence.
- Biliary atresia.
  - Extrahepatic biliary atresia is an obliterative cholangiopathy affecting all or part of the extrahepatic biliary tree. The condition occurs in 1 of 10,000 neonates. The diagnosis is suggested in neonates who remain jaundiced for 6 weeks or more after birth and have pale stools and dark urine.
  - The Kasai procedure (hepatic portoenterostomy with resection of the obliterated bile ducts and re-establishment of biliary drainage to the intestine) can increase survival rates at the early stage. However, progressive intrahepatic bile duct destruction by chronic inflammation, fibrosis, and cirrhosis commonly occurs. Failure of the Kasai procedure is manifested by failure to thrive, recurrent cholangitis, and typical signs of ESLD. These are indications for transplantation.
- Failure of previous liver graft.
  - An important and growing indication for transplantation is the failure of a previous graft. This occurs in the acute setting immediately post transplant arising from technical failures discussed later or chronically because chimeric rejection or disease reoccurrence. Retransplantation can be particularly complex in the chronic setting because of the usual factors associated with reoperative surgery. Overall the results of retransplantation are inferior to that achieved with primary grafts, and each subsequent transplant is associated with an additional decrement in survival.

Patient Selection and Preoperative Consideration

- Patients who experience progressive deterioration or acute decompensation of preexisting chronic liver disease or previously normal patients who suddenly develop fulminant liver failure are candidates for transplantation and should be promptly referred for evaluation to a transplant center.

Assessment of Acute Liver Failure

- The hallmarks of fulminant liver failure include the development of encephalopathy, coagulopathy, and hypoglycemia. Careful neurologic evaluation must determine the stage of hepatic coma. Progression from a state of confusion to one of unresponsiveness is associated with an increased likelihood that brain damage is irreversible. At this stage, assessment must include brain imaging with computed tomography (CT) or magnetic resonance imaging (MRI), and monitoring of intracranial pressure (ICP) should be considered. An attempt should be made to help promote cerebral perfusion (higher than 60 mm Hg) by reducing ICP and maintaining high mean arterial pressure. Irreversible injury is associated with persistent elevation of ICP, which leads to the development of severe brain edema and herniation. Other variables that define the extent of liver injury and predict chances of recovery relate to changes in prothrombin time, levels of factor V, and phosphorous levels and persistence of hypoglycemia. Coagulopathy may be resistant to correction but is best treated with transfusion of fresh frozen plasma. Plasmapheresis may be beneficial in small children in whom administration of large fluid volumes is problematic. Severe hypoglycemia is usually controlled by a dextrose infusion. Interestingly, changes in liver transaminases are not reliable indicators of the potential for recovery.

Operative Complexities and Complications

- Operative bleeding.
  - Excessive bleeding from portal hypertension may occur during hepatectomy and is likely to be accentuated by coagulopathy or adhesions from previous surgery. The removal of the cirrhotic organ, transplantation of a graft with normal function, and correction of coagulopathy by the appropriate use of platelets and fresh frozen plasma best control bleeding during hepatectomy and after reperfusion.
- Thrombosis of the portal vein.
- Hepatic arterial reconstruction.

Post-Transplant Management

Common Complications

- Primary nonfunction (PNF).
  - The mechanisms of immediate graft failure following successful revascularization of the transplanted liver are not completely understood but may relate to donor variables, inadequate preservation, prolonged cold ischemia, or the humoral immune response. This problem is encountered in 2% to 5% of liver grafts. It is characterized by clinical and laboratory findings indicating poor synthetic function and severe hepatocytes injury. The recipient may present postoperatively with progressive hemodynamic

instability, multiorgan system failure, and encephalopathy. Laboratory findings demonstrate worsening acidosis, coagulopathy, and extremely elevated liver enzymes (lactate dehydrogenase [LDH], aspartate transaminase [AST], and alanine transaminase [ALT]). The development of PNF is a surgical emergency can be successfully treated by early retransplantation.

- Intra-abdominal bleeding.
  - The persistence of immediate post-transplant coagulopathy, fibrinolysis, and the presence of multiple vascular anastomoses place these patients at high risk for postoperative bleeding. However, coagulopathy spontaneously corrects itself in the presence of recovering liver graft function and with infusion of platelets. A persistent drop in hemoglobin and the need for transfusion of more than six units of packed red blood cells are usually indications for re-exploration and evacuation of the hematoma. In most cases, removal of the clot will be sufficient to arrest further fibrinolysis and will stop bleeding. Occasionally, it will be necessary to repair bleeding sites.
- Vascular thrombosis.
  - Vascular complications following liver transplantation are more common in the pediatric population and are directly related to the small size of the vessels that are used for reconstruction. The most frequent complication is the occurrence of hepatic artery thrombosis. The pathology can present itself with rapid or indolent worsening of graft function or necrosis of the bile duct and dehiscence of the biliary enteric anastomosis. Early recognition and successful thrombectomy may salvage the graft. However, deteriorating liver function and bile duct necrosis indicate the need for immediate retransplantation.
- Biliary leak.
  - Reconstruction of the biliary system with either duct-to-duct anastomosis or choledochojejunostomy may be complicated with a bile leak, usually secondary to technical error or ischemia of the donor duct. Early leaks can be diagnosed by the appearance of bile in the drains and are confirmed by a T-tube cholangiogram or hepatobiliary iminodiacetic acid (HIDA) scan. Surgical exploration and revision of the anastomosis is mandatory and will solve the problem in most cases. Ischemic bile duct injury secondary to early hepatic artery thrombosis is an indication for retransplantation.
- Infections.
  - Infections remain the most significant complications in liver transplantation and are responsible for most of mortalities

in the early postoperative period. There seems to be a direct correlation among the preoperative status of the recipient, the pattern of recovery after transplantation, and the incidence of bacterial and fungal infections.

Immunologic Aspects of Liver Transplantation

● The relatively low immunogenicity of liver allografts and the unique ability of the liver to regenerate are probably the main reasons for the excellent long-term outcome. Good results are achieved when graft and recipient are ABO blood group compatible. Preoperative HLA matching does not appear to be necessary. Most recipients are treated with combination therapy, which includes a calcineurin inhibitor (cyclosporine or tacrolimus) along with prednisone, with or without azathioprine or MMF. The protocols are adjusted for a rapid taper of the steroids within the first 3 to 6 months after surgery and significant reduction in the calcineurin inhibitor. Long-term maintenance of immunosuppression seems to be necessary in most recipients because complete cessation of immunosuppression carries significant risk for the development of acute and chronic rejection.

Acute Rejection

● T-cell–mediated acute rejection is seen at a rate of 30% to 50% within the first 6 months after transplantation, most often within the first 10 days. Its clinical presentation is variable and may include the development of fever, abdominal pain, and elevated liver enzymes and bilirubin.
● Most rejection episodes are responsive to the administration of high-dose steroids. More potent monoclonal or polyclonal anti–T-cell antibodies are effective against steroid-resistant rejection, leading to the reversal of the acute episode in greater than 90% of the recipients.

Chronic Rejection

● This type of rejection is seen months or years after transplantation. It is manifested by poor synthetic liver function and hyperbilirubinemia. It is usually characterized histologically by paucity of the bile ducts; thus it is often described as "vanishing bile duct syndrome." The etiology for this phenomenon is not well understood and may be related to a humoral reaction involving antibodies and fibrogenic cytokines. The treatment for chronic rejection is limited, and some of these patients may be considered as candidates for retransplantation.

Recurrent Disease

- Replacement of the liver may not permanently cure recipients of their original disease. Recurrence of viral hepatitis is likely within a short time after transplantation in infected recipients.
- Most liver transplant recipients who survive the immediate post-transplant period enjoy full functional recovery. However, restoration of a fully functional status depends on the patient's preoperative condition, an appropriate support system, and his or her attitude to rehabilitation.

Long-Term Results

- UNOS registry data on nearly 30,000 liver transplants demonstrate impressive long-term survival. At 10 years, patient and graft survival for adults is 59% and 51%, respectively. The results in children are even better with 78% of patients and 63% grafts surviving at 10 years.
- Morbidity and mortality following orthotopic liver transplantation is directly correlated with the recipient preoperative status and the immediate function of the liver allograft. A higher mortality has been reported for recipients whose UNOS status was categorized as urgent and in those who had multiorgan system failure. Other variables associated with decreased survival include older age group, ventilator dependency, the need for dialysis, and retransplantation. Controversy exists whether scarce livers should be used under these circumstances, because there would be greater chance of their long-term function in patients less seriously ill. However, the rationale for continuing to offer the procedure to these high-risk patients is based on their inability to survive if a transplant is not performed.

PANCREATIC TRANSPLANTATION

- The purpose of pancreas transplantation is normalization of the diabetic recipient's blood glucose, thus preventing eventual microvascular complications, a goal unlikely to be possible with exogenous insulin therapy. The outcome of pancreas transplantation in the 1960s and 1970s was far inferior to that with other organs (frequent fatalities and less than 20% graft survival). However, because of improvements in surgical technique and immunosuppression, the results of the procedure have progressively improved to the level of other transplants. The usual candidates for pancreas transplants are patients with diabetic nephropathy who are obligated to chronic immunosuppression to prevent rejection of a kidney allograft. Ironically, those diabetics who have no renal or other complications of their disease would be the ones most likely to benefit from the procedure because, if it were carried out at that stage, it would be likely to prevent microvascular complications. However, most diabetologists have been reluctant to recommend pancreatic transplantation in nonuremic diabetics because it would obligate them to chronic immunosuppression.

Indication for Pancreas Transplantation and Patient Selection

- Because insulin is effective therapy for most diabetics (except for its failure to prevent eventual microvascular complications), pancreas transplantation is not considered a life-saving procedure unless the patient is experiencing episodes of severe hypoglycemic unawareness. Thus, in considering pancreas transplantation, the requisite dangers of a major operation and lifelong immunosuppression must be balanced against the possible benefits. The evidence is now convincing that optimizing exogenous insulin therapy favorably influences microvascular complications. That successful pancreas transplantation would also do so is based on softer evidence, although the assumption seems quite safe that the even better control of hyperglycemia associated with this method would provide optimal protection from complications. Microvascular sequelae, such as ocular, neurologic, and renal disabilities, will eventually occur in more than 50% of diabetics on insulin therapy. Thus, the possibility of achieving glucose homeostasis by pancreas transplantation and avoiding microvascular complications is very attractive to patients, including many with advanced complications in whom objective analysis of the risks and benefits does not support its use. It is important for patients to understand that advanced complications (e.g., blindness, pregangrenous extremities, end-stage nephropathy) will not be reversed.
- Because of the prevalence in diabetics of microvascular disease, especially in the coronary arteries, evaluating the risks of major surgery is especially important. Indeed, one of the most common causes of pancreas transplant failure is death from myocardial infarction.
- Uremic type I diabetics who are candidates for cadaver donor kidney transplants are the most usual patients to be considered for pancreas transplantation, which is most often carried out simultaneously with the kidney transplant.

Also appropriate for pancreas transplantation are diabetics who harbor a previously transplanted functioning kidney allograft because they are already committed to immunosuppression. In nonuremic diabetics who either do not need a kidney transplant or have not previously had one, the indications for pancreas transplantation are controversial. However, extremely labile diabetics who are at substantial risk from repeated episodes of dangerous hypoglycemia should be considered for transplantation even if they are not uremic.

- Between 1988 and 2000, 10,562 pancreas transplants were performed: 83% of these were simultaneous pancreas kidney transplants (SPK), 12% pancreas after kidney, and only 5% pancreas alone transplants. In other parts of the world, 93% of pancreas transplants were performed simultaneously with a kidney transplant.

Biologic Factor Influencing the Outcome of Pancreas Transplantation

- Histocompatibility matching.
  - That donor-recipient histocompatibility is advantageous for pancreas transplants has been shown by the somewhat superior outcome of the 142 living related donor pancreas transplants that had been reported as of October 2001 compared with cadaveric pancreas grafts. Despite this immunologic advantage of related donors, they have been used in only 0.8% of pancreas transplants because of the potential risks to the donor.
  - For cadaveric transplants, the advantage of matching is subtle. Analysis of the results from 1997 to 2001 indicated no benefit of HLA matching for simultaneous pancreas kidney grafts, although the pancreas after kidney and pancreas alone transplant there was slightly better survival for HLA-A and B matching but surprisingly not for the HLA-DR matching.
- Immunosuppression.

Rejection

Prevalence and Severity

- Whether human vascularized pancreas allografts are more or less vulnerable to rejection than vascularized allografts of other organs is a difficult question, especially because the pancreas is a composite organ with distinct exocrine and endocrine components, which may not be equally subject to rejection. Rejection of a kidney and pancreas transplanted simultaneously from the same donor is often manifested at the same time. However, either organ may undergo earlier or more severe rejection. In patients who receive pancreas and kidney transplants, rejection episodes tend to be more frequent than in those receiving only a kidney. However, pancreatic graft loss from rejection is more frequent if the pancreas alone is transplanted (PTA) than if both kidney and pancreas are transplanted.

Diagnosis of Rejection

- The early diagnosis of pancreatic allograft rejection is particularly important because physiologic evidence of islet damage (hyperglycemia) is a late indicator of rejection. Once islet damage is advanced, it is often difficult or impossible to reverse it by intensifying immunosuppression. The importance of identifying early rejection has led to exploration of a number of methods, such as imaging techniques and blood and urine tests. None of these has proved to be very reliable. Thus, in the effort to recognize early rejection, a combination of nonspecific indicators are used. These include increases in serum amylase, lipase, and anodal trypsinogen; decreases in urinary amylase (in the case of bladder-drained allografts); impaired function of a concomitantly transplanted kidney allograft; biopsy of the kidney or pancreas allograft; and finally, hyperglycemia.

- Histologic evidence of rejection is, of course, the most definitive indicator of rejection. Biopsy of the concomitantly transplanted kidney or the duodenum associated with the pancreas may be helpful, but most specific of all is a biopsy of the pancreatic allograft itself, which can be obtained by ultrasound guided transcutaneous or transcystoscopic techniques. If necessary, open biopsies can also be performed safely.

Treatment of Rejection Episodes

- Although early initiation of antirejection therapy is more important in pancreas than in kidney transplantation, the treatment of rejection episodes is similar to that used for kidney allograft rejection—high-dose steroids and anti–T-cell antibodies.

Autoimmune Recurrence

- In addition to rejection, an immunologic threat to pancreas transplants is the autoimmune response to islets, which was responsible for elimination of the native pancreatic beta cells. In the case of kidney transplants, an analogous vulnerability of transplanted kidneys was noted in the early 1960s when patients with glomerulonephritis were found to be subject to autoimmune damage of the transplanted kidney even if rejection was avoided by using an identical twin donor.

Complications of Pancreas Transplantation

- Pancreas transplant patients are susceptible to the complications common to all immunosuppressed patients (e.g., infection, malignancy, steroid-induced osteonecrosis). In addition, they are subject to several nonimmunologic complications specific to this type of transplant.

Vascular Thrombosis

- The most common nonimmunologic cause of failure of pancreas allograft failure is vascular thrombosis. This complication is most frequent during the first 7 days. It almost always results in loss of the graft and is responsible for about 70% of technical failures. The reported incidence of this complication varies from 10% to 30%. Its etiology appears to be the relatively sluggish blood flow to the pancreas, estimated as only 1% of cardiac output, compared with the rapid blood flow through kidney, heart, or liver transplants.

Allograft Pancreatitis

- Allograft pancreatitis in the early post-transplant period occurs in 10% to 20% of recipients. Predisposing factors are donor abnormalities (hemodynamic instability, vasopressor administration), procurement injury, perfusion injury (excessive pressure or volume), ischemic damage during preservation, and reperfusion injury. In severe pancreatitis, compromised pancreatic microcirculation causes necrosis and then arterial thrombosis.

Fistula and Abscess

- Extravasation of pancreatic juice from the pancreatic anastomosis is a more serious complication in enteric drained than in bladder-drained allografts. During an era of more danger-ous immunosuppression this accounted for a substantial difference in survival from the two methods between 1987 and 1992 (for bladder-drained pancreas transplants, survival was 75% compared with only 54% for those enterically drained).

Urologic Complications

● Urologic complications, such as urethritis, urethral disruption, hematuria, and recurrent urinary tract infections, are quite common in bladder-drained recipients. These problems, and bicarbonate losses, are the major disadvantages of this technique. Urethritis often resolves after a period of Foley catheter drainage, but, if not, enteric conversion is required to prevent scarring or disruption of the urethra. Hematuria may sometimes respond to simple bladder irrigation. If it persists, fulguration of the bleeding site may be effective; if not, enteric conversion is necessary.

Results of Pancreas Transplantation

Impact on Metabolic Defects of Diabetes

● Successful pancreatic transplantation restores normoglycemia and normal levels of hemoglobin A_{1c}. The response to glucose challenge and to intravenous arginine and secretin is also normalized.
● Although systemic venous drainage of the graft via the donor's iliac vein has been the standard method, several groups have evaluated the alternative of directing the venous effluent into the recipient's portal vein. Because this is the physiologic route, there has been speculation that it would have a metabolic advantage. It does in fact prevent hyperin-sulinemia. However, the procedure is more complex, and there is little evidence that it has a meaningful advantage.

Graft Survival

● After disappointing outcomes during the early years of pancreas transplantation, patient and graft survival rates for the procedure now approach those of other solid organ transplants. From December 1966 to August 2002 more than 17,800 pancreas transplants were reported to the International Pancreas Transplant Registry. For the more than 12,900

United States transplant patients, transplant reporting was complete because since 1988 it has been mandatory for all centers in this country to submit regular reports on their activity and outcomes. In the most recent registry report, of August 31, 2002 the 1997 to 2001 cases were analyzed. Patient's survival at 1 year was greater than 95%.

Recipient Category

- SPK recipients were the largest category, accounting for 83% of U.S. transplants.
- One-year patient and pancreas graft survival rates were 95% and 83%, respectively. Fortunately, kidney graft survival (92%) was not compromised by combining this procedure with a pancreas transplant.

Impact of Duct Management Technique

- In the United States, bladder drainage was until recently by far the most common technique for duct management because of its relative safety and because it facilitates early diagnosis of rejection by serial measurement of urinary amylase, which decreases if the graft suffers immunologic damage.
- Unfortunately, the bladder-drainage technique carries its own urologic and metabolic morbidities including cystitis, urethritis, and chronic acidosis from bicarbonate loss. In fact, in 15% of bladder-drained transplants, these problems are serious enough to warrant enteric conversion within 3 years.
- Although in earlier years bladder-drainage grafts fared substantially better, from 1997 to 2001, 1-year graft survival of SPK transplants was nearly the same for bladder-drained (85%) versus enteric drained (82%); complications remained somewhat more common in enteric-drained grafts (11% vs 8%).

Impact of Pancreas Transplantation on the Microvascular Complications

- Neuropathy.
- Retinopathy.
- Nephropathy.
- Whereas these studies strongly suggest that pancreas transplantation may improve diabetic retinopathy, nephropathy, and neuropathy, no controlled or randomized studies have yet confirmed these. Whether transplantation can also

prevent diabetic complications in otherwise unaffected patients, as tight insulin control has been shown to do, has not been investigated because pancreas transplantation, before the onset of any complications, is rarely if ever performed. Therefore, the potential benefits of pancreas transplantation over other forms of intensive diabetic treatment cannot be fully assessed at this time, although it seems likely that the optimal control of blood glucose possible from a pancreas transplant would be the optimal prophylaxis for microvascular complications.

TRANSPLANTATION OF ISOLATED PANCREATIC ISLETS

● With the report in the year 2000 of seven consecutive successful human islet transplants by the investigator of Edmonton, a new era appears to have begun for this field. Within 3 years of this report almost 300 islet transplants have been performed worldwide. The results of these transplants are much better than before. One-year islet graft survival rates in many of the approximately 30 centers performing them are comparable to that of pancreas transplantation. If this persists, islet transplantation will gradually assume a greater role in treatment of patients with type I diabetes.

Clinical Islet Transplantation

● Isolation methods.
● Surgical technique and complications.
   ● In human transplants, the islets have usually been transplanted by embolization to the liver via the portal vein.
   ● Although most patients tolerate the inoculation of intraportal islets, severe complications have been reported in a few, including portal vein thrombosis and disseminated intravascular coagulation. These complications are probably related to rapid infusion of insufficiently pure islet preparations containing large amounts of enzymatically rich acinar tissue.
● Metabolic factors influencing success.
● Islet autotransplantation.
   ● Transplantation of pancreatic fragments to diabetics was attempted (unsuccessfully) as early as 1893. Modern human islet transplantation began in 1977 when Sutherland and colleagues at the University of Minnesota performed an intraportal autotransplant of islets in a patient who was undergoing a near-total pancreatectomy for the persistent pain of chronic pancreatitis.

- Since then, more than 20 institutions have reported a combined series of 170 human islet autotransplants to the International Registry.
- Because the islets were autologous, rejection was not a possibility, and because these patients were not type 1 diabetics, there was no concern over recurrent autoimmune damage. In these patients, the incidence of insulin independence after 2 years was 34%.
- In autograft recipients, who received at least 300,000 islets, 74% were insulin independent after 2 years.
- Islet allografts after total pancreatectomy for patients with malignant disease.
- Islet allografts for insulin-dependent diabetes.
- Autoimmune damage of islet allografts.
- Fetal islet allografts and xenografts.
- Postoperative monitoring for rejection.

INTESTINAL TRANSPLANTATION

- The introduction of intravenous hyperalimentation by Dudrick and associates in 1968 allowed long-term survival of patients with complete intestinal failure who would previously have died rapidly. However, total parenteral nutrition (TPN) severely affects quality of life and may be associated with a number of highly morbid and sometimes fatal complications.
- An alternative to lifelong intravenous nutrition is restoration of enteral absorptive function by intestinal replacement. The earliest experimental transplants of the intestine performed by Lillehei in the 1960s indicated that success of intestinal grafts would be more difficult to achieve than that reported for other solid organ grafts. In fact, it was not until the availability of cyclosporine that even occasional success was achieved. However, since then the results have greatly improved.
- Nearly equal numbers of small intestine (SI) and liver-small intestine (LI) grafts have been reported, whereas only a few of multivisceral (MV) grafts have been done (about 10% of the total).
- The most frequent etiology of intestinal failure is the "short gut" syndrome, which follows extensive resection for intestinal ischemia or disease. At present, the most common indication for intestinal replacement is inability to sustain successful TPN because of lack of intravenous access sites or because of severe complications from chronic TPN, such as liver failure. That successful intestinal transplantation allows resumption of normal oral intake would make intestinal

transplantation the preferred method of therapy for intestinal failure, if the risks of this relatively new procedure can be further decreased.

- The principal barrier to widespread application of intestinal replacement at present is the unusually vigorous rejection response elicited by intestinal grafts. Unlike other solid organ grafts such as kidney or liver, which may incite a rejection crisis in 10% to 40% of recipients, 90% to 100% of small bowel grafts undergo rejection crisis within the first 6 months. The reasons for this difference are not entirely clear, but it is assumed that the large amount of gut-associated lymphoid tissue is responsible.

- A uniquely dangerous consequence of intestinal transplantation rejection is the loss of the protective mucosal barrier of the gut, consequent bacterial translocation, and systemic sepsis in an immunocompromised host. Thus, it is not surprising that the most common cause of death after small bowel transplantation is sepsis and multiorgan failure.

Results

- Data from the most recent International Intestinal Transplant Registry accumulated from 33 programs indicate that by February of 1997, 273 transplants had been performed in 260 patients. Forty-one percent of grafts were isolated bowel and 48% included a simultaneous liver graft. Only 11% of grafts were multivisceral. For grafts transplanted since 1995, 1-year graft survival was nearly equivalent in all three groups (SI, 55%; LI, 63%; MV, 63%) as was patient survival.

- The importance of experience was emphasized by the superior results at the University of Pittsburgh. This center has performed more than 165 intestinal transplants. It reported an actuarial patient survival rate of 75% at 1 year, 54% at 5 years, and 42% at 10 years. For the 93 patients transplanted since 1994 results were substantially improved. One-year survival was 78% and 5-year survival was 63%. The improvement was attributed to several changes in the immunosuppressive regimen, including cyclophosphamide anti–IL-2 receptor antibody therapy, and in some recent recipients to administration of donor bone marrow cells to and/or pretransplant irradiation of the graft. If this early success is sustained and is attainable by other groups as well, transplantation would become the preferred therapy for patients with intestinal failure.

CHAPTER 27

TUMOR BIOLOGY
AND TUMOR MARKERS

TUMOR BIOLOGY

- Tumors are characterized by an uncontrolled growth of transformed cells.

How Do Tumors Arise?

- The progression of a single transforming event in a cell toward the formation of a tumor requires multiple mutations that occur in sequence.
- In general, mutated genes in transformed cells include tumor suppressor genes and oncogenes. Both types of genes play an essential role in the regulation of cell cycle progression.

Stimulation of Tumor Development

- Together, tumor cells, extracellular matrix (ECM), stroma, and infiltrate produce factors (autocrine and paracrine factors) that in cell-bound, matrix-bound, or soluble form directly or indirectly influence tumor development.

Paracrine and Autocrine Growth Mechanisms

- Simplified, tumor growth is dependent on the response of tumor cells to paracrine and autocrine factors.

Role of Inflammation in Cancer

- Mechanistically, the cells and factors involved in tumor growth are very similar to those involved in wound healing.

Tumor Progression

- The difference between the growth of tumor at an earlier stage and at later stages may be that, at later stages, more tumor cells have acquired a stimulatory paracrine loop of

375

growth factors as a result of the continuous transformations in tumor cells and the selection for survival.

Intravasation and Extravasation

- It is clear from the variety of processes that tumor progression may involve an increased expression of proteases, decreased expression of protease inhibitors, and enhanced expression of certain ECM–receptor interactions, whereas other matrix–receptor interactions are decreased.
- The clonal and genetic diversity of tumors permits adhesion and detachment from the same matrix.

Outgrowth at Preferred Sites

- Invasion and metastatic spread of tumor cells does not appear to be a random process.

Immune Surveillance

- The data from mouse and human studies combined suggest that immune surveillance of cancer does exist, mediated through immune cells and soluble factors.

Immune Effector Cells

Innate Immune Cells

- Innate immune cells, such as macrophages, dendritic cells, natural killer (NK) cells, cells that resemble NK and T cells (NKT cells), and polymorphonuclear cells (PMNs) characteristically do not need sensitization to respond to an immunogen.

Acquired Immunity

- Acquired immunity is mediated by antigen-specific effector cells that recognize tumor antigens. Tumor-specific antigens have been discovered that are either unique or shared by other tumors, and can be recognized by antibodies or T cells.
- T cells, in contrast to antibodies, may directly lyse tumor cells.
- Whereas CD8$^+$ T cells recognize antigens presented by major histocompatibility complex (MHC) class I molecules, CD4$^+$ T cells are generally MHC class II restricted.

Escape from Immune Surveillance

- Only those transformed cells that have a sufficiently distinct phenotype from normal cells are expected to induce an immune response.

Tumor-Related Immune Escape

- In a growing number of cases, loss of MHC expression has been positively correlated with tumor aggressiveness and metastatic potential.
- Soluble factors secreted by tumor cells may also redirect immune responses, activating immune cells that do not harm tumor cells.

Chemotherapy

- In addition to the direct damage effects, however, certain genes may be triggered that are involved in apoptosis, leading to cell death.
- High levels of *bcl-2* are found in tumor cells and may confer resistance to anticancer drugs.

Radiation Therapy

- Radiation has recently been correlated with the induction of apoptosis.
- Radiation may also induce delays in cell division through interference with the cell cycle processes.

Alternative Treatments

- The primary goal of immune therapy is to restore the imbalance between tumor growth and tumor destruction. The secondary goal of immune therapy is to induce protective immunity.

TUMOR MARKERS

What is a Tumor Marker?

- Tumor markers are molecules that can be detected in blood, body fluids, or tissue of a host with underlying cancer.

Molecular Basis of Tumor Markers

- Tumor markers are a result of genetic alterations that occur in tumor cells that directly or indirectly affect the gene expression pattern of the tumor cells or the surrounding tissue.

- Primary abnormalities that are essential at the tumor initiation stage, and secondary abnormalities that occur later, are thought to play a role during tumor progression.

Chromosomal Translocations

- Chromosomal translocations occur frequently and often nonrandomly.

DNA Methylation

- Hypomethylation may increase gene expression and may also decrease chromosome stability and lead to allelic loss. Hypermethylation, on the other hand, could suppress gene transcription.

Detection Methods of Tumor Markers

Immunologic Detection

- The first and still most commonly used method for the initial diagnosis of cancer is through microscopic evaluation of tissue sections or cytologic preparations.

Cytogenetic Analysis

- Another screening method used primarily to support the diagnosis of hematopoietic cancers is cytogenetic analysis.
- Cytogenetics, especially in solid tumors, is used to identify possible locations of new tumor suppressor genes.

Genetic Analysis

- One such technique is based on gene analysis for detection of mutations in known molecules suspected of carrying a mutation.

Clinical Applications of Tumor Markers

Diagnosis

- Histopathologic classification is essential because not all tumors are equal, and they require differential treatment.

Prognosis

- Thus, factors that determine tumor growth, such as expression of particular growth factor receptors, the rate at which the tumor is growing, metastatic potential mediated through expression of certain receptors for ECM molecules, and sensitivity to therapy, are all important for prognosis.

Monitoring Efficacy of Therapy

- By evaluating levels pretherapy and post-therapy, the clinician can monitor the efficacy of therapy and detect recurrences.

Guiding Choice of Therapy

- Although physicians rely on a number of markers, such as carcinoembryonic antigen (CEA), prostate-specific antigen (PSA), and α-fetoprotein (AFP), to treat patients, they do not necessarily select treatment on the basis of the level of expression.

Prevention of Cancer

- Early screening for the known gene mutations (i.e., before the development of cancer) may permit corrective therapy, such as prophylactic surgery.

Some Tumor Markers Most Frequently Used In Surgical Oncology

- In addition to malignancy, several benign conditions may increase the value of serum markers. Many acute and chronic conditions of the biliary tract result in increased levels of CA19-9. Inflammatory bowel disease, hepatitis and cirrhosis and pregnancy can also give rise to elevated AFP levels. Benign conditions such as pregnancy, menstruation, endometriosis, pelvic inflammatory disease, hepatitis, cirrhosis and renal failure may increase CA125 levels (Table 27–1).

TABLE 27–1. Tumor Markers in Clinical Application

Tumor Marker	Type of Molecule	Tumor Type	Type of Application	Nonmalignant Conditions with Elevated Levels
(CEA)	Glycoprotein	Stomach, liver, pancreas, breast and colorectal cancer	Prognosis and monitoring therapeutic response	Hepatitis, cirrhosis, jaundice, COPD, inflammatory bowel disease, smoking
CA 19-9	Mucin type glycoprotein	Pancreas cancer	Diagnosis, prognosis and monitoring therapeutic response	Hepatitis, cirrhosis, sclerosing cholangitis and extrahepatic biliary stasis
AFP	Oncofetal glycoprotein	Liver and testicular cancer	Diagnosis, prognosis and monitoring therapeutic response	Hepatitis, cirrhosis, pregnancy, inflammatory bowel disease
PSA	Oncofetal glycoprotein	Prostate cancer	Screening, diagnosis, prognosis and monitoring therapeutic response	BPH, prostatic massage or biopsy
β-HCG	Trophoblastic protein	Choriocarcinoma, hydatiform mole and invasive mole	Diagnosis, prognosis and monitoring therapeutic response	Pregnancy
CA 125	Ovarian cell surface protein	Ovarian cancer	Prognosis and monitoring therapeutic response	Pregnancy, endometriosis, menstruation, jaundice and pancreatitis

CA 15-3	Membranes of breast cancer cells	Breast cancer	Prognosis	Cirrhosis, hepatitis and benign breast disease
Prostatic acid phosphatase	Prostate cellular protein	Prostate cancer	Prognosis and monitoring therapeutic response	BPH, dermatological disorders
5-Hydroxyindoleacetic acid	Peptide metabolite of indoleacetic acid	Carcinoid	Diagnosis	
Calcitonin	Hormone	Medullary thyroid cancer	Diagnosis, prognosis and monitoring therapeutic response	
Metanephrine	Catecholamine metabolite	Pheochromocytoma	Diagnosis, prognosis and monitoring therapeutic response	

CEA, Carcinoembryonic antigen; CA, carcinoma antigen; AFP, α-fetoprotein; PSA, prostate-specific antigen; β-HCG, beta-human chorionic gonadotropin; COPD, chronic obstructive pulmonary disease; BPH, benign prostatic hypertrophy.

CHAPTER 28

MELANOMA AND CUTANEOUS MALIGNANCIES

MELANOCYTES

● Positioned along the basement membrane at the dermal-epidermal junction, these cells are exposed to carcinogenic stimuli which result in malignant transformation to become melanoma.

MELANOMA

Introduction

● Melanoma accounts for only 4% to 5% of all skin cancers but causes the majority of deaths from skin malignancies.
● In 2003, there were 54,200 new cases diagnosed and 7,600 deaths from melanoma.
● The lifetime probability of developing melanoma is 1 in 57 for males and 1 in 81 for females.
● The median age of diagnosis is in the range of 45 to 55 years.
● Exposure to sunlight increases the risk of developing melanoma.
● Ultraviolet A (UVA) and ultraviolet B (UVB) cause different patterns of effect in the skin; however, both are considered to be carcinogenic. UVB induces the effects of sunburn and increase melanin production and is the most carcinogenic part of the UV spectrum.
● Additional factors that increase the risk for development of melanoma include the dysplastic nevus syndrome, xeroderma pigmentosum, a history of nonmelanoma skin cancer, and a family history of melanoma.
● Congenital nevi, dysplastic nevi (DNs), Spitz nevi, and familial patterns all raise the risk of developing melanoma.
● A DN is a large (6 to 15 mm) pigmented flat skin lesion with indistinct margins and variable color.
● The common features of melanoma are summarized in the mnemonic ABCDE: Asymmetric outline, changing irregular Borders, variation in Color, Diameter greater than 6 mm, and

Elevation. In early melanoma, the changes may be limited to two or three features.

- These amelanotic lesions appear as raised papules, which can be pink, red, purple, or of normal skin colors.
- In summary, any changing skin lesion should be carefully evaluated, and clinicians should have a low threshold to perform a diagnostic biopsy.

Unknown Primary Melanoma

- Unknown primary melanoma accounts for less than 2% of all melanoma cases and less than 5% of all patients who present with metastatic melanoma.
- A thorough search for the primary lesion.
- In the case of a lymph node metastasis, a completion regional lymph node dissection is performed.
- Less than 10% of melanomas arise in the eye, mucosal surfaces, and unknown primary sites.
- Melanomas arising on the mucous membranes occur on the head and neck (oral cavity, oropharynx, nasopharynx, and paranasal sinuses), anal canal, rectum, and the female genitalia.

Biopsy

- These tumors should be excised to negative margins.
- Biopsies should be full thickness into the subcutaneous tissues. For small lesions, an excisional biopsy is commonly performed, which includes a narrow (1 to 2 mm) margin of surrounding skin.
- Shaved biopsies
  - Should not be used when melanoma is suspected.
- The biopsy removes the full thickness of skin taking a layer of the underlying fatty tissue and all of the visible tumor.
- A punch biopsy or excision of a segment of the lesion is appropriate.
- The biopsy should be full thickness and include a margin of adjacent normal skin if possible.
- Biopsy excisions on the extremities should be closed longitudinally to maximize the possibility for a primary wound closure.

Histologic Types

- Histologically, melanoma is divided into four major types based on growth pattern and location. These forms are lentigo maligna melanoma (LMM), superficial spreading melanoma (SSM), acral lentiginous melanoma (ALM), and nodular melanoma (NM).

Lentigo Maligna Melanoma

- It occurs most commonly in older individuals with sun-damaged skin and presents as a flat darkly pigmented lesion with irregular borders and a history of slow development.

Superficial Spreading Melanoma

- Common histologic type is SSM.
- Flat pigmented lesion growing in the radial pattern.

Acral Lentiginous Melanoma

- Confined to the subungual areas and the glabrous skin of the palms and soles.

Nodular Melanoma

- Approximately 15% develop a vertical growth pattern early.

Classification

- Clark and associates described a classification of melanoma based on the extent of tumor invasion relative to the anatomic layers of the skin.
- Breslow described a system based on measuring the vertical thickness of the tumor in millimeters.
- A complete pathologic report of a cutaneous melanoma should include the following: Breslow thickness, presence or absence of ulceration, Clark level, status of the surgical margins, histologic type, presence or absence of satellitosis, and presence or absence of regression. The report may also describe tumor infiltrating lymphocytes, lymphovascular invasion, vertical growth phase, neurotropism, and mitotic rate.
- Staging for melanoma uses the tumor-node-metastasis (TNM) system of classification as defined by the American Joint Committee on Cancer staging system for cutaneous melanoma (Box 28–1).

Treatment

- The patient presenting with melanoma should undergo a systematic evaluation for metastatic disease.

Box 28-1. American Joint Committee on Cancer TNM Melanoma Classification—2002

Primary Tumor (T)

TX Primary tumor cannot be assessed (e.g., shave biopsy or regressed melanoma)

T0 No evidence of primary tumor

Tis Melanoma *in situ*

T1 Melanoma ≤1.0 mm in thickness with or without ulceration

T1a Melanoma ≤1.0 mm in thickness and level II or III, no ulceration

T1b Melanoma ≤1.0 mm in thickness and level IV or V or with ulceration

T2 Melanoma 1.01–2 mm in thickness, with or without ulceration

T2a Melanoma 1.01–2.0 mm in thickness, no ulceration

T2b Melanoma 1.01–2.0 mm in thickness, with ulceration

T3 Melanoma 2.01–4.0 mm in thickness, with or without ulceration

T3a Melanoma 2.01–4.0 mm in thickness, no ulceration

T3b Melanoma 2.01–4.0 mm in thickness, with ulceration

T4 Melanoma >4.0 mm in thickness, with or without ulceration

T4a Melanoma >4.0 mm in thickness, no ulceration

T4b Melanoma >4.0 mm in thickness, with ulceration

Regional Lymph Nodes (N)

NX Regional lymph nodes cannot be assessed

N0 No regional lymph node metastasis

N1 Metastasis in one lymph node

N1a Clinically occult (microscopic) metastasis

N1b Clinically apparent (macroscopic) metastasis

N2 Metastasis in two or three regional nodes or intralymphatic regional metastasis without nodal metastases

N2a Clinically occult (microscopic) metastasis

N2b Clinically apparent (macroscopic) metastasis

N2c Satellite or in-transit metastasis *without* nodal metastasis

N3 Metastasis in four or more regional nodes, or matted metastatic nodes, or in-transit metastasis or satellites, with metastasis in regional nodes(s)

Distant Metastasis (M)

MX Distant metastasis cannot be assessed

M0 No distant metastasis

M1 Distant metastasis

M1a Metastasis to skin, subcutaneous tissues, or distant lymph nodes

M1b Metastasis to lung

M1c Metastasis to all other visceral sites or distant metastasis at any site associated with an elevated serum lactic dehydrogenase

- A history focused on constitutional, central nervous system, pulmonary, gastrointestinal (GI), and soft tissue symptoms.
- When present, all symptoms and signs of metastasis require further radiologic evaluation. Clinical stage 0 and stage I patients do not require any further tests. Stage II and III patients may have a chest x-ray examination and serum lactate dehydrogenase (LDH) level determined; however, these are rarely abnormal in the asymptomatic patient.
- From many retrospective studies, it was clear that the risk of local recurrence and overall survival rates were related to tumor thickness. Four randomized studies were carried out to test whether narrow margins of excision could achieve the same results as wide margins. The current guidelines for wide local excision (WLE) (Table 28–1) are based on these studies.
- In most cases, the margin for a WLE is measured from the edges of the biopsy scar.
- The incision is made through the skin and subcutaneous tissues to the level of the superficial fascia.
- In many cases, the resulting wound can be closed by elevation and advancement of skin edges or the use of local skin flaps.
- Most mucosal melanomas are locally extensive before becoming symptomatic.
- Tumors should be resected with histologically clear margins; however, there is no evidence that wide local excisions increase the chance for cure.
- After WLE of the primary tumor, the most common sites of first recurrence are regional (lymph nodes, in-transit metastases, and local recurrences).
- Line of Sappey.
- As prognostic factors became better understood, it was postulated that patients with thin tumors (<1 mm thickness) would have a low risk of metastases at any site and that patients with thick tumors (>4 mm thickness) had a high risk of distant

TABLE 28–1. Recommended Margins for Surgical Resection of Primary Melanoma

Tumor Thickness (mm)	Margin Radius (cm)*
In situ	0.5
<1.0	1.0
1–2	2.0
>2.0	≥2.0

*Recommended margins may be adjusted to accommodate anatomic or cosmetic circumstances.

and regional metastases. In contrast, patients with intermediate thickness melanoma (1 to 4 mm) would have an elevated
risk of nodal metastases without a high risk of distant disease.

- Four phase III prospective, randomized trials have failed to
  provide convincing evidence to support elective lymph
  node dissection (ELND).

- The development of the sentinel lymph node concept ended
  one debate over ELND, changed clinical management, and
  opened a new series of questions about the tumor biology
  of melanoma.

- Blue dye injected intradermally at the primary site to show that
  the first blue node in the regional lymphatic basin(s) was
  the node that would contain a metastasis if any tumor were
  present. This node was termed the sentinel lymph node (SLN).

- Early reports showed several important findings: (1) using a
  combination of isotope lymphatic mapping, an intraoperative hand-held gamma probe, and intraoperative blue dye,
  the SLN could be identified in more than 95% of cases;
  (2) there was great anatomic variation resulting in drainage
  to multiple or uncommon sites; (3) a detailed pathologic
  analysis of the node using step sections enabled detection of
  micrometastases that could be missed by the standard techniques; (4) in most cases a positive sentinel node was the
  only positive node; (5) there were no prognostic factors that
  accurately identified a subpopulation of SLN-positive patients
  not requiring completion lymphadenectomy; and (6) when
  regional nodal metastases appear after a negative SLN biopsy
  (SLNB), in most cases micrometastases can be found in the
  original SLN by further histologic sectioning and examination.

- SLNB has rapidly become the standard of care for patients
  with tumors 1 mm or greater in thickness to accurately stage
  the disease and provide guidance for treatment planning.

- The therapeutic benefit is now being evaluated in the
  Multicenter Selective Lymphadenectomy Trial (MSLT) in
  which patients with melanomas greater than 1 mm in thickness were randomized to undergo wide local excision alone
  or wide local excision plus sentinel lymph node biopsy.

- Sunbelt Melanoma Trial.

- After the primary treatment of melanoma, the pattern of
  recurrences is predictable based on the same factors used to
  estimate survival (tumor thickness, ulceration, and lymph
  node status).

- The most common sites of initial recurrence are local and
  regional. Patients should be informed about the common
  symptoms and signs of recurrence so that they can report
  important changes arising between scheduled examinations.

- A complete skin examination is performed with inspection and palpation of the primary site and skin surfaces leading to regional nodal basins.
- Approximately 80% of patients who develop melanoma are cured of their disease. Recurrent disease appears locally, regionally, systemically, or in a combination of these sites.

Regional Nodal Recurrence

- Regional nodal metastases are the most common site of first recurrence in patients who undergo WLE alone.
- If positive, complete resection of the nodal basin will control regional disease in a large proportion of patients.
- Even with a single palpable nodal metastasis, the 5-year survival rate is 40% to 50%.

Local and Regional Recurrences

- True local recurrence (N2c, stage III) is defined as tumor appearing in the skin or subcutaneous tissues within a 5-cm radius of the primary wide excision site.
- Local recurrence risk has been reported to be 0.2% for primary tumors less than 0.76 mm, 2% for those 0.76 to 1.49 mm, 6% for lesions 1.5 to 3.99 mm, and 13% for thick melanomas greater than 4 mm.

Distant Metastases

- The most common sites of initial distant metastases are in the brain, lung, and liver and less commonly in the skin, bone, and other GI tract sites. The prognosis varies significantly with the site of first metastases (Table 28–2).
- In most cases, metastases appear at multiple sites simultaneously.

TABLE 28–2. One-Year Survival Rates for Patients with Distant Metastases

Stage	Metastatic Site(s)	Approximate 1-Year Survival (%)
M1a	Skin, subcutaneous tissues, lymph nodes	60
M1b	Lung	55
M1c	Other visceral sites	40

- Occasionally patients will develop metastases that are apparently isolated to a single site. These patients should be evaluated for surgical resection because the long-term disease-free survival rate after metastasectomy is reported in the range of 10% to 20%.
- Most of the increase in the incidence of melanoma is comprised of thin melanomas with an excellent prognosis. Unfortunately, the number of deaths from melanoma is also rising. Although melanoma has been reported to metastasize to almost any tissue site, the most common areas are lung, liver, bone, and brain. The most commonly used drug for systemic therapy is dacarbazine (DTIC), which has a response rate of 15% to 30%; however, complete responses are very rare.
- Doubling of the response rate has been observed with cisplatin, vinblastine, and DTIC (CVD) combined with interferon alfa or interleukin 2 or a combination of these two biologics.
- The combination of CVD + interferon + interleukin 2 (frequently called biochemotherapy) has a response rate of 50% and a complete response rate of 15%; however, several trials of this combination have not resulted in a significant prolongation in survival.

Adjuvant Systemic Therapy

- In the mid-1990s the Food and Drug Administration approved interferon α2b for adjuvant therapy in treating patients with nodal metastases or thick melanomas in whom the expected survival rate is less than 50%.
- Subsequent randomized trials of interferon therapy have failed to confirm the initial observation. An updated analyses of randomized trials in addition to a meta-analysis do not show a consistent benefit for interferon adjuvant therapy. At present, stage IIc and III patients should be evaluated for and invited to participate in randomized clinical trials of adjuvant therapy, when available.

CUTANEOUS MALIGNANCIES: NONMELANOMA SKIN CANCER

- Squamous cell carcinoma (SCC) and basal cell carcinoma (BCC) are the most common types of malignant neoplasms in the world.
- The current predictions are that one in five Americans will develop this disease during his or her lifetime.

Squamous Cell Carcinoma

- The causes of SCC include the following: sunlight, susceptible phenotype, compromise of immunity, environmental conditions, and diseases. Sunlight is thought to be the major causative factor because most SCCs occur on the sun-exposed surfaces of the head and neck.

- UVB is thought to be the form of UV radiation causing this disease.

- It is postulated that UV radiation affects the skin in two ways that result in an increased incidence of SCC. There is a direct carcinogenic effect on frequently dividing keratinocytes in the basal layer of the epidermis. Unrepaired mutations result in tumor promotion and growth. The second mechanism relates to the depression of the cutaneous immune surveillance response, which in turn inhibits tumor rejection.

- Chronic conditions of the skin such as burn scars (Majolin's ulcer), draining sinuses, infections, and ulcers can predate the development of SCCs. Previously healed wounds that break down or chronic wounds that will not heal should be biopsied for the presence of SCC.

- Impaired immunity, especially cell-mediated immunity, is a well established cause of SCCs of the skin.

- Chronically immunosuppressed patients are those undergoing organ transplantation.

- Human papillomavirus, an infection associated with immunosuppression, is proposed as a causative factor of SCCs. Most SCCs begin with a proliferation of keratin cells in the basal layer of epidermis, which appear as red or pink areas, clinically termed actinic keratoses (AKs) (solar keratoses).

- AKs have many features in common with SCC *in situ* microscopically.

- Bowen's disease appears histologically as SCC *in situ* and may vary from small lesions less than 1 cm to large areas of the anogluteal region.

- Invasive SCCs are palpable scaling lesions that become ulcerated centrally and have elevated edges.

- Most SCCs can be treated locally with excellent results (see treatment options). Recurrence is associated with tumor size, degree of differentiation, depth of invasion, perineural involvement, immune status of the patient, and anatomic site.

- The first site of metastases is usually in regional lymph nodes.

Basal Cell Carcinoma

- In contrast to SCCs and AKs, there is no precursor skin lesion for BCCs.

- BCCs grow in distinct patterns described as nodular, pigmented, cystic, and superficial. The nodular growth pattern is characterized by a well-defined, elevated lesion with a waxy appearance. As the lesion grows, it develops "pearly" opalescent nodules along the margins. A central depression with umbilication is a classic sign.
- Cystic BCCs.
- Superficial BCCs (20%) are more macular.
- The white scarring varieties of this growth pattern are termed morpheaform.

Treatment

- AKs and the precursor lesions of SCC are most often treated with cryotherapy; however, alternate treatments include topical 5-fluorouracil, electrodesiccation, curettage, CO_2 laser, dermabrasion, and chemical peel. A tissue biopsy is indicated when the AK is raised or recurrent after topical therapy.
- High-risk factors (Table 28–3). Considerations include size, location, primary versus recurrent, histology, and individual patient factors.
- Standard surgical excision is the preferred treatment for most SCCs and BCCs.

TABLE 28–3. Nonmelanoma Skin Cancer: Risk Factors for Local Recurrence Based on Characteristics of the Primary Tumor

Factor	Low Risk	High Risk
Location		
Trunk and extremities	<20 mm	≥20 mm
Forehead and neck	<10 mm	≥10 mm
Central face	<6 mm	≥6 mm
Borders	Well defined	Poorly defined
Incidence	Primary	Recurrent
Immunosuppression	Negative	Positive
Prior radiation therapy/ chronic inflammation	Negative	Positive
Rapid growth rate	Negative	Positive
Neurologic symptoms	Negative	Positive
Differentiation	Well	Moderate or poorly defined
Perineural/vascular invasion	Negative	Positive

Modified from National Comprehensive Cancer Network Practice Guidelines in Oncology, *www.nccn.org*.

- An alternative surgical approach is the use of Mohs micrographic excision (MME) in which there is a high rate of local tumor control with the use of horizontal frozen sections.
- MME is ideal under high-risk conditions and for anatomic areas where it is important to preserve as much tissue as possible such as around the eye, nose, mouth, and ear.
- Cryotherapy is best suited for small superficial lesions and can be expected to have local control rates of greater than 90%.
- Radiation therapy is highly effective in the treatment of BCC and SCC especially for preserving wide areas of skin in the head and neck region. Radiation is also useful in treating areas that are at high risk for recurrence after extensive surgical excision.

Other Tumors

Cutaneous Angiosarcoma (AS)

- Cutaneous AS is a rare aggressive soft tissue sarcoma derived from blood or lymphatic endothelium. It is most often seen on the face and scalp of older white men.
- Arise in irradiated tissues.
- Flat, painless, often pruritic macule or plaque with a red, blue, or purple color.
- Treatment consists of resection with histologically negative margins and radiation therapy to the involved field.

Dermatofibrosarcoma Protuberans (DFSP)

- DFSP is a low-grade sarcoma arising from dermal fibroblasts.
- Treatment consists of wide local excision with 3- to 4-cm margins.

Extramammary Paget's Disease (EMPD)

- EMPD is a rare form of adenocarcinoma arising from apocrine glands of the skin most commonly in the perianal area, vulva, and scrotum.
- Erythematous plaque but may also be white or depigmented with crusts and scaling.
- In most cases EMPD is confined to the epidermis and is well controlled with excision. When invasion of the deeper structures appears, the disease becomes increasingly difficult to control and the mortality rate increases to ~50%. Because EMPD is also associated with an increased risk of simultaneous internal malignancies of the genitourinary and GI tracts

(~40%), a complete workup should include a survey of these locations.

Kaposi's Sarcoma (KS)

- KS, a low-grade soft tissue malignancy, arises from lymphatic vascular endothelial cells in the skin.
- Often seen in patients with acquired immunodeficiency syndrome (AIDS) and other immunosuppressed states such as organ transplantation.
- HHV-8 has been identified as the causative agent.
- Symptomatic skin lesions can be treated with radiation therapy, intralesional injection of chemotherapeutic agents, cryotherapy, or excision.

Merkel Cell Carcinoma (MCC)

- MCC, derived from neuroendocrine cells, is histologically indistinguishable from small cell carcinoma arising in the lung or any other site.
- SLN biopsy has been used successfully to identify patients with occult regional lymphatic metastases (10% to 30%); however, there is no evidence that patients benefit other than by improved regional tumor control. Involved field radiation.

CHAPTER 29

SOFT TISSUE SARCOMAS AND BONE TUMORS

SOFT TISSUE SARCOMAS

- Soft tissue sarcomas are rare and unusual neoplasms, accounting for about 1% of adult human cancers and 15% of pediatric malignancies.

Predisposing Factors and Molecular Genetics

- In most patients, no specific etiologic agent is found. Multiple predisposing factors have been identified (Box 29–1). Genetic syndromes such as neurofibromatosis, familial adenomatous polyposis, and the Li-Fraumeni syndrome have all been shown to be associated with the development of soft tissue sarcoma. Ionizing radiation and lymphedema are well-established but uncommon antecedents to the development of soft tissue sarcoma.
- Genetic alterations that play a role in the development of soft tissue sarcoma segregate into two major types. The first type consist of sarcomas with specific genetic alterations that include simple karyotypes, including fusion genes resulting from reciprocal translocations and specific point mutations such as *KIT* mutations in gastrointestinal stromal tumors (GISTs) and *APC*/β-catenin mutations in desmoid tumors. The second type consists of sarcomas with nonspecific genetic alterations and typically complex unbalanced karyotypes, representing numerous genetic losses and gains.
- In addition to serving as very specific and powerful diagnostic markers, fusion genes resulting from translocations encode chimeric proteins that are important determinants of tumor biology, acting as abnormal transcription factors that alter the transcription of multiple downstream genes and pathways.

Pathologic Evaluation

- There are more than 50 histologic subtypes, many of which are associated with distinctive clinical, therapeutic, or prognostic features.

Box 29–1.   Predisposing Factors for Sarcomas

GENETIC PREDISPOSITION
Neurofibromatosis (von Recklinghausen's disease)
Li-Fraumeni syndrome
Retinoblastoma
Gardner's syndrome (familial adenomatous polyposis)

RADIATION EXPOSURE
Ortho- and megavoltage therapeutic radiation

LYMPHEDEMA
Postsurgical
Postirradiation
Parasitic infection (filariasis)

TRAUMA
Post parturition
Extremity

CHEMICAL
2,3,7,8-Tetrachlorodibenzodioxin (TCDD)
Polyvinyl chloride
Hemachromatosis
Arsenic

- To summarize the most commonly found are liposarcoma, malignant fibrous histiocytoma (MFH), and leiomyosarcoma (Fig. 29–1). Histopathology is anatomic site dependent: the common subtypes in the extremity are liposarcoma or MFH, in the retroperitoneal location liposarcoma and leiomyosarcoma are the most common histiotypes, and in the visceral location, GISTs are found almost exclusively (Fig. 29–2).
- Sarcoma histiotype is generally an important determinant of prognosis and a predictor of distinctive patterns of behavior, because none of the existing grading systems is ideal and applicable to all tumor types. Biologic behavior is currently best predicted based on histologic type, histologic grade, tumor size, and depth.
- In a postoperative nomogram based on a database of 2136 adult patients from Memorial Sloan-Kettering Cancer Center (MSKCC), histologic type was found to be one of the most important predictors of sarcoma-specific death with malignant peripheral nerve sheath tumors having the highest risk of mortality.

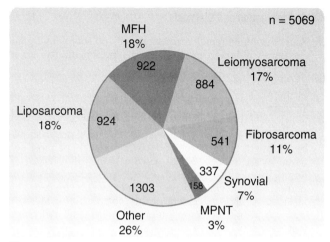

FIGURE 29–1. Histopathologic subtype distribution of 5069 patients with soft tissue sarcoma treated at Memorial Sloan-Kettering Cancer Center from July 1, 1982 through June 30, 2002. These data include extremity, trunk, visceral, and retroperitoneal tumors. MFH, malignant fibrous histiocytoma; MPNT, malignant peripheral nerve tumor.

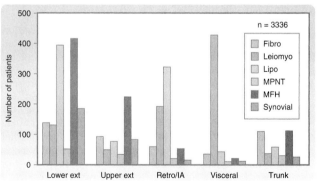

FIGURE 29–2. Site-specific histopathologic subtype distribution of 2336 patients with soft tissue sarcoma treated at Memorial Sloan-Kettering Cancer Center from July 1, 1982 through June 30, 2002. MFH, malignant fibrous histiocytoma; MPNT, malignant peripheral nerve tumor.

Clinical Evaluation and Diagnosis

- Patients with extremity sarcoma usually present with a pain-less mass, although pain is noted at presentation in up to 33% of patients.
- Physical examination should include assessment of the size of the mass and its relationship to neurovascular and bony structures. Generally, in an adult, any soft tissue mass that is symptomatic or enlarging, any mass that is larger than 5 cm, or any new mass that persists beyond 4 weeks should be biopsied. Biopsy technique is important. For most soft tissue masses, an incisional or core biopsy is usually pre-ferred. Ideally, the initial diagnostic procedure should be performed at a center where the patient will be treated. This facilitates proper placement of the biopsy site (or incision) and also avoids the complications and diagnostic difficulties that can arise if such biopsy samples are handled infre-quently. Limb masses are generally best sampled through a longitudinal incision so that the entire biopsy tract can be excised at the time of definitive resection. The incision should be centered over the mass in its most superficial location.
- Excisional biopsy is recommended only for small cutaneous or subcutaneous tumors, usually smaller than 3 cm in size, in which a wide re-excision (if required) is usually straight-forward.
- Tru-Cut biopsy can be then advocated as the first step in the diagnostic armamentarium. The ease of performance, low cost, and low complication rate make this technique attrac-tive. Should tissue be inadequate or there be any indecision, then open linearly placed incisional biopsy is indicated. Biopsy should be only indicated if the actual treatment will be altered by a definitive diagnosis.
- Patients with intra-abdominal or retroperitoneal sarcomas often experience nonspecific abdominal discomfort and gastrointestinal symptoms before diagnosis. The diagnosis is usually suspected on finding a soft tissue mass on abdominal computed tomography (CT) or magnetic resonance imaging (MRI) scan. Fine-needle aspiration biopsy or CT-guided core biopsy has a limited role in the routine diagnostic evaluation of these patients. Needle or core biopsy is indicated if abdominal lymphoma is strongly suspected as part of the differential diagnosis. In most patients, exploratory laparot-omy should be performed and the diagnosis made at oper-ation, unless the patient is clearly unresectable or will be undergoing preoperative investigational treatment.

Evaluation of Extent of Disease

- All patients require a thorough history and physical examination. MRI examination is the usually preferred procedure of choice for imaging extremity soft tissue masses. MRI enhances the contrast between tumor and adjacent structures and provides excellent three-dimensional definition of fascial planes.
- Once the diagnosis and grade are known, evaluation for sites of potential metastasis can be performed. Lymph node metastases occur in less than 3% of adult soft tissue sarcoma. For extremity lesions, the lung is the principal site for metastasis of high-grade lesions; for visceral lesions, the liver is the principal site. Thus, patients with low-grade extremity lesions require a chest x-ray examination, and the majority of those with high-grade lesions require a chest CT scan. Patients with visceral lesions should have their livers imaged as part of the initial abdominal CT or MRI scan.

Staging

- Current staging systems focus on histologic grade of the tumor, size of the primary tumor, and presence or absence of metastasis. Histologic grade is a major prognostic determinant and is based on degree of mitosis, cellularity, presence of necrosis, differentiation, and stromal content. Various grading systems exist, all of which should be considered as categories in a histologic spectrum. For therapeutic planning, the broad categories of low (Grades I or II) and high (Grades III or IV) grade suffice. Clearly such arbitrary decisions may be difficult, but they facilitate practical management of the patient. Low-grade lesions are assumed to have a low (<15%) risk of subsequent metastasis, and high-grade lesions have a high (>50%) risk of subsequent metastasis.
- Size has historically been considered a less important determinant of biologic behavior, but large lesions can be associated with late recurrence. Unequivocal characterization of grade is difficult in large lesions, especially in tumors that can reach 2 or 3 kg. Conversely, very small, high-grade lesions less than 5 cm in maximal diameter have limited risk for metastatic disease if treated appropriately at the first encounter.

Management

- Algorithms for management are shown in Figures 29–3 and 29–4. Surgical excision remains the dominant modality of curative therapy for all soft tissue sarcomas. Whenever

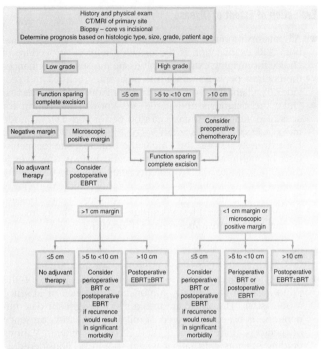

■ FIGURE 29–3. Algorithm for management of primary (with no metastases) extremity or trunk soft tissue sarcoma, using a biologic rationale (i.e., size and grade of tumor). BRT, brachytherapy; CT, computed tomography; EBRT, external beam radiation therapy; MRI, magnetic resonance imaging.

possible, function- and limb-sparing procedures should be performed. As long as the entire tumor is removed, less radical procedures have not been demonstrated to adversely affect local recurrence or outcome. The surgical objective should be complete removal of the tumor with negative margins and maximal preservation of function. When possible, tumors should be excised with 1 to 2 cm of normal tissue, because of the propensity for local, unappreciated spread. Conversely, deliberate sacrifice of major neurovascular structures can generally be avoided, provided the surgeon pays meticulous attention to dissection.

● In retroperitoneal and visceral lesions, operation remains the dominant method of therapy with the most important

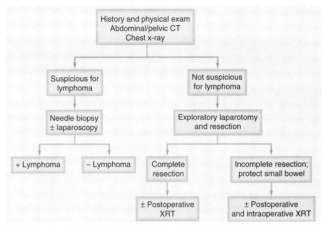

■ FIGURE 29–4. Algorithm for management of primary retroperitoneal or visceral soft tissue sarcoma. Fine-needle aspiration biopsy is not routinely used. CT, computed tomography; XRT, x-ray therapy.

prognostic factors for survival being completeness of resection and grade. Despite an aggressive surgical approach local control is still a major problem, and multifocal, unresectable tumors recur in many patients, particularly those with liposarcoma.

Treatment of Recurrent Disease

● Given the limitations and toxicities associated with cytotoxic chemotherapy, emphasis has been to develop novel drugs against rational drug targets such as the KIT receptor tyrosine kinase, which is constitutively activated in most GISTs. GISTs are mesenchymal neoplasms showing differentiation toward the interstitial cells of Cajal and are typically characterized by the expression of the receptor tyrosine kinase KIT (CD117). Recent studies have established that activating mutations of KIT are present in up to 92% of GISTs and likely play a key role in the development of these tumors. Along with mitotic activity, histologic subtype, and size, the type and location of KIT mutation is prognostic for survival in patients with GIST. Imatinib (STI571: Gleevec, Novartis Pharma) is a competitive inhibitor of BCR-ABL, KIT, and PDGFR tyrosine kinases. In preclinical studies, imatinib was active against mutant isoforms of KIT commonly found in

GIST. A recently completed phase II trial has shown substantial response rates and clinical benefit of imatinib in patients with advanced and metastatic GIST, a group typically highly resistant to convention adriamycin and ifosfamide based chemotherapy.

Prognostic Factors and Results

- The important prognostic factors for local recurrence were age greater than 50, recurrent disease at the time of presentation, microscopically positive surgical margins, and the histologic subtypes fibrosarcoma and malignant peripheral nerve tumor (MPNT).
- For distant recurrence, large tumor size, deep location, high histologic grade, recurrent disease at presentation, leiomyosarcoma, and nonliposarcoma histology were all independent adverse prognostic factors as was depth. For disease-specific survival, large tumor size, high grade, deep location, recurrent disease at presentation, histologic subtypes leiomyosarcoma and MPNT, and microscopically positive margins were all adverse prognostic factors.

Long-term Follow-up

- It is essential to emphasize that long-term follow-up for all patients with soft tissue sarcoma is important. A recent analysis of long-term follow-up for patients followed more than 5 years showed that approximately 9% of patients disease-free at the end of 5 years would go on to have further recurrence of the primary extremity sarcoma.

Summary

- In extremity lesions, one third of patients develop locally recurrent disease, with a median disease-free interval of 18 months. Treatment results for localized extremity local recurrence may approach those for primary disease. Isolated pulmonary metastases may be resected with 20% to 30% 3-year survival rates following complete resection. In patients with retroperitoneal and visceral sarcoma, complete resection remains the dominant factor in outcome. As opposed to extremity sites, local recurrence in this site is a common cause of death. Patients with unresectable pulmonary metastases or extrapulmonary metastatic sarcoma have a uniformly poor prognosis and are best treated with systemic chemotherapy.

BONE TUMORS

- Bone tumors have a low incidence but a high significance.
- Diagnosis and treatment is multidisciplinary.
- Biopsy is needed if imaging is not diagnostic.
- Biopsy should be performed by surgeon who will treat.

Clinical Features

- Pain.
  - Slow-growing, benign tumors—often not painful but may be tender.
  - Malignant tumors and aggressive benign tumors—usually painful.
  - Increased pressure within a rigid compartment.
  - Break through cortex with stretch of periosteum.
  - Tumor pain may be worse at night.
  - Mechanical component made worse by weight bearing— structural insufficiency, may herald a fracture.
- Coincidental findings are common.
  - 30% of patients report antecedent history of trauma.
  - Often concomitant degenerative joint disease—do not let this cloud the diagnosis.
  - If symptoms do not resolve predictably—re-evaluate.
- Palpable mass.
- Painful or restricted joint movement.
- Tenderness.
- Joint effusion.
- Rare vascular or neurologic findings.
- Lymph nodes rarely involved—points toward infection or lymphoma as a cause.
- History and physical examination.
  - Exclude infection.
  - Exclude congenital condition.
  - Evaluate for primary sites as a source for metastatic disease.
  - Family history.

Benign Tumors

- Solitary osteochondroma.
  - Most common benign tumor.
  - 50% develop about the knee.
  - Excision is reserved for symptomatic lesions and lesions growing after skeletal maturity.
  - Prophylactic excision is rarely indicated because surgical risks exceed the risk of sarcomatous degeneration.

- Giant cell tumors.
  - Most worrisome benign, aggressive bone tumor.
  - 65% occur at distal femoral or proximal tibial epiphysis.
  - Approximately 3% metastasize.
  - Lytic lesion.
- Chondroblastoma.
  - Similar to giant cell tumor in distribution.
  - Occur in skeletally immature patients.
  - Have a rim of reactive bone.
- Aneurysmal bone cysts.
  - Benign aggressive tumors that may develop as secondary lesions on top of other bone tumors.
  - Diaphyseal or metaphyseal distribution.
- Unicameral bone cysts.
  - Common lytic lesion.
  - Predilection for proximal humerus and femur.
  - Often present with a fracture.

Malignant Tumors

Sarcomas

- Rare, 2100 cases per year in the United States.
- Osteogenic sarcoma (OS).
  - Most common primary bone malignancy.
  - Accounts for one third of bone sarcomas.
  - Approximately 50% occur above the knee, most commonly at the metaphysis.
- Other spindle-cell neoplasms.
  - Chondrosarcoma.
  - MFH.
  - Fibrosarcoma.
  - Occur most commonly in older patients.
- Ewing's sarcoma.
  - Typically occur in young patients (80%).
  - Diaphyseal tumor in more than 50%.
  - Common in femur and pelvis.
  - Most common tumor of the fibula.

Metastatic Deposits

- Most common type of bone malignancy.
- Breast, renal, lung, and prostate cancers are most common primary sites of origin.

Lymphoma

- May develop as a primary bone tumor.
- Commonly found in the femur.
- Generous biopsy necessary for cytogenetics and lymphoma tissue markers.

Multiple Myeloma

Diagnostic Studies

- Conventional biplane radiography—most specific diagnostic test.
- Blood tests.
  - Sedimentation rate—nonspecific and frequently elevated.
  - Alkaline phosphatase—elevated in 85% of OS and most patients with Paget's disease of the bone.
  - Lactate dehydrogenase (LDH)—elevated in round-cell tumors and lymphoma, level corresponds to tumor burden.
  - Protein electrophoresis—abnormal in multiple myeloma.
  - Calcium and parathyroid hormone level—elevated with brown tumors.
- CT scan—best to evaluate cortical bone.
- MRI—useful to evaluate for soft tissue and marrow involvement.
- Whole-body ^{99m}Technetium pyrophosphate bone scan—essential for staging and screening for multicentric disease.
- CT chest—to evaluate for pulmonary metastasis.
- Biopsy—necessary to establish definitive diagnosis.
- Positron emission tomography (PET) scan—investigational but may prove useful.

Biopsy Technique

- Needle biopsy if radiograph is diagnostic.
- Open biopsy if radiograph is nondiagnostic.
- No preoperative antibiotics (so microorganisms can be recovered).
- No compression bandage.
- ± tourniquet.
- Incision.
  - Small, extensile incision.
  - Biopsy incision planned to be in continuity with the definitive resection incision.
- Soft tissue biopsy if possible.

- X-ray localization when necessary.
- Frozen section to check for adequacy of specimen.
- Cultures should be taken.
- Absolute hemostasis is mandatory.
- Drain (if necessary) in line with the definitive incision.
- Protect from weight bearing—reduces risk of pathologic fracture.

Staging

- Staging defines the extent and the behavior of the lesion.
- Benign lesions: (1) indolent; (2) active, thins cortex; (3) aggressive, transcends cortex.
- Malignant lesions: (I) low grade; (II) high grade, (A) <8 cm; (B) ≥8 cm; (III) metastatic.

Treatment of Primary Tumors

- Types of excision and margin of excision.
  - Intralesional margin—passes through the tumor (e.g., curettage).
  - Marginal margin—courses through the layer of reactive inflammatory tissue around the tumor.
  - Excisional biopsy—goes through the pseudocapsule, almost always leaves tumor behind.
  - Wide excision—removes tumor and some surrounding normal tissue, characteristic of most limb-sparing en bloc resections.
  - Radical margin—removes the entire soft tissue and bone compartment that contains the tumor.

Benign Tumors

- Treatment of benign giant cell tumors is exemplary of treatment methods used for benign tumors.
- Curettage and bone grafting—approximately 50% recurrence rate.
- Wide excision—cures most cases but has greater morbidity and reconstructive difficulty.
- Modern treatment methods—attempt to reduce recurrence and increase preservation of function.
  - Full exposure of tumor.
  - Aggressively eliminate bony involvement with curettage and burr débridement.
- Use adjuvants to improve tumor control.
  - Cryotherapy.
  - Acrylic cement—cement polymerization kills tumor cells.

- Consider prophylactic internal fixation to reduce risk of pathologic fracture.
- En bloc resection with joint reconstruction for treatment failures.
- Recurrence rate is less than 10% with these methods.

Malignant Tumors

- Oncologic goals take precedence over reconstructive (or functional) goals.
- Limb-preserving surgery is appropriate for more than 85% of cases.
- Indications for amputation.
  - Inability to obtain an adequate margin and maintain a useful limb.
  - Widespread contamination of the field by previous surgery.
  - Fracture.
  - Infection.
  - Anticipated loss of vascular of nervous supply that cannot be restored.
- Disadvantages of amputation.
  - Psychologic burden of limb loss.
  - Expense of prosthetic limbs.
  - Increased cardiac demand and O_2 consumption for lower extremity amputees to ambulate.
  - Phantom pain.
- Types of reconstructive procedures to facilitate limb preservation.
  - Autogenous grafts.
  - Taken from the patient's own body.
  - Separate instruments necessary.
  - Bone to permanent biologic solution.
- Rotationplasty.
  - Used for young patients.
  - Knee is excised.
  - Lower leg is rotated 180 degrees.
  - Tibia is fused to the femur.
  - Ankle joint then serves as a knee joint.
  - Rather than a high above knee amputation (AKA), patients function as they would with a below knee amputation (BKA), suitable for a prosthesis.
- Endoprosthetic replacement.
  - Usually used for joint reconstruction.
  - Provides immediate skeletal stability and restoration of function.

- Infections are difficult to treat and may require amputation.
- Greater use may increase likelihood of loosening of the endoprosthesis.
- Allografts.
  - Banked bone from cadaveric donors.
  - Infectious risk.
  - Preservation by freezing and so forth reduces immunogenicity but may diminish strength of the graft.
  - Complications include fracture, nonunion, and infection.
- Alloprosthetic composite reconstruction.
  - Combination of biologic and manmade materials.
  - Works well but frequently degenerate and need to be replaced.
- Arthrodesis.
  - Produces a pain-free, stable limb.
  - Very useful for the hip and wrist.
  - Knee—excellent for walking but poor for sitting or driving.
  - Few patients and doctors select this option.

Adjuvant Therapy

- Chemotherapy—multiagent therapy is now standard of therapy for OS and Ewing's tumor.
- Radiation therapy—primary bone malignancies are relatively radiation resistant.

Specific Types of Malignant Tumors and Their Treatment

Osteogenic Sarcoma

- Most common bone sarcoma.
- Commonly affected sites—distal femur, proximal tibia, and proximal humerus.
- Bimodal peak of incidence—adolescence and around age 60.

Types and Grade

- Primary OS ("conventional").
  - Most common form.
  - High grade—highly malignant.
  - Arises in medullary canal.
  - Metastasizes in more than 80% of patients treated by surgery alone.
- Secondary OS.
  - Common in older patients (accounts for more than 50% of cases in patients older than 60).

- Arises in Paget's disease, bone infarct, fibrous dysplasia, or previously radiated bone.
- Juxtacortical OS.
  - Typically seen on posterior aspect of femur.
  - Tumor arises from external surface of bone.
  - Usually low grade with a favorable prognosis.
  - Some may invade medullary canal and metastasize early.

Treatment

- Low-grade OS—greater than 90% survival with wide surgical excision alone, no need for chemotherapy.
- High-grade OS—surgical excision with multiagent chemotherapy.
- Chemotherapy.
  - Active agents: doxorubicin, platinum, high-dose methotrexate plus leucovorin rescue and ifosfamide.
  - Multiagent chemotherapy is superior to single-agent therapy.
  - Neoadjuvant therapy may result in significant shrinking of tumors.
  - Response to neoadjuvant therapy correlates with prognosis.
- Metastatic disease.
  - Poor prognosis—11% 5-year survival.
  - Aggressive treatment with surgery for metastases and chemotherapy can extend survival.

Ewing's Tumor

- Malignant small round cell tumor of bone.
- Half as common as OS.
- Occurs more frequently in young individuals.
- Cause related to a reciprocal translocation—t(11,22)(q24,q22).
  - Causes EWS to F-1 fusion protein formation.
  - Fusion proteins activate or repress genes that lead to neoplastic transformation.

Clinical Manifestations

- Pain and swelling.
- Rapid tumor growth.
- Some patients demonstrate constitutional symptoms or pathologic fractures.

Diagnosis

- "Onion-skin" periosteal changes.
- Lytic bone lesions—"moth-eaten" appearance.

- Soft tissue mass adjacent to bone.
- Elevated LDH—correlates with burden of disease.

Staging

- Stage I—solitary intraosseous tumor.
- Stage II—solitary tumor with extraosseous extension.
- Stage III—multicentric skeletal involvement.
- Stage IV—distant metastases.

Treatment

- Multiagent chemotherapy—improves survival but local therapy is needed also.
- Chemotherapy is usually given as induction therapy before performing surgical resection. Response to therapy is predictive of local control.
- Definitive local therapy—surgery, radiation therapy, or both.
  - Surgery offers better local control than radiation alone.
  - Unsure if radiation therapy adds anything to local control in patients who have had resection with negative margins.
  - Radiation useful for inaccessible sites.

METASTATIC BONE DISEASE

- More than one third of patients diagnosed with a primary malignancy will develop bony metastasis.
- Bone metastases outnumber primary bone cancers 100 to 1.

Epidemiology

- Breast, prostate, lung, and kidney cancer are the most common site of primary.
- Any cancer can metastasize to the bone.
- Metastases may occur to any bone, but femur, humerus, and vertebrae are most clinically significant.
- Most metastases are found in metaphyses of long bones, frequently multiple.
- Surgical treatment for a pathologic fracture is needed for approximately 9% of patients with metastasis to bones.

Pathogenesis

- Bone metastases are hematogenous in origin.
- Batson's plexus.

- Network of interconnecting veins around vertebrae.
- Influences distribution of blood flow and metastases.
- Implantation from marrow vasculature into cortex.
- Factors influencing metastatic progression.
  - Angiogenesis—important in progression of bone metastasis.
  - Growth factors—influence tumor growth.
  - Cytokines—help destroy local bone and stimulate tumor growth.
  - Osteoclasts—cells mediating bone lysis.

General Considerations

- Pain is the principle symptom.
- Type of lesion.
  - Osteolytic—lung and renal cell cancer.
  - Osteoblastic—prostate and breast cancer.
  - Mixed lytic and blastic—breast cancer.
  - Bone scan—efficient way to screen the whole body.
  - Blood tests usually not of much help.
  - Metastases weakened bone causing mechanical and biologic pain.
  - Biopsy weakens the bone and predispose to pathologic fracture.
  - Restoration of strength may take 6 weeks after treatment.
  - Unknown primary workup includes CT of chest, abdomen, and pelvis and possible PET scan.

Treatment Goals

- Treatment is with palliative intent.
- Primary goals—comfort and independence.
- Most patients without a fracture do not require surgery.
- Fractures are best treated operatively with resection and stabilization.
- Imaging may identify areas at imminent risk for fracture—these should be treated prophylactically (Table 29–1).
- Adjuvant therapies may affect healing postoperatively.

Surgery

- Remove metastatic deposits when repairing a pathologic fracture.
- Radiation should be used as adjuvant.
- Control of the proximal and distal fracture fragments is essential.

TABLE 29–1. Scoring System to Predict Rate of Pathologic Fracture

Variable	Points		
	1	**2**	**3**
Site	Upper extremity	Lower extremity	Pertrochanteric
Pain	Mild	Moderate	Mechanical
Radiograph	Blastic	Mixed	Lytic
Size (% of shaft)	0–33	34–67	68–100

Score	Patients (n)	Fracture Rate (%)
0–6	11	0
7	19	5
8	12	33
9	7	57
10–12	18	100

- Placement of an intramedullary rod is generally more effective than plating for long-term palliation.
- Amputation may be reserved for intractable pain, treatment failures, or an unreconstructable extremity lesion.

Radiation Therapy

- Arrests local tumor growth and permits functional improvement in most patients.
- Effective.
  - 70% of patients experience pain relief within 2 weeks.
  - 90% of patients experience pain relief within 3 weeks.
- Durable response—55% to 70% of patients treated do not develop recurrent pain.
- Will not effectively treat fractures.

Systemic Therapy

- All of the following classes of drugs may have a role in the management of metastatic disease to the bone.
  - Chemotherapy.
  - Hormonal therapy.
  - Bisphosphonates.

CHAPTER 30

HEAD AND NECK

- Numerous noncancerous changes to the squamous epithelium can be seen in the upper aerodigestive tract. Leukoplakia, which describes any white mucosal lesion, and erythroplasia, describing any red mucosal lesion, are both clinical descriptions and should not be used as diagnostic terms.

- Erythroplakia is more often indicative of an underlying malignant lesion.

- Of the sites arising from the aerodigestive tract, laryngeal cancer remains the most common newly diagnosed site and the most common cause of death (Table 30–1). Although there clearly remains a male predominance in aerodigestive tract malignancies, the ratio of male to female has been steadily decreasing because of a direct association between tobacco as a causative agent and the increased incidence of female smokers. Tobacco abuse increases the odds ratio of developing laryngeal cancer by 15.1, whereas alcohol abuse carries an odds ratio of 2.11. Combined abuse of alcohol and tobacco is not additive in terms of odds ratio but is multiplicative. Worldwide, incidence rates of cancer in the head and neck vary, usually in association with alcohol and tobacco use.

- Rates are increasing in most other regions of the world.

- According to the National Cancer Data Base, squamous cell carcinoma (head and neck squamous cell carcinoma [HNSCC]) is the most common head and neck malignant diagnosis (55.8%), followed by adenocarcinoma (19.4%) and lymphoma (15.1%).

- It is estimated that between 3 (early onset nasal cancer) to 11 (laryngeal cancer) separate gene mutations are required to allow a head and neck tumor to develop.

- Carcinogenesis in HNSCC also includes the development of second primary tumors, with patients having a 3% to 7% yearly incidence of secondary lesions in the upper aerodigestive tract, esophagus, or lung. A synchronous second primary lesion is defined as a tumor detected within 6 months of the index tumor. The occurrence of a second primary lesion greater than 6 months after the initial lesion is referred to as metachronous. There is debate as to whether second lesions represent reseeding of the primary tumor or genetically

TABLE 30–1. Head and Neck Cancer 2002 Statistics: Upper Aerodigestive Tract

Site	Estimated Incidence			Estimated Deaths		
	Both Sexes	Male	Female	Both Sexes	Male	Female
Tongue	7100	4700	2400	1700	1100	600
Mouth	9800	5200	4600	2000	1100	900
Pharynx	8600	6500	2100	2100	1500	600
Other oral cavity	3400	2500	900	1600	1200	400
Larynx	8900	6900	2000	3700	2900	800

From Jemal A, Thomas A, Murray T, et al: Cancer statistics, 2002. CA Cancer J Clin 52:23–47, 2002.

separate lesions caused by the field-cancerization effect resulting from carcinogen exposure.

- Fourteen percent of HNSCC patients will develop a second primary in the aerodigestive tract over the course of their lifetime, with more than half of these lesions occurring within the first 2 years of the index tumor. Because of the incidence of either second lung primaries or metastatic lung lesions, both a posterior-anterior and lateral chest x-ray (CXR) are obtained at the time of diagnosis and annually for the patient's post-treatment cancer surveillance.

- If the computed tomography (CT) criteria of nodes with central necrosis or size greater than 1.0 cm is used to determine positivity, only 7% of pathologically positive lymph nodes would be missed and these smaller nodes are most often in necks with more extensive disease.

- The most common sites of distant spread are the lungs and bones, whereas hepatic and brain metastases occur less frequently. The risk of distant metastases is more dependent on the nodal staging than on the primary tumor size.

- Patients with HNSCC are initially evaluated in a similar manner regardless of the site of tumor. Patient histories focus on symptomatology of the tumor, including duration of symptoms, detection of masses, location of pain, and the presence of referred pain. Special attention is paid to numbness, cranial nerve weakness, dysphagia, odynophagia, hoarseness, disarticulation, airway compromise, trismus, nasal obstruction, epistaxis, or hemoptysis. Alcohol and tobacco use histories are obtained.

- Direct laryngoscopy and examination under anesthesia are commonly performed as part of the evaluation of HNSCC.

These procedures allow the physician to evaluate tumors without patient discomfort and with muscle paralysis and to evaluate the oropharynx, hypopharynx, and larynx and obtain biopsies. Pathologic confirmation of cancer is mandatory before initiating treatment.

- The cervical lymphatic nodal basins contain between 50 to 70 lymph nodes per side and are divided into seven levels.

- Patterns of lymphatic drainage generally occur from superior to inferior and follow predictable patterns based on the primary site. Primary tumors from the lip and oral cavity generally metastasize to the nodes in levels I, II, and III, although skip metastases may occur to lower levels.

- Tumors in the oropharynx, hypopharynx, and larynx most commonly metastasize to levels II, III, and IV.

- Tumors of the subglottis, thyroid, hypopharynx, and cervical esophagus spread to levels VI and VII. In addition to the lower lip, the supraglottis and lateral pharynx have high incidences of bilateral metastases.

- The therapeutic options for patients diagnosed with HNSCC include surgery, radiation therapy, chemotherapy, and combination regimens. In general, early-stage disease (stage I or II) is treated by either surgery or radiation. Late-stage disease (stage III or IV) is best treated by a combination of surgery and radiation, chemotherapy and radiation, or all three modalities, depending on the site of the primary. Because surgery was the first therapeutic option available to physicians, it has the longest track record of the three options and established the head and neck surgeon as the leader of the treatment team for HNSCC. Photon irradiation is superior to surgery in eradicating microscopic disease and is an excellent option to surgery for early lesions. Tonsil, tongue base, and nasopharyngeal primary tumors are especially responsive to photon irradiation.

- Radiation therapy is not as effective in treating tumors with large-volume, low-grade neoplasms, or tumors in close proximity to the mandible, resulting from the risk of osteoradionecrosis. The loss of salivary function with irradiation of the oral and oropharyngeal cavity can be very disabling to patients and its impact should not be minimized in the decision-making process.

- All modifications of neck dissection are described in relation to the standard radical neck dissection (RND), which removes nodal levels I through V, the sternocleidomastoid muscle (SCM), the internal jugular vein (IJ), cranial nerve XI, the cervical plexus, and the submandibular gland. Preservation of the SCM, IJ, or cranial nerve XI in any combination is referred to as a modified radical neck dissection (MRND), and the structures preserved are specified for nomenclature. A modified neck dissection may also be referred to as a Bocca neck dissection after the surgeon who demonstrated that not only is the MRND equally as effective in controlling neck disease as an RND when structures are preserved that are not directly involved in tumor but only that the functional outcomes of the patients after MRND are superior to RND. Although resection of the SCM muscle or one IJ is relatively nonmorbid, loss of cranial nerve XI leaves a denervated trapezius muscle that can cause a painful chronic frozen shoulder.

- Either an RND or MRND can be performed for removal of detectable nodal disease. Preservation of any of levels I through V during a neck dissection is referred to as a selective neck dissection (SND) and is based on the knowledge of the patterns of spread to neck regions.

LIP

- Most lip cancers occur on the lower lip (90% to 95%) and less often on the upper lip (2% to 7%) and commissures (1%). The most common group to develop lip cancer are white men aged 50 to 80. Sun exposure and pipe smoking are associated with lip cancer. Whereas SCC is the most common lip cancer (90%), the most common cancer of the upper lip is basal cell carcinoma.
- Early-stage disease may be treated with surgery or radiation with equal success. Local surgery (wide local excision) with negative margin control of at least 3 mm is the preferred treatment, with a supramyohyoid neck dissection for tumors with clinically negative necks but deeper primary invasion or size greater than 3 cm.
- The goals of lip reconstruction include recreating oral competence, cosmesis, and maintenance of dynamic function while allowing adequate access for oral hygiene.
- SCC accounts for 90% of the tumors located in these subsites, with a male predominance in the fifth and sixth decades of life. There is a close association with alcohol and tobacco abuse.

ORAL CAVITY

- Treatment of oral tongue cancers is primarily surgical, with wide local excision and negative margin control. The development of cervical metastases is related to the depth of invasion, perineural spread, advanced T stage, and tumor differentiation. Infiltration of more than 5 mm into the tongue musculature has been shown by several investigators to increase the incidence of occult cervical metastases.

- Split-thickness skin grafts (STSGs), primary closure, or healing by secondary intention of larger tongue defects often results in tongue tethering. Thin, pliable, fasciocutaneous flaps (e.g., the radial forearm free-flap) are the preferred reconstructive technique for such defects.
- Determining mandibular invasion is of utmost importance in preoperative planning.
- Treatment of floor of mouth lesions is primarily surgical with excision of involved tongue or mandible as necessary to obtain negative margins. Removal of bone with soft tissue in continuity is commonly referred to as a "commando" or composite resection.
- Primary radiation therapy for mandibular tumors is not a viable option for treatment because of the high likelihood of osteoradionecrosis and the poor response of involved bone to radiation therapy treatment.
- Necrotizing sialometaplasia is a benign, self-limiting process of minor salivary glands that has a predilection for the palate and can clinically mimic a malignancy.
- Torus palatini are benign exostosis of the midline hard palate that may require surgery if they interfere with denture wearing.

OROPHARYNX

- Ninety percent of tumors of the oropharynx are SCCs. Other tumors include lymphoma of the tonsils or tongue base or salivary gland neoplasms arising from minor salivary glands in the soft palate or tongue base. Presenting symptoms include sore throat, bleeding, dysphagia and odynophagia, referred otalgia, and voice changes including a muffled quality or "hot potato" voice. Trismus suggests involvement of the pterygoid musculature.
- Treatment of oropharyngeal SCC has focused increasingly on conservation therapy with chemotherapy and radiation.
- Surgery is necessary for primary disease, which involves the mandible, and resectable recurrent disease and has a role in very early, superficial tumors that do not justify a full course of radiation.

HYPOPHARYNX

- Hypopharyngeal tumors present as a chronic sore throat, dysphagia, referred otalgia, and a foreign body sensation in the throat. A high index of suspicion should be maintained because similar symptoms may be seen with the more common gastroesophageal reflux disease. In advanced disease, patients may develop hoarseness from direct involvement of the arytenoid, the recurrent laryngeal nerve, or the paraglottic space. The rich lymphatics that drain the hypopharyngeal region contribute to the fact that 70% of patients with hypopharyngeal cancer present with palpable lymphadenopathy.

- Treatment of hypopharyngeal cancer yields poor results compared with other sites in the head and neck, presumable because of the late presentation of disease. For early lesions confined to the medial wall of the piriform or posterior pharyngeal wall, radiation or chemoradiation is effective as a primary treatment modality.

LARYNX

- The most common treatment of hypopharyngeal cancer is laryngopharyngectomy and bilateral neck dissections, including the paratracheal compartments, with adjuvant radiation therapy.
- The estimated 5-year laryngeal preservation rate is 35%, and induction chemotherapy appears to decrease the rate of death by distant metastases.
- For staging purposes, the larynx is divided into three regions: the supraglottis, the glottis, and the subglottis. The supraglottis is composed of the epiglottis, the laryngeal surfaces of the aryepiglottic folds, the arytenoids, and the false vocal folds.
- This plane is also the superior border of the glottis, which is composed of the superior and inferior surfaces of the true vocal folds, and extends inferiorly from the true vocal folds 1 cm in thickness.
- The innervation of the larynx includes the superior laryngeal nerve, which supplies the cricothyroid and inferior constrictor muscles and contains afferent sensory fibers from the mucosa of the false vocal folds and piriform sinuses. The recurrent laryngeal nerve supplies motor innervation to all the intrinsic muscles of the larynx and sensation to the mucosa of the true vocal folds, the subglottic region, and adjacent esophageal mucosa. The normal functions of the larynx are to provide airway patency, protect the tracheobronchial tree from aspiration, provide resistance for Valsalva and cough, and allow for phonation.

- Glottic tumors will often present early with hoarseness because the vibratory edge of the true vocal fold is normally responsible for the quality of voice and is sensitive to even small lesions.
- In comparison to glottic tumors, supraglottic lesions are relatively indolent and present at a later stage of disease.
- Bulky tumors of the epiglottis will often present with a hot potato or muffled voice quality.
- The most common malignant lesion of the larynx is SCC, which is often classified into SCC *in situ,* microinvasive SCC, or invasive SCC.
- The staging system for laryngeal cancers is based on subsite involvement and vocal fold mobility.
- CT scanning is routinely performed for laryngeal lesions and images the preepiglottic and paraglottic regions and the extent of cartilage involvement, as well as determines direct extension into the deep neck structures.
- Tumors confined to the glottis only rarely present with regional disease (4%), and positive nodes when present are most often ipsilateral.
- Poor prognostic factors include size, nodal metastasis, perineural invasion, and extracapsular spread.
- Successful treatment of low-grade lesions includes close follow-up with repeat office or operative laryngoscopy and strict smoking cessation.
- In general, conservation of the larynx in early-stage disease is key, which can be accomplished with either laryngeal preservation surgery or with radiation. Later stage disease, which is still confined to the larynx, is more commonly treated with chemoradiation therapy with total laryngectomy used for salvage.
- If the decision is to undergo nonsurgical therapy, the patient must be able to complete the full course of radiation therapy, which usually includes 5 to 7 weeks of continuous daily therapy visits. Previous irradiation is a contraindication to further radiation. Finally, the patient must be able to follow-up reliably for years to come because recurrences may be indolent and difficult to detect.
- The combination of chemotherapy and radiation for advanced stage disease (Stage III and IV) was first brought into the mainstream with the Veterans Administration larynx trial in 1991. Induction chemotherapy followed by radiation therapy was found to have equal 2-year survival as total laryngectomy with postoperative radiation therapy while being able to preserve the larynges of 64% of patients.

- For patients who present with disease extending outside the larynx, who fail conservative therapy (although some failures may still be amenable to conservation surgery), or who are not otherwise candidates for organ-preserving strategies, total laryngectomy is still commonly performed.
- Lastly, the tracheo-esophageal puncture (TEP) is a surgically created conduit between the tracheal stoma and the pharynx made either at the time of laryngectomy or secondarily. This conduit is fitted with a one-way valve that allows passage of air posteriorly from trachea to pharynx but prevents food and liquid to enter anteriorly into the airway.

NASAL CAVITY AND PRONASAL SINUSES

- Tumors of the nasal cavity and paranasal sinuses tend to present at a late stage because their presenting symptoms are often attributed to more mundane etiologies. Symptoms include epistaxis, nasal congestion, headache, and facial pain.
- Because respiratory epithelium can differentiate into squamous or glandular histologies, SCC and adenocarcinoma represent two of the most common sinonasal cancers.
- Staging is partly dependent on local spread of tumor. "Ohngren's line" extends from the medial canthus to the mandibular angle. Maxillary tumors superior to Ohngren's line have a poorer prognosis compared with those inferior to the line because of the proximity to the orbit and cranial cavity.
- Lymph node metastases are in general uncommon (15%), and elective neck dissection or radiation of a clinically negative neck is most often unwarranted.
- The standard treatment for sinonasal malignancies is surgical resection, with postoperative radiation or chemoradiation for high-grade histologies or advanced local disease.

NASOPHARYNX

- Clinical presentation of nasopharyngeal tumors include symptoms of nasal obstruction, serous otitis with effusion with associated conductive hearing loss, epistaxis, and nasal drainage. Symptoms of cervical mass, headache, otalgia, trismus, and cranial nerve involvement suggest malignancy. Examination of the nasopharynx was historically performed with the mirror and has been greatly improved with the use of either rigid or flexible nasopharyngoscopes in the office.

- Angiofibromas are vascular lesions found exclusively in males, usually presenting during puberty, and are commonly referred to as juvenile nasopharyngeal angiofibromas (JNAs).
- Treatment is based on radiation therapy both to the primary site and bilateral necks. With the addition of cisplatin and 5-fluorouracil, the rate of distant metastases decreases and both disease-free and overall survival increases.

EAR

- Neoplasms of the pinna are most often related to sun-exposure and are basal cell carcinomas and SCCs.
- SCC is the most common cancer of the temporal bone.
- Treatment of malignancies of the pinna are treated similarly to skin cancers elsewhere on the face.

SALIVARY GLANDS

- The major salivary glands include the parotid glands, the submandibular glands, and the sublingual glands. There are also approximately 750 minor salivary glands scattered throughout the submucosa.
- Most neoplasms arise in the parotid gland (70%), whereas tumors of the submandibular gland (22%) and sublingual gland and minor salivary glands (8%) are less common. The ratio of malignant to benign tumors varies by site as well: parotid gland 80% benign, 20% malignant; submandibular gland and sublingual gland 50%:50%; minor salivary glands 25% benign, 75% malignant.
- Numerous non-neoplastic diseases commonly affect the salivary glands. Sialadenitis is an acute, subacute, or chronic inflammation of a salivary gland. Acute sialadenitis commonly affects the parotid and submandibular glands and can be caused by bacterial (most frequently *Staphylococcus aureus*) or viral (mumps) infection. Chronic sialadenitis results from granulomatous inflammation of the glands commonly associated with sarcoidosis, actinomycosis, tuberculosis, or cat-scratch disease. Sialolithiasis is the accumulation of obstructive calcifications within the glandular ductal system, more common in the submandibular gland (90%) than in the parotid (10%). When the calculi become obstructive, stasis of saliva may cause infection creating a painful, acutely swollen gland.
- Salivary gland neoplasms most often present as slow-growing, well-circumscribed masses. Symptoms of pain, rapid growth,

nerve weakness and paresthesias, and signs of cervical lymphadenopathy and fixation to skin or underlying muscles suggest malignancy. When the presenting symptom is complete unilateral facial paralysis, Bell's palsy may be misdiagnosed as the etiology, and it is important to remember that all Bell's palsy patients will show some improvement in facial movement within 6 months of the onset of weakness.

- Pleomorphic adenomas account for 40% to 70% of all tumors of the salivary glands, most commonly occurring in the tail of the parotid.
- Shelling out of pleomorphic adenomas is to be avoided because it has been shown to correlate with increased rates of recurrence. The facial nerve should not be sacrificed in removing a benign lesion.
- Mucoepidermoid carcinoma is the most common malignant tumor of the parotid gland and can be divided into low-grade and high-grade tumors.
- Adenoid cystic carcinoma (ACC) constitutes 10% of all salivary neoplasms, with two thirds occurring in the minor salivary glands.
- An indolent growth pattern and a relentless propensity for perineural invasion characterize ACC.
- Treatment of salivary gland malignancies is en bloc surgical excision. Radiation therapy is administered postoperatively for high-grade malignancies demonstrating extraglandular disease, perineural invasion, direct invasion of surrounding tissues, or regional metastases.

NECK AND UNKNOWN PRIMARY

- The workup of a neck mass is different in children than it is in adults because of differing etiologies. Cervical masses are common in children, and most often represent inflammatory processes or congenital abnormalities.
- The most common etiology of cervical adenopathy is viral upper respiratory tract infections. The associated lymphadenopathy generally subsides within 2 weeks, although mononucleosis lymphadenopathy may persist for 4 to 6 weeks.
- In the adult, neck masses more often represent malignancies than in children. *Persistent masses larger than 2 cm in size represent cancer in 80% of cases.*
- Fine needle aspiration (smaller than 22 gauge) is performed as one of the initial steps in the workup of neck masses with an overall accuracy of 95% for benign neck masses and 87% for malignant masses.

- In all cases of metastases to the neck, lymphadenectomy as treatment is valuable only in cases of SCC, salivary gland tumors, melanoma and thyroid carcinoma. Otherwise, removal of metastatic lymph nodes is indicated for diagnosis only, and systemic treatment must be initiated for treatment.
- The branchial cleft apparatus, which persists after birth, may give rise to a number of neck masses. First branchial cleft cysts present in the preauricular or submandibular areas, are intimately associated with the external auditory canal and parotid gland, and may require dissection of the facial nerve during excision. Second and third branchial cleft cysts and tracts present anterior to the sternocleidomastoid muscle and often become symptomatic following upper respiratory tract infections.
- Carotid body tumors or chemodectomas are more properly referred to as paragangliomas and arise from the branchiomeric paraganglia at the carotid body. Tumors are usually benign, unifocal, and nonhereditary and present as a nonpainful mass at the carotid bifurcation and have a characteristic "lyre" sign on carotid arteriogram.
- Tumors of the parapharyngeal space are distinguished by their location; either prestyloid, usually of salivary gland origin, or post-styloid, usually vascular or neurogenic in origin.

TRACHEOTOMY

- Tracheotomy is most commonly used today in patients requiring prolonged mechanical ventilation to reduce the risk of damage to the larynx, to assist ventilation and pulmonary hygiene, and to improve patient comfort and oral care. There is no hard rule as to how long a translaryngeal endotracheal tube can be left in place. Some laryngologists recommend conversion to tracheotomy after 3 days of intubation, whereas most use 2 to 3 weeks as a limit.
- Preoperative assessment should include a history of previous tracheotomy or neck surgery, laryngeal pathology, bleeding difficulties, or cervical spine injuries. Perioperative complications of tracheotomy include bleeding, aspiration, pneumothorax and pneumomediastinum, recurrent laryngeal nerve injury, and hypoxia. Long-term problems include formation of granulation tissue both at the skin and within the trachea, collapse of tracheal cartilage and airway obstruction, and tracheo-innominant artery and tracheo-esophageal fistulas.
- Although the traditional open tracheotomy technique is still primarily used and preferred, recently the percutaneous

tracheotomy has gained in use. There are reports of both increased and decreased complication rates with the percutaneous technique compared with the open technique.

VOCAL CORD PARALYSIS

- More appropriately termed vocal cord immobility, loss of vocal cord function remains a common occurrence. The recurrent laryngeal nerve supplies all laryngeal musculature except for the cricothyroid muscle, which is supplied by the superior laryngeal nerve. Paralysis of the laryngeal muscles may occur from a lesion in the central nervous system (CNS) or more commonly with peripheral nerve involvement (90%).

- Approaches to the cervical spine should generally be performed from the left to reduce traction injury to the recurrent nerve because right-sided approaches have been associated with a higher rate of laryngeal nerve injuries.

- Injury to the recurrent laryngeal nerve will result in vocal fold paresis or paralysis. The patient with unilateral vocal cord immobility may present with hoarseness, ineffective cough, dysphagia, aspiration, or airway compromise or may be completely asymptomatic based on their ability to compensate. Definitive diagnosis is made through laryngoscopy, and subtle weakness may require stroboscopic examination. Etiologies of paralysis include surgical trauma (most commonly thyroidectomy); malignancies of the thyroid, mediastinum, esophagus, or larynx; mediastinal compression; viral neuropathy; collagen vascular disease; sarcoidosis; diabetic neuropathy; and many other reported causes. The etiology remains unknown in 20% of patients. Because recreating volitional abduction and adduction of the vocal cord is not currently feasible, the goal of treatment entails creating sufficient medialization of the involved vocal cord to allow for efficient voicing and cough and to reduce hoarseness and aspiration.

RECONSTRUCTION

- Perhaps the area of head and neck surgery that has undergone the most advancement in the past 25 years is reconstruction, fueled largely by the advent of microvascular free-flaps.

- Cosmetic deformities are most obvious in the head and neck area. Functional deficits not only occur with speech and swallowing but also affect eyelid function, oral competence, and maintenance of a nasal and oral airway. General principles include reconstructing underlying bony framework, replacing skin with skin of matching quality, minimizing scar visibility and contracture, and reconstructing in zones of facial units. Skin should be matched by color, thickness, and hair-bearing units where possible.

- A spectrum of reconstructive options exists with healing by secondary intention and primary closure at one end and extensive reconstruction such as microvascular free-flaps at the other. Which option is selected depends on the location and severity of the defect, the overall health of the patient, the available donor sites for flaps, the status of the tissue adjacent to the defect (irradiated, infected, previously operated), and the functionality of the area to be reconstructed.
- Skin grafts are most commonly used in the oral cavity, ear, or maxillectomy defects, as well as coverage for donor sites like the radial forearm and fibular free-flaps and the deltopectoral flap. Skin grafts are completely dependent for nutrition on the tissue over which they are placed and can heal well over muscle, perichondrium, and periosteum.
- Full-thickness skin grafts (FTSG) are characterized by a better color match, texture, contour, and less contracture but decreased success rates compared with STSGs. Commonly used donor sites include the postauricular, the upper eyelid, and the supraclavicular fossa skin.
- Local skin flaps have excellent tissue match because of their proximity to the defect. Commonly used designs include the advancement, rotation, transposition, rhomboid, and bilobed flaps.
- Perhaps the regional flap with the most significant effect on head and neck reconstruction was the introduction of the pectoralis myocutaneous flap in 1978. Based on the pectoral branch of the thoracoacromial artery, the artery pierces the pectoralis muscle from the deep surface. A skin paddle designed over the muscle or simply the muscle itself may be transferred to reconstruct defects up to the nasopharynx.
- A free-flap entails removal of composite tissue from a distant site along with its blood supply, and reimplantation of the vasculature in the reconstructive field. Although the first successful human microvasculature transfer was a jejunal interposition flap in 1959, the modern era of microvasculature reconstruction did not take rise until the 1970s with improvements in instrumentation and technique. Today's selection of donor sites allows the benefit of choosing between sites with large-caliber, long vascular pedicles that are anatomically consistent.

- Complete loss of a free tissue transfer should occur in less than 5% of cases.
- The radial forearm has emerged as the workhorse of soft tissue free-flaps in head and neck reconstruction.
- The most commonly used osseous free-flaps include the fibula.
- The fibular free-flap is based on the peroneal artery and vein and the blood supply to the foot should be investigated before harvesting this flap. Up to 25 cm of fibula may be harvested for mandibular or maxillary reconstruction with an osseous or osteocutaneous harvest, with minimal donor site morbidity.
- In 1998, the first successful human laryngeal transplantation was performed with microvascular reconstruction. Not only was the larynx transplanted but also the pharynx, thyroid, parathyroids, and trachea.

CHAPTER 31

DISEASES OF THE BREAST

ANATOMY

- The mature breast lies cushioned in adipose tissue between the subcutaneous fat layer and the superficial pectoral fascia (Fig. 31–1).
- Within the loose areolar fat of the axilla are a variable number of lymph nodes.
- To standardize the extent of axillary dissection, the axillary nodes are arbitrarily divided into three levels.
- Lymphatic channels are abundant in the breast parenchyma and dermis.
- Knowledge of major nervous structures in the axilla is required to avoid their sacrifice during surgery.

Microscopic Anatomy

- The mature breast is composed of three principal tissue types: (1) glandular epithelium, (2) fibrous stroma and supporting structures, and (3) fat.
- The glandular apparatus of the breast is composed of a branching system of ducts, roughly organized in a radial pattern, spreading outward and downward from the nipple-areolar complex (see Fig. 31–1).
- At the opposite end of the ductal system and after progressive generations of branching, the ducts end blindly in clusters of spaces that are called *terminal ductules* or *acini.*
- Under the luminal epithelium, the entire ductal system is surrounded by a specialized myoepithelial cell of ductal epithelial origin that has contractile properties and serves to propel secretion of milk toward the nipple.

BREAST DEVELOPMENT AND PHYSIOLOGY

Development and Physiology

- Ill-defined masses in premenopausal women are correctly observed through the course of one or two menstrual cycles.

427

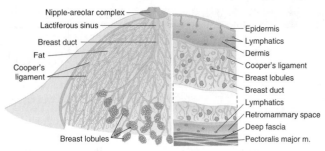

■ FIGURE 31–1. Cut-away diagram of the mature resting breast. The breast lies cushioned in fat between the overlying skin and the pectoralis major muscle. Both the skin and retromammary space under the breast are rich with lymphatic channels. Cooper's ligaments, the suspensory ligaments of the breast, fuse with the overlying superficial fascia just under the dermis, coalesce as the interlobular fascia in the breast parenchyma, and then join with the deep fascia of breast over the pectoralis muscle. The system of ducts in the breast is configured like an inverted tree, with the largest ducts just under the nipple and successively smaller ducts in the periphery. After several branching generations, small ducts at the periphery enter the breast lobule, which is the milk forming glandular unit of the breast.

- Risks of hormone replacement therapy include increased rates of breast cancer, myocardial infarction, pulmonary emboli, stroke, and gallbladder disease. The increased risk of breast cancer was observed after 5 years of combined estrogen and progesterone (Prempro) use and was not observed in women who had undergone hysterectomy and who were taking estrogen without progesterone replacement.

Fibrocystic Changes

- Fibrocystic condition (FCC), previously referred to as *fibrocystic disease,* represents a spectrum of clinical, mammographic, and histologic findings and is present in one of its many forms in up to 90% of women.

Breast Pain

- Usually it is of functional origin and uncommonly is it a symptom of breast cancer.

- For those women with breast pain and an associated palpable mass, the presence of the mass should be the focus of evaluation and treatment. For patients without a mass, the evaluation should be guided by whether the pain is cyclical or noncyclical.
- Normal ovarian hormonal influences on breast glandular elements frequently produce *cyclical mastalgia*.
- *Noncyclical mastalgia* is more likely to be the result of a nonbreast etiology or of a specific significant breast condition.

Abnormal Development and Physiology

Absent or Accessory Breast Tissue

- In contrast, accessory breast tissue (polymastia) and accessory nipples (supernumerary nipples) are both common.

Gynecomastia

- Hypertrophy of breast tissue in men is a common clinical entity for which there is frequently no identifiable cause.

Nipple Discharge

- Nipple discharge is common and is rarely associated with an underlying carcinoma.
- The most common cause of spontaneous nipple discharge from a single duct is a solitary intraductal papilloma in one of the large subareolar ducts directly under the nipple.

Galactocele

- A galactocele is a milk-filled cyst that is round, well circumscribed, and easily movable within the breast.

DIAGNOSIS OF BREAST DISEASE

History

Physical Examination

- Edema of the skin, frequently accompanied by erythema, produces a clinical sign known as peau d'orange.
- Inflammatory carcinoma.

Fine-Needle Aspiration

Breast Imaging

- *Mammography* is the most sensitive and specific imaging test currently available, although 10% to 15% of clinically evident breast cancers have no mammographic correlate.
- Magnetic resonance imaging (MRI) sensitivity for invasive cancers approaches 100% but is only 60% at best for ductal carcinoma *in situ* (DCIS). Specificity remains low, with significant overlap in the appearance of benign and malignant lesions.

Screening Mammography

- The underlying principle of a screening strategy is the assumption that earlier detection will reduce mortality and morbidity rates.
- A meta-analysis using a Bayesian random effects model was used to evaluate the effectiveness of screening mammography after 14 years of observation. In the analysis of all age groups, screening mammography reduced the risk of breast cancer by 16% (relative risk [RR] = 0.84: confidence interval [CI], 0.77 to 0.91). Among women age 50 and older, this risk reduction was 15% (RR = 0.85; CI, 0.73 to 0.99) with the inclusion of the Canadian trial and 22% (RR = 0.78: CI, 0.67 to 0.96) with exclusion of this study. For women ages 40 to 49, screening mammography reduced the risk of breast cancer by 15% (RR = 0.85: CI, 0.73 to 0.99).
- At present, screening mammography should be offered annually to women age 50 and older, and at least biennially in women age 40 to 49 with the screening interval made on an individual basis and considering the risk factors for breast cancer. Younger women with a significant family history, histologic risk factors, or a history of prior breast cancer should be offered annual screening.

Diagnostic Mammography

- *Diagnostic mammography* is performed when there is a breast abnormality on clinical examination or screening mammography. It includes magnifications and compression imaging in addition to the mediolateral oblique (MLO) and craniocaudal (CC) views obtained with screening mammography and is frequently supplemented by ultrasound.

IDENTIFICATION AND MANAGEMENT OF THE HIGH-RISK PATIENT

Risk Factors for Breast Cancer

Age

- Age is probably the most important risk factor that clinicians use in everyday clinical practice.

Histologic Risk Factors

- Lobular carcinoma *in situ* (LCIS) is not a breast cancer but rather a histologic marker for increased breast cancer susceptibility, estimated at slightly less than 1% per year longitudinally.
- A 5-year course of tamoxifen provides a 56% reduction in breast cancer risk.
- The relative risk of cancer in women with *atypical ductal or lobular hyperplasia* was 4.4 times the risk of development of breast cancer in a control population of women.

Family History and Genetic Risk Factors

- Genetic factors are estimated to cause 5% to 10% of breast cancer cases.
- *BRCA1*
  - It accounts for up to 40% of familial breast cancer syndromes. In addition to an increased breast cancer risk, those with this mutation are also at increased risk for ovarian cancer (15% to 45%); colon cancer; and, for men, prostate cancer.
- *BRCA2* accounts for up to 30% of familial breast cancer and is associated with increased breast cancer risk in males. Those with the mutation have a risk of ovarian cancer of up to 20% and increased risks for prostate, laryngeal, and pancreatic cancers.

Reproductive Risk Factors

- Reproductive milestones that increase a woman's lifetime estrogen exposure are thought to increase her breast cancer risk and include menarche before age 12, first live child-birth after age 30, nulliparity, and menopause after age 55.

Exogenous Hormone Use

- For 1000 healthy postmenopausal women taking combined estrogen and progesterone for 10 years, when compared with those taking placebo, there were 8 more cases of breast cancer, 8 more strokes, 8 more pulmonary emboli, and 7 more events from coronary heart disease. In addition, there were 6 fewer cases of colon cancer and 5 fewer hip fractures. The study is still ongoing for women who previously underwent hysterectomy and were randomized to estrogen alone versus placebo. Hormone replacement therapy in the form of estrogen and progesterone is currently recommended for less than 5 years in efforts to ameliorate menopausal symptoms.

Risk Assessment Tools—The Gail Model

Management of the High-Risk Patient

- In practice, reproductive risk factors alone are insufficient to place a woman in the high-risk category for breast cancer. However, a strong family history suggestive of a genetic mutation or a previous breast biopsy demonstrating LCIS, atypical ductal hyperplasia, or atypical lobular hyperplasia can significantly raise a woman's breast cancer risk and prompt concern or treatment.

Close Surveillance

- Recommendations for women in a breast-ovarian cancer syndrome family include monthly breast self examination beginning at age 18, semiannual clinical breast examination beginning at age 25, and annual mammography beginning at age 25 or 10 years before the earliest age of onset of a family member.
- Genetic counseling should be offered to those with a strong family history or early-onset breast and ovarian cancer, including a discussion of genetic testing for *BRCA1* and *BRCA2* mutations.

Chemoprevention for Breast Cancer

- Tamoxifen is an estrogen antagonist with proven benefit for the treatment of estrogen hormone receptor positive breast cancer. Furthermore, tamoxifen reduces the incidence of second-primary breast cancer in the contralateral breast of women who received the drug as adjuvant therapy for a first breast cancer.
- Tamoxifen treatment for 5 years was not devoid of complications. In the tamoxifen treatment arm, endometrial cancers resulting from the estrogen-like effects of the drug on the

endometrium were increased by a factor of about 2.5. Pulmonary embolism (RR = 3) and deep venous thrombosis (RR = 1.7) were also more common.

Prophylactic Mastectomy

Prophylactic mastectomy probably reduces the chance of breast cancer in high-risk women by 90%. However, women who are screened by mammograms annually have an overall 80% chance of surviving the occurrence of breast cancer. Coupled with penetrance figures in the range of 50% to 60% for mutation carriers, the chance of dying of breast cancer for carriers of *BRCA1* or *BRCA2* mutations is approximately 10%, without undergoing preventive mastectomy.

BENIGN BREAST TUMORS AND RELATED DISEASES

Breast Cysts

- Cysts within the breast are fluid-filled, epithelium-lined cavities that may vary in size from microscopic to large, palpable masses containing as much as 20 to 30 mL of fluid.
- The management of palpable cysts is straightforward; needle aspiration is both diagnostic and therapeutic.

Fibroadenoma and Related Tumors

Fibroadenoma (adenofibroma) is a benign tumor composed of stromal and epithelial elements.

Juvenile Fibroadenoma and Giant Fibroadenoma

Hamartoma and Adenoma

These tumors are benign proliferations of variable amounts of epithelium and stromal supporting tissue.

Breast Abscess and Infections

Breast abscess commonly occurs in the subareolar breast tissue and may be recurrent and difficult to treat.

Papilloma and Related Ductal Tumors

- Solitary intraductal papillomas are true polyps of epithelium-lined breast ducts.

- Papillomas under the nipple and areolar complex often present with bloody nipple discharge.
- Papillomatosis refers to epithelial hyperplasia that commonly occurs in younger women or is associated with fibrocystic change.

Sclerosing Lesions

Sclerosing Adenosis

Adenosis refers to an increased number of small terminal ductules or acini. It is frequently associated with a proliferation of stromal tissue producing a histologic lesion, sclerosing adenosis, which can simulate carcinoma both grossly and histologically.

Radial Scar

Radial scar belongs to a group of related abnormalities known as complex sclerosing lesions.

Fat Necrosis

As with the other sclerosing abnormalities, fat necrosis can mimic cancer by producing a mass, a density lesion on mammography that can calcify, and surrounding distortion of the normal breast architecture.

PATHOLOGY OF BREAST CANCER (BOX 31-1)

Noninvasive Breast Cancer

Noninvasive neoplasms are broadly divided into two major types: LCIS and DCIS (or intraductal carcinoma).

Invasive Breast Cancers

- Clinicians and pathologists broadly divide invasive breast cancers into *lobular* and *ductal* histology.
- Invasive ductal cancer, or infiltrating ductal carcinoma, is the most common presentation of breast cancer, accounting for 50% to 70% of invasive breast cancers.
- Invasive lobular carcinoma accounts for 10% to 15% of breast cancer.

Box 31–1. Classification of Primary Breast Cancer

NONINVASIVE EPITHELIAL CANCERS
Lobular carinoma *in situ* (LCIS)
Ductal carcinoma *in situ* (DCIS) or intraductal carcinoma
  Papillary, cribriform, solid, and comedo types

INVASIVE EPITHELIAL CANCERS (percentage of total)
Invasive loublar carcinoma (10–15)
Invasive ductal carcinoma
  Invasive ductal carcinoma, NOS (50–70)
  Tubular carcinoma (2–3)
  Mucinous or colloid carcinoma (2–3)
  Medullary carcinoma (5)
  Invasive cribriform (1–3)
  Invasive papillary (1–2)
  Adenoid cystic carcinoma (1)
  Metaplastic carcinoma (1)

MIXED CONNECTIVE AND EPITHELIAL TUMORS
Phyllodes tumors, benign and malignant
Carcinosarcoma
Angiosarcoma

NOS, nothing otherwise specified.

Other Tumors Primary to the Breast

- Phyllodes tumors.
- Angiosarcoma.

STAGING BREAST CANCER

It is important to recognize that staging systems represent abbreviations to describe a heterogeneous disease and a clinical continuum from the earliest malignancy to fatal metastasis. In 2002, the American Joint Committee on Cancer (AJCC) issued its revised tumor-lymph node-metastasis (TNM) classification system. This system is based on the description of the primary tumor (T), the status of regional lymph nodes (N), and the presence of distant metastases (M).

MODERN SURGICAL TREATMENT FOR BREAST CANCER

Brief Introduction to Breast Cancer

Surgical Procedures Past and Present

- A change in surgical practice occurred in the mid-1970s, with an abrupt shift from radical mastectomy to modified radical mastectomy.
- Current estimates of conservative breast procedures range between 40% and 60%.

Radical Mastectomy

In the radical mastectomy, the breast and underlying pectoralis muscles are sacrificed and regional lymph nodes along the axillary vein to the costoclavicular ligament (Halsted's ligament) are removed.

Modern Mastectomy

- These procedures include total or simple mastectomy and the modified radical mastectomy.
- Mastectomy refers to complete removal of the mammary gland, including the nipple and areola.
- Division of the gland from the axillary contents defines the extent of a simple mastectomy. Extension of the operation under the pectoralis major muscle and extending up to the axillary vein, removing the axillary lymph nodes, is called a modified radical mastectomy.

Wide Local Excision and Primary Radiation Therapy

- Excision of the primary tumor with preservation of the breast has been referred to by many names, including partial mastectomy, segmentectomy, or lumpectomy.
- Surgery to remove ipsilateral lymph nodes (axillary node dissection) continues to evolve in the United States.
- Therefore, *conservative breast surgery* or *breast preservation* usually refers to wide local excision of the primary tumor, whole breast radiation, and a separate axillary dissection and/or sentinel node biopsy.

Older Surgical Trials of Local Therapy for Operable Breast Cancer

- A final update of protocol B-04 was published in 2002 with complete 25-year follow-up for the entire study. No significant differences in either overall survival or disease-free survival were noted for 1079 clinically node-negative patients treated by random allocation to radical mastectomy, total mastectomy plus nodal radiation, or total mastectomy and delayed axillary dissection.

The Shift to Breast-Conserving Procedures

- The concept of breast-conserving treatment (BCT) refers to wide excision of the cancer leaving the breast largely intact, with or without postsurgical radiation therapy and with or without surgery on axillary nodes.

Clinical Trials Comparing Breast Conservation with Mastectomy

- Seven prospective clinical trials have randomized more than 4500 patients to various surgical strategies, all of which include a mastectomy arm and a breast-preserving arm. Six trials using modern radiotherapy are listed in Table 31–1, including survival figures and rates of ipsilateral breast recurrences.
- A total of 1851 patients were randomized to receive a modified radical mastectomy, a lumpectomy alone, or a lumpectomy with postoperative radiation to the breast but without an extra boost to the lumpectomy site.
- Overall survival was the same in all three randomly assigned arms, with about 46% of women surviving at 25 years.
- At 20 years of follow-up, 14.3% of women treated with lumpectomy and radiation suffered a recurrence of cancer in the treated breast and 39.2% of women treated only with lumpectomy suffered a recurrence (p = .001 for the difference).
- For women treated by BCT, follow-up of the breast should be continued for an indefinite period of time; there is no point at which women with a conserved breast reach a baseline level of breast cancer risk.
- The Italian trial used more extensive surgery and advocated use of a quadrantectomy.
- Seven hundred one women were randomly divided to receive radical mastectomy (349) versus quadrantectomy plus postoperative radiation (352 received BCT).
- At 20 years of follow-up, deaths resulting from breast cancer occurred in 24.3% of the women treated by radical mastectomy and in 26.1% of women treated by quadrantectomy (p = .8).

TABLE 31-1. Prospective Trials Comparing Mastectomy with Lumpectomy Plus or Minus Radiation

Surgical Trial	No. of Patients (n)	Maximum Tumor Size (cm)	Systemic Therapy	Follow-up (yr)	Survival (%) Lumpectomy and Radiation	Survival (%) Mastectomy	Local Recurrence (radiation) (%)
NSABP B-06[1]	1851	4	Yes	20	47	46	14*
Milan Cancer Institute[2]	701	2	Yes	20	44	43	8.8*
Institute Gustave-Roussy[3]	179	2	No	10	73	65	13
National Cancer Institute, U.S.[4]	237	5	Yes	10	77	75	16
European Organization for Research and Treatment of Cancer (EORTC)[5]	868	5	Yes	10	65	66	17.6
Danish Breast Cancer Group[6]	905	None	Yes	6	79	82	3

[1]Data from Fisher B, Anderson S, Bryant J, et al: Twenty-year follow-up of a randomized trial comparing total mastectomy, lumpectomy, and lumpectomy plus irradiation for the treatment of invasive breast cancer. N Engl J Med 347:1233, 2002.

[2]Data from Veronesi U, Cascinelli N, Mariani L, et al: Twenty-year follow-up of a randomized study comparing breast-conserving surgery with radical mastectomy for early breast cancer. N Engl J Med 347:1227, 2002.

[3]Data from Arriagada R, Le M, Rochard F, et al: Conservative treatment versus mastectomy in early breast cancer: Patterns of failure with 15 years of follow-up data. J Clin Oncol 14:1558, 1996.

[4]Data from Jacobson J, Danforth D, Cowan K, et al: Ten-year results of a comparison of conservation with mastectomy in the treatment of stage I and II breast cancer. N Engl J Med 332:907, 1995.

[5]Data from van Dongen J, Voogd A, Fentiman I, et al: Long-term results of a randomized trial comparing breast-conserving therapy with mastectomy: European Organization for Research and Treatment of Cancer 10801 Trial. J Natl Cancer Inst 92:1143–1150, 2000.

[6]Data from Blichert-Toft M, Rose C, Andersen J, et al: Danish randomized trial comparing breast conservation therapy with mastectomy: Six years of life-table analysis. Danish Breast Cancer Cooperative Group. J Natl Cancer Inst Monogr 11:19, 1992.

*Includes only women whose excision margins were negative.

- Failure in women younger than 45 years was 1% per year, whereas for older women the failure in the breast was 0.5% per year.
- The trial compared modified radical mastectomy to a lumpectomy and postoperative breast radiation (BCT).
- Local failure rates in the BCT group depended on a microscopically complete excision (clear lumpectomy margins).
- One hundred seventy nine patients were randomly allocated to receive either modified radical mastectomy or a complete tumorectomy (lumpectomy) with a generous 2-cm margin of normal tissue around the cancer.
- No differences were observed between the two surgical groups for risk of death, metastases, contralateral breast cancer, or local-regional recurrence at 15 years of follow-up time.
- The National Cancer Institute (NCI) began a trial in 1979 to compare lumpectomy, axillary dissection, and postoperative radiation therapy to modified radical mastectomy.
- No differences were seen in overall survival rates at 10 years (75% for patients receiving lumpectomy and 77% for patients in the mastectomy arm).
- The risk of relapse in the treated breast appears constant over time and was between 1% and 2% per year after treatment.
- For patients treated in the last 25 years of the 20th century, 10-year survival for stage I breast cancer is 75% to 80% and for stage II breast cancer overall survival is 50% to 60% and is not influenced by the choice of breast conservation in place of mastectomy.
- The incidence of contralateral breast cancer is not increased in women assigned to receive radiation.
- The following are guidelines for counseling patients about breast conservation.

Postsurgical Radiation Therapy

- Recent studies have caused reassessment of radiation therapy to the chest wall and lymph nodes following mastectomy.
- Chest wall and node irradiation after mastectomy reduces the odds of local or regional recurrence.
- Many centers now recommend chest wall and nodal irradiation after mastectomy for patients with multiple positive nodes (e.g., >3 nodes positive), for patients with extranodal extension of breast cancer, and for patients with large cancers or very aggressive histology (e.g., diffuse vascular invasion).

Sentinel Lymph Node Biopsy

- Defined as the first node to receive lymphatic drainage from the site of the primary tumor.
- This technique is contraindicated for patients with suspicious palpable axillary adenopathy, prior axillary surgery, and locally advanced disease and in the pregnant or lactating woman. There are insufficient data to advocate its use for patients with multicentric breast cancers or following neo-adjuvant chemotherapy.
- The acceptance of sentinel node biopsy depends on the false-negative rate of the procedure, that is, the chance that positive nodes will be found in the axilla if the sentinel node is negative.
- In a cohort of 2046 patients with a positive sentinel node, 873 (43%) had at least one additional positive node.
- In a cohort of 2046 patients with a positive sentinel node, 873 (43%) had at least one additional positive node.
- When the sentinel node contains metastatic disease, the likelihood of additional nodes also containing metastatic disease is directly proportional to the size of the breast primary, the presence of lymphatic vascular invasion, the size of the lymph node metastasis, and, if the node metastasis is a micrometastasis (<2 mm), whether the micrometastasis was detected by hematoxylin and eosin or by immunohistochemistry.

Ductal Carcinoma in Situ or Intraductal Carcinoma

- In women undergoing annual mammography, DCIS represents 20% to 40% of newly diagnosed breast cancers and presents as clustered calcifications without an associated density in 75% of these patients, as calcifications coexisting with an associated density in 15%, and as a density alone in 10%.
- The breast cancer mortality rate following treatment by total mastectomy is 1% and represents the standard against which breast conservation techniques are compared.

Mastectomy in DCIS

In current practice, reasons to select total mastectomy for treatment of DCIS include (1) mammographically identified multicentric disease, (2) diffuse suspicious mammographic calcifications suggestive of extensive in-breast disease, (3) persistent positive margins after re-excision(s), (4) unacceptable cosmesis to obtain negative margins, and (5) a patient not motivated to preserve her breast. Contraindications to breast radiation include (1) prior radiation to the breast region, (2) the presence of collagen vascular disease (sclero-derma or active lupus), and (3) first or second trimester pregnancy.

Breast Conservation in DCIS

- For patients choosing breast conservation, factors that reduce the risk of local recurrence include the excision of the tumor to an adequate margin, the use of postexcision radiation, and the use of tamoxifen in patients with estrogen receptor (ER)-positive disease.
- Local recurrence after excision of intraductal carcinoma is reduced by 50% by the use of radiation to the ipsilateral breast.
- Furthermore, if an ipsilateral breast tumor recurs, in half of patients it recurs as DCIS and in the other half it recurs as an invasive cancer. Of those patients whose recurrences are an invasive tumor, a proportion of these patients are found to have positive axillary nodes and a smaller proportion develop metastatic disease.

Role of Axillary Dissection and Sentinel Node Biopsy in DCIS

- Therefore, for patients with small mammographically detected *in situ* tumors, axillary dissection is not recommended. For women with larger tumors, particularly if mastectomy is required, sentinel node mapping or a level I axillary dissection to evaluate the lymph nodes should be considered.
- In addition, when a patient is proceeding directly from a core needle biopsy diagnosis of DCIS to mastectomy, sentinel node mapping should be considered.

Role of Tamoxifen in DCIS

- The addition of tamoxifen to lumpectomy and radiation decreased the incidence of ipsilateral breast cancer by 31% (risk reduction predominantly for invasive cancer recurrence—47%). Subsequent contralateral breast cancer was reduced by 47% (with reduction seen predominantly with *in situ* cancer—68%), and cancer on either side was reduced by 37%.
- The question has been raised as to whether the benefit of tamoxifen is restricted to women with ER-positive lesions.

- With a median follow-up of 8.7 years, those who were ER-positive experienced a 59% reduction of first events if taking tamoxifen compared with placebo (RR = 0.41, p = .0002). For those whose lesions were ER-negative, a statistically significant difference in event rates was not observed between the two groups, although the number of events were small (RR = 0.80, 95% CI = 0.41 to 1.56, p = .51, number of events = 36).

Treatment of Locally Advanced and Inflammatory Breast Cancer

- Neoadjuvant chemotherapy.
- Inflammatory breast cancer.

TREATMENT OF SPECIAL CONDITIONS

Paget's Disease

- Paget's cells do not invade through the dermal basement membrane and, therefore, are a form of carcinoma *in situ*.
- More than 97% of patients with Paget's disease have an underlying breast carcinoma.
- For patients considering breast preservation, presurgical evaluation should include evaluation for occult multicentric disease with mammography with retroareolar spot compression views. Some advocate breast MRI.

Male Breast Cancer

- Risk factors include age (exponential increase with age) and those that may be related to abnormalities in estrogen and androgen balance, including testicular disease (undescended testes, congenital inguinal hernia, orchiectomy, orchitis, testicular injury), infertility, obesity, and cirrhosis. Other factors include benign breast conditions (nipple discharge, breast cysts, breast trauma) and radiation exposure. Risk factors related to a genetic predisposition include Klinefelter syndrome (47, XXY karyotype), family history, and Jewish ancestry. *BRCA2* mutations predispose men to breast cancer.
- Histologically, 90% of male breast cancers are invasive, with most being ductal carcinomas. Approximately 80% are ER positive, 75% progesterone receptor (PR) positive, and 35% overexpress HER2/neu.
- Most men with breast cancer (50% to 97%) present with a breast mass, with the differential diagnosis including

gynecomastia, primary breast carcinoma, metastatic carcinoma to the breast, sarcoma, and breast abscess.
- When matched for age and stage, survival is similar to that in women.

Angiosarcoma

- Metastasis to regional nodes is extraordinarily rare; the usual mode of spread is hematogenous, most commonly to the lungs and bone and less commonly to abdominal viscera, brain, and even the contralateral breast.
- Skin punch biopsy of a single nodular lesion may be insufficient to secure a diagnosis, and a second larger biopsy may be needed.
- In the absence of metastatic disease at presentation, surgery to negative margins, most commonly involving a simple or radical mastectomy, frequently with a split-thickness skin graft or myocutaneous flap required to secure negative skin margins. In the past, radical surgery offered the only hope of cure. Axillary dissection is neither necessary nor helpful, with the exception of the rare patient with concomitant axillary adenopathy.
- After diagnosis, local progression in skin and distant progression most frequently to the lungs and bones occurs rapidly. Within 2 years, there is a 90% mortality.

Phyllodes Tumor (Cystosarcoma Phyllodes)

- A phyllodes tumor is differentiated from the fibroadenoma by the presence of stromal overgrowth, and its diagnosis is qualified by indication of its malignancy (25%), of its benignity (60%), or whether it has indeterminate characteristics, a so-called borderline lesion (15%), with this differentiation made based on the lesion's stromal characteristics.
- Metastases occur in 20% of malignant lesions and in less than 5% of benign lesions.
- Cytology is unreliable in differentiating a low-grade phyllodes tumor from a fibroadenoma.
- Excision with a 1-cm minimum negative margin is advocated.
- In a review of seven series reporting 332 patients, axillary metastases were present in 3 (0.9%) of the patients.
- Local recurrences are usually seen within the first few years of surgery, at the site of the original excision and are inversely correlated with the width of the negative resection margin. There is an unacceptable local recurrence rate, regardless of histologic type or tumor size, if the lesion is enucleated.

CHEMOTHERAPY AND HORMONE THERAPY FOR BREAST CANCER

- Current thinking places the metastatic event early in the progression of breast cancer, probably before the finding of a mass for most patients.
- Metastatic disease is the principal cause of death resulting from breast cancer.

Interpreting Results of Clinical Trials

- To estimate the survival curve for any group of people, investigators use the life-table method (also called the actuarial method).
- The concept of proportional benefit is important when evaluating adjuvant chemotherapy or hormonal therapy for breast cancer; only a small proportion of treated patients benefit from receiving postoperative adjuvant treatments.
- A popular way to express the difference between control and experimental groups is to cite the proportional reduction in treatment failures.

Adjuvant Chemotherapy for Operable Breast Cancer

- The first trials of prolonged postoperative chemotherapy in operable breast cancer were started by the National Surgical Adjuvant Breast Project (NSABP) in 1972 and by the National Cancer Institute of Italy (NCI-Milan) in 1973.
- The results from these two trials are similar and convincingly positive for women undergoing chemotherapy who are younger than 50 years.

Meta-Analysis of Adjuvant Chemotherapy for Breast Cancer

- Although clinically worthwhile, the benefits of adjuvant systemic therapy for operable breast cancer are modest and in the range of a 20% to 30% reduction in the odds of recurrence or death.
- With respect to adjuvant chemotherapy, information from 30,000 women in 69 trials was collected.
- The meta-analysis conducted by the Early Breast Cancer Trialists' Collaborative Group (EBCTCG) provides principles about adjuvant chemotherapy but recognizes that treatment decisions involve consideration of the benefit and the adverse side effects of treatments.

Newer Approaches in Chemotherapy for Breast Cancer

- Dose intensity.
  - Dose intensity is defined as the amount of drug given over an interval of time (milligrams of delivered dose/meter squared/unit of time); more intense regimens give a higher dose in a shorter interval than less intense regimens.
- New agents.
  - Thus, it appears that the addition of an agent, which is "non-cross resistant," can kill additional cancer cells when an increased dose of the same drug may be unable to do so.
  - Trastuzumab (Herceptin; Genentech, Inc.) is a humanized murine monoclonal antibody raised against the erbB-2 or HER2 surface receptor.
- Neoadjuvant chemotherapy for operable breast cancer.
  - Neoadjuvant chemotherapy refers to chemotherapy (systemic therapy) given in addition to surgery or radiation (local therapies), which precedes local treatments.

Hormonal Therapy for Breast Cancer

Steroid Hormone Receptors

- Reproductive and certain other sensitive tissues possess high-affinity protein receptors for estrogen and progesterone.
- Activation of ERs leads to the induction of numerous cellular genes, including those that may encode critical enzymes and secreted peptide growth factors.
- The presence of ERs predicts clinical response to all types of endocrine therapies, both additive and ablative.
- The presence of both receptors in a tumor is associated with almost an 80% chance of favorably responding to hormone addition or blockade (Table 31–2).
- Tamoxifen can replace oophorectomy in premenopausal women with ER-positive metastatic cancer, and it is considered the drug of first choice in both premenopausal and postmenopausal patients with ER- or PR-positive cancers.

Adjuvant Hormonal Therapy for Operable Breast Cancer

The first modern trial of adjuvant tamoxifen was begun in Copenhagen in 1975.

Meta-Analysis of Adjuvant Tamoxifen for Breast Cancer

The overview from the Early Breast Cancer Trialists' Collaborative Group looked at 42,000 women participating in

TABLE 31–2. Relationship Between Steroid Receptor Status of Breast Tumor and Patients' Objective Response to Endocrine Therapy

Steroid Receptor Status*			
ER⁺, PgR⁺	ER⁺, PgR⁻	ER⁻, PgR⁻	ER⁻, PgR⁺
137/174	55/164	17/165	5/11
(78%)	(34%)	(10%)	(45%)

*Number of patients responding to treatment/number of women with receptor status designated.
Based on the collective paper presented at the National Institutes of Health (NIH) Consensus Development Conference on Steroid Receptors in Breast Cancer (Proceedings of the NIH Consensus Development Conference, 1980).
From Donegan WL, Spratt JS (eds): Cancer of the Breast. Philadelphia, WB Saunders, 1988.
ER, estrogen receptor; PgR, progesterone receptor.

63 randomized trials, in which tamoxifen was compared with placebo or no treatment. Statistically significant benefits for both node-positive and node-negative women were discovered.

Adjuvant Ovarian Ablation

● One surprising result of the overview process was to rekindle interest in ovarian ablation as an effective adjuvant for operable breast cancer in premenopausal women.

Aromatase Inhibitors as Adjuvant Therapy

● Several clinical trials are introducing selective aromatase inhibitors (SAIs) into adjuvant therapy and comparing these agents against tamoxifen, the current standard for adjuvant therapy of ER-positive breast cancer after local treatment.

Summary of Adjuvant Therapy for Operable Breast Cancer

● Adjuvant chemotherapy is likely to benefit nearly all patients with invasive breast cancers, and hormonal adjuvants probably benefit all breast cancer patients with ER- or PR-positive cancers.

TREATMENT OF METASTATIC DISEASE

● When breast cancer recurs, it is generally thought to be incurable, with a median life expectancy between 18 and 24 months.

- Systemic therapy can extend life and improve quality of life during the metastatic phase of breast cancer. This is particularly true for hormone-sensitive metastatic breast cancer.
- Tamoxifen is the first choice among the antiestrogens for patients with metastatic, hormone-sensitive breast cancer.
- At some point in the treatment of most patients with metastatic breast cancer, chemotherapy is indicated.
- One exciting discovery is the monoclonal antibody against the HER-2 (ErbB2) receptor protein, trastuzumab, which has recently been approved for use in metastatic breast cancer.

CHAPTER 32

BREAST RECONSTRUCTION

PATIENT SELECTION

- Young healthy patients with early-stage disease are the best candidates for reconstruction.
- Because of the multitude of different reconstructive options available, all women should at least be presented with the options (Box 32–1).

TIMING

- Physician support for immediate reconstruction is based on the absence of medical contraindications.
- Early reconstruction after mastectomy reduces the emotional impact, improves ability to provide breast symmetry because the skin flaps are pliable and not contracted, makes it easier to preserve the inframammary crease (IMC), and is more cost-effective.
- There is no statistically significant difference in complication rates after immediate versus delayed breast reconstruction.

SURGICAL PLANNING

- Ablative surgical planning as early as the breast biopsy is performed can improve the reconstructive outcome.
- The biopsy can be made in or very near the nipple-areola complex in most cases.
- Skin-sparing mastectomy can be performed whenever feasible; only the nipple-areola complex may need to be excised.
- Additional incisions can be added to help with the dissection, such as a lateral extension of the periareolar incision for access to a large mammary gland or a separate incision in the axillary crease for the lymphadenectomy.
- A skin-sparing mastectomy, with the skin flaps shaved too thin leads to tissue necrosis and loss of breast skin over the flap or implant.
- Care should be taken to avoid disrupting the IMC; preoperative marking of the IMC helps.

Box 32–1.   Factors Affecting Choice of Reconstruction Procedures

Patient Factors
Age
    Medical conditions
    Previous abdominal or thoracic surgeries
    Coronary artery disease
    Chronic obstructive pulmonary disease
    Medications
    Chronic corticosteroid use
    Obesity
Body morphology
Occupation
Social activities
Financial resources
Support systems
Expectations/desires

Disease Factors
Stage of disease
Type of tumor
Need for adjuvant therapy

Miscellaneous Factors
Experience of the surgeon
Availability of equipment (e.g., microscope)
Religious beliefs regarding blood transfusions
Blood banking facilities

- In large or very ptotic breasts, alternative skin incisions can be planned.
- A breast reduction type of skin incision using the keyhole type pattern provides excellent exposure of the breast mound and adequate exposure for the axillary dissection.
- For a contralateral breast reduction or mastopexy, the standard elliptical mastectomy incision provides less symmetry.
- The keyhole (pattern of Wise) incision design affords skin excision in the horizontal and vertical planes.

SURGICAL OPTIONS

- Symmetry is ultimately more important to a successful outcome than anything else.

- The reconstructive plan must accommodate not only the size and shape of the opposite breast but also the position on the chest wall; the location of the IMC; the height, size, and color of the nipple-areolar complex; and the amount of breast ptosis.
- Reconstructive options can be divided into two main types: those that use autogenous tissue and those that require alloplastic material.
- The choice of procedure for a given patient is affected by her age, health, contralateral breast size and shape, her

---

Box 32–2. Options for Breast Reconstruction

Autogenous
    Abdominal-based flaps
    TRAM
        Single pedicle
        Double pedicle
        Free flap*
        Deep inferior epigastric perforator flap*
    Upper abdominal horizontal flap
    Vertical abdominal flap
    Tubed abdominal flap
  Latissimus dorsi musculocutaneous flap
  Gluteal flap*
    Superior-based
    Inferior-based
  Rubens flap*
  Thoracoepigastric flap
  Lateral thigh flap*
  Breast-splitting procedure†
Alloplastic
    Silicone gel implant
    Silicone implant with saline fill
        Smooth wall
        Textured wall
        Round shaped
        Anatomic shaped
    Silicone injection†
Combination procedures
    Latissimus dorsi flap with implant
    TRAM flap with implant

TRAM, transverse rectus abdominis myocutaneous.
*Require microsurgical procedure.
†Historical note only.

personal preference, and the expertise of the reconstructive surgeon (Box 32–2).

- The most significant complication that can occur is the delay of initiation of adjuvant therapy.
- Partial or complete flap loss, wound breakdown, and infection are all reasons why chemotherapy or radiation therapy would be delayed.
- Survival in patients who have undergone reconstruction is no different than in patients who have undergone mastectomy alone.

Breast Reconstruction with Implants

- Breast implants can provide a technically simple means of achieving breast symmetry, pose a minimal risk, and are appropriate for patients requiring bilateral breast reconstruction in which excellent symmetry can be achieved.
- Unilateral mastectomy patients with small breasts and minimal ptosis can also benefit.
- Placement of the implant in a submuscular plane beneath the pectoralis major, superior portion of rectus abdominis, and serratus anterior muscles provides better protection against implant extrusion and a decreased risk for capsular contracture and implant displacement.
- Complications include exposure, extrusion, or infection of the implants.
- Long-term problems also include asymmetry, capsular contracture, malposition of the implant, rupture, and pain.
- The breast implant may be used for thin patients who have inadequate abdominal and back soft tissue for use with the transverse rectus abdominis or latissimus dorsi myocutaneous flaps.
- Women expected to receive radiotherapy have a relative contraindication to reconstruction with implants because of increased risk for capsular contracture and inelastic skin (Box 32–3).

Latissimus Dorsi Myocutaneous Flap

- This flap is ideally suited for single-stage reconstruction for women with small- to medium-sized breasts and a moderate degree of breast ptosis.
- Blood supply comes from the thoracodorsal artery, which provides musculocutaneous perforating vessels.
- In some women who do not require a modified radical mastectomy and in whom the resultant segmental resection is

---

Box 32–3. Implant Reconstruction

Indications
Bilateral reconstruction
Patient requesting augmentation in addition to reconstruction
Patient not suited for long surgery
Lack of adequate abdominal tissue
Patient unwilling to have additional scars on either back
    or abdomen
Small breast mound with minimal ptosis

Relative Contraindications
Young age (may need implant replacement multiple times)
Patient unwilling to follow up
Very large breast
Very ptotic breast

Contraindications
Silicon allergy
Implant fear
Previous failed implants
Need for adjuvant radiation therapy

---

enough to cause significant breast deformity, the latissimus
dorsi flap can be extremely useful in restoring breast contour.
- If the breast volume requirements exceed the available
  tissue from this region, a breast implant can be used to augment the reconstruction (Box 32–4).
- Patients who have had previous surgery in the back or the
  axilla (lateral thoracotomies) and those with a history of

Box 32–4. Latissimus Dorsi Reconstruction

Indications
Small breast
Minor breast ptosis
Abdominal donor site unavailable (e.g., scars, lack of tissue)
Salvage of previous breast reconstruction

Relative Contraindications
Planned postoperative radiation therapy
Bilateral reconstruction
Significant breast ptosis

Contraindications
Previous lateral thoracotomy
Very large breast in patient who does not desire reduction

radiation therapy to the axilla should be discouraged from undergoing this form of reconstruction.

- One of the disadvantages of this technique is that simultaneous harvesting of the flap while the mastectomy is being performed is not possible.
- Inset of the flap necessitates the repositioning of the patient before breast shaping and closure, unless both are performed in the lateral decubitus position, which results in mild inconvenience to the operating staff, delays the operation, and raises the theoretical consideration of contamination and increased rates of infection.

Transverse Rectus Abdominis Myocutaneous (TRAM) Flap

- In its original description, an ellipse of skin from the upper abdomen was used; this design was later modified to be placed over the lower abdomen to take advantage of the larger amount of adipose tissue, the more favorable scar location, and longer pedicle for ease of transposition. (Box 32–5).
- One of the advantages of this technique is the diversity of configurations available.
- The flap can be harvested as a single- or a double-pedicle flap, using the deep superior epigastric blood supply; it may also be harvested as a free flap based on the deep inferior epigastric vessels.

Box 32–5.   Transverse Rectus Abdominis Muscle Flap Reconstruction

Indications
Breasts of all sizes
Breast ptosis

Relative Contraindications
Smoking
Abdominal liposuction
Previous abdominal surgery
Pulmonary disease
Obesity

Contraindications
Previous abdominoplasty
Patient unable to tolerate 4- to 6-week recovery period
Patient unable to tolerate longer procedure

- In patients who are obese, having larger tissue requirements, or with a history of upper abdominal scars, use of the free inferiorly based TRAM flap is considered more reliable; the free TRAM flap is also advocated for patients who smoke.
- Donor-site complications can include abdominal wall laxity, diastasis, abdominal skin necrosis, umbilical malposition, seroma, and severe pain.
- Many surgeons use mesh to close the abdominal wall defect caused by the elevation of the muscle flap; others close the defect by approximating the fascia.
- Breast complications include partial or complete flap loss and fat necrosis.

Other Options for Autologous Breast Reconstructions

Free Gluteal Flap

- The free gluteal flap has been used for breast reconstruction as a myocutaneous flap based on either the inferior or the superior gluteal vessels.
- Because of the technical complexity and complications, including sciatica, seroma, unfavorable scar location, and asymmetrical buttock contour, this option is a secondary choice.

Rubens Flap

- The Rubens flap, based on the circumflex iliac vessels, is elevated with a full thickness of tissue over the hip and underlying musculature, including the oblique and transverse muscles.
- Because this reconstructive procedure is limited in bulk and skin envelope and often requires a balancing procedure on the contralateral hip, it is not usually considered as a first option.

Nipple-Areola Reconstruction

- Nipple-areola complex reconstruction is performed as a second stage.
- Proper position of the nipple may not be able to be determined until 2 to 3 months after the initial surgery.
- The nipple is created from local flaps on the breast mound.
- Within 12 months, most undergo at least a 50% reduction in projection.

- The pigmented areola was originally reconstructed with split-thickness skin grafts from the hyperpigmented upper medial thigh, labia majora, or retroauricular regions; this has been replaced with medical tattooing performed 3 to 4 weeks after nipple creation.

OUTCOME

- No study has been able to demonstrate any difference in survival between patients undergoing breast reconstruction and those with mastectomy alone.

MANAGEMENT OF CONTRALATERAL BREAST

- The challenge of breast reconstruction requires not only creating a natural-appearing breast but also achieving breast symmetry.
- Breast reconstruction occasionally requires an additional procedure on the contralateral breast, matching preexisting ptosis and larger contralateral breast size.
- A reduction mammoplasty, mastopexy, or implant insertion may be required to optimize the breast reconstruction to achieve optimal symmetry.

CHAPTER 33

THYROID

ANATOMIC CONSIDERATIONS

Embryology

- These include the thyroglossal duct cysts and fistulas, which result from retained tissue along the thyroglossal duct.
- Recurrent laryngeal nerve.
  - The recurrent laryngeal nerves ascend on either side of the trachea, and each lies just lateral to the ligament of Berry as they enter the larynx.
  - The motor function of the recurrent laryngeal nerve is abduction of the vocal cords from the midline.
- Superior laryngeal nerve.
- Blood supply.
- Lymphatic system.
- Parathyroid glands.
  - The superior and inferior parathyroid glands have a single end artery, which supplies them medially from the inferior thyroid artery.

PHYSIOLOGY OF THE THYROID GLAND

- Cells derived from the neural crest are called *C cells* and migrate into the thyroid during embryologic development.

Iodine Metabolism

- The thyroid gland is responsible for storing 90% of the total-body iodide at any given time, leaving less than 10% existing in the extracellular pool.
- Thyroid hormone synthesis.
  - This rapid and metabolically active process results in the storage of about 2 weeks' worth of thyroid hormone within the organism under normal circumstances.

Regulation of Thyroid Hormone Secretion

- Thyroid stimulating hormone (TSH).
- Triiodothyronine (T_3) and thyroxine (T_4).

- Thyroglobulin.
- Calcitonin.
  - Basal or stimulated calcitonin levels are sensitive markers for primary or recurrent medullary carcinoma of the thyroid (MCT).

Peripheral Action of Thyroid Hormones

- In the periphery, T_4 is relatively inactive compared with T_3.
- In adults, the half-life of T_4 is about 7 days because of the efficient and significant degree of binding to carrier proteins.

Inhibition of Thyroid Synthesis

- Drugs—Propylthiouracil (PTV); methimazole (Tapazole).
- Iodine.
- Steroids.
- Beta-blockers.

Tests of Thyroid Function

- Evaluation of the pituitary-thyroid feedback loop.
- Serum T_3 and T_4 levels.
- Calcitonin.
- Radioactive iodine uptake.
- Thyroid autoantibody levels.

Radiologic Evaluation of the Thyroid

- Thyroid scintigraphy.
- Thyroid ultrasound.

DISORDERS OF THYROID METABOLISM—BENIGN THYROID DISEASE

Hypothyroidism

- Metabolic consequences of iodine deficiency.
- Postirradiation hypothyroidism.
- Postsurgical hypothyroidism.
- Pharmacologic hypothyroidism.
  - Cytokines.
  - Lithium.
  - Amiodarone.
  - Antithyroid drugs.

- Peripheral tissue hormone resistance.
- Clinical presentation and diagnosis of hypothyroidism.
  - Fatigue, headache, weight gain, dry skin, brittle hair and muscle cramps. Severe progression of disease can result in cardiovascular symptoms including hypertension, pericardial effusions and pleural effusions. Abdominal distension and constipation are signs of severe hypothyroidism. Anemia may occur in 12% of cases.
  - Diagnosis.
  - Treatment.

Thyroiditis

- Acute suppurative thyroiditis.
- Hashimoto's thyroiditis.
- Subacute thyroiditis.
- Reidel's struma.

Hyperthyroidism

Graves' Disease (Diffuse Toxic Goiter)

- Clinical presentation.
  - The patient with classic Graves' disease usually has a visibly enlarged neck mass consistent with a goiter. Accompanying clinical thyrotoxicosis and exophthalmos complete the classic triad of the disease. Hair loss, myxedema, gynecomastia, and splenomegaly can accompany the clinical presentation. Physical examination is remarkable for an enlarged palpable thyroid with bilateral and central enlargement. With increased vascularity, a bruit is often heard. Tracheal compression can result in airway-obstructive symptoms, although **acute compression with respiratory distress is exceedingly rare.**
- Diagnosis. Increased levels of T_3 and T_4; decreased or undetectable levels of TSH.
- Treatment.
  - There have been three classic methods to treat Graves' disease: radioiodine ablation, surgery, and antithyroid medication.
  - Radionuclide therapy, ^{131}I 10–15 mCi.
  - Antithyroid medication.
  Medical treatment of patients with severe thyrotoxicosis initially starts with beta-blockers such as propranolol, which is specifically effective in treating tachycardia.

- Thyroid resection.
Complete ablation of thyroid tissue requires a total thyroidectomy, which is associated with the highest rates of hypoparathyroidism and recurrent laryngeal nerve damage.

Toxic Nodular Goiter-Toxic Adenoma

Nontoxic Goiter

- Multinodular goiter.
- Substernal goiter.
  - Most substernal goiters can be approached through a cervical incision.
- Special considerations for the patient with goiter.
  - If the patient has a history of pain and night sweats, a diagnosis of a lymphoma should be considered.

WORKUP AND DIAGNOSIS OF THE SOLITARY THYROID NODULE

Presentation

- Exposure to radiation, especially during childhood, is associated with an increased prevalence of thyroid nodules, and malignancy, particularly between the late teenage years and early 20s.
- Diagnostic evaluation—PE and ultrasound (Fig. 33–1).
- Laboratory evaluation.

Radionucleic Scan

- Hot or cold nodule.

Fine-Needle Aspiration (FNA)

- A series of 561 FNA biopsy results reported an 86% sensitivity rate at 91% specificity. The accurate diagnosis of a benign lesion has significantly decreased surgery rates on patients with thyroid nodules. Additionally, preoperative FNA is replacing the use of intraoperative frozen-section analysis of pathology.
- The finding of a malignant diagnosis of FNA is associated with a high accuracy rate, approaching 100%. Certain discrete cytologic characteristics of papillary carcinoma allow the use of FNA to be extremely accurate in its diagnosis. The diagnosis of follicular carcinoma cannot be made with FNA (Table 33–1).

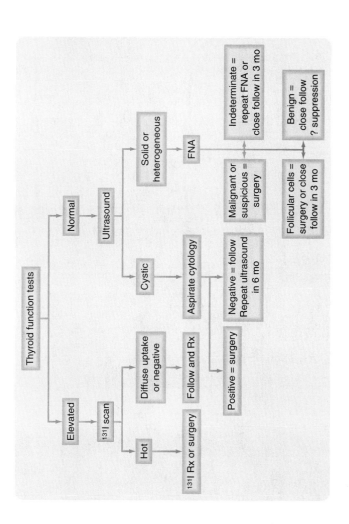

TABLE 33-1. Thyroid Nodules

Diagnosis	Factors Associated with Diagnosis	Factors that Confirm Diagnosis	Factors Associated with Worse Prognosis
Benign			
Colloid	Multinodular goiter FNA shows colloid and Macrophages	Surgery	—
Hyperfunctioning nodule	Hyperthyroidism	Iodine 131 Scan	—
Malignant			
Papillary carcinoma	Radiation exposure Previous surgery for papillary carcinoma "Follicular cells" by FNA	FNA or surgery	Male gender, age >40 yr, size >3 cm, tall cell variant
Follicular carcinoma		Permanent section pathology	Male gender, age >40 yr, size >3 cm, poorly differentiated cell type
Medullary carcinoma	MEN types 2a and 2b Elevated calcitonin level	Calcitonin levels *ret* oncogene	MEN type 2b and sporadic
Anaplastic carcinoma	Rapid progression of tumor mass Pain, hoarseness	FNA Surgery	Diagnosis

FNA, fine-needle aspiration; MEN, multiple endocrine neoplasia.

Decision Making and Treatment

THYROID MALIGNANCIES

Thyroid Oncogenesis

- Oncogene activators.
  - *ras* gene family.
  - *RET* proto-oncogene.
  - Thyroid-stimulating hormone receptor.
  - Tyrosine kinase receptors.
- Tumor suppressor genes.
  - *p53.*

Different Thyroid Cancer

- Age at diagnosis turns out to be the most important clinical prognosic finding; diagnosis at ages younger than 40 is an important prognostic factor of long-term survival.

Papillary Carcinoma

- Papillary carcinoma is the most common of the thyroid neoplasms and is usually associated with an excellent prognosis.
- The association of irradiation and thyroid cancer has been known for years.
- Treatment—Surgical resection.

Follicular Carcinoma

- The histologic diagnosis of follicular thyroid carcinoma (FTC) depends on the demonstration of what would appear to be normal follicular cells occupying abnormal positions, including capsular, lymphatic, or vascular invasion.
- Treatment—Surgical resection.

OTHER THYROID MALIGNANCIES

Hürthle Cell Carcinoma

- Subtype of FTC with similar prognosis.
- Treatment—Surgical resection.

Medullary Carcinoma

- MCT is associated with the secretion of a biologic marker, calcitonin.
- Sporadic or Familial (MEN type 2A or 2B).
- Treatment—Total thyroidectomy.

Anaplastic Thyroid Cancer

- Less than 1% of all thyroid malignancies.
- Rapid growth.
- Treatment—Nonsurgical external beam radiation therapy and chemotherapy.

Lymphoma

- Rare.
- Treatment—With systemic chemotherapy.

CHAPTER 34

PARATHYROID GLAND

HISTORICAL ASPECTS

EMBRYOLOGY AND ANATOMY

- The superior parathyroid glands arise from branchial pouch IV, and the inferior parathyroids arise from III.
- The inferior glands are more likely to be found in an ectopic location than the superior glands.
- The vascular supply to the parathyroid glands is usually from the inferior thyroid artery, but it can arise from the superior thyroid artery or from anastomoses between these vessels.

NORMAL PARATHYROID PHYSIOLOGY

- The intact molecule and N-terminal fragment have half-lives of minutes, whereas the C-terminal fragment has a half-life of hours. Normally, parathormone (PTH) secretion is inversely related to levels of serum ionized calcium and 1,25-dihydroxyvitamin D.

PARATHYROID PATHOPHYSIOLOGY

Hypoparathyroidism

- The earliest manifestations are numbness and tingling in the circumoral area and the fingers. Mental symptoms such as anxiety or confusion can occur. Tetany may develop, characterized by carpopedal spasms, convulsions, or laryngospasm (which can be fatal).
- If there is concomitant hypomagnesemia, it is difficult to correct the hypocalcemia until the magnesium level has been corrected.

Primary Hyperparathyroidism

- The finding of an elevated plasma level of PTH does not in itself establish the diagnosis of hyperparathyroidism (HPT).

One must evaluate the PTH level as a function of the serum calcium concentration. Patients with increased serum concentrations of both calcium and PTH generally have HPT.

- HPT in pregnancy.
  - When the diagnosis is made, the mother should undergo operation, if possible during the second trimester.
- Neonatal primary HPT and familial hypocalciuric hypercalcemia (FHH).
  - Neonatal primary HPT and FHH are caused by a defect in the gene coding for the calcium-sensing receptor.
  - This benign condition manifests later in life as an elevation in the calcium set point causing an elevated serum calcium and mildly elevated serum PTH without complications of primary HPT. This disease can be distinguished from primary HPT by a low 24-hour urine calcium measurement.
- Hyperparathyroid crisis.
  - The management of severe hypercalcemia addresses four main goals—to correct dehydration, to enhance renal excretion of calcium, to inhibit bone resorption, and to treat the underlying disorder.

Hyperparathyroidism—Secondary and Tertiary

- As glomerular filtration rate falls, the renal production of 1,25-dihydroxyvitamin D_3 decreases, which then reduces intestinal calcium absorption to create a negative calcium balance. A compensatory increase in PTH secretion keeps serum calcium near normal by mobilizing calcium from bone. PTH secretion is further stimulated by hyperphosphatemia (via a phosphorus-specific receptor) and a decrease in ionized calcium (from reduced solubility caused by hyperphosphatemia).
- Tertiary hyperparathyroidism (tertiary HPT) follows long-standing secondary HPT when the chronically stimulated parathyroid glands act independently of the serum calcium concentration.

Parathyroid Carcinoma

- In about 50% of patients with parathyroid carcinoma, the involved parathyroid gland is palpable, a finding rarely observed in patients with benign primary HPT.

SURGICAL MANAGEMENT OF HYPERPARATHYROIDISM

Primary Hyperparathyroidism: Operative Versus Nonoperative Management

- There is general agreement that most *symptomatic* patients should undergo parathyroidectomy.
- The indications for operation in asymptomatic patients were outlined as follows: (1) significant hypercalcemia (serum calcium 1 mg/dL above the upper limit of normal reference range); (2) significant hypercalciuria (24-hour urinary calcium excretion 400 mg); (3) creatinine clearance reduced by 30% compared with age-matched subjects; (4) decreased bone density at the lumbar spine, hip, or distal radius (as determined by dual-energy x-ray absorptiometry) that is more than 2.5 standard deviations below peak bone mass (t-score <−2.5); (5) age younger than 50 years; and (6) patients for whom medical surveillance is either not desirable or not possible.

Operative Approaches for Primary Hyperparathyroidism: Standards and Developments

- Critical in determining the next sequence of maneuvers is the inference of which gland is missing—the superior or the inferior—based on proper identification of normal glands already found. As the RLN obliquely bisects the lateral view of the trachea and esophagus, the inferior gland should generally be located anterior and caudal to this plane (Fig. 34–1). The superior parathyroid gland should be located posterior and cranial to this plane.
- There is contralateral symmetry of superior glands in approximately 80% of patients (inferior in 70%); thus, the location of a gland on one side can lead to discovery of a difficult to find gland on the other.
- By far, the most common location is into a paraesophageal or retroesophageal position descending toward the posterior mediastinum; it is here that the adenoma is often obvious to the palpating finger of the surgeon before it is visible. A truly intrathyroidal superior parathyroid gland very rarely exists, and thyroid lobectomy is not routinely indicated for a missing superior adenoma.
- True ectopia (based on embryologic influences) is much more common with inferior parathyroids.

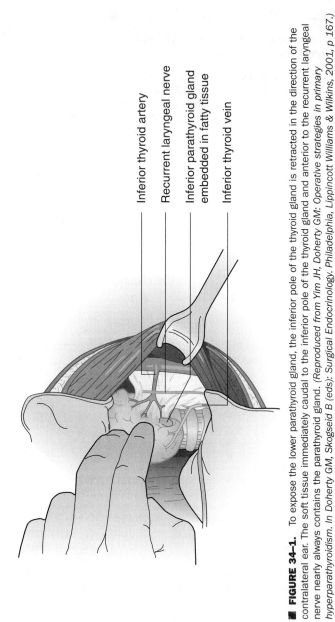

Inferior thyroid artery

Recurrent laryngeal nerve

Inferior parathyroid gland embedded in fatty tissue

Inferior thyroid vein

■ **FIGURE 34-1.** To expose the lower parathyroid gland, the inferior pole of the thyroid gland is retracted in the direction of the contralateral ear. The soft tissue immediately caudal to the inferior pole of the thyroid gland and anterior to the recurrent laryngeal nerve nearly always contains the parathyroid gland. (Reproduced from Yim JH, Doherty GM: Operative strategies in primary hyperparathyroidism. In Doherty GM, Skogseid B (eds): Surgical Endocrinology. Philadelphia, Lippincott Williams & Wilkins, 2001, p 167.)

- If the inferior adenoma is not found, a sequence of the following three maneuvers is undertaken: (1) a full cervical thymectomy is performed, (2) the ipsilateral carotid sheath is opened to visually and manually explore the contents to at least the level of the arterial bifurcation, and (3) the ipsilateral inferior thyroid pole is interrogated with intra-operative ultrasound and/or resected to include the possibility of an intrathyroidal gland.
- The essential change from conventional management is more strategic than it is procedural and can be summarized in two cardinal issues: (1) reliance on preoperative localization of the adenoma by sestamibi scintigraphy or high-resolution ultrasound and (2) intraoperative indication of cure that does not require morphologic assessment of uninvolved normal glands (e.g., intraoperative PTH monitoring [IOPTH]).
- IOPTH monitoring is predicated on the fact that intact PTH has a very short half life (2.5 to 4.5 minutes) and that large decrements can be measured in 10 to 15 minutes.

Persistent or Recurrent Hyperparathyroidism

- Biochemical HPT evident within the first 6 months after exploration is termed *persistent.*
- *Recurrent* disease occurs after 6 months and is often caused by growth of hyperplastic tissue knowingly or unknowingly left behind at the initial operation.
- A wise practice is to offer reoperation when two localization studies are in agreement.
- If a superior gland is suspected, the lateral approach is ideal to establish a less distorted route of access.
- If an inferior parathyroid gland is the target of re-exploration, a low anterior approach reopening the midline raphe exposes the lower thyroid lobes, trachea, and cervical thymus.

Secondary and Tertiary Hyperparathyroidism

- Careful medical management prevents most patients (>90%) from requiring surgical intervention.
- Open skin lesions mandate urgent skin biopsy to establish the diagnosis of calciphylaxis (medial arterial calcification), which requires urgent parathyroidectomy.

Parathyroid Carcinoma

- It is important to recognize parathyroid carcinoma at the initial neck exploration because radical resection of the malignant parathyroid gland, the ipsilateral thyroid lobe, and involved adjacent soft tissue offers the only possibility for cure.

- If disease recurs, reoperation is indicated (including resection of pulmonary and liver metastases) because patients, if untreated, die of uncontrolled hypercalcemia.

CHAPTER 35

ENDOCRINE PANCREAS

- Endocrine cells of the pancreas reside in islets.
  - The A (alpha) cell—glucagon.
  - The B (beta) cell—insulin.
  - The D (delta) cell—somatostatin.
  - The D_2 (delta-2) cell—vasoactive intestinal peptide (VIP).
  - The PP (or F) cell—pancreatic polypeptide (PP).
- Gastrin cells are present normally only in the fetal pancreas.
- Ectopic gastrin cells may give rise to gastrinomas in the pancreas, duodenum, or adjacent structures.
- Tumors of any of these cells may secrete multiple peptides.
- Syndromes produced named for peptide for which symptoms predominate.
- Pancreatic islet tumors rarely produce growth hormone–releasing factor (GRF), adrenocorticotropic hormone (ACTH), and parathyroid hormone-related peptide (PTHrP).
- All pancreatic endocrine tumors are rare, 5 cases per 1 million population per year (Tables 35–1 and 35–2).

ENDOCRINE PHYSIOLOGY

- The chief physiologic function of the endocrine pancreas is regulation of body energy.
- Insulin is the hormone of energy storage.
- Glucagon the hormone of energy release.
- Insulin stores energy by
  - Decreasing blood glucose level.
  - Increasing protein synthesis.
  - Decreasing glycogenolysis.
  - Decreasing lipolysis.
  - Increasing glucose transport into cells (except beta cells, hepatocytes, and central nervous system cells).
- Glucagon releases energy by
  - Increasing blood glucose level via stimulation of glycogenolysis.
  - Stimulating gluconeogenesis and lipolysis.

ISLET CELL TUMORS

- These tumors are rare.

TABLE 35–1. Endocrine Cells of Pancreas and Tumor Syndromes

Cells	Content†	% Islet Cells	Secretory Granule Size (nm)	Tumor Syndromes	Clinical Features	Diagnostic Hormone Levels	% Malignant	% Multiple	MEN 1	At Operation: % Identified/% Resectable
A	**Glucagon** glicentin (TRH, CCK, endorphin, PYY, pancreastatin)	15	225	Glucagonoma	Necrolytic migratory erythema, diabetes, anemia	Normal = <150 pg/mL Tumor = 200–2000 pg/mL	Nearly all	Rare	Few	98/35
B	**Insulin** (TRH, CGRP, amylin, pancreastatin, prolactin)	65	300	Insulinoma	Hypoglycemic symptoms (catecholamine release) plus mental confusion	>5 μU/mL in face of hypoglycemia	10	10	10%	80–100/ >90
D	**Somatostatin** (met-encephalon)	5	200–235	Somatostatinoma	Diabetes, gallstones, steatorrhea	Normal = 10–25 pg/mL Tumor = 100–400 pg/mL	Nearly all	0	—	100/60
D₂	VIP	<1	120	VIPoma (watery diarrhea, hypokalemia, achlorhydria [WDHA] [Verner-Morrison])	High-volume secretory diarrhea, hypokalemia, metabolic acidosis, hypochlorhydria	Normal = <200 pg/mL Tumor = 225–2000 pg/mL	50	Rare	Few	100/70

EC	Substance P and serotonin	<1	325	?	—	—	—	—	—
G*	Gastrin (ACTH-related peptides)	—	300	Gastrinoma (Zollinger-Ellison syndrome)	Abdominal pain with ulcer disease, massive gastric hypersecretion, secretory diarrhea that can be halted by nasogastric aspiration	Normal = <100 pg/mL Tumor = 100–1000 pg/mL Suspicious = >1000 pg/mL With secretin Test, ↑ > 200 pg/mL diagnostic	70	25%	50–85/79 Of the 70%: Pancreatic, <20 duodenal, all Ectopic, 80
PP (F)	Pancreatic polypeptide (met-encephalon, PHI)	15	140	Tumors (PPomas) are without endocrine symptoms	—	—	—	Frequent	—

*Gastrin is present in fetal but not in normal adult pancreatic islets.

ACTH, adrenocorticotropic hormone; CCK, cholecystokinin; CGRP, calcitonin gene-related peptide; MEN1, multiple endocrineneoplasia type l; PHI, peptide histidine isoleucine; PYY, peptide YY; TRH, thyrotropin-releasing hormone; VIP, vasoactive intestinal peptide.

Modified from Bonner-Weir S: Anatomy of the islet of Langerhans. In Samols E (ed): The Endocrine Pancreas. New York, Raven Press, 1991, p 16; and Marx M, Newman JB, Guice KS, et al: Clinical significance of gastrointestinal hormones. In Thompson JC, Greeley GH Jr, Rayford PL, Townsend CM Jr (eds): Gastrointestinal Endocrinology. New York, McGraw-Hill, 1987, p 416.

TABLE 35–2.   Efficacy of Localization of Endocrine Tumors of the Pancreas and Duodenum

Modality	True Positives (%)
Noninvasive	
Ultrasonography	23
Octreotide radioimaging (SRS)*	86
CT	43
MRI	26
Invasive	
Endoscopic ultrasonography	82
Selective angiography	56
Portal venous sampling	76
Provocative angiography†	65

*Rarely for melanoma.
†Calcium for insulinoma; secretin for gastrinoma.
CT, computed tomography; MRI, magnetic resonance imaging; SRS, somatostatin receptor scintigraphy.
Modified from Norton JAL: Neuroendocrine tumors of the pancreas and duodenum. Curr Probl Surg 31:97, 1994.

- Five to 10 cases per 1 million population per year; autopsy rate is said to be 1%.
- Criterion of malignancy is simple; if they metastasize, they are malignant.
- Forty percent of patients with neoplasms may have elevated levels of multiple hormones not all of which produce symptoms.
- Nearly all insulinomas, glucagonomas, and VIPomas occur within the pancreas itself.
- Most gastrinomas occur in the duodenum, with the pancreas a close second.
- Somatostatinomas equally divided between the pancreas and the proximal small bowel.
- Patients with von Recklinghausen's disease may have somatostatinomas or gastrinomas in the duodenum.
- Pancreatic endocrine tumors may occur sporadically or in conjunction with the MEN-1 syndrome.
- Because islet cell tumors in MEN-1 patients are always multiple, preoperative recognition of the MEN-1 status is necessary.
- About 25% of patients with gastrinomas, 10% of those with insulinomas, and lesser percentages of those with glucagonomas and VIPomas have the MEN syndrome.
- Of all MEN-1 patients, more than half have gastrinomas and one out of five has an insulinoma.

- Nearly all MEN-1 patients manifest hyperparathyroidism.
- Any patient with a pancreatic endocrine tumor syndrome should have a measurement of calcium level.
- A general principle is that in MEN-1 patients with islet tumors, hyperparathyroidism should be surgically managed first, by removing all four glands with immediate autograft.

Insulinoma

- Insulinoma is the most common functioning tumor of the pancreas.
- Symptoms of hypoglycemia (symptoms of catecholamine release), mental confusion and obtundation, or both.

Clinical Features and Diagnosis

- The diagnostic hallmark—Whipple triad—symptoms stimulatory fasting.
  - Hypoglycemia (catecholamine release).
  - Low blood glucose level (40 to 50 mg/dL).
  - Relief of symptoms after intravenous administration of glucose.
- The best way to induce hypoglycemia is with fasting; two thirds of patients will experience hypoglycemic symptoms in 24 hours, and nearly all other patients experience symptoms by 72 hours of fasting.
- Self-administration of insulin can be detected because there is no C-peptide or proinsulin.

Localization

- Insulinomas are small (usually <1.5 cm) and usually single (only 10% are multiple and those are usually associated with multiple endocrine neoplasia type 1 [MEN 1] syndrome).
- Usually benign (only 5% to 10% are malignant).
- Somatostatin receptor scintigraphy (SRS) is not highly successful.
- Selective arteriography is 50% to 90% accurate in large series.
- Portovenous sampling in about 75% of cases does provide accurate information on the region of the pancreas from which high levels of insulin are released.
- Intraoperative ultrasound most successful for localization.

Operation

- Treatment for insulinoma is surgical: enucleation.
- The 10% of patients with hyperinsulinism who have the MEN 1 syndrome have multiple islet tumors.

Zollinger-Ellison Syndrome (ZES) (Gastrinoma)

- Second most common islet cell tumor and is the most common symptomatic, malignant endocrine tumor of the pancreas.
- Fifty percent arise in the duodenum.
- Only ovarian cancers can process progastrin to gastrin to bring about ZES.

Clinical Features and Diagnosis

- In 75% of patients with ZES, the gastrinoma is sporadic.
- Twenty-five percent have MEN 1 syndrome.

Box 35–1. Causes of Hypergastrinemia

↑ **STIMULATION OF GASTRIN RELEASE**
Zollinger-Ellison syndrome (gastrinoma)
Antral G cell hyperplasia ± pheochromocytoma
Pyloric obstruction

↓ **INHIBITION OF GASTRIN RELEASE**
Hypochlorhydria or achlorhydria
   Atrophic gastritis
   Pernicious anemia
   Gastric carcinoma
   Vitiligo
   Most important: antisecretory drugs (H_2-receptor
     antagonist and especially proton-pump inhibitors)
Antral exclusion operation
Vagotomy

↓ **CATABOLISM**
Chronic renal failure

UNKNOWN
Rheumatoid arthritis
Small bowel resection (temporary)

Adapted from Townsend CM Jr, Thompson JC: Up-to-date treatment of the patient with hypergastrinemia. Adv Surg 20:161, 1987.

- There is a slight (60%) male predominance.
- The average age of onset is 50 years.
- With MEN 1, onset is usually 10 to 20 years earlier.
- Symptoms caused by peptic acid hypersecretion, with abdominal pain the chief complaint in about 75% of patients.
- Two thirds of patients have diarrhea; 10% to 20% of patients present with diarrhea alone.
- Diarrhea is halted by nasogastric aspiration of gastric secretion, a feature that separates it from all other secretory diarrheas.
- Most patients have peptic ulcers; duodenal are the most common, but jejunal ulceration may be found.
- Most common complications of peptic ulcer are nausea and vomiting in 30%, bleeding in 10%, and perforation in 7%.
- About one third of patients present with signs and symptoms of gastroesophageal reflux disease.
- ZES must be excluded in all patients with intractable peptic ulcer, severe esophagitis, or persistent secretory diarrhea.
- Diagnosis depends on hypergastrinemia in the face of increased secretion of gastric acid; normal of 100 pg/mL.
- Levels of more than 1000 pg/mL are nearly diagnostic of ZES, provided that the patient makes gastric acid.
- Other causes of hypergastrinemia must be ruled out.
- An increase in the gastrin value of more than 200 pg/mL after secretin administration is found in 87% of patients with no false-positive results.
- Clinical clues for patients with ZES are as follows:
  - A virulent peptic ulcer or gastroesophageal reflux disease diathesis.
  - Absence of *Helicobacter pylori* or failure of the peptic ulcer to heal after either anti-*H. pylori* therapy of H_2-blockade.
  - A secretory diarrhea that persists (especially if the diarrhea is halted by nasogastric suction).
  - Signs or symptoms of MEN 1 syndrome (elevated serum calcium, elevated parathormone [PTH], pituitary tumor) (Box 35–1).

Pathology

- At least half originate in the duodenum.
- Sixty percent to 90% are found in the so-called gastrinoma triangle.
- Duodenum is the site of gastrinomas in 45% to 60% of patients.
- Only about one third are malignant.

- Sixty percent to 80% of MEN-1 patients have duodenal gastrinomas.
- Usually metastasize to local nodes (80% have lymph node metastases)
- In general, metastases to the liver occur from large (>3 cm) sporadic pancreatic tumors.
- Lymph node metastases do not appear to be dependent on size or location of the primary tumor (duodenal and pancreatic gastrinomas appear to be equally malignant, with about 50% of the metastases going to lymph nodes).
- The presence or absence of lymph node metastases did not affect survival.
- Most promising localizing method is SRS, which involves radionuclide scanning after inject of radiolabeled octreotide.
- Greater than 90% of gastrinomas have receptors for somatostatin.
- SRS should be the first imaging method used for gastrinoma localization in ZES patients.
- Detection depends on size.
- Direct endoscopy and endoscopic ultrasonography are the most effective preoperative studies for detection of duodenal gastrinomas (Table 35–3).

Operations

- Pharmacologic control of acid secretion has rendered total gastrectomy unnecessary.
- We now operate only for tumor removal.
- Although gastrinomas have a high rate of malignancy, they are more apt to be cured than is cancer of any other abdominal viscus.
- Intraoperative ultrasonography of the pancreas is required.
- Intraoperative endoscopy with transillumination of the duodenal wall facilitates visualization of many duodenal tumors.
- Duodenotomy is essential; much more common proximally than distally (70% are in the first portion, 20% in the second, 10% in the third, and none in the fourth).
- If all apparent tumor is removed, immediate cure rates now approach 90%.
- Nearly half of the patients show symptomatic or biochemical recurrence by 5 years.
- No consensus has yet been achieved in the treatment of patients with ZES and MEN 1.

TABLE 35–3. Comparison of Clinical and Laboratory Characteristics of Patients with a Benign or Malignant Clinical Course with Gastrinoma

Characteristics*	Clinical Course (% all patients)	
	Benign† (n = 140)	Malignant† (n = 45)
Percentage of patients	76	24
Present with liver metastases	0	19
Develop liver metastases	0	5
Gender	Predominantly male (68)	Predominantly female (67)
MEN 1 at initial evaluation	21	Uncommon (6)
Time from onset to diagnosis	Long (mean 5.9 yr)	Short (mean 2.7 yr)
Serum gastrin level‡	Moderately elevated (mean, 1711 pg/mL)	Very elevated (mean, 5157 pg/mL)
Size of primary tumor	Small (≤1 cm)	Large (>3 cm)
Location of primary tumor	Primarily duodenum (66)	Primarily pancreatic (92)
Survival at 10 yr	Excellent (96)	Poor (30)
Flow cytometry of tumor	Low S phase (mean 3.3)	High S phase (mean 5.1)
	High percentage of nontetraploid aneuploid (32)	Low percentage of nontetraploid aneuploid
	Multiple stem line aneuploid rare	Multiple stem line aneuploid frequent (25)

*All characteristics were significantly different (P < 0.0001) between the two groups.
†The benign or nonaggressive course was not associated with the development of liver metastases (n = 140), whereas patients in whom the gastrinoma pursued a malignant or aggressive course had liver metastases either at the initial evaluation (n = 36) or developed liver metastases (n = 9) during follow-up.
‡Normal serum gastrin level <100 pg/mL.
MEN 1, multiple endocrine neoplasia type 1.
From Jensen RT: Gastrin-producing tumors. Cancer Treat Res 89:304, 1997.

- All ZES and MEN 1 patients should undergo parathyroidectomy.
- In the absence of widespread disease, laparotomy is indicated to delay progress of these islet cell tumors.

Verner-Morrison Syndrome (VIPoma)

- VIPomas are endocrine tumors usually arising from pancreatic islets that secrete VIP.
- Syndrome of profound watery diarrhea, hypokalemia, and achlorhydria.
- Secretory diarrhea persists despite fasting and despite nasogastric aspiration (which differentiates it from ZES).
- Constant features are as follows:
  - Diarrhea.
  - Hypovolemia.
  - Hypokalemia.
  - Acidosis.
- Variable features are as follows:
  - Achlorhydria or hypochlorhydria.
  - Hypercalcemia.
  - Hyperglycemia.
  - Flushing with rash.
- The diagnostic triad in Verner-Morrison syndrome is as follows:
  - Secretory diarrhea.
  - High levels of circulating VIP.
  - Pancreatic tumor.
- Diagnosis of VIPoma is unlikely if stool volume is less than 700 mL/day.
- Differential diagnosis is as follows:
  - Laxative abuse.
  - Bacterial and parasitic diarrhea.
  - The carcinoid syndrome.
  - ZES.
- Normal VIP levels are greater than 200 pg/mL, and VIPoma patients have levels ranging from 225 to 2000 pg/mL.
- Localization is often achieved with enhanced computed tomography (CT), magnetic resonance imaging (MRI), or arteriography.
- About 50% of patients have metastatic spread by the time of diagnosis.
- Ten percent of the tumors are intrathoracic.
- Treatment with octreotide should be used to control fluid loss.

- Surgical removal of VIPoma should be attempted in all VIPoma patients.
- Most VIPomas can be excised by pancreatectomy.
- Adrenals and retroperitoneal tissues should be carefully examined if no pancreatic tumor is found.
- Local excision of as much tumor as can be safely removed (debulking) is indicated.

Glucagonoma

- A tumor of islet alpha cells.
- Characteristic skin rash (a necrolytic migrating erythema), diabetes mellitus, anemia, weight loss, and elevated circulating levels of glucagon.
- The syndrome is rare.
- Associated with a low level of amino acids; diagnosis made from the characteristic skin lesion, elevated levels of glucagon, and pancreatic tumor.
- Parenteral administration of amino acids brings about the disappearance of the skin lesions.
- Upper limit of normal for glucagon is 150 to 190 pg/mL; glucagonoma patients have levels of 200 to 2000 pg/mL.
- Islet tumor may be demonstrated by enhanced CT or MRI or by selective angiography.
- Patient should be prepared by administration of total parenteral nutrition containing amino acids, with simultaneous octreotide for symptomatic relief.
- One third of patients have been reported to have thrombotic complications after surgery; perioperative heparin is indicated.
- Treatment is surgical excision of the tumor with aggressive approach to remove the primary and metastatic tumor.
- Cure rate appears to be only 30%.

Somatostatinoma

- Somatostatinoma: fewer than 60 cases have been reported.
- Diagnosis: steatorrhea, diabetes mellitus, hypochlorhydria, and gallstones.
- Features of the syndrome are variable and do not always coincide with predictable effects of high circulating levels of somatostatin.
- Ten percent have symptoms of hypoglycemia.
- Clinical presentation is unpredictable.
- Some duodenal somatostatinomas have been associated with von Recklinghausen's neurofibromatosis.

- Tumors can be localized by CT, MRI, arteriography, and even SRS because somatostatinomas possess functioning somatostatin receptors.
- Treatment is surgical.
  - Seventy percent to 90% of tumors are malignant.
  - Tumors most common in the tail of the pancreas.
  - Debulking of metastatic tumor tissue is indicated.
  - Small duodenal tumors can be treated by local excision.
  - Cholecystectomy should be performed.

Still Rarer Tumors

- GRFomas are associated with the MEN 1 syndrome.
  - Thirty percent of GRF tumors originate in the pancreas, 50% in the lung, and 10% in the small bowel.
  - Forty percent of GRFoma patients have ZES.
  - Forty percent have Cushing's syndrome.
  - ACTH-secreting tumors have other endocrine syndromes, most frequently ZES.
  - Classic symptoms of Cushing's syndrome.
- Neurotensinoma cause the following:
  - Hypokalemia.
  - Weight loss.
  - Hypotension.
  - Cyanosis.
  - Flushing.
  - Diabetes.
- Usually malignant.
- PPomas are associated with high circulating PP levels and no characteristic symptoms.

Nonfunctioning Endocrine Tumors

- Surgical resection should be attempted for cure.
- Sixty percent of tumors are metastatic at the time of diagnosis.
- Prolonged survival is possible even with incurable disease (44% at 5 years).

MEDICAL THERAPY FOR ISLET CELL TUMORS

- Best agent for pharmacologic control of hyperinsulinemia is diazoxide.
- Octreotide therapy has also been effective, although its response rate compared with diazoxide is not yet clear.

- Streptozocin combined with fluorouracil has proved effective in treatment of advanced islet cell carcinoma.
- ZES patients:
  - Proton pump inhibitors have been particularly effective.
  - Dosage adjusted to achieve a gastric acid secretion of less than 10 mEq/hour for the hour before the next dose.
  - For patients with unresectable metastatic disease, long-term antisecretory therapy with proton-pump inhibitor drugs has proved more effective and more reliable than treatment with H_2-receptor antagonists or with octreotide.
  - Long-term use of octreotide has its greatest success in the long-term treatment of VIPoma symptoms.
  - All islet cell tumors except insulinomas (10%) and GRFomas (30%) have a malignancy rate of greater than 60%.
  - Responses to chemotherapy have been variable.

CHAPTER 36

THE PITUITARY AND ADRENAL GLANDS

PITUITARY GLAND

Anatomy and Embryology

- The pituitary is composed of two parts: an anterior lobe or adenohypophysis and the neurohypophysis, which consists of the posterior lobe, neural stalk, and infundibulum.

Histology

- Cell types of the anterior pituitary are classified by their secretory products: lactotrophs produce prolactin (PRL), somatotrophs produce growth hormone (GH), adrenocorticotrophs produce adrenocorticotropic hormone (ACTH), thyrotrophs produce thyroid-stimulating hormone (TSH), and gonadotrophs produce follicle-stimulating hormone (FSH) and luteinizing hormone (LH).

- The neurohypophysis, or posterior pituitary, includes the posterior lobe, the pituitary stalk, and the median eminence. Antidiuretic hormone (ADH) and oxytocin are synthesized in the supraoptic and paraventricular nuclei of the hypothalamus and are transported through axons from these nuclei to the posterior pituitary where the active hormones are released into the capillary circulation.

Physiology

- Anterior pituitary hormone secretion is controlled by the hypothalamus. Axons from the arcuate and other anterior hypothalamic nuclei terminate in the median eminence next to portal capillaries where they release hormones into the hypothalamic-pituitary portal circulation to inhibit or stimulate cells of the anterior pituitary.

- The anterior pituitary secretes three groups of hormones: (1) proopiomelanocortin (POMC)-derived ACTH and beta-lipotropin (β-LPH); (2) the related hormones GH and PRL;

485

and (3) the glycoprotein hormones LH, FSH, and TSH. ACTH controls glucocorticoid production by the adrenal cortex; GH regulates growth and intermediary metabolism; PRL is necessary for lactation; TSH regulates the thyroid; and LH and FSH together control the gonads in males and females. Target gland hormones, in turn, participate in feedback control of the pituitary and hypothalamus.

- ACTH.
- Opioids.
- PRL and GH family.
  - PRL.
  - GH.
- Glycoprotein hormones.
  - TSH.
  - LH AND FSH.
- Neurohypophyseal hormones.
  - ADH (also known as vasopressin) and oxytocin are the two principal hormones secreted by the posterior pituitary.
  - ADH.
  ADH stimulates sodium and chloride reabsorption by epithelial cells of the medullary thick ascending loop of Henle. In addition, ADH enhances permeability to water within the collecting ducts of the medulla.
  Oxytocin stimulates uterine contraction during labor and elicits milk ejection by myoepithelial cells of the mammary ducts during lactation.

Pituitary Tumors

- Pituitary tumors are the most common intracranial neoplasm and account for 10% to 15% of all intracranial tumors.
- Prolactinomas and GH-producing adenomas are the most frequent pituitary tumor types. ACTH-producing adenomas and gonadotroph adenomas are less common, and TSH-producing adenomas are rare.
- Pathogenesis.
- Clinical presentation.
  - Prolactinomas cause galactorrhea and hypogonadism (e.g., amenorrhea and infertility in women and impotence in men). GH-secreting tumors cause gigantism in children and acromegaly in adults. ACTH-producing tumors produce signs and symptoms of hypercortisolism (Cushing's syndrome). Glycoprotein hormone (LH, FSH, and TSH) producing adenomas cause infertility and sexual dysfunction. Pituitary tumors may also cause deficiency of

one or more hormones or may even result in panhypopituitarism.

- Pituitary tumors may also cause symptoms from local mass effects.
- The classic defect, bitemporal hemianopsia, is variable, and other visual defects occur.

- Diagnostic evaluation.
- Diagnostic imaging and localization.
  - Dynamic high-resolution magnetic resonance imaging (MRI) with intravenous gadolinium contrast is the diagnostic imaging modality of choice for patients with suspected pituitary disease.
  - Inferior petrosal sinus (IPS) sampling and venous sampling of the cavernous sinus assist in the evaluation of patients with acromegaly or Cushing's syndrome by localizing GH- or ACTH-secreting pituitary tumors that are undetectable by MRI or computed tomography (CT).
- General approach to management of pituitary disorders.
  - Medical therapy.

  Medical management of pituitary disease serves two purposes: primary or adjuvant treatment for select functioning tumors, and hormone replacement for hypopituitarism. Three classes of agents are available for the treatment of hormone excess resulting from pituitary tumors: (1) dopamine agonists, (2) somatostatin analogues, and (3) hormone receptor antagonists.

  Primary medical treatment of functioning pituitary tumors is generally limited to dopamine receptor agonists (bromocriptine or cabergoline) for the treatment of prolactinomas.
  - Surgical therapy.

  Surgical resection is the primary therapy for pituitary adenomas other than prolactinoma and for pituitary apoplexy unresponsive to medical therapy. A trans-sphenoidal approach is appropriate for more than 95% of pituitary lesions.

  The results of trans-sphenoidal pituitary surgery reflect the expertise of the surgeon, the size of the tumor, and previous therapy. Trans-sphenoidal resection of microadenomas results in remission rates of 70% to 90%.

  Trans-sphenoidal resection of macroadenomas is curative in only 40% to 50% of cases, although visual field abnormalities are improved in 70% to 80% of patients.

  Complication rates for trans-sphenoidal pituitary surgery are low and current mortality rates are less than 0.5%. Major complications such as cerebrospinal fluid (CSF) rhinorrhea, cranial nerve palsy, and vision loss occur in 1.5% of patients. Panhypopituitarism is observed in approximately

3% of operations performed for microadenoma and in a somewhat higher percentage of operations for macroadenoma. Diabetes insipidus occurs in 5% to 30% of cases and is usually transient.

- Radiation therapy.

Radiation therapy is reserved for patients with incompletely resected tumors, with recurrent symptoms after surgery, and for those who refuse surgery or who are a prohibitive surgical risk.

- Diagnosis and management of specific pituitary tumors.
  - Prolactinoma.

Prolactinomas are the most common functioning pituitary tumors, representing 30% to 50% of all pituitary neoplasms.

  - GH-producing adenoma.
  - Corticotropin-producing adenoma.

Corticotropin-producing pituitary adenomas *(Cushing's disease)* comprise 10% to 15% of functional pituitary adenomas. They cause up to 60% to 75% of cases of Cushing's syndrome and are diagnosed in the microadenoma stage in 90% of cases.

  - Gonadotropin-producing adenoma.
  - Thyrotropin-producing adenoma.
  - Nonfunctioning or incidentally discovered pituitary adenomas.

Other Pituitary Disorders

- Posterior pituitary disorders.
- Hypopituitarism.
  - Hypopituitarism may be either selective (partial hypopituitarism) or complete (panhypopituitarism) and may be caused by untreated pituitary adenomas, pituitary radiation or surgery, or head injury.
- Pituitary apoplexy.
- Sheehan's syndrome.
- Empty sella syndrome.

ADRENAL GLAND

Embryology

- Composed of two endocrine glands: adrenal cortex and medulla have distinct embryologic and functional characteristics.
- Cortex arise from coelomic mesoderm adjacent to the urogenital ridge.
- Aberrant tissue may be found near kidney or pelvis along the migration of structures arising from urogenital ridge.

- Neural crest cells migrate to the para-aortic and paravertebral regions, and along the adrenal vein.
- Error in migration may form organ of Zuckerkandl, located usually left of aortic bifurcation near the origin of the inferior mesenteric artery.

Anatomy

- The adrenal glands are bilateral retroperitoneal organs located on the superior-medial aspect of the upper pole of each kidney.
- The normal adrenal cortex is bright yellow and thicker than the red-brown medulla.
- The adrenal glands derive their blood supply from branches of the inferior phrenic artery superiorly, the aorta medially, and the renal artery inferiorly.
- The right adrenal vein drains to the inferior vena cava through a wide but short central vein. The left adrenal vein empties primarily into the left renal vein but may occasionally drain directly to the vena cava.
- Histologically, the adult adrenal cortex is composed of three zones: an outer zona glomerulosa, a middle zona fasciculata, and an inner zona reticularis.
- The adrenal medulla is smaller than the cortex and contributes approximately 10% of the total gland weight.

Adrenal Steroid Biochemistry and Physiology

- Three major biosynthetic pathways lead to the production of glucocorticoids, mineralocorticoids, and adrenal androgens.
- Adrenocortical hormones are synthesized from cholesterol that is either extracted from plasma or synthesized within the adrenal cortex.
- Glucocorticoids.
  - These metabolites are conjugated to glucuronate and excreted in the urine, where they may be measured as 17-hydroxycorticosteroids.
  - The diverse physiologic actions of glucocorticoids center on intermediary metabolism, immune modulation, and regulation of intravascular volume.
  - Prolonged exposure to high levels of endogenous corticosteroids leads to a catabolic state with negative nitrogen balance, proximal muscle weakness, and insulin-resistant diabetes mellitus.
  - Glucocorticoids possess profound anti-inflammatory and immunosuppressive properties.

- Mineralocorticoids.
  - Aldosterone is the major mineralocorticoid in humans.
  - Aldosterone regulates fluid and electrolyte balance by stimulating sodium retention and potassium and hydrogen ion secretion by the distal convoluted tubule of the kidney.
  - The renin-angiotensin system and plasma potassium are the principal regulators of aldosterone secretion.
  - Aldosterone secretion is exquisitely sensitive to changes in serum potassium levels.
- Adrenal sex steroids.
  - Dehydroepiandrosterone (DHEA) is the major C-19 sex steroid produced by the adrenal cortex.

Diseases of the Adrenal Cortex

Cushing's Syndrome

- Cushing's syndrome is ACTH dependent in 80% of cases and ACTH independent in 20% of cases. Causes of ACTH-dependent Cushing's syndrome include ACTH-producing pituitary tumors (Cushing's disease) and ectopic ACTH-producing tumors (most commonly bronchial carcinoids and small cell lung cancer). ACTH-dependent Cushing's syndrome is always associated with bilateral adrenal hyperplasia.
- Signs and symptoms.
  - The presence of central obesity with prominent supra-clavicular fat pads, plethora, wide purple striae on the abdomen and extremities, proximal muscle weakness, and inappropriate osteopenia are relatively specific for Cushing's syndrome and should prompt a workup for hypercortisolism.
- Biochemical evaluation of Cushing's syndrome.
  - The diagnostic evaluation of the patient with suspected Cushing's syndrome should proceed in a stepwise fashion to first determine whether or not the patient has hyper-cortisolism.
  - The next step is to determine whether it is due to ACTH-dependent or ACTH-independent causes. Finally, the source of the Cushing's syndrome should be identified by imaging.
  - The sine qua non of this disorder is the presence of hyper-cortisolism that is insensitive to suppression by adminis-tration of exogenous glucocorticoid.
- Establishing the presence of Cushing's syndrome.

- 24-hour urinary free cortisol. The most useful test in the initial diagnostic evaluation of the patient with suspected Cushing's syndrome is determination of 24-hour urinary free cortisol.
- Overnight low-dose dexamethasone suppression test.
- Late-night salivary cortisol.
- Corticotropin-releasing hormone (CRH)/dexamethasone suppression test.
- Differentiation of ACTH-dependent from ACTH-independent Cushing's syndrome.
  - Plasma ACTH level. Measurement of plasma ACTH levels, which is done using a two-site immunometric assay, is the best test to distinguish ACTH-dependent (pituitary or ectopic ACTH) from ACTH-independent (primary adrenal) causes of Cushing's syndrome.
  - Suppression of plasma ACTH to below 5 pg/mL is characteristic of adrenocortical neoplasms.
  - High-dose dexamethasone suppression test.
  - CRH test.
- Localization of the source of Cushing's syndrome.
- Treatment of Cushing's syndrome.
  - Effective treatment of Cushing's syndrome entails removing the cause of cortisol excess, either a primary adrenal lesion or ectopic and pituitary lesions secreting excessive ACTH.
  - Cushing's disease.
  - Ectopic ACTH syndrome.
- Primary adrenal Cushing's.
  - Adrenal adenoma. Ten percent to 25% of patients with endogenous Cushing's syndrome have a primary adrenal cause.
  - All patients who undergo adrenalectomy for primary adrenal causes of Cushing's syndrome require perioperative and postoperative glucocorticoid replacement, because the contralateral gland is suppressed.
  - Primary adrenal hyperplasia.
  - Adrenocortical carcinoma.
- Subclinical Cushing's syndrome.
- Cushing's syndrome in children.

Primary Hyperaldosteronism

- High levels of circulating plasma aldosterone cause hypokalemia and hypertension.

- The most common cause of primary aldosteronism is an aldosterone-producing adrenal adenoma, which accounts for two thirds of cases.
- Signs and symptoms.
- Patients with primary aldosteronism have moderate to severe diastolic hypertension that is often resistant to medical treatment. Hypokalemia occurs spontaneously in 80% to 90% of patients with this disorder and can usually be induced in those who have a normal potassium by oral sodium loading.
- Diagnosis.
  - Primary aldosteronism should be sought in any hypertensive patient with hypokalemia.
  - Other individuals who should be evaluated for hyperaldosteronism include those with severe hypertension, hypertension refractory to medical therapy, and young age of onset of hypertension.
  - The goals of diagnostic evaluation of the patient with suspected primary aldosteronism are (1) to establish the presence of hyperaldosteronism biochemically and (2) to distinguish surgically correctable aldosterone-producing adrenal adenoma (aldosteronoma) from medically treatable idiopathic cortical hyperplasia.
  - The biochemical diagnosis of primary aldosteronism requires demonstration of elevated aldosterone levels with suppressed plasma renin activity. The initial screening evaluation, therefore, consists of measurement of upright plasma aldosterone concentration (PAC) and plasma renin activity (PRA). A PAC/PRA ratio of greater than 20 to 30 in the setting of a plasma aldosterone level of greater than 15 ng/dL is suggestive of the diagnosis and merits further evaluation to confirm the presence of inappropriate aldosterone secretion. Patients should be off spironolactone for 6 weeks as well as off angiotensin-converting enzyme (ACE) inhibitors before testing.
  - The preferred imaging modality for suspected aldosteronoma is CT because the sensitivity of CT for detecting adrenal lesions greater than 0.5 to 1.0 cm in size is greater than 90%.
  - The presence of a unilateral adenoma 1 cm or larger on CT with a normal contralateral adrenal is strong evidence for the presence of a unilateral aldosteronoma.
  - If the CT shows bilateral adrenal nodularity, a unilateral adrenal lesion less than 1 cm, unilateral adrenal thickening, or bilateral normal adrenals, additional testing is indicated to determine whether a unilateral source for increased aldosterone production is present.

- Sampling of the adrenal veins for aldosterone and cortisol is the preferred method for differentiating unilateral aldosteronoma from idiopathic hyperaldosteronism in cases in which the radiographic imaging is unclear.

Management of Primary Aldosteronism

- Adrenal adenoma. Adrenalectomy for an aldosterone-secreting adenoma results in resolution of hypokalemia in virtually 100% of cases and substantial improvement of hypertension in more than 90%. However, long-term cure of hypertension occurs in only 60% to 70%.
- These tumors are usually small (1 to 2 cm); therefore, laparoscopic adrenalectomy is the preferred approach.
- Bilateral adrenalectomy for adenomas is not recommended because the resulting adrenal insufficiency may be more difficult to manage than the hypertension.
- Idiopathic adrenal hyperplasia and glucocorticoid-remediable aldosteronism.
- Adrenal neoplasms associated with excess sex steroids.
  - Virilizing adrenal tumors. Benign and malignant adrenal cortical tumors may cause virilization by production of excess adrenal androgens, in particular the androgen precursor DHEA.
  - Feminizing adrenal tumors.

Adrenogenital Syndromes

- Congenital adrenal hyperplasia.
- 21-Hydroxylase deficiency.

Adrenocortical Carcinoma

- Background.
  - Most patients (75%) present with Stage III or IV disease (Table 36–1). Syndromes of adrenal hormone overproduction occur in 36% to 60% of adult patients and may include hypercortisolism, hyperaldosteronism, or virilization.
- Diagnosis.
- Management.
  - Complete surgical resection of locally confined tumor is the only chance for cure of adrenocortical carcinoma.
  - Mitotane, or ortho, para DDD is an adrenal cytotoxic agent with limited effectiveness in some patients with adrenocortical carcinoma.

TABLE 36–1. Staging of Adrenocortical Carcinoma

Stage	TNM	Criteria	Percentage of Cases (%)
I	T_1, N_0, M_0	<5 cm; confined to adrenal	2
II	T_2, N_0, M_0	>5 cm; confined to adrenal	19
III	T_3, N_0, M_0 $T_1/T_2, N_1, M_0$	Local invasion or positive nodes	18
IV	$T_3/T_4, N_1, M_0$ Any T/N; M_1	Local invasion and positive nodes or metastases	61

TNM, tumor-node-metastasis classification; subscript numbers represent the level of malignant involvement.
Modified from Pommier RF, Brennan MF: Management of adrenal neoplasms. Curr Probl Surg 28:684, 1991.

Adrenal Insufficiency

- Signs and symptoms.
  - Acute adrenal insufficiency is a medical emergency and should be suspected in stressed patients with a history of adrenal surgery, adrenal insufficiency, or exogenous steroid use.
- Diagnosis.
  - Hyponatremia, hyperkalemia, azotemia, and fasting or reactive hypoglycemia.
  - The rapid ACTH stimulation test is the best test for detection of adrenal insufficiency.
- Management.
  - Intravenous volume replacement with normal or hypertonic saline and dextrose is essential, as is immediate intravenous steroid replacement therapy with 4-mg dexamethasone.
  - Patients who have known adrenal insufficiency or have received supraphysiologic doses of corticosteroid for more than 1 week in the year preceding surgery should receive perioperative stress-dose corticosteroids.

Physiology of the Adrenal Medulla

- Adrenal medullary or chromaffin cells store and secrete several biologically active amines, including dopamine, norepinephrine, and epinephrine.
- Phenylethanolamine-N-methyl transferase (PNMT) is localized exclusively in cells of the adrenal medulla and the organ of Zuckerkandl. Thus, with rare exceptions, epinephrine-secreting tumors arise only in these two sites.

- The physiologic responses to catecholamines are mediated by alpha- and beta-adrenergic receptors on peripheral tissues.

DISEASES OF THE ADRENAL MEDULLA

Pheochromocytoma

- Pheochromocytomas are catecholamine-secreting adrenal tumors that arise from chromaffin cells of the adrenal medulla.
- These tumors may occur in a sporadic or familial manner and are found with increased frequency in screened hypertensive populations.
- The *rule of tens* is a commonly cited description of pheochromocytomas: tumors are bilateral in 10%, extra-adrenal in 10%, familial in 10%, malignant in 10%, and occur in children in 10% of cases.
- The organ of Zuckerkandl is the most common extra-adrenal site of pheochromocytoma.
- Signs and symptoms.
  - Pheochromocytomas present with signs and symptoms of catecholamine excess.
- Diagnosis.
  - Demonstration of increased plasma or urinary levels of catecholamines and their metabolites is the sine qua non for the diagnosis of pheochromocytoma.
  - The measurement of plasma fractionated metanephrines (metanephrine and normetanephrine) has become available as a screening test for the detection of pheochromocytomas.
  - CT and MRI are the two radiologic modalities of choice to localize pheochromocytomas.
- Management of pheochromocytomas.
  - Preoperative management of patients with pheochromocytoma centers on (1) control of hypertension, (2) alpha blockade to prevent intraoperative hypertensive crisis resulting from tumor manipulation and release of catecholamines, and (3) fluid resuscitation to prevent circulatory collapse after removal of the catecholamine-secreting tumor. Alpha-adrenergic blockade is achieved with phenoxybenzamine, starting at a dose of 10 mg twice daily.
  - Beta-adrenergic blockade is indicated in patients who develop tachycardia with alpha blockade or who have tachyarrhythmias or predominately epinephrine-secreting tumors. Beta-blockers may enhance pressor response to endogenous norepinephrine and thus should not be given until adequate alpha blockade has been established.

- Today, CT, MRI, and radionuclide scans permit preoperative localization of tumor in 95% or more of cases, so that the surgical approach may be more directed. In most cases, pheochromocytomas are appropriate for excision using a laparoscopic approach.

Special Issues in Pheochromocytoma

- Hereditary pheochromocytomas.
  - Pheochromocytomas may occur as a component of a variety of inherited endocrine tumor syndromes, including multiple endocrine neoplasia (MEN) type 2, von Hippel-Lindau (VHL) disease, and neurofibromatosis type 1 (NF-1).
  - MEN 2.
  - VHL disease.
  - Neuroectodermal dysplasias.
- Malignant pheochromocytoma.
- Extra-adrenal pheochromocytoma.
  - Extra-adrenal pheochromocytomas, also known as *functional paragangliomas,* can occur at any site in the abdomen where chromaffin tissue is located and have been found in the paravertebral ganglia, the organ of Zuckerkandl, and the urinary bladder.
- Pheochromocytoma in pregnancy.
- Pheochromocytoma in childhood.

Incidental Adrenal Mass

- The prevalence of unsuspected adrenal masses detected in CT scan series has ranged from 1% to 5%.
- Proper evaluation of the patient with an adrenal incidentaloma requires an understanding of the differential diagnosis of adrenal masses, the biochemical profile of hyperfunctioning adrenal tumors, and risk factors for adrenal malignancy. Adrenalectomy is reserved for patients with hyperfunctioning tumors and for potentially malignant lesions.
- The diagnostic evaluation should consist of both a determination of the functional status of the adrenal lesion and an assessment of its malignant potential.
- Nonfunctioning cortical adenomas.
- Nonfunctioning adrenocortical adenomas account for most incidentally discovered adrenal masses in patients with no prior history **of cancer.**
- Adrenocortical carcinoma.
- Adrenocortical carcinomas are rare tumors that are large (>6 cm) and typically exhibit radiographic features suggestive

of malignancy, such as irregular borders, regional lymphadenopathy, or local invasiveness.

- More than 90% of reported adrenocortical carcinomas are greater than 6 cm in diameter and the likelihood that an incidentaloma represents a primary adrenal carcinoma increases with increasing size of the lesion.
- Biochemical evaluation.
  - Biochemical screening for pheochromocytoma in the setting of an adrenal incidentaloma should consist of measurement of plasma fractionated metanephrines or a 24-hour urine collection for catecholamines and metanephrines. Screening for hypercortisolism consists of an overnight, single dose (1 to 3 mg) dexamethasone test.
  - Screening for hyperaldosteronism should consist of measurement of plasma aldosterone concentration and plasma renin activity.
- Biopsy.
  - Fine-needle aspiration (FNA) biopsy is rarely indicated for the evaluation of the patient with an adrenal mass.
- Management.
  - The presence of a hormonally active tumor is an indication for adrenalectomy. In patients with nonfunctional adrenal masses, adrenalectomy should be performed if the tumor is more than 6 cm in diameter or if the imaging features on CT and/or MRI are atypical for an adenoma.

Technique of Adrenalectomy

- A number of different surgical approaches are available for the removal of the adrenal glands.
- The choice of approach in an individual patient depends on the suspected pathology, size of the adrenal lesion, and surgeon experience. Tumors under 6 cm that are likely benign are usually resected using a laparoscopic approach. Large adrenal masses (>10 cm) and suspected primary adrenal malignancies larger than 6 cm should generally be resected using an anterior approach to adequately explore the entire abdomen and to ensure resection with negative margins.

CHAPTER 37

THE MULTIPLE ENDOCRINE NEOPLASIA SYNDROMES

INTRODUCTION

- The familial multiple endocrine neoplasia (MEN) syndromes result from genetic changes in both a tumor suppressor gene and a proto-oncogene. These hereditary cancer syndromes are characterized by the predisposition to neoplastic transformation in multiple target endocrine tissues and pathologic involvement of nonendocrine tissues. The associated endocrine tumors may be benign or malignant and may develop either synchronously or metachronously. Within an affected endocrine target tissue, a diffuse preneoplastic hyperplasia typically precedes the development of microscopic invasion or grossly evident multifocal carcinoma. Importantly, the recent discovery of the specific genetic basis for the MEN types 1 and 2 syndromes has allowed the development of strategies for direct genetic testing and early surgical intervention. Early thyroidectomy is indicated for patients with a genetic diagnosis of MEN 2, with the aim of preventing the subsequent development of regional or distant medullary thyroid carcinoma (MTC) metastases. The optimal early surgical intervention to prevent metastatic spread of the potentially malignant neuroendocrine tumors (NETs) in patients with a genetic diagnosis of MEN 1 is currently more controversial.
- The MEN syndromes are characterized by differing patterns of involvement. In its full expression, MEN 1 is characterized by the concurrence of parathyroid hyperplasia, NETs of the pancreas and duodenum, and adenomas of the anterior pituitary gland. MEN 2A is characterized by the concurrence of MTC, pheochromocytomas, and parathyroid hyperplasia, whereas MEN 2B consists of MTC, pheochromocytomas, mucosal neuromas, and a distinctive *marfanoid habitus.*

MULTIPLE ENDOCRINE NEOPLASIA TYPE 1

Genetic Studies and Pathogenesis

- The *MEN1* disease gene was ultimately identified by positional cloning in 1997. Frequent chromosome deletions involving the *MEN1* locus, termed loss of heterozygosity (LOH), are observed in the DNA from tumor tissue derived from patients with MEN 1 and from mice with an engineered deletion of their *Men1* alleles. This pattern of allelic deletion is consistent with a two-mutational model of oncogenesis, in which *two hits* are required to inactivate both copies of a tumor suppressor gene.
- The *MEN1* gene encodes a 610 amino acid protein product termed menin.
- The menin mRNA transcript is ubiquitously expressed in both endocrine and nonendocrine tissues.
- The menin protein sequence is highly conserved among human, mouse (98%), and rat (97%). However, database analysis of menin protein sequence reveals no significant homology to other known protein families.
- The combination of findings from all current studies has not yielded a clear picture of the mechanisms of menin's tumor suppressor activity or the specific role for menin in endocrine tumorigenesis.
- The combination of findings from all current studies has not yielded a clear picture of the mechanisms of menin's tumor suppressor activity or the specific role for menin in endocrine tumorigenesis.
- Genetic testing is currently available in selected centers with certain limitations.

Clinical Features and Management

- The MEN 1 syndrome is characterized by parathyroid hyperplasia, NETs of the pancreas and duodenum, and adenomas of the anterior pituitary. In addition, bronchial and thymic carcinoids, thyroid nodules, adrenocortical nodular hyperplasia, lipomas, ependymomas, and cutaneous angiofibromas occur with increased frequency in patients with MEN 1.
- The clinical expression of MEN 1 most often develops in the third or fourth decade, with the onset of signs or symptoms being rare before age 10 years. Males and females are affected equally, as predicted by the autosomal dominant inheritance pattern.

- The MEN 1 trait is transmitted with essentially 100% penetrance but with variable expressivity, such that each affected person may exhibit some but not necessarily all of the components of the syndrome. The most common abnormality in MEN 1 is parathyroid hyperplasia, which eventually develops in 90% to 97% of affected individuals. Duodenopancreatic NETs (which carry a malignant potential) and pituitary adenomas occur with variable frequency. The clinical manifestation of NETs of the duodenum and pancreas occurs in approximately 30% to 80% of patients, whereas pituitary tumors become clinically evident in 15% to 50% of affected patients.
- The clinical manifestations of patients with MEN 1 depend on the endocrine tissue involved, the overproduction of a specific hormone, or the local mass effect and malignant progression of the neoplasm.

Parathyroid Glands

- The most common endocrine abnormality in MEN 1 is hyperparathyroidism, occurring in more than 95% of patients.
- Hypercalcemia is usually the first biochemical abnormality detected in patients with MEN 1 and may precede the clinical onset of a pancreatic NET or pituitary neoplasm by several years.
- In general, hyperparathyroidism in patients with MEN 1 has an earlier age of onset and usually causes a milder hypercalcemia than that observed in primary sporadic hyperparathyroidism. The diagnosis is made by measuring serum calcium and parathyroid hormone levels.
- The aim of surgical treatment for hyperparathyroidism in patients with MEN 1 is to achieve the lowest incidence of recurrent hypercalcemia, while minimizing the complication of permanent hypoparathyroidism. Because patients with MEN 1 develop multiglandular disease, there is a significantly higher rate of recurrent or persistent hyperparathyroidism after parathyroidectomy when compared with the results for the treatment of sporadic parathyroid adenoma. The appropriate surgical procedure for patients with MEN 1 is either three-and-one-half gland parathyroidectomy leaving the parathyroid tissue remnant *in situ* in the neck or total four-gland parathyroidectomy with intramuscular autotransplantation of parathyroid tissue into the forearm muscle.
- A transcervical, partial thymectomy should also be performed because of the possibility of an ectopic or supernumerary parathyroid gland within the cranial horns of the

thymus. In general, preoperative imaging tests are not necessary for patients with MEN 1 undergoing initial neck exploration, because appropriate treatment requires bilateral neck exploration and identification of all four glands. Noninvasive imaging tests, such as sestamibi scanning and ultrasound, may be useful for parathyroid localization before reoperative surgery.

Pancreas and Duodenum

- The second most frequent component of MEN 1 is the development of NETs of the duodenum or pancreas. Depending on the method of study, 30% to 80% of patients with MEN 1 develop these tumors.
- The pancreaticoduodenal tumors in patients with MEN 1 cause symptoms either because of hormone oversecretion or the mass effects from tumor growth itself and are characterized by a high malignant potential. Pancreatic NETs that are nonfunctioning or that secrete pancreatic polypeptide are probably the most frequent NETs that occur in patients with MEN 1.
- The most common *functional* NET in patients with MEN 1 is gastrinoma. The presenting signs and symptoms in patients with hypergastrinemia or the Zollinger-Ellison Syndrome (ZES) may include epigastric pain, reflux esophagitis, secretory diarrhea, and weight loss.
- Gastrinoma is diagnosed by the documentation of gastric acid hypersecretion (>15 mEq/L in patients without operation or >5 mEq/L in patients with prior ulcer surgery), associated with elevated fasting levels of serum gastrin (>100 pg/mL.).
- Gastrinomas that develop in patients with MEN 1 are usually malignant, as indicated by the presence of regional lymph node or distant metastases. Gastrinomas were previously thought to be located predominately in the head of the pancreas within the *gastrinoma triangle*. More recent data suggest that gastrinomas in patients with MEN 1 occur most frequently within the wall of the duodenum. Because of the small size of these neoplasms, the primary gastrinoma may not be localized preoperatively by computed tomography (CT) scanning or angiography. Endoscopic ultrasound, although dependent on the operator's experience, has been used successfully to localize gastrinomas within the wall of the duodenum or head of the pancreas.
- The value of surgical resection for intended cure of gastrinoma in patients with MEN 1 is controversial. Although most evidence indicates that patients with ZES and MEN 1 are rarely cured by operation, localized resection of a potentially

malignant NET may be indicated in an attempt to control the tumoral process and prevent subsequent malignant dissemination. The recognition that primary gastrinomas occur frequently in the duodenal wall, combined with efforts to perform an extensive regional lymphadenectomy or even pancreaticoduodenectomy, may improve the success rate of surgery for ZES in the setting of MEN 1.

- The second most common clinically evident pancreatic neuroendocrine neoplasm in patients with MEN 1 is insulinoma. These are usually small (<2 cm) and occur with even distribution throughout the pancreas. Patients typically present with recurrent symptoms of neuroglycopenia: sweating, dizziness, confusion, or syncope. The diagnosis of insulinoma is made by documenting symptomatic hypoglycemia in association with inappropriately elevated plasma levels of insulin and C-peptide during a supervised 72-hour fast. Factitious hypoglycemia, the purposeful administration of insulin or hypoglycemic drugs, must be excluded. Insulinomas may be occult and are infrequently localized by conventional preoperative imaging studies such as CT scanning, ultrasound, magnetic resonance imaging (MRI), or angiography.

- There is no ideal medical therapy for insulinoma; therefore, the preferred treatment is accurate localization and surgical resection of the functioning tumor to correct life-threatening hyperinsulinemia.

- The operative approach includes complete mobilization of the pancreas and careful examination of the gland by inspection and palpation. Intraoperative ultrasound greatly facilitates the identification of small tumors, especially within the pancreatic head or uncinate process. Small, benign insulinomas are amenable to enucleation. Partial pancreatectomy may be required for multiple or potentially malignant tumors. In the event that the insulinoma is not identified despite an exhaustive intraoperative search, blind subtotal pancreatectomy is not recommended.

- Other functional NETs of the pancreas, such as glucagonoma, somatostatinoma, and tumors secreting vasoactive intestinal peptide or pancreatic polypeptide, occur rarely in association with MEN 1.

Pituitary Gland

- Pituitary neoplasms occur in 15% to 50% of patients. Most of these tumors are prolactin-secreting adenomas. Pituitary tumors cause symptoms either by hypersecretion of hormones or compression of adjacent structures. Large adenomas may cause visual field defects by pressure on the optic chiasm or manifestations of hypopituitarism through compression of the adjacent normal gland.

- Pituitary tumors, either functioning or nonfunctioning, may require surgical ablation or irradiation. Bromocriptine (Parlodel), a dopamine agonist and an inhibitor of prolactin secretion, and cabergoline (Dostinex) have been used to treat prolactinomas medically.

Other Tumors

- Bronchial and thymic carcinoids, benign thyroid tumors, benign and malignant adrenocortical tumors, lipomas, ependymomas of the central nervous system (CNS), and facial cutaneous angiofibromas and collagenomas occur with increased frequency in patients with MEN 1.

THE MULTIPLE ENDOCRINE NEOPLASIA TYPE 2 SYNDROMES

Epidemiology and Clinical Features

- The MEN type 2 syndromes include MEN 2A, MEN 2B, and familial, non-MEN medullary thyroid carcinoma (FMTC). These autosomal dominant inherited syndromes are caused by germline mutations in the *RET* gene, on chromosome 10. The hallmark of these syndromes is MTC, which is multifocal, bilateral, and occurs at a young age. In patients affected by MEN 2A, MEN 2B, or FMTC, there is complete penetrance of MTC; all persons who inherit the disease allele develop MTC. Other features of the syndromes are variably expressed, with incomplete penetrance. These features are summarized in Table 37–1.
- In MEN 2A, patients develop multifocal, bilateral MTC, associated with C-cell hyperplasia. Approximately 42% of affected patients develop pheochromocytomas, which may also be multifocal and bilateral, and are associated with adrenal medullary hyperplasia. Hyperparathyroidism develops in 10% to 35% of patients and is due to hyperplasia, which may be asymmetric, with one or more glands becoming enlarged.
- In MEN 2B, as in MEN 2A, all patients who inherit the disease develop MTC. All MEN 2B individuals have mucosal neuromas, and 40% to 50% of patients develop pheochromocytomas. These patients often have a distinct physical appearance with a prominent mid-upper lip, everted eyebrows, multiple tongue nodules, and "marfanoid" body

habitus, with a relatively small torso and long limbs. MEN 2B patients do not develop hyperparathyroidism. MTC in MEN 2B patients presents at a very young age—in infancy—and appears to be the most aggressive form of hereditary MTC, although its aggressiveness may be more related to the extremely early age of onset rather than to the biologic virulence of the tumor.

- FMTC is characterized by the occurrence of MTC without any other endocrinopathies. MTC in these patients has a later age of onset and a more indolent clinical course than MTC in patients with MEN 2A and MEN 2B.

Medullary Thyroid Carcinoma

- MTC originates from the parafollicular cells, or C-cells, of the thyroid.
- In the MEN 2 syndromes, MTC is associated with C-cell hyperplasia,
- Basal and stimulated serum calcitonin levels correlate with tumor burden and are always elevated in patients with palpable thyroid tumors. MTCs may also secrete other hormones, including carcinoembryonic antigen (CEA). Secretory diarrhea and flushing, most often attributed to elevated calcitonin, are the main paraneoplastic manifestations of advanced MTC.
- Early diagnosis in hereditary MTC is critical, because metastases occur in the early stages of disease. Lymph node metastases are rarely present in patients in whom genetic testing established the diagnosis of MEN 2A or FMTC in childhood, when thyroidectomy is performed before the occurrence of a thyroid mass or elevation of calcitonin level.
- MTC spreads within the central compartment to perithyroidal and paratracheal lymph nodes (level VI nodes).
- Within this compartment, spread is commonly bilateral. Upper mediastinal nodes (level VII nodes) are also frequently involved. Further lymphatic spread can also occur to the lateral neck compartment, including jugular (levels II, III, and IV nodes), posterior triangle (level V nodes), and supraclavicular nodes.
- We found that the incidence of central (levels VI and VII) node involvement was extremely high (80%), regardless of the size of the primary tumor. There was also frequent involvement of ipsilateral (75%) and contralateral (47%) level II, III ,and IV nodes (Table 37–2).
- MTC may involve adjacent structures by direct invasion or compression. Structures most commonly affected include the trachea, recurrent laryngeal nerve, jugular veins, and

TABLE 37–1. Clinical Features of Sporadic MTC, MEN 2A, MEN 2B, and FMTC

Clinical Setting	Features of MTC	Inheritance Pattern	Associated Abnormalities	Genetic Defect
Sporadic MTC	Unifocal	None	None	Somatic *RET* mutations in >20% of tumors
MEN 2A	Multifocal, bilateral	Autosomal dominant	Pheochromocytomas, hyperparathyroidism	Germline missense mutations in extracellular cysteine codons of *RET*
MEN 2B	Multifocal, bilateral	Autosomal dominant	Pheochromocytomas, mucosal neuromas, megacolon, skeletal abnormalities	Germline missense mutation in tyrosine kinase domain of *RET*
FMTC	Multifocal, bilateral	Autosomal dominant	None	Germline missense mutations in extracellular or intracellular cysteine codons of *RET*

FMTC, familial medullary thyroid carcinoma; MEN, multiple endocrine neoplasia; MTC, medullary thyroid carcinoma.
Reproduced with permission from Moley JF, Lairmore TC, Phay JE: Hereditary endocrinopathies. Curr Probl Surg 36:653–764, 1999.

TABLE 37–2. Lymph Node Metastases in Palpable Medullary Thyroid Carcinoma

Tumor Size (cm)	No. Patients	Central Metastases	Ipsilateral Metastases	Contralateral Metastases
0–0.9	16	11/16	12/16	5/16
1–1.9	16	13/16	14/16	7/16
2–2.9	13	11/13	7/13	8/13
3–3.9	12	9/12	10/12	8/12
4 cm+	16	14/16	12/16	6/16
Total	73	58/73 (80%)	55/73 (75%)	34/73 (47%)

From Moley JF, DeBenedetti MK: Patterns of nodal metastases in palpable medullary thyroid carcinoma: Recommendations for extent of node dessection. Ann Surg 229:880–888, 1999.

carotid arteries. Invasion of these structures may result in stridor, upper airway obstruction, hoarseness, dysphagia, and bleeding or arterial stenosis or occlusion.
- Distant metastases occur in liver, lung, bone, and other soft tissues.

Pheochromocytoma

- Pheochromocytomas occur in 40% to 50% of MEN 2A and MEN 2B patients.
- Pheochromocytomas arise in adrenal medullary or chromaffin cells that synthesize, store, and secrete catecholamines. These tumors often present with classic signs and symptoms of excess catechol secretion (i.e., hypertension, headache, heart palpitations, anxiety, and tremulousness).
- Pheochromocytomas rarely precede the development of C-cell abnormalities in MEN 2 syndrome. Approximately 10% of MEN 2 patients present with signs or symptoms of pheochromocytomas that precede those of MTC. As with the thyroid C-cells, adrenal medullary cells undergo similar, predictable morphologic changes in the development of a pheochromocytoma. Histologically, the lesion progresses from diffuse hyperplasia to nodular hyperplasia, with nodules greater than 1 cm being defined as pheochromocytomas. In MEN 2, pheochromocytomas are often multifocal, with bilateral tumors occurring in more than half of these patients. As opposed to the sporadic form of the disease, malignant and extra-adrenal pheochromocytomas are very rare within MEN 2 populations.

- Pheochromocytomas may be clinically silent in up to 60% of MEN 2 cases, when they are detected by biochemical testing.

Parathyroid Disease

- Hyperparathyroidism occurs in 10% to 35% of patients with MEN 2A.
- Unlike MEN 1, hyperparathyroidism is rarely the initial presenting problem in patients with MEN 2A. Hyperparathyroidism in MEN 2A is characterized by multiglandular hyperplasia. Fewer than one in five patients have a single parathyroid adenoma.

Phenotypic Features of MEN 2B

- MEN 2B is distinguished by characteristic physical features.
- As described earlier, mucosal neuromas and a marfanoid habitus are present. The mucosal neuromas are unencapsulated, thickened proliferation of nerves that occur principally on the lips and tongue but can also be found on the gingiva, buccal mucosa, nasal mucosa, vocal cords, and conjunctiva. MEN 2B patients can also develop ganglioneuromas of the intestine in the submucosal and myenteric plexus. This results in an extremely large colon. Intestinal dysfunction may manifest early in life with poor feeding, failure to thrive, constipation, or pseudo-obstruction.

Genetics

- Mutations in the *RET* proto-oncogene are responsible for MEN 2A, MEN 2B, and FMTC. This gene encodes a transmembrane protein tyrosine kinase. The mutations that cause the MEN 2 syndromes are activating, gain-of-function mutations that cause constitutive activation of the protein.
- Over 30 mis-sense mutations have been described in patients affected by the MEN 2 syndromes (Table 37–3). Within an affected kindred, a single *RET* mutation is present, and the specific type of mutation is related to the phenotypic expression of the disease within that kindred. The aggressiveness of MTC, and the probability of developing pheochromocytoma and parathyroid disease, is influenced by the specific *RET* mutation in a kindred.
- Patients with MEN 2B most commonly have a germline mutation in codon 918 of *RET* (ATG→ACG), which is in the tyrosine kinase domain. Other mutations have been described

TABLE 37–3. RET Mutations and Associated Clinical Syndromes

Exon	Affected Codon	Affected Amino Acid	Clinical Syndrome	MEN 2 Mutations (%)
10	609	Cysteine	MEN 2A, FMTC, MEN 2A, and Hirschsprung's disease	0–1
10	611	Cysteine	MEN 2A, FMTC	2–3
10	618	Cysteine	MEN 2A, FMTC	3–5
10	620	Cysteine	MEN 2A, FMTC	6–8
11	634	Cysteine	MEN 2A	80–90
11	635	Thr Ser Cys Ala	MEN 2A	<1
11	637	Cys Arg Thr	MEN 2A	<1
13	768	Glutamine	FMTC	0–1
13	790	Leucine	MEN 2A, FMTC	<1
13	791	Tryptophan	FMTC	0–1
14	804	Valine	FMTC, MEN 2A	<1
15	883	Ala → Phe	MEN 2B	<1
15	891	Ser → Ala	FMTC	<1
16	918	Met → Thr	MEN 2B	3–5
16	922	Ser → Tyr	MEN 2B	<1

FMTC, familial medullary thyroid carcinoma; MEN, multiple endocrine neoplasia.

(codon 883 and 922). In contrast to MEN 2A and FMTC, 50% of mutations in MEN 2B patients arise de novo and are not present in the parents.

- There is overlap in the mutations that give rise to MEN 2A and FMTC.
- The exon 16 mutation common in MEN 2B patients has also been identified in approximately 40% of sporadic MTC tumors, where it is assumed to be a somatic, rather than an inherited, mutation in the tumor cells only.

Diagnosis

Medullary Thyroid Carcinoma

- The age of onset and the aggressiveness of MTC may vary considerably, depending on the clinical situation. Sporadic MTC is unilateral and unifocal in most cases, whereas MTC in the MEN 2 syndromes is usually bilateral and multifocal. MTC in MEN 2A often becomes clinically apparent in late childhood or in the teenage years. In FMTC, the tumors are indolent and appear later in life, whereas MTC in MEN 2B presents in infancy or early childhood, with gross evidence of cancer present in children as young as 6 months of age.
- The prognosis of MTC is associated with disease stage at the time of diagnosis.
- Palpable cervical adenopathy is present in more than 50% of patients who present with palpable MTC, and lymph node metastases are present histologically in up to 80%.
- Approximately 12% of patients with palpable MTC present with evidence of distant metastatic disease.
- Approximately 25% of all patients with MTC have MEN 2A, MEN 2B, or FMTC. Because of this, we feel that genetic testing should be considered in all patients who present with MTC. An in-depth family history with close attention to any relatives with severe hypertension or thyroid and adrenal tumors is essential.
- The caregiver should also note any phenotypic physical characteristics that might suggest MEN 2B. If a *RET* mutation is found on genetic screening, first-degree relatives should be tested for the same mutation. Patients found to have a mutation in the *RET* proto-oncogene should have biochemical testing for pheochromocytoma before thyroidectomy.
- Thyroid C-cells and MTC cells secrete calcitonin, which is an invaluable serum marker for the presence of disease in screening and follow-up settings. CEA level is also elevated in more than 50% of patients with MTC. Calcitonin is a more

useful tumor marker for MTC than CEA because of its shorter half-life (days compared with months) and because many MTCs do not secrete CEA. Blood levels of calcitonin may be measured in the basal state or after the administration of the secretagogues calcium and pentagastrin.

- Genetic screening of all individuals in a known MEN 2 kindred is the standard of care. If patients from a kindred with a known mutation are shown not to have inherited the mutation, they need no further follow up. Controversy exists over the management of patients found to have a *RET* mutation with no clinical or biochemical evidence of disease. At present, we recommend in-depth genetic counseling and encourage prophylactic thyroidectomy in childhood for carriers of the mutant gene.

Pheochromocytoma

- Biochemical screening for pheochromocytoma is best done by measurement of plasma or 24-hour urine catecholamines and metanephrines. This test should be done on an annual basis. If testing is negative, no further workup is necessary until the next year. If the test is positive or borderline, imaging is needed to determine if a pheochromocytoma is present.

Parathyroid Disease

- All known MEN 2A carriers should be screened annually for the presence of hyperparathyroidism by serum calcium measurements. Parathyroid hormone levels should be measured if the serum calcium is high or borderline.

Medical and Surgical Therapy

Medullary Thyroid Carcinoma

- Recommended surgical treatment of MTC is influenced by several factors. First of all, the clinical course of MTC is usually more aggressive than that of differentiated thyroid cancer, with higher recurrence and mortality rates. Second, MTC cells do not take up radioactive iodine, and radiation therapy and chemotherapy are ineffective. Third, MTC is multicentric in 90% of patients with the hereditary forms of the disease. Fourth, in patients with palpable disease, more than 70% have nodal metastases. Finally, the ability to measure postoperative stimulated calcitonin levels has allowed assessment of the adequacy of surgical extirpation.

- Preventative thyroidectomy is recommended before age six in patients with MEN 2A and FMTC. Patients with MEN 2B should undergo thyroidectomy during infancy, because of the aggressiveness and earlier age of onset of MTC in these patients.
- In patients without a palpable neck mass who are found to be carriers of a *RET* mutation by genetic testing, total thyroidectomy and central node dissection is recommended. At our institution, total parathyroidectomy with autotransplantation is often done at the same time as total thyroidectomy for MTC. This is because the blood supply to the parathyroids is closely associated with the posterior capsule of the thyroid and with the perithyroidal lymph nodes.
- Other experts in this field attempt to preserve the glands with vascular supply intact during thyroidectomy for MTC. Parathyroidectomy with autotransplantation should be done in all patients with gross parathyroid enlargement or biochemical evidence of parathyroid disease at the time of operation for MTC.
- In patients with MTC who present with a palpable thyroid mass, the risk of more extensive nodal metastatic disease is increased.
- Metastatic involvement of cervical lymph nodes is present in more than 75% of patients with palpable MTC tumors. Based on this observation, our recommendation for patients who present with palpable MTC is total thyroidectomy, parathyroidectomy with autotransplantation, central neck dissection, and ipsilateral level II to V node dissection.
- A systematic approach to the removal of all nodal tissue in these patients has been reported to improve recurrence and survival rates when compared retrospectively to procedures in which only grossly involved nodes were removed.

Persistent or Recurrent Disease

- Patients who present with palpable MTC often have elevated calcitonin levels following primary surgery, indicating residual or recurrent MTC. Currently, there is no defined role for chemotherapy or radiation therapy in these patients. Reoperation for patients with recurrent disease can be done with curative or palliative intent. Evidence of distant metastases is a contraindication to surgery unless some palliative benefit can be identified. Two such indications are to prevent invasion or compression of the airway and to debulk large tumors that cause profuse, intractable diarrhea secondary to hormone secretion. If no evidence of distant metastases is found in a patient who has not had previous cervical node dissections, re-exploration of the neck with completion of node dissection is an option for patients with persistent or recurrent elevations of calcitonin.

- Diagnostic laparoscopy with direct examination of the liver is extremely useful in detecting distant metastases in these patients before reoperation on the neck. In one series, liver metastases were identified by laparoscopy in 25% of patients with persistent elevation of calcitonin levels despite negative CT or MRI scanning of the liver.

- If laparoscopy and imaging studies show no evidence of metastatic disease, re-exploration of the neck is considered to remove residual nodal tissue. The operative strategy in these reoperations is to remove all residual thyroid and nodal tissue in at-risk areas that was not removed at the previous operation, guided by the previous operative records, pathology reports, and imaging studies. Reoperation resulted in normalization of the calcitonin level in one third of patients in a study from our institution. Long-term follow-up of these patients is in progress to determine if these responses are durable.

Pheochromocytoma

- Partial or complete adrenalectomy is recommended in patients with MEN 2A and MEN 2B who are found to have a pheochromocytoma. It is important to medically stabilize the patient before surgery to avoid any perioperative events resulting from excessive catechol secretion. Preoperative alpha blockade is achieved by administration of phenoxybenzamine (40 to 200 mg/day) for 5 days to 2 weeks before surgery. The dose is titrated to the lowest blood pressure tolerated by these patients without symptomatic relative hypotension.

- Traditionally, controversy has existed as to whether unilateral or bilateral adrenalectomy should be performed for unilateral tumors. In a series at our institution, the results of unilateral and bilateral adrenalectomies were compared. Nearly one fourth of patients undergoing bilateral adrenalectomy experienced at least one episode of acute adrenal insufficiency requiring hospitalization. Two of these patients died from episodes of adrenal insufficiency. Of the patients who had unilateral adrenalectomies, 52% developed contralateral pheochromocytomas after a mean interval of 12 years. Conversely, 48% of patients remained disease free by biochemical and symptomatic standards during a mean interval of 5 years. Based on these results, it is our practice to perform resection of the involved adrenal only and to maintain yearly biochemical screening thereafter.

● Patients with MEN 2A and MEN 2B may be ideally suited to the laparoscopic approach, because the pheochromocytomas arising in these syndromes are rarely malignant and almost never extra-adrenal. Pheochromocytomas may be successfully removed by unilateral or bilateral laparoscopic adrenalectomy provided the adrenal tumors are small, confined to the adrenal gland(s), and accurately localized preoperatively by high-resolution CT or MRI scanning, and the patient is adequately prepared pharmacologically.

Parathyroid Disease

● The need for isolated parathyroidectomy in MEN 2 patients is rare. As discussed previously, we usually perform routine total parathyroidectomy with autotransplantation at the time of thyroidectomy, regardless of gross appearance of the parathyroid glands. Should hyperparathyroidism occur at a later time in these patients with forearm grafts, surgical removal of a portion of the graft can be done under local anesthetic in an outpatient setting. If, at the time of the initial neck exploration, the parathyroids are left *in situ,* subsequent development of hyperparathyroidism requires re-exploration of the neck with identification and removal of all four glands followed by autotransplantation.

Complications and Postoperative Care

● In thyroidectomy for MEN 2 related MTC, the complications include injury to the recurrent laryngeal nerve, hypocalcemia secondary to parathyroid damage, and compromise of the airway secondary to hematoma formation.

● After total thyroidectomy with parathyroid autotransplantation, it is necessary to supplement calcium, vitamin D, and thyroid hormone. Calcium and vitamin D supplementation is withdrawn 4 to 8 weeks postoperatively as the parathyroid grafts begin to function.

● The long-term postoperative care for MEN 2 patients demands a close and lifelong relationship between the care provider and the patient. Yearly screenings for MTC recurrences and other manifestations of the syndrome must still be conducted. After thyroidectomy for MTC, calcitonin levels should be documented in the immediate postoperative period and should be followed closely. If a patient is found to have persistent or elevated calcitonin level postoperatively, an extensive physical examination and imaging workup for focal and metastatic disease must be conducted, as outlined in the previous section.

- In patients who have undergone adrenalectomy for pheochromocytoma, routine yearly plasma or 24-hour urine screens must be performed to rule out a contralateral tumor. If catecholamines or metanephrines become elevated, MRI or CT imaging should be repeated to localize the tumor.

Prognosis

- MTC in the MEN 2 syndromes is usually indolent and slow-growing, but it is lethal in most patients with distant metastases. Patients with MEN 2A and FMTC have a better long term outcome than patients with MEN 2B or sporadic tumors. Within these clinical settings, however, there is variation. In the MEN 2 population, with the relatively recent widespread use of genetic screening modalities and related changes in treatment for patients identified by these methods, long-term prognosis has yet to be established.

Conclusions

- The identification of mutations in the *RET* proto-oncogene associated with MEN 2A, MEN 2B, and FMTC has led to a new paradigm in surgery—the performance of an operation based on the result of a genetic test. Prophylactic thyroidectomy based on direct mutation analysis appears to be curative in MEN 2A and FMTC patients when they are screened at a young age. The application of meticulous reoperative strategies for persistent hypercalcitoninemia, combined with more accurate staging studies, have led to better patient selection for surgery and improved outcome.

CHAPTER 38

ESOPHAGUS

ANATOMY

- Striated muscle of upper esophagus is derived from the caudal branchial arches and is innervated by the vagus nerve.
- Smooth muscle of the lower esophagus arises from splanchnic mesenchyme and is supplied by a visceral nerve plexus derived from neural crest cells.
- Hollow tube of muscle approximately 25 to 30 cm long, beginning at C6 and ending at T11; penetrates the diaphragm at T10 and joins the cardia of the stomach.
- Mucosal-lined muscular tube that lacks a serosa and is surrounded by a layer of loose fibroalveolar adventitia.
- Divided into four segments.
  - Pharyngoesophageal.
  - Cervical.
  - Thoracic.
  - Abdominal.
- Cricopharyngeal sphincter is unique to the gastrointestinal (GI) tract because it does not consist of a circular ring of muscle, but rather it is a bow of muscle connecting the two lateral borders of the cricoid cartilage.
- Although the cervical esophagus is a midline structure positioned posterior to the trachea, it tends to course to the left of the trachea and is, therefore, more easily approached surgically through a left-sided neck incision.
- The diaphragmatic esophageal hiatus is a sling of muscle fibers that arise from the right crus in approximately 45% of patients; however, both the left and right crura may contribute to the hiatus.
- The squamocolumnar epithelial junction (ora serrata or Z line), as identified endoscopically, is the most practical definition of the gastroesophageal junction.
- Three distinct areas of anatomic narrowing.
  - Cervical constriction: occurs at the level of the cricopharyngeus sphincter, the narrowest point of the GI tract (14 mm).
  - Bronchoaortic constriction: located at the level of the fourth thoracic vertebra behind the tracheal bifurcation

where the left main stem bronchus and the aortic arch cross the esophagus (15 to 17 mm).
- Diaphragmatic constriction: occurs where the esophagus traverses the diaphragm (16 to 19 cm).

- Nourished by numerous segmental arteries arising from the superior thyroid artery, inferior thyroid artery, and aortic esophageal branches.
- Extensive venous drainage of the esophagus includes the hypopharyngeal, azygous, hemiazygous, intercostal, and gastric veins.
- Has both sympathetic and parasympathetic innervation.
- Meissner and Auerbach plexuses provide an intrinsic autonomic nervous system within the esophageal wall.
- Meissner plexus of nerves is located in the submucosa, whereas the Auerbach plexus is in the connective tissue between the circular and longitudinal muscle layers.
- Has an extensive lymphatic drainage that consists of two lymphatic plexuses, one arising in the mucosa and the other in the muscular layer.

PHYSIOLOGY

- Primary function is to transport swallowed material from the pharynx into the stomach.
- Secondary function is prevention of retrograde flow of gastric contents into the esophagus is prevented by the lower esophageal sphincter (LES).
- Entry of air with each inspiration is prevented by the upper esophageal sphincter (UES), which normally remains closed because of tonic contraction of the cricopharyngeus muscle.
- Swallowing is a complex, rapid series of events.
- Three types of contractions are seen in the esophageal body:
  - Primary peristalsis: progressive and is triggered by voluntary swallowing.
  - Secondary peristalsis: also progressive but is generated by distention or irritation not by voluntary swallowing.
  - Tertiary contractions: nonprogressive (simultaneous) contractions that may occur either after voluntary swallowing or spontaneously between swallows.
- Manometry has defined an elevated distal esophageal resting pressure that is 3 to 5 cm in length, which serves as the barrier against abnormal regurgitation of gastric contents into the esophagus and represents a functional sphincter.
- LES is more accurately referred to as the *LES mechanism* or the *distal esophageal high-pressure zone (HPZ)*.

- Normal resting pressure within the HPZ ranges from 10 to 20 mm Hg, but no absolute HPZ per se indicates either competence or incompetence of the LES mechanism.

DISEASES

Vascular Rings

- Usually become apparent during early adult life as esophageal obstruction.
- Barium swallow or endoscopy reveals a typical constriction of the esophagus at the aortic arch and great vessel, and angiography or magnetic resonance imaging (MRI) usually shows which vessels are involved.
- Definitive treatment, if dysphagia is persistent or progressive, is to divide the vascular ring by a transthoracic procedure.

Esophageal Webs

- Plummer-Vinson syndrome (sideropenic dysphagia) refers to the development of cervical dysphagia in patients with chronic iron-deficiency anemia.
- Cause of dysphagia is usually a cervical esophageal web.
- Treatment consists of esophageal dilatation and correction of the nutritional deficiency.

Lower Esophageal Webs (Schatzki's Ring)

- Occurs at the squamocolumnar epithelial junction and involves only the mucosa and submucosa not the esophageal muscle.
- Many patients with symptomatic rings respond to intermittent esophageal bougienage; other patients with reflux do well with periodic dilatations and antireflux medical therapy.

Esophageal Cysts and Duplications

- Esophageal congenital cysts are created during the embryonic process of separation of the pulmonary tree and the esophagus from their common origin.
- Possibilities of enlargement, infection, and bleeding warrant surgical excision for most patients.
- In addition, the mucosa of the cyst can be stripped away to prevent cyst recurrence or computed tomography (CT)-guided transthoracic aspiration, cytologic evaluation, and follow-up can be used.

Disorders of Esophageal Motility

Motor Disorders of the Body of the Esophagus

- Best viewed as a continuum, with hypomotility (achalasia) at one extreme and hypermotility (diffuse esophageal spasm [DES]) at the other.
- Between these extremes are conditions such as vigorous achalasia, which has elements of both achalasia and DES, and a variety of less clearly characterized examples of neuromotor dysfunction.

Achalasia

- The classic triad of presenting symptoms includes dysphagia, regurgitation, and weight loss.
- Regurgitation of undigested food is common as the disease progresses, and aspiration becomes life threatening.
- Diagnosis.
  - Characteristic appearance on a standard chest x-ray film is a double mediastinal stripe throughout the length of the chest and a retrocardiac air-fluid level in a patient with typical symptoms.
  - Roentgenographic hallmark on barium swallow is the distal bird-beak taper of the esophagogastric junction.
  - Manometric criteria are failure of the LES to relax reflexively with swallowing and lack of progressive peristalsis throughout the length of the esophagus.
  - Esophagoscopy is indicated to evaluate the severity of esophagitis and rule out the possibility of an associated carcinoma, a distal esophageal stricture from reflux esophagitis, or a tumor of the cardia mimicking achalasia (pseudoachalasia).
- Treatment.
  - Definitive treatment requires disruption of the circular layer of smooth muscle within the LES area.
  - Two most widely used and analyzed methods of therapy are forceful dilatation, either pneumatic or hydrostatic, and esophagomyotomy.
  - Results were considered excellent or good in 65% of patients with dilatation and 85% of those after esophagomyotomy.
  - Novel pharmacologic treatment is intrasphincteric botulinum toxin injected into the LES through the flexible esophagoscope but relief is short term (6 to 9 months).
  - Surgical treatment, either open or video-assisted, with division of the circular muscle from the inferior pulmonary

ligament extending 1 cm on to the gastric cordia, offers precise and less traumatic division of the circular muscle layer of the lower esophagus than that achieved through forceful dilatation with surgery.

- Video-assisted thorascopic techniques to accomplish an esophagomyotomy, both laparoscopically and thoracoscopically, have yielded comparable results to the open approach with less postoperative pain and a shorter hospital stay.
- Addition of an antireflux procedure with surgical esophagomyotomy is controversial.
- Esophagectomy for end-stage achalasia should be strongly considered in symptomatic patients with end-stage disease in whom lesser approaches offer little relief.

Diffuse Esophageal Spasm and Related Hypermotility Disorders

- Poorly understood hypermotility disorder in which patients experience chest pain and/or dysphagia as a result of repetitive, simultaneous, high-amplitude esophageal contractions.
- Classic manometric criteria are simultaneous, multiphasic, repetitive, often high-amplitude contractions that occur after a swallow and spontaneously in the smooth muscle portion.
- Diagnostic hallmark is the correlation of subjective complaints with objective evidence of spasm on manometric tracings.
- Nutcracker or super-squeeze esophagus is a hypermotility disorder characterized by extremely high-amplitude (225 to 430 mm Hg) progressive peristaltic contractions, often of prolonged duration.
- Esophageal motor disturbances occur in several collagen vascular diseases, such as dermatomyositis, polymyositis, and lupus erythematosus, but particularly scleroderma.
- Abnormal peristalsis is so common in scleroderma that it is a major diagnostic sign of the disease (Table 38–1).
- Treatment.
  - Response to nitrates is variable but may be dramatic.
  - Esophageal dilation with tapered dilators (50 to 60 French) may relieve dysphagia and chest pain.
  - Although long thoracic esophagomyotomy has been advocated by some surgeons, results are much less favorable (than in achalasia), with success in only 50% to 60%.

TABLE 38–1. Differential Characteristics of Achalasia and Primary Spasm

Characteristic	Achalasia	Vigorous Achalasia	Diffuse Esophageal Spasm	Nutcracker Esophagus
Dysphagia	Common	Common	Rare	Common
Pain	Rare	Common	Common	Common
Barium esophagogram	Abnormal; dilated esophagus, bird-beak taper	Abnormal	Normal caliber "corkscrew" esophagus	Normal contraction progression
Endoscopy	Normal	Normal	Normal	Normal
Motility	Nonrelaxing LES, absent or weak simultaneous contraction after swallowing	Nonrelaxing LES + hypertonic simultaneous, multiphasic contractions after swallowing	Hypertonic simultaneous, multiphasic contractions after swallowing	Normal peristalsis present, very high amplitude and duration of contractions

LES, lower esophageal sphincter.

Esophageal Diverticula

- Epithelial-lined mucosal pouches that protrude from the esophageal lumen.
- Commonly occur at three distinct sites:
  - Pharyngoesophageal (Zenkers) diverticula occur at the junction of the pharynx and esophagus.
  - Parabronchial (midesophageal) diverticula occur near the tracheal bifurcation.
  - Epiphrenic (supradiaphragmatic) diverticula arise from the distal 10 cm of esophagus.
- A *true* diverticulum contains all layers of the normal esophageal wall, including mucosa, submucosa, and muscle, whereas a false diverticulum consists primarily of mucosa and submucosa.
- Pulsion diverticula (pharyngoesophageal and epiphrenic) are false diverticula that arise because elevated intraluminal pressure forces the mucosa and submucosa to herniate through the esophageal musculature.
- Almost all diverticula of the body of the esophagus are of the pulsion variety caused by an underlying motility abnormality.
- Motility studies are necessary as manometric or motility abnormalities are varied and often atypical.
- Treatment is designed to relieve dysphagia, to palliate chest pain, and to protect against aspiration of regurgitated esophageal contents.
- Surgical therapy must address the motor disorder; therefore, esophagomyotomy of the abnormally functioning muscle identified by manometric examination is essential.

Pharyngoesophageal (Zenker's) Diverticula

- A Pulsion diverticulum resulting from a transient incomplete opening in the UES, also referred to as cricopharyngeal achalasia.

Diagnosis

- Asymptomatic initially, often discovered during routine radiographic or endoscopic evaluation.
- Symptomatic patients complain of a vague sensation or sticking in the throat, intermittent cough, excessive salivation, and intermittent dysphagia.

Treatment

- Surgical approach is cervical esophagomyotomy (7 to 10 cm to divide all muscle fibers) and resection of the diverticulum.

Epiphrenic Diverticula

Diagnosis

- Best detected by barium esophagogram; motility studies are necessary.

Treatment

- Surgery is a long extramucosal thoracic esophagomyotomy from beneath the aortic arch through the esophagogastric junction onto the stomach 5 cm.
- The distal extent of the muscle incision and the need for a concomitant antireflux operation is controversial.
- During an antireflux procedure on a myotomized esophagus, a partial fundoplication (Belsey type), rather than a 360-degree Nissen fundoplication, is less likely to produce functional obstruction on long-term follow-up.

Caustic Injury

- Most important element is immediate verification of the etiologic agent and accurate assessment of the depth and extent of injury.
- Caustic injury is manifest by the symptoms of oral pain, drooling, excessive salivation, and inability or refusal to swallow or drink.
- Esophagoscopy is essential because 10% to 30% of patients with no external evidence of burn have been subsequently confirmed by esophagoscopy to have sustained damage.
- Likewise, the stomach must be examined.
- Evidence of significant pharyngeal or laryngeal damage (identified by direct laryngoscopy or as suggested by symptoms of hoarseness, stridor, or dyspnea) demands hospitalization and observation.
- Successful management of acid ingestion with full-thickness injury demands acute surgical intervention, including emergency cervical esophagostomy, esophagogastrectomy, and occasionally duodenectomy (Fig. 38–1).
- Identification of ulcerations, especially when they are circumferential, warrants concern because of the high potential for stricture formation.

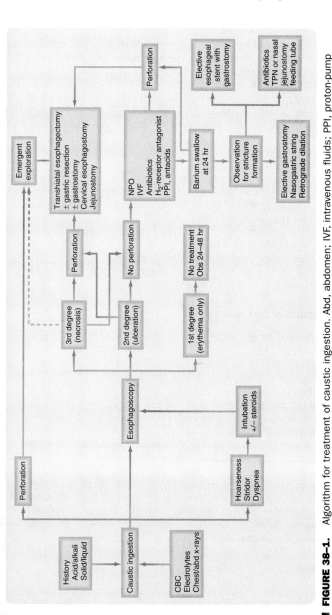

■ **FIGURE 38–1.** Algorithm for treatment of caustic ingestion. Abd, abdomen; IVF, intravenous fluids; PPI, proton-pump inhibitor; TPN, total parenteral nutrition. (*Modified from Zwischenberger JB, Savage C, Bidani A: Surgical aspects of esophageal disease. Am J Respir Crit Care Med 164:1037–1040, 2001.*)

- Should be serially assessed by contrast studies repeated at intervals of 3 weeks.
- Corticosteroid treatment is contraindicated in patients with severe caustic burns that have perforated the esophagus or produced necrosis of the stomach.
- Most frequent complication is stricture formation, which usually develops between 3 and 8 weeks after initial injury.
- Some lesions respond to dilatation without recurrence; others may require placement of intraluminal Silastic stents or, rarely, resection.
- Indications for esophageal resection/reconstruction include the following:
  - An ongoing requirement for dilatation of extensive or multiple strictures for more than 6 months.
  - Failure or refusal of the patient to comply with a schedule for regular dilatations.
  - The presence of a fistula between the esophagus and the tracheobronchial tree.
  - Iatrogenic perforation of the esophagus.
- Long-term complication of esophageal scarring and stricture formation is malignant degeneration.

Perforation of the Esophagus

- Remains a true emergency because delay clearly affects survival.
- Endoscopic procedures are the most common cause, although the frequency is still very low.
- Fiberoptic endoscopy results in a 0.09% incidence of perforation, compared with 0.07% if the procedure is performed with a rigid scope; when dilatation is added, the frequency increases to 0.25%.
- Sclerosis of varices and hydropneumatic dilatations for motor disorders are associated with perforation in 1% to 5% of patients.
- Esophageal rupture induced by straining (Boerhaave's syndrome) is the most common type of spontaneous perforation.
- Perforations from penetrating or blunt trauma are frequently overshadowed by associated injuries and have a poor prognosis if unrecognized.

Diagnosis

- Severe pain is the most consistent symptom, present in 70% to 90% of patients, and usually related to the site of disruption.

- Plain chest x-ray film is suggestive of the diagnosis (blunting of the costophrenic angle) in 90% of patients with perforation; however, immediately after disruption, may be normal.
- Pneumomediastinum, subcutaneous emphysema, mediastinal widening, or a mediastinal air-fluid level must prompt investigation to rule out esophageal perforation.
- Esophagogram reveals the primary site or area of leakage and determines whether the perforation is confined to the mediastinum or communicates freely with the pleural or peritoneal cavities.
- CT of the chest, which can often show the site of perforation, is used when the presentation is atypical.
- Esophagoscopy can be helpful during a procedure but can easily miss a perforation and can enlarge the hole (Fig. 38–2).

Treatment

- Treatment of esophageal perforation is directed toward fluid resuscitation, control of sepsis, operative drainage of the mediastinum and pleural cavity, suture repair of the esophagus, and reinforcement of the suture line with vascularized tissue, especially muscle.
- Sepsis, shock, pneumothorax, pneumoperitoneum, mediastinal emphysema, and respiratory failure are all absolute indications for rapid surgical intervention.
- Principles of repair include a local esophagomyotomy proximal and distal to the tear to expose the entire mucosal defect, débridement of the mucosal defect, closure over a bougie, and reapproximation of the muscle.
- Reinforcement with vascularized tissue and side drainage reportedly decreases incidence of fistulas (13%) and mortality (6%) compared with treatment by simple primary repair (fistula, 39%; mortality, 25%).
- Delay in diagnosis makes repair more difficult because of friability and necrotic tissue at the site of the tear; primary repair may still be possible, but cervical diversion or drainage, gastric diversion or drainage, enteral feeding tube or jejunostomy, wide mediastinal drainage, and wrapping of the esophagus with a vascularized muscle flap may have to be considered.
- When extensive mediastinitis and sepsis are present from continued contamination, resection of the esophagus with delayed reconstruction may be necessary.
- Postoperative care includes control of infection and enteral or parenteral hyperalimentation until healing of the tear is demonstrated by barium swallow.

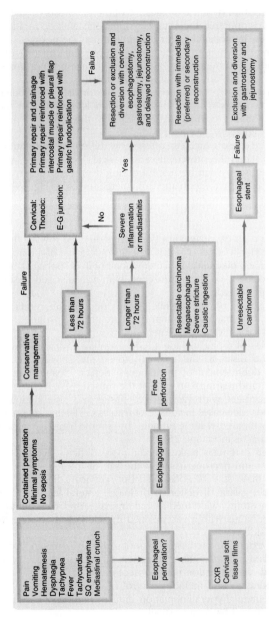

■ **FIGURE 38–2.** Algorithm for treatment of esophageal perforation. *(Modified from Zwischenberger JB, Savage C, Bidani A: Surgical aspects of esophageal disease. Perforation and caustic injury. Am J Respir Crit Care Med 164:1037–1040, 2001.)*

Tracheoesophageal Fistula (Acquired)

- Long-term intubation accounts for most acquired, nonmalignant tracheoesophageal fistulas (TEFs) because of either overinflation of the cuff or placement of a small tracheostomy tube necessitating overinflation of the cuff to provide airway sealing.
- Operative closure is necessary because spontaneous closure is rare.

Benign Esophageal Tumors

- Benign tumors of the esophagus are rare.
- Approximately 60% are leiomyomas, 20% are cysts, and 5% are polyps.

Leiomyomas

Diagnosis

- Esophageal symptoms prompt performance of a barium swallow and/or an endoscopic examination.
- Barium swallow appearance is distinctive because the well-localized mass has a smooth surface and distinct margins and is not circumferential.
- During endoscopy, the mucosa is intact, and the extrinsic mass narrows the lumen but can easily be displaced and passed with the esophagoscope.

Treatment

- As a general rule, excision of symptomatic benign tumors or cysts or those larger than 5 cm is advised.
- Operative technique for excision of esophageal cyst is identical to that for benign tumor.
- The tumor is located and overlying longitudinal esophageal muscle is split in the direction of its fibers to reveal the mass which is gently dissected away from contiguous tissues and underlying mucosa.

Esophageal Cancer

- Represents 4% of newly diagnosed cancers in North America.
- Most present with locally advanced (stage T_3 and/or N_1) disease.
- Heavy smoking and drinking combine to increase the risk 25- to 100-fold.

- Ninety-five percent of esophageal cancers worldwide are squamous cell carcinomas, which arise from the mucosa of the esophagus.
- Notorious for aggressive biologic behavior; infiltrates locally, involves adjacent lymph nodes and metastasizes widely by hematogenous spread.
- Lack of esophageal serosal layer tends to favor local tumor extension.
- Tumors of the upper and middle thirds infiltrate the tracheobronchial tree, aorta, and left recurrent laryngeal nerve as it loops around the aortic arch, whereas lower-third tumors may invade the diaphragm, pericardium, or stomach.
- Extensive mediastinal lymphatic drainage, which communicates with cervical and abdominal collateral vessels, is responsible for the finding of mediastinal, supraclavicular, or celiac lymph node metastasis in at least 75% of patients.
- Prognosis for patients with invasive squamous cell carcinoma is poor; the overall 5-year survival for patients with treated tumors is 5% to 12%.
- Extraesophageal tumor extension is present in 70% of cases at the time of diagnosis, and the 5-year survival is only 3% when lymph node metastases are present, compared with 42% when no lymph node spread has occurred.
- The incidence of adenocarcinoma has doubled over the last decade which strongly correlates with a rise in Barrett's metaplasia, suggesting a possible link to untreated or silent gastroesophageal reflux.
- Seven percent of the U.S. population suffers from symptomatic gastroesophageal reflux disease (GERD), and 2% to 15% of those patients with chronic reflux disease develop Barrett's esophagus (metaplastic columnar epithelium replaces the distal squamous mucosa thought to be attributable to prolonged exposure of the distal esophageal mucosa to gastroesophageal reflux).
- Barrett's esophagus is of clinical importance because adenocarcinoma occurs in patients with Barrett's esophagus at a rate 30 to 40 times greater than that of the general population; adenocarcinoma is now the most common cell type in the United States.

Diagnosis

- Symptoms are insidious, beginning as nonspecific retrosternal discomfort or indigestion, followed by dysphagia and weight loss.

- Patients complain of "food getting stuck" often at the location of the lesion.
- Dysphagia always warrants esophagoscopy to rule out carcinoma.
- Likewise, esophagoscopy and biopsy are mandatory in every patient with esophageal stenosis or when white finger-like plaques (Barrett's esophagus) are present.
- Accuracy of the combination of brush cytology and biopsy is more than 97%.

Staging

- Critical step in determining which therapeutic option is appropriate.

Lymph Nodes (N Stage)

- Advances in imaging technology have greatly changed the preoperative staging schema.
- Lymph node involvement may be assessed by endoscopic ultrasound, CT, positron emission tomography (PET), or video-assisted thoracoscopy and laparoscopy.
- Endoscopic ultrasound and CT can then be used for image-directed fine-needle aspiration of mediastinal or celiac nodes.
- Video-assisted thoracoscopy and laparoscopy have been found to be accurate, although invasive, lymph node staging techniques (~90% to 94%).
- Surgical exploration with lymph node sampling definitively stages esophageal cancer patients when necessary (Table 38–2).
- Lymph node metastases from primary esophageal tumors along the extensive esophageal lymphatics are common.

TABLE 38–2. Accuracy of Staging Techniques

Modality	T Accuracy (%)	N Accuracy (%)	M Accuracy (%)
Computed tomography	49–60	39–74	85–90
Endoscopic ultrasound	76–92	50–88	66–86
Magnetic resonance imaging	96	56–74	
Positron emission tomography		48–76	71–91
Thoracoscopy or laparoscopy		90–94	

- Celiac nodal involvement is common in patients with esophageal cancer (up to 46%) and also predicts a poor prognosis.

Treatment

- Curative efforts include surgery, chemotherapy, radiation, or a combination of these techniques; however, despite multitudes of clinical trials and retrospective reviews, no treatment modality alone has proved superior.
- Current trials have focused on radiation and chemotherapy with or without resection.

Palliative Treatment

- Is appropriate when patients are too debilitated to undergo surgery or have a tumor that is unresectable because of extensive invasion of vital structures, recurrence of resected or irradiated tumor, and/or metastases.
- Depending on the perceived life expectancy, palliation includes dilatation, stent placement, photodynamic therapy, radiotherapy with or without chemotherapy, and/or laser therapy; none of these methods have proven superior.

Curative Treatment

- At best, only 50% of patients are eligible for curative resection at presentation.
- If an esophagectomy is indicated, three major technical approaches are available:
  - A transthoracic esophagectomy.
  - Transhiatal esophagectomy without a thoracotomy.
  - An en bloc radial esophagectomy.
- No consensus has been formed on the preferred technique, but transthoracic esophagectomy is preferred by most thoracic surgeons.
- Regardless of technique, an R0 resection (i.e., a complete macroscopic and microscopic removal of tumor) is required for a surgical resection to achieve the highest cure rate.

Reconstruction after Esophagectomy

- After a portion of the esophagus is removed, or after complete esophagectomy, a conduit must be established for alimentary continuity.

- Stomach, colon, and jejunum have all been successfully used as esophageal substitutes, but the stomach appears to be the conduit of choice because of ease in mobilization and its ample vascular supply.

Radiation Therapy

- Patients who undergo external-beam radiation therapy, used alone in the treatment of esophageal carcinoma, have only a 5% to 10% 5-year survival, so this therapy is not considered curative.

Chemotherapy

- Used as a single modality in the treatment of esophageal cancer is the least effective strategy.
- Surgery implemented after chemotherapy, appears to be slightly better than with radiation therapy alone or with chemoradiotherapy alone (median survival ranges from 4 to 32 months).
- Cisplatin-based chemotherapeutic regimens have modestly improved median survival.
- Surgery can be used in conjunction with radiation therapy or chemotherapy to rid local and regional areas of residual malignancy, to yield a complete histologic response rate of 25% to 30%.
- In trials involving induction radiation therapy and chemotherapy, survival rates are dramatically increased (5-year survival rates approach 60%) when no residual cancer is found in the tumor specimen; overall, however, chemotherapy/radiation/surgery shows no improvement in survival over surgery alone.

Barrett's Esophagus

Diagnosis

- Can be found in 10% to 15% of patients who have endoscopic examinations for symptoms of GERD.
- Carcinogenesis may involve activation of proto-oncogenes, dysfunction of tumor suppressor genes, or both.
- True dysplasia represents a neoplastic alteration of the columnar epithelium and is widely regarded as the precursor of invasive malignancy.
- Prevalence of adenocarcinoma at time of diagnosis is approximately 8%.

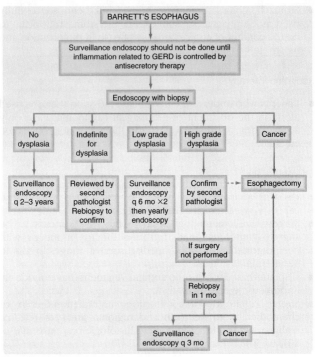

■ **FIGURE 38–3.**   Management algorithm for Barrett's esophagus.

Treatment

● Patients undergoing surgery for carcinoma *in situ* or confirmed high-grade dysplasia should have an esophagectomy that includes the entire columnar-lined esophageal segment (Fig. 38–3).

CHAPTER 39

HIATAL HERNIA AND GASTROESOPHAGEAL REFLUX DISEASE

GASTROESOPHAGEAL REFLUX DISEASE (GERD)

- The lower esophageal sphincter has the primary role of preventing reflux of the gastric contents into the esophagus. The sphincter is a unique physiologic entity, as opposed to an anatomic structure, that is located just cephalad to the gastroesophageal junction and is clearly identifiable as a zone of high pressure during manometric evaluation as the sensing device passes from the stomach into the esophagus. Several factors contribute to the high-pressure zone.

Endoscopy

- The value of the study is in its ability to exclude other diseases, especially a tumor, and to document the presence of peptic esophageal injury.

Manometry

- The pertinent information to be gained from the manometry tracings concerns the function of the lower esophageal sphincter and the esophageal body.

pH Monitoring

- The gold standard for diagnosing and quantifying acid reflux is the 24-hour pH test.

Esophagogram

- The true value of the study is to determine the external anatomy of the esophagus and the proximal stomach.

Medical Management—Proton Pump Inhibitors

- These drugs act by irreversibly binding the proton pump in the parietal cells of the stomach, thus effectively stopping gastric acid production. The maximal effect occurs after approximately 4 days of therapy, and the effects will linger for the life of the parietal cell. Thus, the acid suppression will persist for 4 to 5 days after therapy has ended. For this reason, the patient should be off therapy for 1 week before being evaluated with pH monitoring.

Surgical Therapy

- The indications for surgical therapy have changed somewhat with the advent of proton pump inhibitors. Certainly, patients with evidence of severe esophageal injury (ulcer, stricture, or Barrett's mucosa) and incomplete resolution of symptoms or relapses while on medical therapy are appropriate to consider for operative intervention. Other patients with a long duration of symptoms or those in whom symptoms persist at a young age should be considered for operative treatment initially. In these patients, operative therapy should be considered an alternative to medical therapy rather than a treatment of last resort.

360-Degree Wrap (Left Crus Approach)

- Once the esophagus is mobilized, the crura are reapproximated posteriorly with heavy permanent sutures to allow the easy passage of a 52-French bougie (Fig. 39–1). The posterior aspect of the fundus is then passed behind the esophagus from left to right. The wrap is created over a length of 2.5 to 3 cm with three or four interrupted permanent sutures (Fig. 39–2).
- With the bougie removed, the wrap is anchored to the esophagus and the right crus at the hiatus.

Endoscopic Therapy

- Recently, several endoscopic techniques have been developed for the treatment of GERD.

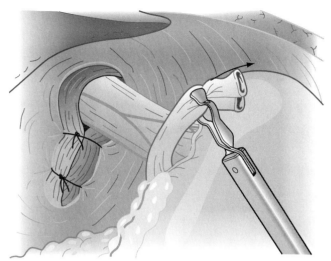

■ FIGURE 39–1. Posterior crural closure is performed with heavy permanent suture. Note how the peritoneum and, thus, the phrenoesophageal membrane are incorporated into the closure. The exposure is facilitated by displacement of the esophagus to the left and anterior.

- At the time of this writing each of these approaches should be considered experimental and longer follow-up is needed before recommending their widespread use.

Symptomatic and Objective Results

Symptom response to the operative treatment of gastro-esophageal reflux disease is excellent. Most authors report response rates of 90 to 94%.

Complications

- Reported in 3% to 10% of patients. Many of the complications are minor and are related to surgical intervention in general (urinary retention, wound infection, venous thrombosis, and ileus). Others are related specifically to the procedure or the approach (splenic injury, hollow viscus perforation, dysphagia, and pneumothorax).
- Operative.
- Postoperative.
- Failures.

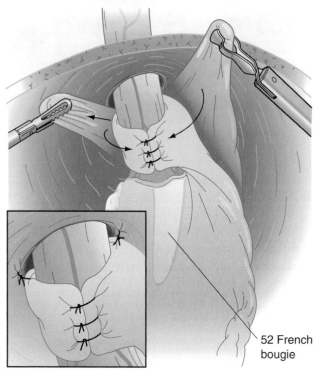

■ FIGURE 39–2. The wrap is fashioned with fundus over a length of 2.5 to 3 cm. The bougie is placed after the first suture of wrap is secured to ensure a "floppy" fundoplication. The wrap is secured to the diaphragm with right and left coronal sutures *(inset)*.

- Strictures.
  - The most effective therapy for peptic stricture of the esophagus is an antireflux procedure. Although there is evidence to support effective symptom control with endoscopic dilation and proton pump inhibitor maintenance therapy, operative treatment results in fewer dilations per patient.

Barrett's Esophagus

- If Barrett's esophagus is found, multiple biopsies are necessary to exclude cancer or dysplasia, which may indicate a tendency toward the development of adenocarcinoma.

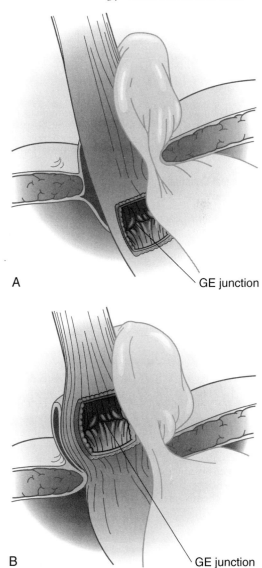

A

GE junction

B

GE junction

■ **FIGURE 39–3.** Two (out of three) types of hiatal hernia. Type 2 is known as a rolling hernia *(A)*, and Type 3 is referred to as a mixed hernia *(B)*. GE, gastroesophageal.

- Regardless of the impact of an antireflux procedure on the evolution of Barrett's esophagus, the patients should still be examined endoscopically for surveillance of metaplasia after the operation is performed.

Short Esophagus

- By mobilizing the esophagus well into the mediastinum, a 2- to 3-cm segment of esophagus can usually be placed into the abdomen without tension. However, if this cannot be accomplished, a Collis gastroplasty may be performed.

Extraesophageal Symptoms

- A relatively new area of study in GERD is the involvement of the respiratory tract. Symptoms of hoarseness, laryngitis, cough, wheezing, and aspiration may occur when patients have high proximal reflux. Pulmonary fibrosis has also been associated with high gastroesophageal reflux.

PARAESOPHAGEAL HERNIAS

- Paraesophageal hernias, Type II or Type III (Fig. 39–3A and B), are less commonly encountered in surgical practice than GERD.
- Because of these risks and early reports of Belsey and Hill, most for decades have recommend repair of these hernias when detected regardless of symptoms. Recent evidence, however, suggests that the risk of acute strangulation is around 1% per year. Therefore we, and many others, recommend surgical intervention only for younger patients (<60 years) and those with significant symptoms.
- The most common symptoms include intermittent dysphagia for solids that result from episodes of acute gastric or esophageal obstruction, abdominal and chest pain secondary to visceral torsion, gastrointestinal bleeding from mucosal ischemia, and heartburn.

CHAPTER 40

ABDOMINAL WALL, UMBILICUS, PERITONEUM, MESENTERIES, OMENTUM, AND RETROPERITONEUM

ABDOMINAL WALL

Embryology

- The abdominal wall begins to develop in the earliest stages of embryonic differentiation from the lateral plate of the intraembryonic mesoderm. At this stage, the embryo consists of three principal layers: an outer protective layer termed ectoderm, an inner nutritive layer termed endoderm, and the mesoderm. The intraembryonic mesoderm becomes segmented into mesodermal somites or myotomes from which proliferating cells grow into the developing abdominal wall or somatopleure.

- At this early stage, the lining of the coelomic cavity communicates broadly with the lining outside the body cavity. As the embryo enlarges and the abdominal wall components grow toward one another, the ventral open area bounded by the edge of the amnion becomes smaller. This results in the development of the umbilical cord as a tubular structure containing the yolk stalk (omphalomesenteric duct), allantois, and the fetal blood vessels that pass to and from the placenta.

- By the end of the third month of gestation, the body walls have closed except at the umbilical ring.

Anatomy

- There are nine layers to the abdominal wall: skin, subcutaneous tissue, superficial fascia, external oblique muscle, internal oblique muscle, transversus abdominis muscle,

541

endoabdominal or transversalis fascia, extraperitoneal or preperitoneal adipose and areolar tissue, and peritoneum.

Subcutaneous Tissues

● The subcutaneous tissue consists of Camper's and Scarpa's fascia. Camper's fascia is the superficial layer that contains the bulk of the subcutaneous fat; Scarpa's fascia is a denser layer of fibrous connective tissue contiguous with the fascia lata of the thigh.

Muscle and Investing Fascias

● The muscles of the anterolateral abdominal wall include the external and internal oblique and the transversus abdominis. These flat muscles enclose much of the circumference of the torso and give rise anteriorly to a broad, flat aponeurosis investing the rectus abdominis muscles (i.e., rectus sheath). The external abdominal oblique muscles are the largest and the thickest of the flat abdominal wall muscles. They originate from the lower seven ribs and course in a superolateral to inferomedial direction.

● At the midclavicular line, the muscle fibers give rise to a flat, strong aponeurosis that passes anteriorly to the rectus sheath to insert medially into the linea alba.

● The inguinal ligament is the lower, free edge of the external oblique aponeurosis under which pass the femoral artery, vein, and nerve and the iliacus, psoas major, and pectineus muscles.

● The internal abdominal oblique muscle originates from the iliopsoas fascia beneath the lateral half of the inguinal ligament, from the anterior two thirds of the iliac crest and the lumbodorsal fascia. Its fibers course in a direction opposite to those of the external oblique (i.e., inferolateral to superomedial). The uppermost fibers insert into the lower five ribs and their cartilages. The central fibers form an aponeurosis at the semilunar line that, above the semicircular line (of Douglas), is divided into an anterior and posterior lamella that envelope the rectus abdominis muscle. Below the semicircular line, the aponeurosis of the internal oblique muscle courses anteriorly to the rectus abdominis muscle as a part of the anterior rectus sheath.

● The transversus abdominis muscle is the smallest of the muscles of the anterolateral abdominal wall. It arises from the lower six costal cartilages, the spines of the lumbar vertebra the iliac crest, and the iliopsoas fascia beneath the lateral third of the inguinal ligament. The fibers course transversely to give rise to a flat aponeurotic sheet that passes posterior to the rectus abdominis muscle above the semicircular line and anterior to this muscle below it.

- The transversalis fascia covers the deep surface of the transversus abdominis muscle and with its various extensions forms a complete fascial envelope around the abdominal cavity.
- The transversalis fascia is responsible for the structural integrity of the abdominal wall, and, by definition, a hernia results from a defect in the transversalis fascia.
- The rectus abdominis muscles are paired muscles that appear as long, flat triangular ribbons wider at their origin on the anterior surfaces of the fifth, sixth, and seventh costal cartilages and the xiphoid process than at their insertion on the pubic crest and pubic symphysis. Each muscle is composed of long, parallel fascicles interrupted by three to five tendinous inscriptions.
- The rectus abdominis muscles are contained within a fascial sheath, the rectus sheath, which is derived from the aponeuroses of the three flat abdominal muscles. Superior to the semicircular line of Douglas the fascial sheath completely envelopes the rectus abdominis muscle with the external oblique and the anterior lamellae of the internal oblique aponeuroses passing anterior to the rectus abdominis and the aponeuroses from the posterior lamellae of the internal oblique muscle, the transversus abdominis muscle, and the transversalis fascia passing posterior to the rectus muscle. Below the semicircular line, all of these fascial layers pass anteriorly to the rectus abdominus muscle except for the transversalis fascia. In this location the posterior aspect of the rectus abdominis muscle is covered only by transversalis fascia, preperitoneal areolar tissue, and peritoneum.
- The rectus abdominis muscles are held closely in apposition near the anterior midline by the linea alba. The linea alba consists of a band of dense, crisscross fibers of the aponeuroses of the broad abdominal muscles.

Preperitoneal Space and Peritoneum

- The preperitoneal space lies between the transversalis fascia and the parietal peritoneum and contains adipose and areolar tissue. The inferior epigastric artery and vein course through this space before entering the rectus sheath at a level just above the hypogastrium.
- This space also contains the remnants of three fetal structures that are apparent during laparotomy or laparoscopy.

These include (1) the medial umbilical ligaments, which are the vestiges of the fetal umbilical arteries; (2) the median umbilical ligament, which is a midline fibrous cord representing the remnant of the fetal allantoic stalk (or urachus); and (3) the falciform ligament of the liver, which is a peritoneum-covered projection of extraperitoneal adipose tissue extending from the umbilicus to the liver. The round ligament or ligamentum teres is contained within the free margin of the falciform ligament and represents the obliterated umbilical vein coursing from the umbilicus to the left branch of the portal vein.

- The parietal peritoneum is the innermost layer of the abdominal wall. It consists of thin layer of dense, irregular connective tissue covered on its inner surface by a single layer squamous mesothelium.

Vascular Supply

- The anterolateral abdominal wall receives its arterial supply from the last six intercostals and four lumbar arteries, the superior and inferior epigastric arteries and the deep circumflex iliac arteries.
- The venous drainage of the anterior abdominal wall follows a relatively simple pattern in which the superficial veins above the umbilicus empty into the superior vena cava by way of the internal mammary, intercostal, and long thoracic veins. The veins inferior to the umbilicus (i.e., the superficial epigastric, circumflex iliac and the pudendal veins) converge toward the saphenous opening in the groin to enter the saphenous vein and become tributary to the inferior vena cava.
- The lymphatic supply of the abdominal wall follows a pattern similar to the venous drainage. Those lymphatic vessels arising from the supraumbilical region drain into the axillary lymph nodes while those arising from the infraumbilical region drain toward the superficial inguinal lymph nodes.

Innervation

- The anterior rami of the thoracic nerves follow a curvilinear course forward in the intercostal spaces toward the midline of the body.
- Thoracic nerves 7 to 12 pass behind the costal cartilages and lower ribs to enter a plane between the internal oblique muscle and the transversus abdominis. The seventh and eighth nerves course slightly upward or horizontally to reach

the epigastrium, whereas the lower nerves have an increasingly caudal trajectory. As these nerves course medially they provide motor branches to the abdominal wall musculature. Medially, they perforate the rectus sheath to provide sensory innervation to the anterior abdominal wall. The anterior ramus of the 10th thoracic nerve reaches the skin at the level of the umbilicus, and the 12th thoracic nerve innervates the skin of the hypogastrium.

- The ilioinguinal and iliohypogastric nerves often arise in common from the anterior rami of the 12th thoracic and first lumbar nerves to provide sensory innervation to the hypogastrium and lower abdominal wall.

Congenital Abnormalities

Umbilical Hernias

- Umbilical hernias may be classified into three distinct forms: (1) omphalocele, (2) infantile umbilical hernia, and (3) acquired umbilical hernia.

Omphalocele

- An omphalocele is a funnel-shaped defect in the central abdomen through which the viscera protrude into the base of the umbilical cord. It is caused by failure of the abdominal wall musculature to unite in the midline during fetal development. The umbilical vessels may be splayed over the viscera or pushed to one side. In larger defects, the liver and spleen may lie within the cord along with a major portion of the bowel. These large hernias are cover by peritoneum and, more superficially, amnion. There is no skin covering these defects. These lesions are associated with a high incidence of concomitant congenital anomalies.
- Gastroschisis is another defect of the abdominal wall presenting at birth in which the umbilical membrane has ruptured allowing the intestine to herniate outside the abdominal cavity. The defect is nearly always to the right of the umbilical cord and the intestine is not covered with skin or amnion. Concomitant congenital anomalies occur in only about 10% of patients.

Infantile Umbilical Hernia

- Infantile umbilical hernias appear within a few days or weeks after the stump of the umbilical cord has sloughed.

It is caused by a weakness in the adhesion between the scarred remains of the umbilical cord and the umbilical ring. In contrast to omphalocele, the infantile umbilical hernia is covered by skin. Generally, these small hernias occur in the superior margin of the umbilical ring. They are easily reducible and become prominent when the infant cries. Most of these hernias resolve within the first 24 months of life and complications such as strangulation are rare. Operative repair is indicated for those patients in whom the hernia has persisted beyond the age of 3 or 4 years.

Acquired Umbilical Hernia

- In this condition, an umbilical hernia develops at a time remote from closure of the umbilical ring. This hernia occurs most commonly at the upper margin of the umbilicus and results from weakening of the cicatricial tissue that normally closes the umbilical ring.
- In contrast to infantile umbilical hernias, acquired umbilical hernias do not spontaneously resolve but instead gradually increase in size. The dense fibrous hernia ring at the neck of this hernia makes strangulation of herniated intestine or omentum an important complication.

Abnormalities Resulting from Persistence of the Omphalomesenteric Duct

- During fetal development, the midgut communicates widely with the yolk sac.
- Over time, communication between the yolk sac and the intestine becomes obliterated and the intestine resides free within the peritoneal cavity. Persistence of part or all of the omphalomesenteric duct results in a variety of abnormalities related to the intestine and abdominal wall.
- Persistence of the intestinal end of the omphalomesenteric duct results in an abnormality known as Meckel's diverticulum. These congenital diverticula arise from the antimesenteric border of the small intestine, most often the ileum. They are found in about 2% of the population and may be associated with inflammation, perforation, hemorrhage, or obstruction.
- The omphalomesenteric duct may remain patent throughout its course producing an enterocutaneous fistula between the distal small intestine and the umbilicus. This condition presents with the passage of meconium and mucus from the umbilicus in the first days of life. Because of the risk

of mesenteric volvulus around a persistent omphalomesenteric duct, these lesions should be promptly treated with laparotomy and excision of the fistulous tract. Persistence of the distal end of the omphalomesenteric duct results in an umbilical polyp, which is a small excrescence of omphalomesenteric ductal mucosa at the umbilicus. Such polyps resemble umbilical granulomas except that they do not disappear after silver nitrate cauterization. They suggest the presence of a persistent omphalomesenteric duct or umbilical sinus and are most appropriately treated by excision of the mucosal remnant and underlying omphalomesenteric duct or umbilical sinus if present. Umbilical sinuses result from the persistence of the distal omphalomesenteric duct. The morphology of the sinus tract may be readily delineated by a sinogram. Treatment involves excision of the sinus. Finally, the accumulation of mucus in portion of a persistent omphalomesenteric duct may result in the formation of a cyst that may be associated with either the intestine or the umbilicus by a fibrous band. Treatment consists of excision of the cyst and the associated persistent omphalomesenteric duct.

Abnormalities Resulting from Persistence of the Allantois

- The allantois is the cranial most component of the embryologic ventral cloaca. The intraabdominal portion of the allantois is termed the urachus and connects the urinary bladder with the umbilicus, whereas the extra-abdominal part of the allantois is contained within the umbilical cord. At the end of gestation, the urachus is converted into a fibrous cord which courses between the extraperitoneal urinary bladder and the umbilicus as the median umbilical ligament. Persistence of a part or all of the urachus may result in the formation of a vesicocutaneous fistula with the appearance of urine at the umbilicus, an extraperitoneal urachal cyst presenting as a lower abdominal mass, or an urachal sinus with the drainage of a small amount of mucus. Proper treatment is excision of the urachal remnant with closure of the bladder, if necessary.

Acquired Abnormalities of the Abdominal Wall

Diastasis Recti

- Diastasis recti refers to a thinning of the linea alba in the epigastrium and is manifested in a midline protrusion of the anterior abdominal wall. The transversalis fascia is intact and hence this is not a hernia.

● Appropriate management consists of reassurance of the patient and the family regarding the innocuous nature of this condition.

Anterior Abdominal Wall Hernias

● Epigastric hernias occur at sites through which vessels and nerves perforate the linea alba to course into the subcutaneum. Through these openings extraperitoneal areolar tissue and, at times, peritoneum may herniate into the subcutaneous tissue. Although these hernias are often small, they may produce significant localized pain and tenderness resulting from direct pressure of the hernia sac and its contents on the nerves emerging through the same fascial opening.

● Spigelian hernias occur through the fascia in the region of the semilunar line and present with localized pain and tenderness and rarely a palpable mass. The hernia sac is often small, tends to remain beneath the external oblique aponeurosis, and is only rarely palpable. Sonography of the abdominal wall or computed tomography (CT) with thin cuts through the abdomen, after careful marking of the suspected site, may be diagnostic. Treatment consists of simple operative closure of the fascial defect.

Rectus Sheath Hematoma

● Bleeding into the rectus sheath may result from blunt or penetrating injuries to the abdominal wall, including needle punctures during paracentesis or injections, violent contraction or stretching of the rectus muscle during sneezing or coughing, or less commonly spontaneously in patients receiving anticoagulants.

● Above the semicircular line, the rectus sheath tamponades the bleeding, thus limiting expansion of the hematoma. In this instance, localized abdominal pain and tenderness are relatively early findings. Below the semicircular line, the posterior rectus muscle is covered only by the transversalis fascia and the readily distensible preperitoneal layer of fatty areolar tissue. This allows expansion of the hematoma to a much larger size before the occurrence of symptoms. Most rectus sheath hematomas occur in the lower abdomen.

● Abdominal pain is the most common symptom associated with rectus sheath hematomas. It is often severe in nature and exacerbated by movements that require muscular contraction of the abdominal wall. Physical examination will demonstrate tenderness over the rectus sheath, often with voluntary guarding. A diffuse mass, or fullness, may be noted in thin patients; however, in others this will not be discernible.

- Ultrasonography or CT will confirm the presence of the hematoma and localize it to the abdominal wall in nearly all cases. The management of patients with rectus sheath hematomas depends on the etiology and the nature of the hematoma (i.e., whether there is evidence of continued hemorrhage or the hematoma is stable). In general, coagulopathies should be corrected; however, continued anticoagulation of selected patients may be prudent depending on the indications for anticoagulation and the seriousness of the hemorrhage. For patients in whom the hematoma is stable, pain medication and avoidance of abdominal wall muscular strain is usually sufficient. Progression of the hematoma necessitates operative evacuation and hemostasis.

Malignancies of the Abdominal Wall

- The two most common primary malignancies of the abdominal wall are desmoid tumors and sarcomas.

Desmoid Tumor

- Desmoid tumor, sometimes referred to as aggressive fibromatosis, is an uncommon neoplasm that occurs sporadically or as part of an inherited syndrome, most notably, familial adenomatous polyposis (FAP). The tumor may arise from fascia or muscle and has been classified as superficial (fascial) or deep (musculoaponeurotic). The superficial disease, also known as Dupuytren's fibromatosis, is slow growing, small in size, and rarely involves deeper structures. Deep fibromatosis has a relatively rapid growth rate, often attains a large size, has a high rate of local recurrence, and involves the musculature of the trunk and extremities. Desmoid tumors are also classified as extra-abdominal (e.g., shoulder girdle), abdominal wall, and intra-abdominal (mesenteric and pelvic desmoid). Most spontaneous desmoid tumors occur at the shoulder girdle or the abdominal wall, whereas intra-abdominal desmoids, especially mesenteric desmoids, are more common in patients with FAP.
- In the general population, desmoid tumors occur with a frequency of 2.4 to 4.3 cases per million people; this risk is increased 1000-fold in patients with FAP. Typically, abdominal

wall desmoid tumors occur in young women during gestation or, more frequently, within a year of childbirth.

- There is also often a temporal association between the development of this neoplasm and an antecedent history of abdominal trauma or operation.

- Patients with desmoid tumors present with a painless enlarging mass. Local symptoms may arise from compression of adjacent organs or neurovascular structures. Magnetic resonance imaging (MRI) provides information regarding the extent of the disease and its relationship to intra-abdominal organs.

- After MRI, an incisional biopsy or a core needle biopsy should be performed.

- The treatment of abdominal wall desmoids is complete resection with a tumor-free margin. Even with tumor-free margins the local recurrence rate approaches 40%. Although multiple local recurrences are unfortunately common, systemic metastases are extremely rare. The role for radiation therapy in the management of desmoid tumors either as an adjunct to surgery or as primary treatment is evolving.

- Antiproliferative agents and cytotoxic chemotherapy have been used to palliate the aggressive nature of desmoid tumors with variable results. The two most widely used groups of noncytotoxic drugs are nonsteroidal anti-inflammatory drugs (NSAIDS) and antiestrogens.

Abdominal Wall Sarcoma

- Truncal sarcomas (including both chest and abdominal wall) account for about 10% of sarcomas. Histologic subtypes include liposarcoma, fibrosarcoma, rhabdomyosarcoma, leiomyosarcoma, and malignant fibrous histiocytoma. The clinical behavior of these tumors is determined more by anatomic site, grade, and size than by specific histologic pattern. Similar to desmoid tumors, abdominal wall sarcomas present as a painless mass.

- Clinical characteristics that suggest an abdominal wall malignancy are (1) nonreducible lesions arising from below the superficial fascia, (2) size greater than 5 cm, (3) recent increase in size, (4) fixation to the abdominal wall, and (5) fixation to organs in the abdomen.

- MRI will provide information regarding the location and extent of these neoplasms and involvement of contiguous structures. However, definitive diagnosis requires biopsy, which may be performed with a core needle or by incision.

- The treatment for these malignancies is resection with a tumor-free margin. Reconstruction of the abdominal wall defect may be accomplished primarily, with myocutaneous flaps, or with prosthetic meshes, depending on the site and extent of resection.

Symptoms of Intra-abdominal Diseases Referred to the Abdominal Wall

- Abdominal pain may be categorized as visceral, somatoparietal, and referred. Visceral pain is caused by stimulation of visceral nociceptors by inflammation, distention, or ischemia. The pain is dull in nature and poorly localized to the epigastrium, periumbilical regions, or hypogastrium depending on the embryonic origin of the organ involved. Inflammation of the stomach, duodenum, and biliary tract (derivatives of the embryonic foregut) localizes visceral pain to the epigastrium. Stimulation of nociceptors in midgut derived organs (i.e., small intestine, appendix, and right colon) cause the sensation of pain in the periumbilical region, whereas inflammation or distention of hindgut-derived organs (left colon and rectum) causes hypogastric pain. The pain is felt in the midline because these organs transmit sympathetic sensory afferents to both sides of the spinal cord. The pain is poorly localized because the innervation of most viscera is multi-segmental and contains fewer nerve receptors than highly sensitive organs such as the skin. The pain is often characterized as cramping, burning, or gnawing and may be accompanied by secondary autonomic effects such as sweating, restlessness, nausea, vomiting, perspiration, and pallor.
- Somatoparietal pain arises from inflammation of the parietal peritoneum and is more intense and more precisely localized than visceral pain. The nerve impulses mediating parietal pain travel within the somatic sensory spinal nerves and reach the spinal cord in the peripheral nerves corresponding to the cutaneous dermatomes from the sixth thoracic to the first lumbar region. Lateralization of parietal pain is possible because only one side of the nervous system innervates a given part of the parietal peritoneum.
- Referred pain.

PERITONEUM AND PERITONEAL CAVITY

Embryology

Anatomy

- The peritoneum consists of a single sheet of simple squamous epithelium of mesodermal origin, termed mesothelium, lying on a thin connective tissue stroma. The surface area is 1.0 to 1.7 m^2, approximately that of the total body surface area.

- The peritoneal membrane is divided into parietal and visceral components. The parietal peritoneum covers the anterior, lateral, and posterior abdominal wall surfaces and the inferior surface of the diaphragm and the pelvis. The visceral peritoneum covers most of the surface of the intra-peritoneal organs and the anterior aspect of the retro-peritoneal organs.

- The peritoneal cavity is subdivided into interconnected com-partments or spaces by 11 ligaments and mesenteries. The peritoneal ligaments or mesenteries include the coronary, gastrohepatic, hepatoduodenal, falciform, gastrocolic, duo-denocolic, gastrosplenic, splenorenal, and phrenicocolic ligaments and the transverse mesocolon and small bowel mesentery. These structures partition the abdomen into nine potential spaces: right and left subphrenic, subhepatic, supramesenteric and inframesenteric, right and left paracolic gutters, pelvis, and lesser space. These ligaments, mesenter-ies, and peritoneal spaces direct the circulation of fluid in the peritoneal cavity and thus may be useful in predicting the route of spread of infectious and malignant diseases.

Physiology

- The peritoneum is a bidirectional, semipermeable mem-brane that controls the amount of fluid within the peritoneal cavity, promotes the sequestration and removal of bacteria from the peritoneal cavity, and facilitates the migration of inflammatory cells from the microvasculature into the peri-toneal cavity.

- The circulation of fluid within the peritoneal cavity is driven in part by the movement of the diaphragm. Intercellular pores in the peritoneum covering the inferior surface of the diaphragm.

- Communicate with lymphatic pools within the diaphragm. Lymph flows from these diaphragmatic lymphatic channels via subpleural lymphatics to the regional lymph nodes and ultimately the thoracic duct.

- Contraction of the diaphragm during inhalation propels the lymph through the mediastinal lymphatic channels into the thoracic duct. It is postulated that this "diaphragmatic pump" drives the movement of peritoneal fluid in a cephalad direc-tion toward the diaphragm and into the thoracic lymphatic vessels.

Ascites

Pathophysiology and Etiology

- Ascites is the pathologic accumulation of fluid within the peritoneal cavity. The principal causes of ascites formation and their pathophysiologic basis are listed in Box 40–1. Cirrhosis is an important cause of ascites in the United States.
- Ascites occurs in the absence of cirrhosis in about 15% to 20% of patients. Increased portal venous pressure resulting from obstruction of the portal venous system in the absence of cirrhosis causes the transudation of fluid across the mesenteric and intestinal wall into the peritoneal cavity. A similar pressure-based mechanism is operative in instances of cardiac failure, although in the latter cases there is also profound sodium and water retention resulting from the release of vasopressin and activation of the renin-aldosterone and sympathetic nervous systems.

Clinical Presentation

- The diagnosis of ascites is made on the basis of the medical history and the appearance of the abdomen. Risk factors for hepatitis or cirrhosis should be carefully sought by questioning patients about alcohol or intravenous drug use, blood transfusions, sex with a member of the same sex, acupuncture, tattoos, or ear or body piercing. Long-standing obesity is associated with nonalcoholic steatohepatitis, an important cause of cirrhosis in the United States.
- A full, bulging abdomen with dullness of the flanks on percussion is consistent with the presence of ascites.
- Physical evidence of cirrhosis should be sought including palmar erythema, large dilated abdominal wall collateral veins, and multiple spider angiomata. Patients with cardiac ascites should have impressive jugular venous distention and other evidence of congestive heart failure.

Ascitic Fluid Analysis

- Paracentesis with ascitic fluid analysis is the most rapid and cost-effective method of determining the etiology of ascites. Paracentesis should be performed and ascitic fluid analyzed in all patients with new onset of ascites. The occurrence of symptoms, signs, or laboratory evidence of infection (e.g., abdominal pain or tenderness, fever, encephalopathy, hypotension, renal failure, acidosis, or leukocytosis) in patients with

---

Box 40–1.   Principal Causes of Ascites Formation Categorized According to Their Underlying Pathophysiology

Portal Hypertension
Cirrhosis
Noncirrhotic
  Prehepatic portal venous obstruction
    Chronic mesenteric venous thrombosis
    Multiple hepatic metastases
  Posthepatic venous obstruction
    Budd-Chiari syndrome

Cardiac
Congestive heart failure
Chronic pericardial tamponade
Constrictive pericarditis

Malignancy
Peritoneal carcinomatosis
  Primary peritoneal malignancies
    Primary peritoneal mesothelioma
    Serous carcinoma
  Metastatic carcinoma
    Gastrointestinal carcinomas (e.g., gastric, colonic, and
      pancreatic cancer)
    Genitourinary carcinomas (e.g., ovarian cancer)
Retroperitoneal obstruction of lymphatic channels
  Lymphoma
  Lymph node metastases (e.g., testicular cancer,
    melanoma)
  Obstruction of the lymphatic channels at the base of the
    mesentery
  Gastrointestinal carcinoid tumors

Miscellaneous
Bile ascites
  Iatrogenic after operations of the liver and/or biliary tract
  Traumatic after injuries to the liver and/or biliary tract
Pancreatic ascites
  Acute pancreatitis
  Pancreatic pseudocyst
Chylous ascites
  Disruptions of retroperitoneal lymphatic channels
    Iatrogenic during retroperitoneal dissections

Box 40–1. **Principal Causes of Ascites Formation Categorized According to Their Underlying Pathophysiology—cont'd**

Retroperitoneal lymphadenectomy
Abdominal aortic aneurysmorrhaphy
Blunt or penetrating trauma
Malignancy
Obstruction of retroperitoneal lymphatic channels
Obstruction of lymphatic channels at the base of the mesentery
Congenital lymphatic abnormalities
Primary lymphatic hypoplasia
Peritoneal infections
Tuberculous peritonitis
Myxedema
Nephrotic syndrome
Serositis in connective tissue disease

---

ascites should also prompt paracentesis with ascitic fluid analysis.

● Abdominal paracentesis can be performed safely in most patients including those with cirrhosis and mild coagulopathy.

● Paracentesis is performed most commonly in the lower abdomen with the left lower quadrant preferred over the right. Ultrasound guidance may be particularly useful in obese patients and in those with laparotomy scars and potential intra-abdominal adhesions.

● The most valuable laboratory tests on ascitic fluid include the cell count and differential and the ascitic fluid albumin and total protein concentrations. The leukocyte count in uncomplicated cirrhotic ascites is usually less than 500 cells/mm^3 with about half of these cells being neutrophils. More than 250 neutrophils/mm^3 of ascitic fluid suggests an acute inflammatory process, the most common of which is spontaneous bacterial peritonitis (SBP). In this instance, both the total white blood cell count and the absolute neutrophil count are elevated, and neutrophils usually account for more than 70% of the total cell count.

● The serum–ascites albumin gradient (SAAG) is the most reliable method to categorize the various causes of ascites. The SAAG is calculated by measuring the albumin concentration of serum and ascitic fluid specimens and subtracting the ascitic fluid value from the serum value. If the SAAG is greater than or equal to 1.1 g/dL, the patient has portal hypertension; a SAAG less than 1.1 g/dL is consistent with the absence of portal hypertension.

- The accuracy of this measurement in predicting the presence or absence of portal hypertension is about 97%.

Management of Ascites in Cirrhotics

- For those patients in whom alcohol is an important factor in the pathogenesis of their cirrhosis, it is important to convince the patient to stop drinking alcohol. Over a period of months, abstinence can allow healing of the reversible component of their liver disease and the ascites may resolve or become more responsive to medical management. The mainstays of medical management of ascites are dietary sodium restriction and diuretics.

Management of Refractory Ascites in Cirrhotics

- Refractory ascites refers to that which is unresponsive to sodium restriction and high-dose diuretic treatment, a situation occurring in less than 10% of patients with ascites resulting from cirrhosis. Current therapeutic options these patients includes liver transplantation, serial therapeutic paracentesis, transjugular intrahepatic portosystemic stent shunt, and peritoneovenous shunts.

Chylous Ascites

- Chylous ascites is the collection of chyle in the peritoneal cavity and may result from one of three principal mechanisms: (1) obstruction of the major lymphatic channels at the base of the mesentery or the cisterna chyli with exudation of chyle from dilated mesenteric lymphatics, (2) direct leakage of chyle through a lymphoperitoneal fistula due to abnormal or injured retroperitoneal lymphatic vessels, and (3) exudation of chyle through the walls of retroperitoneal megalymphatics without a visible fistula or thoracic duct obstruction.
- In adults, the most common cause of chylous ascites is an intra-abdominal malignancy producing obstruction of the lymphatic channels at the base of the mesentery or in the retroperitoneum. Lymphoma is the most common malignancy associated with chylous ascites.
- In children, chylous ascites is most often due to congenital lymphatic abnormalities such as primary lymphatic hypoplasia resulting in lower extremity lymphedema, chylothorax, and

chylous ascites. Chylous ascites may also result from division or injury of the retroperitoneal lymphatics during operative procedures such as aortic procedures and retroperitoneal lymph node dissections. Finally, blunt and penetrating traumatic injuries are also important causes of chylous ascites, particularly in children.

- Patients with chylous ascites most often present with painless abdominal distention. Malnutrition and dyspnea occur in about 50% of cases. Paracentesis yields a characteristic milky-appearing ascitic fluid with a high protein and fat content. The SAAG will be less than 1.1 mg/dL and the triglyceride level will be greater than that of plasma, often two to eight times that of plasma.

- Management of patients with chylous ascites includes the maintenance or improvement of nutrition, reduction in the rate of chyle formation, and correction of the underlying disease process.

- Paracentesis may be used to temporarily relieve the dyspnea and abdominal discomfort associated with chylous ascites; however, repeated paracentesis leads to hypoproteinemia and malnutrition. Experience with peritoneovenous shunts to treat chylous ascites has generally been disappointing because of a variety of complications not the least of which is rapid shunt occlusion by the highly viscous chyle. Surgical exploration of the abdomen and the retroperitoneum is recommended for those patients failing to improve with nonoperative management, an occurrence in as many as 50% to 66% of patients.

Peritonitis

- Peritonitis is inflammation of the peritoneum and peritoneal cavity and is most commonly due to a localized or generalized infection. Primary peritonitis results from bacterial, chlamydial, fungal, or mycobacterial infection in the absence of a perforation of the gastrointestinal tract, whereas secondary peritonitis occurs in the setting of gastrointestinal perforation.

Spontaneous Bacterial Peritonitis

- SBP is defined as a bacterial infection of ascitic fluid in the absence of an intra-abdominal, surgically treatable source of infection. Although most commonly associated with cirrhosis, SBP may also occur in patients with nephrotic syndrome and less commonly congestive heart failure. It is extremely rare for patients in whom the ascitic fluid has a high protein concentration to develop SBP, such as those with peritoneal carcinomatosis. The most common pathogens in adults with SBP are the aerobic enteric flora *Escherichia coli* and *Klebsiella pneumoniae.* In children with nephrogenic or hepatogenic ascites, Group A *Streptococcus, Staphylococcus aureus,* and *Streptococcus pneumonia* are common isolates.

- The diagnosis of SBP is made initially by demonstrating greater than or equal to 250 neutrophils/mm^3 of ascitic fluid in a clinical setting consistent with this diagnosis (i.e., abdominal pain, fever, and/or peripheral leukocytosis in a patient with low-protein ascites). It is very unusual to document bacterascites on Gram stain of ascitic fluid and delay of appropriate antibiotic management until the ascitic fluid cultures grow bacterial isolates risks the development of overwhelming infection and death.

- Broad-spectrum antibiotics, such as a third-generation cephalosporin, should be started immediately in patients suspected of having ascitic fluid infection. These agents cover about 95% of the flora most commonly associated with SBP.

- If the setting, symptoms, ascitic fluid analysis, or response to therapy are atypical, repeat paracentesis may be helpful in detecting secondary peritonitis. Multiple bacterial isolates, particularly of gram-negative enteric organisms, combined with a poor response to antibiotic therapy, suggests the presence of secondary peritonitis.

- The immediate mortality risk resulting from SBP is low, particularly if recognized and treated expeditiously. However, the development of other complications of hepatic failure including gastrointestinal hemorrhage or hepatorenal syndrome contribute to the death of many of these patients during the hospitalization in which SBP is detected. The occurrence of SBP is an important landmark in the natural history of cirrhosis with 1- and 2-year survival rates are about 30% and 20%, respectively.

Tuberculous Peritonitis

- Between 1953 and 1985 the number of cases of tuberculosis declined by about 5% per year. Since 1985, the numbers of cases of tuberculosis has increased dramatically especially in Hispanics, African Americans, immigrants, refugees, and individuals with acquired immunodeficiency syndrome (AIDS).

- Most cases of tuberculous peritonitis result from reactivation of latent peritoneal disease that had been previously established hematogenously from a primary pulmonary focus.

About one sixth of cases are associated with active pulmonary disease.

- Abdominal swelling resulting from ascites formation is the most common symptom, occurring in more than 80% of instances. Fever, weight loss, and abdominal pain are also commonly reported. Only about half of these patients will have an abnormal chest radiograph. The tuberculin skin test is positive in most cases. The ascitic fluid SAAG is less than 1.1 g/dL. Microscopic examination of the ascitic fluid will show erythrocytes and an increased number of leukocytes, most of which are lymphocytes.

- The diagnosis is best made by laparoscopy with directed biopsy of the peritoneum. This will provide a presumptive diagnosis in nearly 90% of cases. Laparotomy or laparoscopy will demonstrate multiple whitish nodules (<5 mm) scattered over the visceral and parietal peritoneum. Histologic examination will demonstrate caseating granulomas in nearly 90% of cases.

- Microscopic examination of ascitic fluid for acid-fast bacilli will identify the organism in less than 3% of cases. Similarly the frequency of positive ascites culture for *Mycobacterium tuberculosis* occurs in less than 20% of instances. Furthermore, it may take up to 8 weeks for the culture to yield definitive information, thus limiting its diagnostic usefulness.

- The treatment of peritoneal tuberculosis is antituberculous drugs. Drug regimens useful in treating pulmonary tuberculosis are also effective for peritoneal disease; isoniazid and rifampin daily for 9 months is a commonly used and effective regimen.

Peritonitis Associated with Chronic Ambulatory Peritoneal Dialysis (CAPD)

- In the United States, about 8% of patients with chronic renal failure undergo peritoneal dialysis. Peritonitis is one of the most common complications of CAPD, occurring with an incidence of approximately one episode every 1 to 3 years. Patients present with abdominal pain, fever, and cloudy peritoneal dialysate containing more than 100 leukocytes/mm^3 with more than 50% of the cells being neutrophils. Gram stain will detect organisms in only about 10% to 40% of cases. About 75% of infections are due to gram-positive organisms with *Staphylococcus epidermidis* accounting for 50% of cases. *S. aureus,* gram-negative enteric organisms, and fungal species are also important causes of peritonitis associated with CAPD.

- Peritonitis associated with CAPD is treated by the intraperitoneal administration of antibiotics with an appropriate antibacterial spectrum (e.g., first-generation cephalosporins). Ultimately, the most appropriate regimen must be based on the antibiotic sensitivities of the specific causative agents. Recurrent or persistent peritonitis requires removal of the dialysis catheter and resumption of hemodialysis.

Malignant Neoplasms of the Peritoneum

- Malignant neoplasms of the peritoneum may be classified as primary or secondary depending on the site of origin of the tumor. Primary malignancies of the peritoneum are rare and include malignant mesothelioma and its subtypes, serous tumors, malignant tumors of other Mullerian types, desmoplastic small round cell tumor, and sarcomas. Most malignancies of the peritoneum are transperitoneal metastases from a carcinoma of the gastrointestinal tract (especially the stomach, colon, and pancreas), the genitourinary tract (most commonly, ovarian), or, more rarely, an extra-abdominal site (e.g., breast). In its advanced stage, where metastatic cancer deposits diffusely coat the visceral and parietal peritoneum, these peritoneal metastases are referred to as carcinomatosis.

Malignant Peritoneal Mesothelioma

- The most common primary malignant peritoneal neoplasm is malignant mesothelioma.
- Patients present with abdominal pain, ascites, and weight loss. Fifty percent to 70% of patients will have a history of asbestos exposure.
- CT will demonstrate mesenteric thickening, peritoneal studding, hemorrhage within the tumor, and ascites. At laparotomy the ascitic fluid ranges from a serous transudate to a viscous fluid rich in mucopolysaccharides. The neoplasm tends to involve all peritoneal surfaces producing large masses of tumor. In contrast to pseudomyxoma peritonei, local invasion of intra-abdominal organs, such as the liver, intestine, bladder, and abdominal wall, is the rule.
- Complete surgical resection is rarely possible and most commonly operative intervention is used to provide palliation for intestinal obstruction.
- Intraperitoneal chemotherapy, including the use of cisplatin and mitomycin C, have been reported but with very limited success.

Pseudomyxoma Peritonei

- Pseudomyxoma peritonei is a rare malignant process of the peritoneal cavity that characteristically arises from a ruptured ovarian or appendiceal adenocarcinoma. In this disease, the peritoneum becomes coated with a mucus-secreting tumor that fills the peritoneal cavity with tenacious, semisolid mucus. Large, loculated cystic masses may also form within the abdomen.

- Pseudomyxoma peritonei is most prevalent in women between 50 and 70 years of age. It is often asymptomatic until very late in its course.

- Symptoms include abdominal pain and distention and numerous nonspecific symptoms. Physical examination reveals a distended abdomen with nonshifting dullness. On occasion, a palpable abdominal mass may be present, especially in tumors of appendiceal origin. CT may demonstrate posterior displacement of the small intestine, loculated collections of fluid density material, and scalloping of intra-abdominal organs resulting from extrinsic pressure of adjacent peritoneal implants. At laparotomy liters of yellowish- gray colored mucoid material are present on the omental and peritoneal surfaces.

- The management of these patients includes drainage of the mucus and intraperitoneal fluid and cytoreduction of the primary and secondary tumor implants including peritonectomy and omentectomy. For those tumors originating from an appendiceal adenocarcinoma, a right colectomy should be also performed. Ovarian malignances should be treated with total abdominal hysterectomy and bilateral salpingooophorectomy and cytoreduction.

- Postoperative adjuvant therapy has included the use of intraperitoneal 5-fluorouracil, mitomycin C, and cisplatin as well as intraperitoneal mucolytics, such as dextran sulphate and plasminogen activator (urokinase). Although the tumor will recur in approximately two thirds of patients, the slow progression of the disease results in 5- and 10-year survival rates of 50% and 20%, respectively.

MESENTERY AND OMENTUM

Embryology and Anatomy

Physiology

- The omentum and the intestinal mesentery are rich in lymphatics and blood vessels. The omentum contains areas with high concentrations of macrophages that may aid in the removal of foreign material and bacteria. Furthermore, the omentum becomes densely adherent to intraperitoneal sites of inflammation often preventing free peritonitis during instances of intestinal gangrene or perforation (e.g., acute diverticulitis or acute appendicitis).

Diseases of the Omentum

Omental Cysts

- Omental cysts are unilocular or multilocular cysts containing serous fluid that are thought to arise from congenital or acquired obstruction of omental lymphatic channels. They are lined by a lymphatic endothelium similar to that of cystic lymphangiomas. Most commonly omental cysts are discovered in children or young adults. Small cysts are often asymptomatic and discovered at the time of laparotomy for an unrelated problem, whereas larger cysts may present as a palpable abdominal mass. Uncomplicated cysts usually lie in the lower midabdomen and are freely moveable, smooth, and nontender. Complications are more common in children and include torsion, infection, or rupture.
- Ultrasound or CT will show a fluid-filled mass with internal septations, the differential diagnosis of which includes cysts and solid tumors of the mesentery, peritoneum, and retroperitoneum including desmoid tumors. Ultimately, the diagnosis is made by excision of the cyst and histologic examination of the wall. Local excision is curative.

Omental Torsion and Infarction

- Torsion of the greater omentum is defined as the axial twisting of the omentum along its long axis causing ischemia. This condition requires the omentum to be fixed in one point with the remainder of the structure redundant and free within the peritoneal cavity. If the twist is tight enough (or the venous obstruction is of sufficient duration) arterial inflow will become compromised leading to infarction and necrosis.
- Omental torsion occurs twice as often in men as women and is most frequent in patients in their fourth or fifth decade of life. Patients present with the acute onset of severe abdominal pain, which is localized to the right side of the abdomen in 80% of patients. Nausea and vomiting may be present but are not a predominant finding in these patients. There may be a moderate leukocytosis and the patient's temperature is

often normal or only slightly elevated. Physical examination demonstrates localized abdominal tenderness with guarding suggesting peritonitis. A mass may be palpable if the involved omentum is sufficiently large.

- Often the patient's clinical presentation will justify laparotomy at which time free serosanguineous fluid, a congested and inflamed portion of the omentum, and the absence of another pathologic condition will suggest the occurrence of omental torsion. Treatment consists of resection of the involved omentum and correction of any related condition.

Omental Neoplasms

- Primary malignancies of the omentum are extremely rare events and when they do occur they are most commonly of soft tissue origin. A more common scenario is involvement of the omentum by metastatic tumor spread transperitoneally from an intra-abdominal carcinoma. In an advanced stage, the omentum becomes replaced by the metastatic tumor resulting in the descriptive term "omental cake."

Omental Grafts and Transpositions

Diseases of the Mesentery

Mesenteric Cysts

- The most common non-neoplastic mesenteric cysts are termed mesothelial cysts based on the ultrastructure of the cells lining the cyst. The cysts contain either chyle or a clear serous fluid and may occur in the mesentery of either the small intestine (60%) or the colon (40%). These cysts occur most commonly in adults with a mean age of 45 years and are twice as common in women than in men. Depending on the size of the cyst, patients may present with complaints of abdominal pain, fever, and emesis. A midabdominal mass may be palpable on examination of the abdomen. The diagnosis can usually be made preoperatively with ultrasonography or CT. Enucleation of the cyst at laparotomy is curative and can usually be accomplished because the mesenteric blood vessels and the intestinal wall are usually not adherent to the cyst wall.

Acute Mesenteric Lymphadenitis

- Acute mesenteric lymphadenitis is a syndrome of acute right lower quadrant abdominal pain associated with mesenteric lymph node enlargement, and a normal appendix. Generally, the diagnosis is made on exploration of the abdomen of a patient suspected of having acute appendicitis at which time a normal appendix and enlarged mesenteric lymph nodes are discovered. This syndrome occurs most commonly in children and young adults and occurs with equal frequency in males and females.

- The symptom complex associated with acute mesenteric lymphadenitis is similar to acute appendicitis and includes the acute onset of periumbilical pain that shifts to the right lower quadrant over time. Physical examination demonstrates right lower quadrant tenderness with abdominal wall muscular rigidity and rebound tenderness. Nausea, vomiting, and anorexia may also be present but are not dominant symptoms. Generally, the patient's temperature and white blood cell count are normal or only slightly elevated.

- The diagnosis is made at the time of operation for presumed acute appendicitis at which time a normal appearing appendix is found with enlarged mesenteric lymph nodes. Excision of an enlarged lymph node with culture and nodal histology may provide information regarding the etiology but is not routinely used.

Mesenteric Panniculitis

- Mesenteric panniculitis is an inflammatory disease of the adipose tissue of the mesentery.

- The small bowel mesentery is most frequently involved although the mesocolon may also be affected. Grossly the disease is characterized by a thickened, hard, rubbery, or nodular mesentery or by multiple mesenteric masses of this consistency. The process most often involves the root of the small bowel mesentery and frequently encompasses the mesenteric vessels. In advanced cases, mesenteric venous and lymphatic obstruction may be present.

- Mesenteric panniculitis occurs most commonly in the fifth decade of life, but it has been reported in persons of nearly all ages. The disease is twice as common in males as females. Most patients present with abdominal pain, vomiting and abdominal swelling occur less commonly. Other complaints include anorexia, weight loss, constipation, diarrhea, and rectal bleeding. An abdominal mass is palpable in about half of patients; abdominal tenderness and/or distention, fever, and evidence of peritoneal irritation are present in a small number of cases.

- Laparotomy or laparoscopy with biopsy of the involved mesentery remains necessary for definitive diagnosis.
- Mesenteric panniculitis requires treatment only infrequently. Resection or bypass is necessary only in those instances associated with bowel obstruction. The prognosis in mesenteric panniculitis is good with lethal disease reported only rarely. In general abdominal pain continues or recurs in about 25% of patients after diagnosis.

Intra-abdominal (Internal) Hernias

Mesocolic (or Paraduodenal) Hernias

- Mesocolic hernias are unusual congenital hernias in which the small intestine herniates behind the mesocolon. They result from abnormal rotation of the midgut and have been categorized as either right or left. A right mesocolic hernia occurs when the prearterial limb of the midgut loop fails to rotate around the superior mesenteric artery. This results in the majority of the small intestine remaining to the right of the superior mesenteric artery. Normal counterclockwise rotation of the cecum and proximal colon into the right side of the abdomen and its fixation to the posterolateral peritoneum causes the small intestine to become trapped behind the mesentery of the right side of the colon. The ileocolic, right colic, and middle colic vessels lie within the anterior wall of the sac and the superior mesenteric artery courses along the medial border of the neck of the hernia.
- It is postulated that the left mesocolic hernia occurs as a consequence of *in utero* herniation of the small intestine between the inferior mesenteric vein and the posterior parietal attachments of the descending mesocolon to the retroperitoneum. The inferior mesenteric artery and vein are integral components of the hernia sac. About 75% of mesocolic hernias occur on the left side.
- The most common clinical presentation is that of small intestinal obstruction in which patients may present with symptoms of either acute or chronic small bowel obstruction. Barium radiographs will demonstrate displacement of the small intestine to the left or the right side of the abdomen. CT with intravenous contrast may demonstrate displacement of the mesenteric vessels.
- The operative management of patients with a right mesocolic hernia involves incision of the lateral peritoneal reflections along the right colon with reflection of the right colon and

cecum to the left. The entire gut then assumes a position simulating that of nonrotation of both the prearterial and postarterial segments of the midgut. Opening the neck of the hernia will injure the superior mesenteric vessels and fail to free the herniated bowel.

- The operative management of patients with a left mesocolic hernia consists of incision of the peritoneal attachments and adhesions along the right side of the inferior mesenteric vein with reduction of the herniated small intestine from beneath the inferior mesenteric vein. The vein is then allowed to return to its normal position on the left side of the base of the mesentery of the small intestine. The neck of the hernia may be closed by suturing the peritoneum adjacent to the vein to the retroperitoneum.

Malignancies of the Mesentery

- Similar to the peritoneum and omentum, the most common neoplasm involving the mesentery is metastatic disease from an intra-abdominal adenocarcinoma. This may result from the direct invasion of the primary tumor (or its lymphatic metastases) into the mesentery or from the transperitoneal spread of the malignancy into the mesentery. Distortion and fixation of the mesentery by the tumor itself or by the resultant desmoplastic reaction may cause intestinal obstruction. The most common primary malignancy of the mesentery is a desmoid tumor.

Mesenteric Desmoid

- Mesenteric desmoid accounts for less than 10% of sporadic desmoid tumors; however, it is a particularly common tumor in patients with FAP. In this group of patients, 70% of the desmoid tumors are intra-abdominal and one half to three fourths of these involve the mesentery. The association between desmoid tumor and FAP is particularly strong in that subset of patients with Gardner's syndrome. Patients with FAP and family history of desmoid tumors have a 25% chance of developing a desmoid tumor.
- Although mesenteric desmoid tumors tend to be aggressive, there is considerable variability in their growth rate during the course of the disease. In fact, the biology of intra-abdominal desmoid may be characterized by initial rapid growth followed by stability or even regression. However, mesenteric desmoid, by virtue of its relationship to vital structures and its ability to infiltrate adjacent organs, may cause significant

complications, including intestinal obstruction, ischemia and perforation, hydronephrosis, and even aortic rupture. Despite these complications the overall 10-year survival for patients with intra-abdominal desmoids can be as high as 60% to 70%.

- The treatment of choice is complete resection of tumor with margins free of the malignancy. The recurrence rate following resection has been reported to be between 60% and 85%. Given the high likelihood of recurrence and prolonged survival even in the setting of advanced disease, some authors have suggested that a trial of watchful waiting along with minimally toxic agents such as sulindac and antiestrogen therapy may be the best strategy, particularly in patients with minimal symptoms.

RETROPERITONEUM

Anatomy

Retroperitoneal Operative Approaches

- The aorta, vena cava, iliac vessels, kidneys, and adrenal glands may be approached operatively through the retroperitoneal space.
- Specific operative procedures performed through the retroperitoneum include extirpative procedures such as adrenalectomy and nephrectomy and aortic aneurysmorrhaphy and renal transplantation. The advantages to this approach over a transabdominal approach includes (1) less postoperative ileus facilitating a more rapid resumption of a diet, (2) no intra-abdominal adhesions thus decreasing the likelihood of subsequent small bowel obstruction, (3) less intraoperative evaporative fluid losses with less dramatic intravascular fluid shifts, and (4) fewer respiratory complications such as atelectasis and pneumonia.

Retroperitoneal Abscesses

- Retroperitoneal abscesses may be classified as primary if the infection results from hematogenous spread or secondary if it is related to an infection in an adjacent organ. The conditions associated with the development of retroperitoneal abscesses are shown in Table 40–1. Infections originating from the kidney and gastrointestinal tract most commonly underlie the development of retroperitoneal abscesses. Renal causes include infections related to renal lithiasis or previous urologic operative procedures. Gastrointestinal causes include appendicitis, diverticulitis, pancreatitis, and Crohn's disease.

TABLE 40–1.   Etiology and Relative Frequency of Retroperitoneal Abscesses

Etiology	Frequency (%)
Renal diseases	47
Gastrointestinal diseases, including diverticulitis, appendicitis, and Crohn's disease	16
Hematogenous spread from remote infections	11
Abscesses complicating operative procedures	8
Bone infections, including tuberculosis of the spine	7
Trauma	4.5
Malignancies	4
Miscellaneous causes	3

These data were compiled from three retrospective reviews of 134 patients treated between 1971 and 2001.

- The bacteriology of retroperitoneal abscesses is related to the etiology. Infections originating from the kidney are often monomicrobial and involve gram-negative rods such as *Proteus mirabilis* and *E. coli*. Retroperitoneal abscesses associated with diseases of the gastrointestinal tract involve *E. coli, Enterobacter* species, enterococcus, and anaerobic species such as *Bacteroides*. These infections often involve numerous bacterial species including gram-negative bacilli, enterococcus, and anaerobic species. Patients with infections from hematogenous spread are most commonly monomicrobial and related to *Staphylococcal* species. Tuberculosis of the spine is an important cause of retroperitoneal abscesses in immunocompromised individuals and those immigrating from underdeveloped countries.
- The most common symptoms include abdominal or flank pain (60% to 75%), fever and chills (30% to 90%), malaise (10% to 22%), and weight loss (12%). Patients with psoas abscesses may have referred pain to the hip, groin, or knee. The duration of symptoms is often greater than 1 week. Patients with retroperitoneal abscesses frequently have concurrent, chronic illnesses such as renal lithiasis, diabetes mellitus, human immunodeficiency virus infection, or malignancies.
- CT will demonstrate a low-density mass within the retroperitoneum with surrounding inflammation.
- Treatment of retroperitoneal abscesses includes appropriate antibiotics and adequate drainage. Many reports have demonstrated the efficacy of CT-guided drainage in managing this aspect of the treatment. In one recent study, 86% of

abscesses resolved with this approach. Operative drainage through a retroperitoneal approach is indicated for those lesions not amenable to percutaneous drainage or those lesions that fail percutaneous drainage.

Retroperitoneal Hematomas

- Retroperitoneal hematomas most commonly occur after blunt or penetrating injuries, in the setting of abdominal aortic or visceral artery aneurysms, with acute or chronic anticoagulation or fibrinolytic therapy.
- Patients present with abdominal or flank pain that may radiate into the groin, labia, or scrotum. Clinical evidence of acute blood loss may be present depending on the volume of blood lost and the rapidity in which the patient bled. A palpable abdominal mass may be present, as well as physical evidence of ileus. The complete blood count may provide evidence of subacute or chronic blood loss or platelet deficiency. The prothrombin and partial thromboplastin time may demonstrate a coagulopathy. Microscopic hematuria is a common finding on urinalysis. CT will establish the diagnosis by demonstrating a high-density mass in the retroperitoneum with surrounding stranding in the retroperitoneal tissue planes.
- Patients who develop retroperitoneal hematomas as a result of anticoagulation are best managed by the restoration of circulating blood volume and correction of the underlying coagulopathy. In rare circumstances, arteriography with embolization of a bleeding artery or operative exploration is required to stop the bleeding.

Retroperitoneal Fibrosis

- Retroperitoneal fibrosis is an uncommon inflammatory condition characterized by the proliferation of fibrous tissue in the retroperitoneum. Seventy percent of cases are idiopathic (termed Ormond's disease), whereas 30% are associated with various drugs (most notably, ergot alkaloids or dopaminergic agonists), infections, trauma, retroperitoneal hemorrhage or retroperitoneal operations, radiation therapy, or primary or metastatic neoplasms. Many of the idiopathic cases are associated with inflammatory abdominal aortic aneurysms or vasculitis syndromes. The fibrosis is usually confined to the central and paravertebral spaces between the renal arteries and sacrum and tends to encase the aorta, inferior vena cava, and ureters. The process usually begins at the level of the aortic bifurcation and spreads cephalad.

● Patients present with a vague constellation of symptoms including abdominal or flank pain, weight loss, malaise, and hypertension. Scrotal or leg edema caused by lymphatic obstruction may also be present. Laboratory tests will often provide evidence of renal insufficiency and anemia. Other laboratory abnormalities include an elevated erythrocyte sedimentation rate and an elevated C-reactive protein. The diagnosis is based on the patient's history and intravenous urography demonstrating hydronephrosis and hydroureter associated with delayed excretion and medial deviation of the ureters. Most commonly the disease is bilateral although unilateral cases do occur. CT without intravenous contrast will show a fibrous plaque that is usually isodense or slightly hyperdense compared with surrounding muscle.

● MRI of early benign retroperitoneal fibrosis may show areas of high signal intensity on T2-weighted images because of the abundant fluid content and hypercellularity associated with the acute inflammation. In the mature and quiescent stage of benign retroperitoneal fibrosis, the low signal intensity on both T1- and T2-weighted images is similar to that of psoas muscle.

● Malignant retroperitoneal fibrosis may result from direct spread of malignant cells entrapping the ureter or to multiple metastases causing a severe desmoplastic reaction in the retroperitoneum. Hence, differentiating malignant from benign fibrosis is important and requires multiple biopsies from the retroperitoneal fibrotic tissue.

● Primary, idiopathic retroperitoneal fibrosis is treated with ureteral stenting and immunosuppression including methylprednisolone, azathioprine, or penicillamine. Others have reported success with tamoxifen. Most secondary cases of retroperitoneal fibrosis are treated with midline transperitoneal ureterolysis with wrapping the ureter with an omental flap or lateral retroperitoneal ureteral transposition.

Retroperitoneal Malignancies

● Malignancies in the retroperitoneum may result from (1) extracapsular growth of a primary neoplasm of a retroperitoneal organ such as the kidney, adrenal, colon, or pancreas; (2) development of a primary germ cell neoplasm from embryonic rest cells; (3) development of a primary malignancy of the retroperitoneal lymphatic system (e.g., lymphoma); (4) metastases from a remote primary malignancy into a retroperitoneal lymph node (e.g., testicular cancer); and (5) development of a malignancy of the soft tissue of the retroperitoneum including sarcomas and desmoid tumors. The most common primary malignancy of the retroperitoneum is a sarcoma.

Retroperitoneal Sarcoma

- Most patients with retroperitoneal sarcomas present with an asymptomatic abdominal mass, often after the primary tumor has reached a considerable size. Abdominal pain is present in half of patients and less common symptoms, depending on the location of the tumor and the specific organs involved, include gastrointestinal hemorrhage, early satiety, nausea and vomiting, weight loss, and lower extremity swelling. Symptoms related to nerve compression by the tumor, such as lower extremity paresthesia and paresis, have also been associated with retroperitoneal sarcoma. CT and MRI will provide important information regarding size and precise location of the primary tumor and its relationship to major vascular structures, as well as the presence or absence of metastatic disease. Preoperative imaging studies will provide important clues to the diagnosis and hence a histologic diagnosis of sarcoma by CT-guided core biopsy is usually reserved for those lesions with a significant likelihood to be lymphoma or germ cell tumor.

- The goal of sarcoma treatment is the complete *en bloc* resection of the tumor and any involved adjacent organs. Lymph node metastases by sarcoma is rare (<5%), and hence radical lymphadenectomy is not indicated unless there is gross evidence of lymph node involvement at the time of resection. The most important prognostic variable is the ability to resect the neoplasm with a tumor-free resection margin (Table 40–2).

- Local recurrence after complete resection of retroperitoneal sarcoma is common, occurring in 40% to 80% of cases. There is no difference in the rate of local recurrence when comparing high-grade and low-grade sarcomas; however, the median time to recurrence is much shorter in high-grade than in low-grade sarcoma (15 months vs 42 months). Patients with high-grade sarcoma also have a higher risk for systemic disease and death than do those patients with low-grade sarcoma.

TABLE 40–2.   Outcomes in the Primary Resection of Retroperitoneal Sarcoma

Study	No. of Patients	Resectability (%)	Local Recurrence at 5 Yr (%)	Survival at 5 Yr (%)	Median Survival (mo)
Lewis et al, 1998	278	83	41	NR	72
Alvarenga et al, 1991	120	25	80	29	NR
Singer et al, 1995	83	NR	NR	54*	NR
Karakousis et al, 1996	57	100	42	66	NR

NR, not reported.
*Reported at 12 years.
From Lewis JJ, Leung D, Woodruff JM, Brennan ME: Retroperitoneal sarcoma: analysis of 500 patients treated and followed at a single institution. Ann Surg 228:355–365, 1998; Alvarenga JC, Ball AB, Fisher C: Limitations of surgery in the treatment of retroperitoneal sarcoma. Br J Surg 78:912–916, 1991; Singer S, Corson JM, Demmetri GD: Prognostic factors predictive of survival for truncal and retroperitoneal soft tissue sarcoma. Ann Surg 222:185–195, 1995; and Karakousis CP, Velez AF, Gerstenbluth R: Resectability and survival in retroperitoneal sarcomas. Ann Surg Oncol 3:150–158, 1996.

CHAPTER 41

HERNIAS

- A hernia is *reducible* when its contents can be replaced within the surrounding musculature, and *irreducible* or *incarcerated* when it cannot be reduced. A *strangulated* hernia.
- Richter s hernia.
- An *external* hernia protrudes through all layers of the abdominal wall, whereas an *internal* hernia is a protrusion of intestine through a defect within the peritoneal cavity.
- Inguinal hernias are classified as either *direct* or *indirect*.

INCIDENCE

- Both indirect inguinal and femoral hernias occur more commonly on the right side.
- Femoral hernias have the highest rate of strangulation (15% to 20%) of all hernias.

CLASSIFICATION OF GROIN HERNIAS

- Direct
- Indirect

DIAGNOSIS OF GROIN HERNIAS

- A bulge in the inguinal region remains the main diagnostic finding in most groin hernias.

EXAMINATION OF THE INGUINAL AREA FOR HERNIAS

- Patient standing, facing physician, who should sit.
- Visual inspection can reveal a loss of symmetry.
- Valsalva s maneuver or a cough may accentuate the bulge.
- Fingertips placed on abdominal wall while patient performs Valsalva s maneuver.
- Fingertip then placed in inguinal canal and Valsalva s maneuver repeated.
- Differentiation between indirect and direct hernias not essential.
- Examine in supine position, repeating above steps.

MANAGEMENT

Nonoperative Management of Inguinal Hernia

Most surgeons recommend operation upon discovery of an inguinal hernia, because the natural history of a groin hernia is that of progressive enlargement and weakening, with the potential for incarceration and strangulation.

Operative Repair of Inguinal Hernias

- Anterior repairs.
  - Anterior repairs are the most common operative approach for inguinal hernias.
- Iliopubic tract repair.
- Shouldice repair.
- Bassini repair.
- Cooper ligament (McVay) repair.
- The tension-free repair with mesh has become the dominant method of inguinal hernia repair.
- Posterior approaches.
- Preperitoneal repair.
- Laparoscopic management of inguinal hernias.

FEMORAL HERNIA

- A femoral hernia produces a mass or bulge *below* the inguinal ligament.

SPECIAL PROBLEMS

- Sliding hernia.
  - The primary danger associated with a sliding hernia is the failure to recognize the visceral component of the hernia sac before injury to the bowel or bladder.
- Recurrent hernias.
  - Recurrences after anterior hernia repair using mesh are best managed by a posterior approach and placement of a second prosthesis.
- Strangulated hernias.
- Bilateral hernias.

UMBILICAL HERNIA

- Umbilical hernias in adults are largely acquired. These hernias occur more frequently in women and in patients with conditions that result in increased intra-abdominal pressure, such as pregnancy, obesity, ascites, or abdominal distention.

EPIGASTRIC HERNIA

- Incisional and ventral hernia.
- Incisional hernias occur as a result of excessive tension and inadequate healing of a previous incision, which is often associated with surgical site infections.

UNUSUAL HERNIAS

- Spigelian hernia.
  - A Spigelian hernia occurs through the Spigelian fascia, which is composed of the aponeurotic layer between the rectus muscle medially and the semilunar line laterally. Nearly all Spigelian hernias occur at or below the arcuate line.
- Obturator hernia.
- Lumbar hernia.
- Interparietal hernia.
- Sciatic hernia.
- Perineal hernia.

COMPLICATIONS

- Surgical site infection.
  - Most would agree that there is no need to use routine antimicrobial prophylaxis for hernia repair.
- Nerve injuries.
  - Laparoscopic nerve injuries are minimized by not placing any tacks or staples below the lateral portion of the ilio-pubic tract.
- Ischemic orchitis.
- Injury to the vas deferens and viscera.
- Hernia recurrence.
- Quality of life.

CHAPTER 42

ACUTE ABDOMEN

- The term *acute abdomen* designates symptoms and signs of intra-abdominal disease usually treated best by surgical operation.
- Abdominal pain accounts for 5% to 10% of all emergency department visits or 5 to 10 million patient encounters in the United States annually.
- Hospitalized patients may develop abdominal pain during the course of their illness making diagnosis and treatment more difficult.

ANATOMY AND PHYSIOLOGY

Developmental Anatomy

- The developmental anatomy of the abdominal cavity and of its viscera determines normal structure and influences the pathogenesis and clinical manifestations of most abdominal diseases.
- When visceral inflammation irritates the parietal peritoneal surface, localization of pain occurs. Maneuvers that exacerbate this irritation then intensify the pain. The many "peritoneal signs" useful in the clinical diagnosis of the acute abdomen originate in this fashion.
- Sensory afferents involved with intraperitoneal abdominal pain transmit dull, sickening, poorly localized pain of more gradual onset and protracted duration.
- Cutting, tearing, crushing, or burning usually does not produce pain in the abdominal viscera. However, stretching or distention of the peritoneum produces pain. Bacterial or chemical peritoneal inflammation produces visceral pain, as does ischemia.
- *Visceral pain* is dull and poorly localized, usually in the epigastrium, periumbilical region, or suprapubic region, and it usually does not lateralize well.
- The *parietal* or *somatic pain* associated with intra-abdominal disorders may be more intense and precisely localized. *Referred pain* is perceived at a site distant from the source of stimulus.

Peritoneal Pathophysiology

- This loss of fluid from the circulation may lead to dehydration and may produce the clinical signs of resting or orthostatic hypotension and tachycardia.
- Thus, subdiaphragmatic, subhepatic, paracolic, or pelvic fluid collections can accompany visceral perforation.
- The fibrinous surface thus created, aided by decreased intestinal movement, causes adherence between bowel and omentum and effectively walls off inflammation.
- *Primary* or *spontaneous peritonitis* can occur as a diffuse bacterial infection without an obvious intra-abdominal source of contamination.
- The more common secondary peritonitis results from perforation, infection, or gangrene of an intra-abdominal organ, usually of the gastrointestinal tract.
- The syndrome of poorly localized intra-abdominal infection, an altered microbial flora, progressive organ dysfunction, and high mortality define tertiary peritonitis.
- Physical findings of patients with peritonitis are abdominal tenderness, guarding, and rebound tenderness.

CLINICAL DIAGNOSIS

History and Present Illness

- *Pain* is the focal issue in the evaluation of the patient suspected of having an acute abdomen.
- In an evaluation of the location of the pain, the concept of referred pain becomes important.
- Migratory pain shifting from one place to another can give insight into the diagnosis.
- The initial manifestations of the acute abdomen and the evolution of the pain syndrome may give some insight into the cause of the pain.
- The quality, severity, and periodicity of the pain may provide clues to the diagnosis.
- *Radiation of pain* or referral of pain may help in diagnosis.
- Generally, patients with abdominal pain requiring surgical treatment experience the pain before vomiting occurs.
- Most patients with acute abdominal pain have no desire to eat.
- A careful menstrual history is important in women with abdominal pain.

- Corticosteroids also immunosuppress patients and obscure the manifestations of acute intra-abdominal disease.

Physical Examination

- Examination of the abdomen always begins with inspection, with particular attention to scars, hernias, masses, or abdominal wall defects.
- *Palpation* is a crucial step in evaluating the patient with acute abdominal pain.
- The detection of increased abdominal muscle tone during palpation is called *guarding*.
- *Rebound tenderness* is also a sign of peritonitis.

Laboratory Testing

- Intra-abdominal inflammation can produce elevation in the white blood cell count, although this is not always true.
- Measurements of serum amylase and lipase may help in the evaluation of upper abdominal pain by giving evidence of pancreatitis.
- Women of childbearing age who have acute abdominal pain or hypotension should have measurement of the serum or urine beta-human chorionic gonadotropin concentration.

Diagnostic Imaging

- An upright chest x-ray film can detect under the diaphragm as little as 1 mL of air injected into the peritoneal cavity.
- The characteristics of small bowel obstruction include multiple air-fluid levels in dilated, centrally located loops of intestine with visible valvulae conniventes and an absence or paucity of colon gas. Obstructed colon usually appears as peripherally located distended bowel with haustral markings. If the ileocecal valve is incompetent, colon obstruction will cause distention of the distal small bowel.
- The radiographic findings of paralytic ileus include excessive distention and fluid with gas distributed from stomach to rectum.
- Although history and physical examination provide essential information in evaluating patients with the acute abdomen, modern imaging techniques, including ultrasound and computed tomography (CT), can lead to an anatomic diagnosis in most cases.

CLINICAL MANAGEMENT

Differential Diagnosis

- Because appendicitis is a common disease, it must remain in the differential diagnosis of any patient with persistent abdominal pain, particularly right lower quadrant pain.

Decision to Operate

- Certain indications for surgical treatment exist. For example, definite signs of peritonitis such as tenderness, guarding, and rebound tenderness support the decision to operate (Fig. 42–1). Likewise, severe or increasing localized abdominal tenderness should prompt an operation. Patients with abdominal pain and signs of sepsis that cannot be explained by any other finding should undergo operation. Those patients suspected of having acute intestinal ischemia should be operated on after complete evaluation.
- Patients presenting with abdominal pain and free intra-abdominal gas seen on x-ray film warrant operation except for limited exceptions (Fig. 42–2).
- Some patients with clear findings of the acute abdomen may be treated without surgical operation.

Preoperative Preparation

- Unstable patients must have more careful evaluation and resuscitation before one proceeds to surgical intervention.

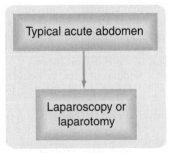

■ FIGURE 42–1.   Patients with unrelenting abdominal pain, tenderness, guarding, and rebound should undergo laparoscopy or laparotomy following suitable resuscitation and preparation.

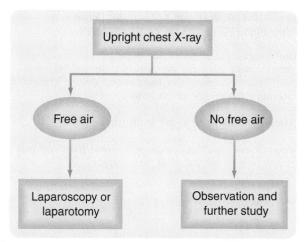

FIGURE 42-2. Most patients with free air in the peritoneal cavity should undergo laparoscopy or laparotomy following suitable resuscitation and preparation.

ACUTE VISCERAL ISCHEMIA

- Abdominal pain out of proportion to the abdominal physical findings should raise a question about this diagnosis.

ACUTE ABDOMINAL PAIN

During Pregnancy

- Appendicitis occurs once in 1500 pregnancies, evenly distributed in the trimesters.
- Cholecystectomy has been performed in 3% to 8% of 10,000 pregnancies.

The Patient in the Medical Intensive Care Unit

- Patients in the medical intensive care unit who develop abdominal pain while undergoing treatment for another primary condition pose a common and very difficult management challenge.

ACQUIRED IMMUNODEFICIENCY SYNDROME (AIDS), IMMUNOSUPPRESSION, AND THE ACUTE ABDOMEN

● The diagnosis and treatment of acute abdominal pain in patients with immune deficiency pose special problems. One must recognize the immunosuppressed patient and determine the degree of immunosuppression.

NONSURGICAL CAUSES OF ACUTE ABDOMINAL PAIN

● Many diseases produce acute abdominal pain and may be treated best by means other than surgery.

CHAPTER 43

ACUTE GASTROINTESTINAL HEMORRHAGE

- In the United States, 1% to 2% of acute hospital admissions are for patients requiring evaluation and treatment of gastrointestinal hemorrhage. Although the overall mortality rate for these patients ranges from 5% to 12%, the mortality rate in patients with persistent or recurring hemorrhage approaches 40%. Mortality is linked not only to the degree of hemorrhage but also, more importantly, to the coexisting medical conditions in the patient with hemorrhage.

- More than 85% of major bleeding episodes can be linked to one of four diagnoses: peptic ulcer disease, variceal hemorrhage, colonic diverticulosis, or angiodysplasia.

- Only advancing age appears to be a risk factor for hemorrhage that applies across the full spectrum of bleeding conditions of the intestinal tract. Up to half of patients with acute gastrointestinal hemorrhage are older than 60 years.

- In all patients, regardless of bleeding source, successful initial management requires that the treating physician be mindful of the potential severity of gastrointestinal hemorrhage. Appropriate resuscitation to restore volume and red blood cell deficits is critical in patients with major hemorrhage. This resuscitation phase must be followed by rapid diagnosis of the source of bleeding. Thereafter, institution of appropriate specific therapies may be offered to effect successful management.

INITIAL EVALUATION AND TREATMENT OF PATIENTS WITH ACUTE GASTROINTESTINAL HEMORRHAGE

- Initial management of a patient with acute gastrointestinal hemorrhage has four primary goals: (1) comprehensive patient assessment, with attention to hemodynamic status and identification of significant medical comorbidities; (2) institution of appropriate resuscitation and monitoring;

(3) identification of the major source of gastrointestinal bleeding; and (4) institution of specific therapeutic interventions to stop or control the bleeding.

Goal 1: Initial Patient Assessment

History and Physical Examination

- The essential elements to be ascertained are the characteristics of the bleeding, the onset and duration of bleeding (hours or days antecedent), the associated symptoms, the use of concurrent medications.

Characteristics of Bleeding

- Acute gastrointestinal hemorrhage can present with hematemesis (vomiting of blood or bloody gastric contents), melena (passage of dark tarry or maroon stool), or hematochezia (passage of bright red blood from the rectum).
- Gastrointestinal bleeding that is slow or intermittent is usually not evident to the patient hence the term *occult* is associated with this pattern of blood loss. Such patients present to primary care venues with secondary signs of slow blood loss, such as anemia or fatigue.
- Hematemesis is diagnostic of upper gastrointestinal bleeding, that is, bleeding from the esophagus, stomach, or duodenum. Rarely, hematemesis may result from brisk hemorrhage from the nasal passages or pharynx when the patient swallows large volumes of blood.
- Melena can be indicative of either upper or lower gastrointestinal hemorrhage. Melena may also represent bleeding from lesions in the small bowel or right colon. Hematochezia is the characteristic sign of colonic hemorrhage and reflects rapid elimination of blood from the bowel. Ten percent of patients with very rapid upper gastrointestinal hemorrhage may also have a history of hematochezia and syncope.

Associated Symptoms

- A history of orthostatic dizziness or syncope indicates rapid and profound blood loss. Antecedent dyspepsia is suggestive of peptic ulcer disease; crampy abdominal pain is more consistent with upper gastrointestinal bleeding, whereas hematochezia is usually painless. Antecedent vomiting may suggest Mallory-Weiss tears; weight loss raises the possibility of malignancy.

Medications

- The risk for gastrointestinal ulceration and hemorrhage is elevated in patients taking salicylates or nonsteroidal anti-inflammatory drugs (NSAIDs).

Past Medical History

- A history of dysphagia or reflux esophagitis, recent gastrointestinal distress with vomiting, peptic ulceration, *Helicobacter pylori* infection, liver disease, alcohol abuse, inflammatory bowel disease, intestinal polyps, diverticulosis, or malignancy may point to the source of bleeding. Equally important is identification of comorbid medical conditions that alter the patient s ability to respond to hemorrhage. Complications and mortality are much more likely to occur in patients with a history of renal insufficiency, atherosclerotic cardiovascular disease, congestive heart failure, chronic respiratory conditions, preexisting liver disease, or central nervous system disability.

Physical Examination

- The major initial objective of the physical examination is to determine the degree of blood loss and volume depletion.
- Orthostatic vital signs should be checked in all patients not in shock by allowing the patient to sit up with the legs dangling for a period of 5 minutes.
- These signs are less reliable in elderly patients, who may show exaggerated postural changes or blunted changes in heart rate or are more likely to be using beta-blocker medication. All patients showing a volume deficit of greater than 20% of blood volume require prompt and aggressive resuscitation.

Initial Laboratory Assessment

- All patients with gastrointestinal hemorrhage should have basic laboratory testing, including hemoglobin and hematocrit, coagulation profile, liver function tests, serum electrolytes, and renal function. The initial hematocrit may not reflect the actual degree of hemorrhage.
- The finding of initial hemoglobin of less than 10 g per 100 mL is associated with an increased risk for morbidity and mortality. A specimen should also be sent to the blood bank for type and crossmatching.

Goal 2: Resuscitation

- Based on the estimated volume deficit, rapid restoration of intravascular volume is indicated. All patients with gastrointestinal hemorrhage should have two large-bore intravenous lines for administration of lactated Ringer s solution. Urine output should be monitored with a Foley catheter. Patients in shock should receive prompt transfusion of packed red blood cells if immediate response to electrolyte solutions is not evident. Patients with major hemorrhage; elderly patients; and patients with significant comorbidities including cardiac, pulmonary, hepatic, or renal insufficiency should be monitored with central venous or pulmonary artery catheters.
- Patients with massive hematemesis and mental obtundation are at high risk for pulmonary aspiration. These and hemodynamically unstable patients should have endotracheal intubation performed to protect the airway.

Goal 3: Identification of Source of Bleeding

- Successful management of a patient with acute gastrointestinal hemorrhage requires knowledge of the site of bleeding.
- Patients with hematemesis, melena, or hematochezia require emergency upper endoscopy by an endoscopist capable of therapeutic intervention. Airway protection may require endotracheal intubation.
- Patients presenting with melena and hematochezia without a history of hematemesis should have a nasogastric tube inserted to examine the gastric contents. Findings of blood-tinged secretions, coffee grounds, or guaiac-positive fluid should prompt upper endoscopy. Patients with melena and hematochezia with hemodynamic instability should have initial emergency upper endoscopy.
- Hemodynamically stable patients with hematochezia and patients with melena with a negative upper gastrointestinal examination may be presumed to have acute lower gastrointestinal hemorrhage.

Goal 4: Institution of Specific Therapy

- After resuscitation and identification of the source of bleeding, specific therapy can be instituted. For the 15% of patients with ongoing gastrointestinal hemorrhage and hemodynamic instability, the time interval until this intervention should be less than 2 hours, and all measures to provide ongoing support to avoid shock should be used during the interval.

ACUTE UPPER GASTROINTESTINAL HEMORRHAGE

Definition and Incidence

● Upper gastrointestinal bleeding is defined as bleeding from a source proximal to the ligament of Treitz. Acute upper gastrointestinal hemorrhage is a common and potentially deadly condition accounting for roughly 85% of hospital admissions for gastrointestinal bleeding. Peptic ulcer disease remains the most common cause, responsible for half of bleeding episodes. Esophageal and gastric varices secondary to portal hypertension of alcoholic cirrhosis constitutes the next most frequent source, identified in 10% to 20% of patients. Acute mucosal lesions, broadly characterized as gastritis or duodenitis, are observed in 15% to 30% of patients with hemorrhage in both urban and nonurban settings.

Clinical Presentations

● Hematemesis and melena are the most frequent clinical findings in significant upper gastrointestinal bleeding. However, massive bleeding from an upper source may be associated with hematochezia.

Endoscopy

● Endoscopy in the setting of acute hemorrhage carries specific risks compared with elective endoscopy.
● Arterial desaturation during the procedure occurs four times as frequently in patients undergoing emergency compared with elective upper endoscopy. Patients with hypotension have a decreased level of consciousness and are at increased risk for pulmonary aspiration.
● Careful airway protection is mandatory, and elective orotracheal intubation is often appropriate for these patients. Despite the risks, endoscopy is essential.

Bleeding Peptic Ulcer

● Of patients with peptic ulcer disease, 5% have hemorrhage as the initial manifestation of the condition, and up to 20% of patients with peptic ulcers develop bleeding at least once.
● Of ulcer deaths in the elderly, 80% occur as a consequence of an episode of acute hemorrhage.

Pathogenesis

- Bleeding ulcer is caused by acid-peptic erosion into the submucosal or extraluminal vessels.
- Patients using NSAIDs have a 15% to 20% greater risk for bleeding ulcer than patients with *H. pylori* infection, and NSAID use may be an independent indicator of adverse outcome. Only 1% to 2% of patients with ulcer disease develop the condition as a result of acid hypersecretion caused by gastrin-secreting endocrine tumors of the gastrointestinal tract (Zollinger-Ellison syndrome).

Clinical Prognostic Features

- Organ-specific complications, need for emergency surgery, and death are the primary factors cited as adverse outcomes after acute upper gastroduodenal hemorrhage. The primary factors associated with poor outcome are severe magnitude (rate and volume) of the initial hemorrhage; persistence or recurrence of major hemorrhage during the hospitalization for the acute hemorrhage; advanced age, generally older than 60 years; and presence of medical comorbid conditions.

Prognostic Findings at Endoscopy

- The actual appearance of the ulcer at endoscopy is the most important predictor of rebleeding. Ulcers generally have one of five appearances: a clean ulcer base; a flat, pigmented spot, which may be purple, brown, or black, on the ulcer surface; an adherent clot; a visible vessel, which appears as a smooth surfaced or tubular protuberance on the smooth ulcer surface; or active bleeding with either spurting blood, continuous oozing, or oozing around an adherent clot. The latter four appearances are considered to be stigmata of hemorrhage. The probability of rebleeding can be estimated based on this endoscopic appearance: a clean ulcer base rarely bleeds; a flat pigmented spot ulcer bleeds again in about 10% of patients; an adherent, nonbleeding clot carries a rebleeding risk of about 20%; and a visible vessel carries a rebleeding risk of 40% to 80%.

Therapeutic Interventions

- Endoscopic therapy can be used to arrest active ulcer bleeding and to prevent rebleeding in patients with ulcers at high risk for rebleeding (FI, FIIa, and FIIb ulcers). Several endoscopic devices can deliver the thermal energy required to achieve coagulation. Transendoscopic bipolar electrocoagulation and heater probe therapy can decrease rebleeding rates and the need for surgical intervention by up to 50%.

- Injection therapy is an equally effective nonthermal method to secure hemostasis.
- Rebleeding rates are reduced by half, relative to those ulcers with similar characteristics not subjected to endoscopic therapy.
- Endoscopic therapy fails in about 20% of patients, manifest as either failure to control hemorrhage on initial presentation or as early recurrent hemorrhage.

Surgical Therapy

- Surgery is ultimately required in roughly 10% of patients with bleeding ulcer. Surgery is indicated for patients with active hemorrhage not responsive to endoscopic measures, significant recurrent hemorrhage after endoscopic treatment, an ongoing transfusion requirement, or transfusion requirements exceeding six units of packed red blood cells in a 24-hour interval. Given the now extensive successful experience with endoscopic therapy, surgery is generally reserved for those patients in whom endoscopic measures have failed as the primary intervention, assuming expert endoscopy is readily available.
- Clinical judgment is essential in deciding who will benefit from surgical intervention at what time. Early definitive surgical intervention is clearly indicated for patients in whom primary endoscopic therapies fail. It is also clear that elderly patients with lesions at highest risk for rebleeding fair better with early definitive operation than with episodes of recurrent hemorrhage as a result of failed repeated efforts at hemostasis.
- Choice of operation.
  - The goal of surgical intervention in bleeding peptic ulcer is to control hemorrhage.
- Bleeding duodenal ulcer.
  - Operative intervention for bleeding duodenal ulcer requires direct exposure of the ulcer in the duodenum by way of duodenotomy or duodenopyloromyotomy. Because these ulcers are typically located on the posterior duodenal wall, direct suture ligation with a nonabsorbable suture suffices in most patients to arrest bleeding.
- Bleeding gastric ulcer.
  - Up to 10% of gastric ulcers prove to be a gastric adenocarcinoma or lymphoma. In addition, rebleeding rates for gastric ulcer treated with simple ligation approach is 30%.

Therefore, ideally, the surgical procedure should include ulcer excision.

- Ulcers of the incisura, antrum, and distal body of the stomach should be managed with distal gastrectomy and Billroth I or II reconstruction.
- Ulcer surgery in patients with *H. pylori* infection.
  - A role for definitive antisecretory ulcer surgery is clear in the setting of hemorrhage from peptic ulcer in patients taking NSAIDs who must continue this therapy. Some gastroenterologists and surgeons have questioned the need for definitive antiulcer surgery in patients with *H. pylori*—associated ulcer disease. A definitive judgment cannot be made at this time. A role for excluding a definite antisecretory procedure in perforated duodenal ulcer is supported by a recent study showing that, in *H. pylori* infected patients with perforated duodenal ulcers, those treated with *H. pylori* therapy after closure alone had significantly less ulcer recurrence than those treated with closure and omeprazole alone.

Bleeding Caused by Portal Hypertension

- Bleeding from esophagogastric varices is responsible for one third of all deaths in patients with cirrhosis and portal hypertension. Up to 90% of cirrhotic patients develop esophageal varices, and 25% to 30% of these develop hemorrhage. The mortality risk from each episode of hemorrhage approaches 25%. After bleeding has occurred, repeated hemorrhage develops in 70% of patients.

Treatment of Acute Variceal Hemorrhage

- Hemorrhage from varices in cirrhotic patients is a potentially highly lethal event. The clinical presentation includes massive hematemesis, melena, and occasionally hematochezia. Hemodynamic instability is common. Initial management calls for prompt resuscitation with particular attention to correction of volume deficit, coagulopathy, and airway management. Patients with poor liver function as reflected by Child s classification system are at high risk for mortality. Treatment in an intensive care unit (ICU) is imperative.
- Emergency endoscopy is required to evaluate the source of bleeding.
- Endoscopy is necessary both to confirm the source of bleeding and to allow endoscopic therapy. Both variceal

sclerotherapy and rubber band ligation are effective endo-scopic measures.

- Concomitant treatment with vasoactive drugs is indicated. The somatostatin analogue octreotide, given by continuous intravenous infusion, offers the best efficacy and safety profile. Somatostatin decreases splanchnic blood flow thereby decreasing portal and variceal pressure without eliciting coronary vasoconstriction.
- Endoscopic therapy and somatostatin infusions are effective in arresting hemorrhage in 80% to 90% of cases.
- If sclerotherapy is ineffective, a Sengstaken-Blakemore tube should be inserted.
- The patient with acute variceal hemorrhage who continues to bleed after endoscopic and medical therapies have been applied can be considered for transjugular intrahepatic shunt (TIPS) or emergency surgical decompression of the portal circulation.
- In most reported series, emergency decompressive surgery for patients (procedures discussed in Chapter 51) with uncontrolled hemorrhage carries an operative mortality rate in excess of 50%. This reflects the fact that ongoing hemor-rhage is more likely to occur in patients with poor liver function (Child s Class C).
- The risks for early and late mortality after variceal hemor-rhage are largely determined by the patient s liver function at the time of hemorrhage.

Acute Gastric Mucosal Lesions

- Acute gastric mucosal lesions (AGMLs) include a broad cate-gory of acute erosive mucosal conditions that develop in critically ill patients. Also known as *stress gastritis, acute mucosal ischemia, erosive gastritis,* or *stress ulceration,* these conditions share a common epidemiology and clinical pres-entation. They are characterized by stigmata of mucosal injury evidenced by mucosal pallor, petechiae, and erosions. The lesions can be distributed throughout the gastric mucosa but are predominately identified in the body of the stomach. Bleeding is the clinical presenting sign in critically ill patients. The bleeding may be massive and life threatening. Prompt correction of the factors leading to the critical illness is the most important priority in management.
- Patients at risk for non—NSAID-associated AGML include virtually all critically ill patients in medical and surgical ICUs. Particular risk factors include sepsis, respiratory failure, hemodynamic instability, coma following head injury or

intracranial operation, burns covering greater than 35% of body surface area, multiple trauma, cardiopulmonary bypass, and coagulopathy.

- The pathogenesis of AGML is related to a combination of both gastric acid and activated pepsin injuring the gastric mucosa and is exacerbated by mucosal ischemia secondary to hypoperfusion.

Prophylaxis

- AGML can be prevented by any of several strategies. The most widely applied methods involve neutralization of the contents in the gastric lake.
- Again, pH monitoring is required to ensure efficacy because acid hypersecretion may be present in these patients, rendering conventional dosing inadequate.
- With these observations, the current recommendation regarding stress ulceration calls for gastric neutralization with either histamine-2 (H_2)-receptor antagonists or proton-pump inhibitors.

Diagnosis and Treatment

- AGMLs in hospitalized patients are heralded by gastrointestinal bleeding evidenced by hematemesis, nasogastric aspiration of blood or coffee ground—like material, or an unexplainable drop in hematocrit.
- Emergency evaluation with upper endoscopy, a procedure that should be completed in the ICU, is indicated. Careful attention to prevent aspiration and hypovolemia during the procedure is mandatory.
- Findings at endoscopy are characterized by diffuse petechiae, superficial erosions, and mucosal pallor. If a solitary site of bleeding is identified, endoscopic therapy, such as thermal or bipolar electrocoagulation, fibrin glue application, or injection therapy, is appropriate. Frequently, however, bleeding is too diffuse to allow endoscopic therapy. In this case, aggressive medical management with transfusion and component therapy to correct coagulation defects and anemia is indicated. Measures to correct hypoperfusion, hypovolemia, and gastric acid neutralization are also important elements of management.
- The role of angiography in stress ulceration is limited to diffuse, unremitting hemorrhage.
- Surgery is rarely used to treat AGML.

- In the few patients that do come to surgery, the goal of surgery is hemostasis. At laparotomy, a generous gastrotomy is made to evaluate the sites of hemorrhage. In the unlikely finding of a single bleeding site or bleeding from only a few small sites, oversewing of these sites and truncal vagotomy and drainage are appropriate. Unfortunately, multiple sites are usually found, leaving only subtotal or near-total gastrectomy with Roux-en-Y gastrojejunostomy as the only viable option.

Mallory-Weiss Tears

- About 10% of cases of upper gastrointestinal hemorrhage are caused by Mallory-Weiss tears. The lesion is characterized by a tear in the proximal gastric mucosa near the esophagogastric junction. The clinical presentation is typified by an antecedent history of vomiting, retching, or coughing followed by hematemesis.
- Up to 10% of patients may have bleeding of sufficient magnitude to have hematochezia and hypotension as presenting signs. Up to 90% of these lesions stop bleeding spontaneously without specific intervention. Patients with cirrhosis and portal hypertension with coagulopathy are at greatest risk for morality, which overall averages 3%.
- Endoscopic therapy by either injection or thermal energy is efficacious in patients with active bleeding.
- Surgery is rarely required for control of hemorrhage. If bleeding fails to stop after endoscopic therapy, laparotomy for oversewing of the mucosal tear through a high gastrotomy is appropriate.

Unusual Causes of Acute Upper Gastrointestinal Hemorrhage

Esophageal Sources

- The esophagus is the source of major hemorrhage in fewer than 3% of patients admitted for evaluation of acute upper gastrointestinal hemorrhage. The most common causes are infectious esophagitis, gastroesophageal reflux disease, Barrett s epithelium, malignancy (including adenocarcinomas and squamous carcinomas), medication-induced erosions, Crohn s disease, and radiation. Patients with human immunodeficiency virus infection and other immunocompromised patients are at particular risk for infectious esophagitis.
- If active hemorrhage is identified, endoscopic electrocoagulation or heater probe therapy is usually effective in stopping

hemorrhage, at least temporarily while definitive management is planned.

Dieulafoy's Lesion

- Dieulafoy s vascular malformations are rare causes of acute upper gastrointestinal hemorrhage. The lesions are unusually large submucosal or mucosal vessels found in the gastric mucosa, most commonly along the lesser curvature in the mid-stomach.
- Bleeding occurs when superficial erosion into the vessel occurs, resulting in brisk, voluminous hemorrhage that ceases spontaneously. Endoscopic diagnosis is difficult because the lesion is rarely associated with an obvious ulcerated lesion.
- If a lesion is definitively identified, the site should be marked endoscopically with India ink injection to allow precise surgical resection.
- Recurrent hemorrhage is common; often, several episodes occur before accurate diagnosis.
- Appropriate definitive management calls for wedge resection of the gastric wall.

Aortoenteric Fistula

- Aortoenteric fistula is an uncommon condition in which an inflammatory tract develops between the aorta and the gastrointestinal tract. The fistula may develop as a primary process resulting from infectious aortitis or inflammatory aortic aneurysm or as a secondary process following aortic replacement with a synthetic graft for treatment of abdominal aortic aneurysm. The secondary aortoenteric fistulas are by far the more common cause, and this complication may develop in up to 1% of patients after aortic aneurysm repair.
- Emergency upper endoscopy is mandatory for all patients with suspected aortoenteric fistula. If endoscopy is negative, computed tomography to look for evidence of inflammation at the aortic anastomosis is indicated. Others advocate emergency angiography, including lateral views, to identify the small mycotic aneurysm that is frequently present. Angiography should be pursued in all patients with negative computed tomography scans.
- In patients with exsanguinating hemorrhage, emergency laparotomy with control of the proximal aorta is indicated. Effective surgical management calls for removal of the

aortic graft and extra-anatomic vascular bypass to restore distal aortic flow.

ACUTE LOWER GASTROINTESTINAL HEMORRHAGE

Definition and Incidence

- Acute lower gastrointestinal bleeding is hemorrhage arising distal to the ligament of Treitz. The colon is the source of hemorrhage in more than 95% to 97% of cases, with the remaining 3% to 5% arising in small bowel sites. Lower gastrointestinal bleeding accounts for about 15% of major episodes of gastrointestinal hemorrhage and hence is much less common than upper gastrointestinal bleeding. The incidence of lower gastrointestinal bleeding increases with age, reflecting the parallel increase in acquired lesions responsible for colonic bleeding: diverticulosis and angiodysplasias.

Clinical Presentation

- The hallmark of acute lower gastrointestinal hemorrhage is hematochezia; passage of bloody stool, blood, or blood clots per rectum.

Causes

- Validating the source of an episode of hemorrhage from the colon is more problematic.
- Therefore, it is important to have a clear understanding of the significance of findings on diagnostic evaluation and to keep in mind the limited certainty that may accompany some of these findings. The direct observation of a bleeding lesion or findings of stigmata of recent hemorrhage at endoscopy are required to establish a definitive diagnosis.

Diverticulosis

- Colonic diverticulosis represents the most common source of lower gastrointestinal hemorrhage, responsible for 40% to 55% of cases of hemorrhage in most series.
- The anatomic basis for bleeding is thought to be asymmetric rupture of intramural branches (the vasa recta) of the marginal artery at the dome of the diverticulum or at its antimesenteric margin. It appears likely that luminal traumatic factors, including impacted fecaliths with abrasion of

the vessels, lead to hemorrhage. Hemorrhage is rarely associated with the inflammation of clinical diverticulitis.

- Diverticular hemorrhage ceases spontaneously in up to 90% of patients.

Angiodysplasia

- Angiodysplasias are responsible for 3% to 20% of cases of acute lower intestinal bleeding. Angiodysplasias, also referred to as *arteriovenous malformations,* are small ectatic blood vessels in the submucosa of the gastrointestinal tract. The overlying mucosa is often thin, and superficial erosion at the site of an angiodysplasia has been observed on histologic examination of surgical or autopsy specimens.
- Angiodysplasias are evident on colonoscopy as red, flat lesions about 2 to 10 mm in diameter. Lesions may appear stellate, oval, sharp, or indistinct. Colonoscopy is the most sensitive method to identify angiodysplasias, although angiography is also able to identify these lesions.
- On angiography, angiodysplasias appear as ectatic, slowly emptying veins or as arteriovenous malformations with brisk, early venous filling.

Neoplasia

- Typically, bleeding from these lesions is slow.
- Juvenile polyps are the second most common cause of hemorrhage in patients younger than the age of 20.

Inflammatory Conditions

- Hemorrhage complicates the course of ulcerative colitis in up to 15% of cases. Crohn s disease is less likely to cause massive colonic hemorrhage and occurs in roughly 1% of patients with this condition.

Vascular Causes

- Vasculitides, mesenteric ischemia, or ischemic colitis.

Hemorrhoids

- Hemorrhoids are usually noted on physical examination in more than half of patients with lower gastrointestinal hemorrhage. However, the hemorrhage can be attributed to these lesions in fewer than 2% of cases. Unless unequivocal signs of bleeding are evident on anoscopy, investigation of the patient for another source of lower intestinal bleeding should be pursued.

Uncommon Causes

- Solitary rectal ulcer, Dieulafoy s lesion of the colon, portal colopathy, NSAID s, intussusception, or bleeding following colonoscopic biopsy or polypectomy.

Initial Assessment

- The initial history and physical examination are directed to determining the potential source of the hemorrhage and the severity of initial hemorrhage.
- Physical examination should include measurement of orthostatic vital signs in patients without overt shock. All patients should be resuscitated, as outlined in the previous section. Pertinent findings on physical examination may include scars from previous abdominal incisions, the presence of abdominal masses, or skin and oral lesions suggestive of polyposis syndromes. Stigmata of cirrhosis suggestive of bleeding from hemorrhoids or varices secondary to portal hypertension should be considered.
- A nasogastric tube should be inserted to look for blood or coffee ground—like material to exclude an upper gastrointestinal source. In patients with hematochezia and hemodynamic instability, emergency upper endoscopy is required.

Diagnosis

- The three options for primary diagnostic testing are colonoscopy, selective visceral angiography, and technetium-99m (^{99m}Tc)-labeled red blood cell scintigraphy.

Colonoscopy

- Recognition that most episodes of hemorrhage cease spontaneously and that stigmata of bleeding are subtle has led to efforts to perform colonoscopy as early as possible in the course of evaluation.
- It is important that incidental lesions, such as blood clots in multiple diverticular orifices, nonbleeding arteriovenous malformation, nonbleeding polyps, and nonbleeding diverticula, are not concluded to be the site of recent hemorrhage. Hemorrhage can be attributed only to lesions with clear stigmata of bleeding.

- Patients presenting with massive lower gastrointestinal hemorrhage are poor candidates for emergency colonoscopy.

Selective Visceral Angiography

- Mesenteric arteriography has been widely used in the evaluation and treatment of patients with lower gastrointestinal hemorrhage. Selective injection of radiographic contrast into the superior mesenteric or inferior mesenteric arteries identifies hemorrhage in patients bleeding at a rate of 0.5 mL/minute or greater. The study can accurately identify arterial hemorrhage in 45% to 75% of patients if they are actively bleeding at the time of contrast injection.
- About 10% of patients develop a complication of angiography. Major complications include stroke, renal failure, femoral artery thrombosis, lower extremity immobilization, and hematoma formation. Given that most patients with lower gastrointestinal hemorrhage are older than 60 years, medical comorbidities, including vascular disease and renal insufficiency, may place these patients at high risk for the procedure. Hence, angiography is reserved for patients with evidence of significant ongoing hemorrhage.

Technetium-99m Red Blood Cell Scintigraphy

- ^{99m}Tc red blood cell scintigraphy has met with mixed success in the diagnosis of lower gastrointestinal hemorrhage.
- If bleeding is present at the time of injection and initial imaging, ^{99m}Tc red blood cell scans can accurately identify a source of bleeding in up to 85% of cases. If bleeding is not active at the time of the initial study, or if delayed bleeding occurs, subsequent imaging to detect the luminal isotope can be inaccurate because of the sporadic movement of the tracer in the gut lumen. The study is accurate in only 40% to 60% of patients, little better than a 50:50 ratio, to isolate bleeding to the left or right colon. Hence, patients in whom a surgical resection is anticipated to control recurrent or persistent hemorrhage should have the bleeding confirmed with either a positive angiogram or a positive colonoscopy. The red blood cell scans serve primarily to target the subsequent confirmatory study.

Treatment

Endoscopic Treatment

- Efforts at endoscopic control of diverticular hemorrhage may precipitate more significant bleeding. In contrast, angiodysplasias are readily treated with endoscopic measures. Acute bleeding can be controlled in up to 80% of patients with bleeding angiodysplasias, although rebleeding may develop in up to 15%.

- Endoscopic therapy is also appropriate for patients with bleeding from a recent snare polypectomy site.

Angiographic Treatment

- In patients whose bleeding source is identified by angiography, a trial of angiographic therapy may be appropriate as a perioperative temporizing measure or as a definitive measure for high-risk surgical candidates.
- Given the lack of collateral blood supply to the colonic wall, these procedures may be complicated by colonic infarction heralded by abdominal pain, fever, and sepsis. Hence, like vasoconstrictive therapy, this procedure should be restricted to patients who cannot tolerate surgery or as a temporizing measure in massive hemorrhage in patients for whom a definitive surgical resection is imminent.

Surgery

- Surgery is indicated for patients with ongoing or recurrent hemorrhage.
- Every effort should be made to localize the source of bleeding so that a hemicolectomy can be performed rather than a blind subtotal abdominal colectomy.
- Blind total abdominal colectomy carries significantly higher perioperative morbidity, and associated mortality rates approach 25% in some series.

CHAPTER 44

STOMACH

ANATOMY

Gross Anatomy

- Blood supply
  - The blood supply to the stomach is from the celiac artery. There are four main arteries: the left and right gastric arteries along the lesser curvature and the left and right gastroepiploic arteries along the greater curvature. In addition, a substantial quantity of blood may be supplied to the proximal stomach by the inferior phrenic arteries and by the short gastrics from the spleen. The largest artery to the stomach is the left gastric artery, and it is not uncommon (15% to 20%) for an aberrant left hepatic artery to originate from it.
- Innervation
  - At the gastroesophageal (GE) junction, the left vagus is anterior, and the right vagus is posterior (mnemonic: L,A,R,P).
  - Most (greater than 90%) of the vagal fibers are afferent, carrying stimuli from the gut to the brain.

Gastric Morphology

- The mucosa consists of surface epithelium, lamina propria, and muscularis mucosae. The latter is on the luminal side of the submucosa and is probably responsible for the rugae that greatly increase epithelial surface area. It also marks the microscopic boundary for invasive and noninvasive gastric carcinoma.

Gastric Glandular Organization

- Open-type endocrine cells have their microvilli on the apical membranes, which allows direct contact with gastric contents.
- Closed-type endocrine cells do not have microvilli in contact with the gastric lumen.

- Biopsy specimens taken from the stomach have demonstrated that parietal cells account for 13% of epithelial cells, whereas chief cells account for 44%, mucus cells account for 40%, and endocrine cells account for 3%.

PHYSIOLOGY

General Considerations

- Receptive relaxation refers to the process whereby the proximal portion of the stomach relaxes in anticipation of food intake. This relaxation enables liquids to pass easily from the stomach along the lesser curvature, whereas the solid food settles along the greater curvature of the fundus. In contrast to liquids, emptying of solid food is facilitated by the antrum, which pumps solid food components into and through the pylorus.

Regulation of Gastric Function

Gastric Peptides

Gastrin

Synthesis and Action

- Gastrin is produced by G-cells located in the gastric antrum (Table 44–1).
- Ninety percent of antral gastrin is released as the 17 amino acid peptide, although G-34 predominates in the circulation because its metabolic half-life is longer than that of G-17. The pentapeptide sequence contained at the carboxyl terminus of gastrin is the biologically active component and is identical to that found on another gut peptide, cholecystokinin (CCK).
- The release of gastrin is stimulated by food components contained within a meal, especially protein digestion products. Luminal acid inhibits the release of gastrin. Somatostatin (see later discussion) has paracrine actions on antral G-cells and acts to inhibit gastrin release. In the antral location, somatostatin and gastrin release are functionally linked and an inverse reciprocal relationship exists between these two peptides. Moreover, somatostatin exerts a tonic inhibitory effect on gastrin release and likely mediates the inhibitory effects of luminal acid on gastrin release.

TABLE 44–1. Gastric Cell Types, Location, and Function

Cells	Location	Function
Parietal	Body	Secretion of acid and intrinsic factor
Mucus	Body, antrum	Mucus
Chief	Body	Pepsin
Surface epithelial	Diffuse	Mucus, bicarbonate, prostaglandins (?)
ECL	Body	Histamine
G	Antrum	Gastrin
D	Body, antrum	Somatostatin
Gastric mucosal interneurons	Body, antrum	Gastrin-releasing peptide
Enteric neurons	Diffuse	CGRP, others

CGRP, calcitonin gene-related peptide; ECL, enterochromaffin-like.

Hypergastrinemia

- Hypergastrinemia that results from administration of anti-secretory agents is an appropriate response caused by loss of feedback inhibition of gastrin release by luminal acid.
- Gastrin levels increase inappropriately in patients with gastrinoma (Zollinger-Ellison syndrome).

Somatostatin

Synthesis and Action

- Somatostatin is produced by D-cells and exists endogenously as either the 14 or 28 amino acid peptide. The predominant molecular form in the stomach is somatostatin 14. It is produced by diffuse neuroendocrine cells located in both the fundus and the antrum.
- The principal stimulus for somatostatin release is antral acidification, and acetylcholine from vagal fibers inhibits its release.

Effects of *Helicobacter pylori* on Somatostatin

- Gastrin-releasing peptide.
- Histamine.
  - Histamine may be a necessary intermediary of gastrin and acetylcholine stimulated acid secretion. Histamine is stored in the acidic granules of ECL cells and in resident

mast cells. Its release is stimulated by gastrin, acetyl-choline, and epinephrine following receptor ligand inter-actions on enterochromaffin-like (ECL) cells. In contrast, somatostatin inhibits gastrin-stimulated histamine release through interactions with somatostatin receptors located on the ECL cell.

Gastric Acid Secretion

- Gastric acid secretion by the parietal cell is regulated by three local stimuli: acetylcholine, gastrin, and histamine. These three stimuli account for basal and stimulated gastric acid secretion.

Basal Acid Secretion

- Under basal conditions, 1 to 5 mmol of hydrochloric acid is secreted and this is reduced by 75% to 90% following vago-tomy or administration of atropine.
- Histamine-2 (H_2)-receptor blockade diminishes the magnitude of acid secretion by 90%.
- Basal acid secretion is due to a combination of cholinergic and histaminergic input.

Stimulated Acid Secretion

- Cephalic phase.
  - The cephalic phase originates with the sight, smell, thought, or taste of food, which stimulates neural centers in the cortex and hypothalamus.
  - These higher centers transmit signals to the stomach by the vagus nerves, which release acetylcholine that in turn activates muscarinic receptors located on target cells.
  - Although the intensity of the acid secretory response in the cephalic phase surpasses that of the other phases, it accounts for only 20% to 30% of the total volume of gas-tric acid produced in response to a meal in humans because of the short duration of the cephalic phase.
- Gastric phase.
  - The gastric phase of acid secretion begins when food enters the gastric lumen.
  - In humans, mechanical distention of the stomach accounts for about 30% to 40% of the maximal acid secre-tory response to a peptone meal with the remainder resulting from gastrin release. The entire gastric phase accounts for most (60% to 70%) of meal-stimulated acid output, because it lasts until the stomach is empty.

- Intestinal phase.
  - It accounts for only 10% of the acid secretory response to a meal and does not appear to be mediated by serum gastrin levels.

Cellular Basis of Acid Secretion

- Gastrin receptors.
  - Binding of gastrin to the CCK-B receptor is coupled to the calcium-signaling pathway.
- Muscarinic receptors.
  - This receptor is coupled to increased levels of intracellular calcium.
- Histamine receptors.
  - The H_2 subtype binds histamine to activate adenylate cyclase, which, in turn, leads to an increase in intracellular cyclic AMP levels.
- Somatostatin receptors.
  - Binding of somatostatin with its receptors is coupled to one or more inhibitory guanine nucleotide binding proteins.
  - The ability of somatostatin to exert its inhibitory actions on cellular function is primarily thought to be mediated via inhibition of adenylate cyclase with a resultant reduction in cyclic AMP levels.
- Second messengers.

Activation and Secretion by the Parietal Cell

- During the resting or nonsecreting state, gastric parietal cells store the H/K-ATPase within intracellular tubulovesicular elements.
- The secretion and exchange of hydrogen for potassium, however, does require energy in the form of ATP because hydrogen is being secreted against a gradient of more than a millionfold. Because of this large energy requirement, the parietal cell also has the largest mitochondrial content of any mammalian cell with a mitochondrial compartment representing 34% of its cell volume.
- There is a linear relationship between maximal acid output and parietal cell number.

Pharmacologic Regulation of Gastric Acid Secretion

- Proton pump inhibitors are weak acids with a pKa of 4.0 and, therefore, become selectively localized in the secretory canaliculus of the parietal cell.

- The cysteine residues on the alpha-subunit form a covalent disulfate bond with activated benzimidazoles, which irreversibly inhibits the proton pump.
- These agents have a longer duration of action than the plasma half-life for these agents with intragastric pH being maintained above 3 for 18 hours or more.
- Chronic administration of omeprazole was in fact found to cause ECL hyperplasia that could progress to carcinoid tumors in rats. These tumors were more common in females than in males and occurred only when the rats were at the end of their natural life span.

Other Gastric Secretory Products

- Gastric juice.
- Intrinsic factor.
- Pepsinogen.
  - Group 1 pepsinogens are secreted by chief cells and by mucus neck cells located in the glands of the acid secreting portion of the stomach. Group 2 pepsinogens are produced by surface epithelial cells throughout the acid secreting portion of the stomach, the antrum, and the proximal duodenum.
  - Pepsins become inactivated at a pH greater than 5, although group 2 pepsinogens are active over a wider range of pH values than the group 1 pepsinogens.
- Mucus and bicarbonate.

Motility

Fasting Gastric Motility

- The electrical basis of gastric motility begins with the depolarization of pacemaker cells located in the midbody of the stomach along the greater curvature. Once initiated, slow waves travel at three cycles per minute in a circumferential and antegrade fashion toward the pylorus. In addition to these slow waves, gastric smooth muscle cells are capable of producing action potentials, which are associated with larger changes in membrane potential than slow waves. In comparison to slow waves, which are not associated with gastric contractions, action potentials are associated with actual muscle contractions.
- Myoelectric migrating complex (MMC). Each cycle of MMC lasts 90 to 120 minutes and is made up of four phases (I–IV) of electrical activity.

Postprandial Gastric Motility

- Abnormal gastric motility.
- Gastric emptying studies.

Gastric Barrier Function

- Decreased gastric mucosal blood flow has minimal effects on lesion production until it approaches 50% of normal. When blood flow is reduced by more than 75%, marked mucosal injury results and this is exacerbated in the presence of a luminal acid.

PEPTIC ULCER DISEASE

Epidemiology

- The annual incidence of active ulcer (gastric ulcer and duodenal ulcer) in the United States is about 1.8% or roughly 500,000 new cases per year. In addition, there are approximately 4 million ulcer recurrences yearly.
- During the past couple decades, elective admissions have decreased dramatically, whereas admissions for complications related to ulcer disease have shown little change.
- Hospitalization rates have decreased for duodenal ulcer but have remained stable for gastric ulcer.
- Admissions for bleeding gastric ulcers have increased over the last several years.

Location and Type of Ulcer

- Peptic ulcer disease occurs near mucosal junctions.
- An ulcer by definition extends through the muscularis mucosa in contrast to an erosion, which is superficial to the muscularis mucosa.

Pathogenesis

Helicobacter Pylori Infection

- Ninety percent of duodenal ulcers and roughly 75% of gastric ulcers are associated with *H. pylori* infection.
- One of the most potent producers of urease of any bacteria yet described.
- *H. pylori* can only live in gastric epithelium because only gastric epithelium expresses specific adherence receptors.

- In patients with *H. pylori* infection, basal and stimulated gastrin levels are significantly increased. It appears that the mechanism for this increase is secondary to a reduction in antral D cells.
- Eradication of *H. pylori* leads to an increase in antral D cells and somatostatin with a consequent decrease in gastrin levels.
- Peptic ulcers are also strongly associated with antral gastritis.
- Most cases of histologic gastritis are due to *H. pylori* infection. Interestingly, 25% of patients with an nonsteroidal anti-inflammatory drug (NSAID)-associated ulcer had evidence of a histologic antral gastritis as opposed to 95% in non-NSAID-associated ulcers.
- Once a person is infected, usually in childhood, it is probably for life because spontaneous remission is rare. There tends to be an inverse relationship between infection and socio-economic status.
- *H. pylori* in one household member is associated with a greater chance of infection in other members.
- Developing countries have a higher rate of *H. pylori* infection and this is especially true in children. Multiple studies have demonstrated what appears to be a steady, linear increase in acquisition of *H. pylori* infection with age, especially in the United States and Northern European nations.
- In the United States, normal blood donors have an overall prevalence of about 20% to about 55% with variations by age and ethnicity of the population.
- Limited data are available to estimate the lifetime risk of developing an ulcer in patients with *H. pylori* infection. However, a study by Cullen et al was performed as a serologic study from Australia with a mean period of evaluation of 18 years. During this time frame, 15% of *H. pylori* positive subjects developed verified duodenal ulcer as compared with 3% of seronegative individuals.

Nonsteroidal Anti-Inflammatory Drugs

- The increased risk of bleeding and ulcerations is proportional to the daily dosage of NSAID.
- NSAID ingestion not only causes acute gastroduodenal injury but is also associated with chronic gastroduodenal injury.

Acid

- An adequate level of acid secretion is a prerequisite for duodenal ulcers and their presence is rare in patients who have a maximal acid output of less than 12 to 15 mmol/hour. For type 1 and type 4 gastric ulcers, which are not associated with excessive acid secretion, acid acts as an important cofactor, exacerbating the underlying ulcer damage and attenuating the ability of the stomach to heal.

Duodenal Ulcer Pathophysiology

- Duodenal ulcer is a disease of multiple etiologies. The only relatively absolute requirements are acid and pepsin secretion in combination with either infection with *H. pylori* or ingestion of NSAIDs.
- Mean parietal cell number is increased in duodenal ulcers patients but not in gastric ulcer patients.

Gastric Ulcer Pathophysiology

- Usually present on the lesser curvature near the incisura angularis. Approximately 60% of ulcers are located in this location and are classified as type 1 gastric ulcers. These ulcers generally are not associated with excessive acid secretion.
- Type 2 gastric ulcers are located in the body of the stomach in combination with a duodenal ulcer. These types of ulcers usually are associated with excess acid secretion. Type 3 gastric ulcers are prepyloric ulcers and account for about 20% of the lesions. These ulcers also behave like duodenal ulcers and are associated with hypersecretion of gastric acid. Type 4 gastric ulcers occur high on the lesser curvature near the GE junction.
- Are not associated with excessive acid secretion.
- In the presence of gastric mucosal damage, acid is ulcerogenic even when present in normal or less than normal amounts.

Clinical Manifestations

Duodenal Ulcer

- Abdominal pain.
- Perforation.
  - A hallmark of free perforation is the demonstration of free air underneath the diaphragm on an upright chest x-ray film.
- Bleeding.
  - Bleeding duodenal ulcers account for about 25% of all upper gastrointestinal (GI) bleeding patients who present to the hospital.

- Obstruction.
  - In cases of prolonged vomiting, patients may become dehydrated and develop a hypochloremic hypokalemic metabolic alkalosis; fluid resuscitation requires replacement of the chloride and potassium deficiencies in addition to nasogastric suction for relief of the obstructed stomach.

Gastric Ulcer

- Surgical intervention is required in 8% to 20% of those patients developing complications from their gastric ulcer disease. Hemorrhage occurs approximately 35% to 40% of the time at some point during the course of gastric ulceration.

Zollinger-Ellison Syndrome

- Zollinger-Ellison syndrome is a clinical triad consisting of gastric acid hypersecretion, severe peptic ulcer disease, and non-beta islet cell of the pancreas. The tumors are known to produce gastrin (G-17 and G-34) and are referred to gastrinomas.
- About one half of these gastric tumors are multiple and two thirds are malignant. About one fourth have multiple endocrine neoplasia syndrome (MEN 1) with tumors of the parathyroid, pituitary, and pancreatic islet cells being present.
- The secretin test is probably the most sensitive and specific provocative test.
- If an isolated duodenal wall tumor is present on computed tomography (CT) and or visceral angiography, surgical resection followed by measurement of gastric acid secretion is performed.
- Total gastrectomy is generally obsolete.

Diagnosis

- About 5% of ulcers that appear radiographically benign are malignant.

Helicobacter Pylori Testing

- Serology.
  - Serology is the diagnostic test of choice when endoscopy is not indicated

- This test cannot be used to assess eradication following therapy.
- Urea breath test.
  - Another noninvasive test.
  - This test is based on the ability of *H. pylori* to hydrolyze urea.
  - The test is performed by having the patient ingest a carbon isotope-labeled urea using either C14 or C13.
  - Following ingestion of the carbon isotope, urea will be metabolized to ammonia and labeled bicarbonate if *H. pylori* infection is present. The labeled bicarbonate is excreted in the breath as labeled carbon dioxide which is then quantified.
  - False negatives can occur if the test is done too soon after treatment; thus, it is usually best to test 4 weeks after therapy is finished. The urea breath test is the method of choice to document eradication.
- Rapid urease assay.
  - The method of choice to diagnosis *H. pylori* if endoscopy is used is the rapid urease test.
  - The enzyme urease catalyzes degradation of urea to ammonia and bicarbonate, creating an alkaline environment that can be detected by a pH indicator.
- Histology.
- Culture.
  - Provides the opportunity to perform antibiotic sensitivity testing on isolates should the need arise.
- *H. Pylori* testing summary.

Upper Gastrointestinal Radiography

- The location of a gastric ulcer is of little predictive value in establishing malignancy because benign and malignant ulcers can occur anywhere in the stomach.
- The finding of an ulcer with an associated mass, interrupted, fused, or nodular mucosal folds approaching the margin of the crater or an ulcer with irregular filling defects in the ulcer crater is suggestive of a malignancy.

Fiberoptic Endoscopy

- If multiple biopsies and brushings for cytology are performed, the probability of diagnosing a malignancy is also in excess of 97%.

Treatment

Medical Management

- Antacids.
  - Antacids reduce gastric acidity by reacting with hydrochloric acid, forming a salt and water to inhibit peptic activity by raising pH.
  - They are most effective when ingested 1 hour after a meal. If taken on an empty stomach, the antacids are emptied rapidly and have only a transient buffering effect.
  - Doses of 200 to 1000 mmol/day.
  - Results in approximately 80% ulcer healing at 1 month.
- H_2-receptor antagonists.
  - Continuous intravenous infusion of H_2-receptor antagonists has been shown to produce more uniform acid inhibition than intermittent administration.
  - Many randomized controlled trials indicate that all H_2-receptor antagonists result in duodenal ulcer healing rates from 70% to 80% after 4 weeks and from 80% to 90% after 8 weeks of therapy.
- Proton pump inhibitors.
  - Proton pump inhibitors also produce more rapid healing of ulcers than standard H_2-receptor antagonists.
  - Proton pump inhibitors have a healing rate of 85% at 4 weeks and 96% at 8 weeks.
  - Proton pump inhibitors require an acidic environment within the gastric lumen to become activated and bind to the proton pump at the secretory canaliculus.
  - Antacids and H_2-receptor antagonists should not be used in combination with proton pump inhibitors.
- Sucralfate.
- Treatment of *H. pylori* infection.
  - The clinician has three major goals when faced with a patient with ulcer disease. First, symptoms need to be relieved; second, the ulcer needs to be healed; and third, one must prevent recurrence.
  - For duodenal ulcers, the recurrence rate following successful healing is roughly 72% if no additional therapy is used. If H_2-receptor antagonists are used as maintenance therapy, patients still have a 25% recurrence rate. However, if *H. pylori* is eradicated, only 2% of the patients have an ulcer recurrence.
  - All patients with gastric or duodenal ulcers who were infected with *H. pylori*, regardless of whether first presentation or recurrence, should be treated. *H. pylori*-infected

ulcer patients receiving maintenance treatment or with a history of complicated or refractory disease should also be treated.

- No reason to consider routine detection or treatment in the absence of ulcers and when it is concluded that NSAID use should not alter treatment.

- For patients with complications such as bleeding or perforation, documentation of eradication was imperative.
- For treatment of active NSAID ulcers, it is best to discontinue the NSAID if at all possible while the ulcer is being treated.
- Switch to the selective cyclooxygenase (COX)-2 inhibitors. Testing should be performed for *H. pylori* and, if present, treatment administered.
- Proton pump inhibitors have been shown to be more effective that H_2-receptor antagonists in patients taking NSAIDs.

Approach to the Patient Bleeding from Peptic Ulcer Disease

- Approximately 80% of upper GI bleeds are self-limited. The overall mortality of 8% to 10% for those who continue to bleed or in whom bleeding recurs has not changed dramatically over the last several decades.
- Mortality increases with age; the American Society for Gastrointestinal Endoscopy (ASGE) study found a mortality of 8.7% for patients 60 years old or younger and 13.4% for those older than 60. The severity of the initial bleed is also an adverse prognostic factor.
- Recurrent bleeding increased the mortality rate from 8% to 30% in one study and from 7% to 44% in another. The onset of bleeding in a hospital was also associated with a higher mortality rate (33%) compared with those who bled outside of the hospital or before admission.
- Stigmata of recent hemorrhage from peptic ulcers also predicts an adverse prognostic sign. These stigmata included a visible vessel on endoscopy, oozing of bright red blood, and fresh or old blood clot at the base of the ulcer.
- Pumping or oozing lesions had a significantly greater mortality (16%) and need for surgery (24%) when compared with those with clot or no blood (mortality 6.7%, surgery 11%).
- The visible vessel is regarded as the one stigmata of recent hemorrhage that is associated with the highest incidence of rebleeding. In patients with a visible vessel, rebleeding has occurred in 56% of patients in one study compared with 8% to those with oozing and 0% of those with no stigmata of recent hemorrhage. Mortality was also limited to those patients with visible vessels.

- When the bleeding is controlled, long-term medical therapy includes antisecretory agents usually in the form of a proton pump inhibitor plus testing for *H. pylori* with treatment if positive. If *H. pylori* is present, documentation of eradication should be performed.
- If the bleeding continues or recurs, surgery may be indicated.

Surgical Procedures for Peptic Ulcer Disease

- Vagotomy decreases peak acid output by approximately 50%, and vagotomy plus antrectomy, which removes the gastrin-secreting portion of the stomach, decreases peak acid output by approximately 85%.
- Truncal vagotomy.
  - Truncal vagotomy is performed by division of the left and right vagus nerves above the hepatic and celiac branches just above the GE junction.
  - There is little difference in the side effects associated with the type of drainage procedure performed.
- Highly selective vagotomy (parietal cell vagotomy).
  - This procedure divides only the vagus nerves supplying the acid-producing portion of the stomach.
  - Two or three branches to the antrum and pylorus should be preserved.
  - Recurrence rates of 10% to 15% are reported for this procedure when performed by skilled surgeons. These compare very favorably or even slightly higher than those reported after truncal vagotomy in combination with pyloroplasty.
  - When the results of this procedure are broken down by the preoperative ulcer site, there appears to be strong data suggesting that prepyloric ulcers are more likely to be associated with recurrence than duodenal ulcers for unclear reasons. As a result, it may not be the procedure of choice for prepyloric ulcers.
- Truncal vagotomy and antrectomy.
  - The recurrence rate for ulceration after truncal vagotomy and antrectomy is approximately 0% to 2% and probably represents the gold standard with regards to recurrence rates.
  - Postgastrectomy and postvagotomy syndromes (see later) that rarely occur following highly selective vagotomy appear in 20% of the patients undergoing this procedure.
- Subtotal gastrectomy.
- Laparoscopic procedures.

Surgical Indications

Intractable Duodenal Ulcer

- Although rarely seen today, intractable duodenal ulcer should be treated by parietal cell vagotomy. Although this can be performed openly, many prefer a laparoscopic approach.

Intractable Gastric Ulcer

- Type 1 gastric ulcer.
  - Malignancy remains a major concern and excision of the ulcer is necessary. Consequently, the distal gastrectomy is probably the best operation in this clinical situation. Re-establishment of intestinal continuity.
  - Billroth I is the preferred choice.
  - Vagotomy usually is not necessary for the type 1 gastric ulcer.
  - It is important to ensure that adequate time has elapsed and appropriate therapy has been administered to allow healing of the ulcer to occur. This includes confirmation that *H. pylori* has been eradicated and that NSAIDs have been eliminated as a potential cause.
- Type 2 or type 3 gastric ulcers.
  - Assuming that the patient has had adequate time to heal their ulcer and *H. pylori* has been eradicated, a distal gastrectomy in combination with vagotomy should be performed.
  - The type of vagotomy performed in combination with the resection could be either a selective or truncal vagotomy.

Bleeding Duodenal Ulcers

- The duodenal bleeding is usually controlled by opening the duodenum and oversewing the ulcer with a U stitch from the vessel, which is usually the pancreaticoduodenal artery or gastroduodenal artery.
- Truncal vagotomy with pyloroplasty is performed.

Bleeding Gastric Ulcers

- For bleeding type 1 gastric ulcers, a distal gastrectomy with Billroth I anastomosis is usually performed.
- For type 2 and type 3 gastric ulcers, distal gastrectomy in combination with vagotomy is indicated.

Perforated Duodenal Ulcers

- Simple patching of the perforation followed by treatment with *H. pylori* is all that is necessary for patients who present with a perforated duodenum secondary to peptic ulcer disease.
- If the patient is known to be *H. pylori*-negative, then an acid-reducing procedure (i.e., truncal vagotomy with pyloroplasty) should be performed.
- For all perforated duodenal ulcer patients who are *H. pylori*-positive, documentation of *H. pylori* eradication with a urea breath test is mandatory and it is paramount that the patients are compliant with their medications to treat *H. pylori*.

Perforated Gastric Ulcer

- For perforated type 1 gastric ulcers that occur in hemodynamically stable patients, distal gastrectomy with Billroth I reanastomosis is usually performed.
- Type 2 and type 3 gastric ulcers, because they behave like duodenal ulcers, can be simply treated with patch closure followed by treatment for *H. pylori*.

Gastric Outlet Obstruction

- All patients with gastric outlet obstruction require preoperative nasogastric decompression for several days, correction of fluid and electrolyte imbalances, antisecretory therapy, and endoscopy with biopsies before surgical intervention.
- The preferred procedure for those patients presenting with a gastric outlet obstruction is parietal cell vagotomy with a gastrojejunostomy. In addition, these patients require therapy for *H. pylori*.

Type 4 Gastric Ulcers

- The surgical treatment depends on the ulcer size, the distance from the GE junction, and the degree of surrounding inflammation. Whenever possible, the ulcer should be excised.

Giant Gastric Ulcers

- Giant gastric ulcers are defined as ulcers with a diameter of 3 cm or greater.
- The incidence of malignancy ranges from 6% to 30% and increases with the size of the ulcer. Giant gastric ulcers have a high likelihood of developing complications.

- The operation of choice is resection including the ulcer bed with vagotomy reserved for type 2 and type 3 gastric ulcers.

Postgastrectomy Syndromes

Postoperative Complications for Peptic Ulcer Disease

- When these postgastrectomy symptoms develop, it has become more apparent that every attempt should be made to avoid reoperation because many of these patients lack a clearly mechanical or physiologic defect and because many of the problems persist despite reoperation.

Postgastrectomy Syndromes Secondary to Gastric Resection

Dumping Syndrome

- Early dumping.
  - The early form of dumping syndrome usually occurs within 20 to 30 minutes following ingestion of a meal and is accompanied by both GI and cardiovascular symptoms.
  - It is more common after partial gastrectomy with the Billroth II reconstruction.
  - It occurs because of the rapid passage of food of high osmolarity from the stomach into the small intestine.
  - The symptoms associated with early dumping syndrome appear to be secondary to the release of several humoral agents.
  - In those situations in which symptoms are prolonged, dietary measures are usually sufficient.
  - Recently, however, the long-acting somatostatin analog octreotide acetate (Sandostatin) has been shown to be highly effective in preventing the development of symptoms, both vasomotor and GI.
  - In the less than 1% of patients who fail to respond to the conservative measures mentioned previously, operative intervention may become necessary.
  - The use of isoperistaltic or antiperistaltic jejunal segments has had the greatest success in dealing with this problem in most centers.
  - Using a 10- to 20-cm loop of jejunum and interposing it between the stomach and small intestine.
- Late dumping.
  - The syndrome of late dumping appears 2 to 3 hours after a meal.

- The basic defect in this disorder is also rapid gastric emptying; however, it is related specifically to carbohydrates being delivered rapidly into the proximal intestine.
- Hyperglycemia triggers the release of large amounts of insulin to control the rising blood sugar.
- Profound hypoglycemia occurs in response to the insulin.
- These patients should be advised to ingest frequent small meals and to reduce their carbohydrate intake. Some patients have found benefit with pectin, either alone or in combination with acarbose.

Metabolic Disturbances

- The most common metabolic defect appearing following gastrectomy is anemia.
- Iron deficiency anemia is more common than vitamin B_{12} deficiency anemia.
- Megaloblastic anemia can also occur following gastrectomy, especially when more than 50% of the stomach is removed, such as that occurring during subtotal gastrectomy.

Postgastrectomy Syndromes Related to Gastric Reconstruction

- Afferent loop syndrome.
  - Afferent loop syndrome occurs as a result of partial obstruction of the afferent limb that is unable then to empty its contents.
  - In the setting of partial obstruction, the intraluminal pressure increases to forcefully empty its contents into the stomach, resulting in bilious vomiting that is often projectile but offers immediate relief of symptoms.
  - In the setting of complete obstruction, necrosis and perforation of the loop can occur because the obstruction is a closed loop.
  - For both forms of afferent loop syndrome, acute and chronic, operation is indicated because it is a mechanical problem not a functional problem. A long afferent limb is usually the underlying problem and treatment, therefore, involves the elimination of this loop.
- Efferent loop obstruction.
  - The most common cause of efferent loop obstruction is herniation of the limb behind the anastomosis in a right to left fashion.
  - Operative intervention is almost always necessary.
- Alkaline reflux gastritis.

- Hepatobiliary iminodiacetic acid (HIDA) scans are usually diagnostic.
- Most of the medical therapies that have been tried to treat alkaline reflux gastritis have not shown any consistent benefit. Thus, for those patients with intractable symptoms, surgery is recommended. The surgical procedure of choice usually means converting the Billroth II anastomosis into a Roux-en-Y gastrojejunostomy.
- Retained antrum syndrome.
  - Because the antral mucosa may extend past the pyloric muscle for a distance of 0.5 cm, the syndrome of retained gastric antrum may occur following partial gastrectomy even if the resection is carried beyond the pyloric sphincter.
  - It can be eliminated if biopsy confirmation of duodenal mucosa is obtained following resection of the proximal duodenum at the time of the Billroth II gastrectomy.
  - A technetium scan may prove helpful in diagnosing retained antrum.

Postvagotomy Syndromes

- Postvagotomy diarrhea.
  - Most patients with postvagotomy diarrhea have their symptoms resolve over time. In those patients who fail to resolve their symptoms, cholestyramine, an anionic exchange resin that absorbs bile salts rendering them unabsorbable and inactive, can significantly diminish the severity of diarrhea.
  - Only in rare cases is operative therapy necessary.
  - The operative procedure of choice is to interpose a 10-cm segment of reverse jejunum 70 to 100 cm from the ligament of Treitz.
- Postvagotomy gastric atony.
  - A mechanical cause of gastric outlet obstruction such as postoperative adhesions, afferent or efferent loop obstruction, and internal herniations must be ruled out.
  - In those patients with a functional gastric outlet obstruction and documented gastroparesis, pharmacotherapy is usually used.
- Incomplete vagal transection.
  - Predisposes the patient to the possible development of recurrent ulcer formation.
  - Either vagus nerve may be incompletely transected during truncal vagotomy, although the right vagus nerve is more frequently transected inadequately than the left.

STRESS GASTRITIS

Pathophysiology

- These stress-induced gastric lesions appear to require the presence of acid.
- Mucosal ischemia is thought to be the main factor responsible for the breakdown of these normal defense mechanisms.

Therapy

- There is little evidence to suggest that endoscopy with electrocautery or heater probe coagulation has any benefit in the therapy of bleeding from acute stress gastritis. However, some studies suggest that acute bleeding can be effectively controlled by selective infusion of vasopressin into the splanchnic circulation via the left gastric artery.
- Although vasopressin may decrease blood loss, it has not been shown to result in improved survival.
- Bleeding that recurs or persists requiring more than 6 units of blood (3000 mL) is an indication for operation.
- Bleeding areas are oversewn.
- Truncal vagotomy and pyloroplasty to reduce acid secretion.

Prophylaxis

- The patients at risk for stress gastritis in the intensive care setting appear to be patients with respiratory failure and who have underlying coagulopathy. For patients who do not have coagulopathy or require mechanical ventilation for less than 48 hours, one study suggested that prophylaxis for stress gastritis was unnecessary.
- Antacids can be administered as prophylaxis for stress gastritis and have an efficacy of 96%.
- There appears to be no significant advantage of H_2 blockers over antacids.
- Sucralfate has also been used for prophylaxis against stress gastritis and like antacids and H_2-receptor antagonists is extremely efficacious in the 90% to 97% range.

GASTRIC NEOPLASIA

Benign Tumors

Gastric Polyps

- Gastric polyps are usually an incidental finding on endoscopy, detected in 2% to 3% of gastroscopic evaluations.

Fundic gland polyps compromise 47% of all gastric polyps and have no malignant potential.

- Hyperplastic polyps are among the most frequently observed polyps and compose 28% to 75% of all gastric polyps. The lesions are typically less than 1.5 cm in size and arise in a setting of chronic atrophic gastritis 40% to 75% of the time.
- Although the hyperplastic polyp itself is non-neoplastic, dysplastic changes may occasionally develop in the polyp. Frank adenocarcinoma is detected in 2% of hyperplastic polyps.
- Adenomatous polyps have a distinct risk for malignancy. They account for 10% of all gastric polyps.
- Gastric adenocarcinoma may be found in 21% of cases, with increased risk with larger size and villous histology.
- Focal carcinomas were found in 6% of flat tubular adenomas and 33% of villous and tubulovillous adenomas.
- Coincident carcinomas have been reported in 8% to 59% of cases.
- Operative excision is recommended for sessile lesions larger than 2 cm, polyps found to have areas of invasive tumors, or polyps that are symptomatic secondary to pain or bleeding. Because of the increased risk of coincident gastric carcinoma, these patients should be followed closely by serial endoscopies.

Ectopic Pancreas

- The incidence of ectopic pancreatic tissue is 1% to 2% in autopsy series with 70% of cases occurring in the stomach, duodenum, and jejunum. Most patients with gastric ectopic pancreatic tissue are asymptomatic, whereas others present with symptoms similar to those of peptic ulcer disease.
- The mass can be visualized on upper GI endoscopy; however, tissue diagnosis can be difficult because of the submucosal location of the rests.
- Pancreatic rests that cause symptoms are treated by surgical excision.

Malignant Tumors

Adenocarcinoma

- Epidemiology
  - Gastric cancer is the 10th most common cancer in the United States.

- It is estimated that 22,000 patients will develop the disease each year and 13,000 of those will die.
- Twice as common in men as it is in women.
- Higher among U.S. black men than white men.
- Increases with age.
- The incidence of adenocarcinoma of the gastric cardia has increased steadily, whereas the incidence of cancer in other anatomic subsites has decreased.
- Risk factors.
  - Epidemiologic studies investigating the role of diet.
  - Diets low in animal protein and fat, high in complex carbohydrates.

Increased Risk

- The consumption of raw vegetables, citrus fruits, and high fiber breads are associated with a lower risk for gastric cancer.
- High levels of nitrates.
- *H. pylori* in drinking water.
- Increased risk for gastric cancer.
- Other factors associated with an increased risk of gastric cancer include low socioeconomic status, cigarette smoking, male gender, *H. pylori* infection.
- Infection with the *cagA* of *H. pylori* strain elicits more mucosal inflammation than *cagA*-negative strains and also confers a greater risk for developing gastric cancer.
- Balfour first reported a correlation between prior gastric surgery for benign disease and the subsequent development of gastric cancer in 1922.
- However, the risk is only observed after a latency of 15 years and is increased in patients operated on for gastric but not duodenal ulcers.
- Patients with pernicious anemia are also at increased risk for developing gastric cancer. The mucosa becomes very atrophic and develops antral and intestinal metaplasia. The relative risk for a patient with pernicious anemia developing gastric cancer is approximately 2.1 to 5.6.
- The presence of gastric polyps can increase a patient's risk of gastric cancer.
- Hyperplastic polyps are benign.
- Presence is associated with an increased risk of gastric cancer because they form in stomachs with established gastritis, a known risk factor for carcinoma.
- Adenomatous polyps carry a distinct risk for the development of malignancy in the polyp.

- The risk for the development of carcinoma is approximately 10% to 20% and increases with increasing size of the polyp.
- The c-*met* proto-oncogene is the receptor for the hepatocyte growth factor and is frequently overexpressed in gastric cancer as are the k-*sam* and c-*erbB2* oncogenes. The inactivation of the tumor suppressor genes *p53* and *p16* have been reported in both diffuse and intestinal-type cancers, whereas adenomatous polyposis coli (*APC*) gene mutations tend to be more frequent in intestinal type gastric cancers.
- Microsatellite instability reflects a gain or loss of repeat units in a germline microsatellite allele, indicating the clonal expansion that is typical of a neoplasm.
- Pathology.
  - Ninety-five percent of all malignant gastric neoplasms are adenocarcinomas.
  - The Borrmann classification system was developed in 1926 and remains useful today for the description of endoscopic findings. The Borrmann system divides gastric carcinoma into five types depending on the lesion's macroscopic appearance (Fig. 44–1).
  - The original histologic classification system was developed by Borders in 1942. Borders classified gastric carcinomas according to the degree of cellular differentiation, independent of morphology, and ranged from 1 (well differentiated) to 4 (anaplastic).

Borrmann's classification

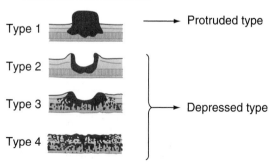

FIGURE 44–1. Bormann pathologic classification of gastric cancer based on gross appearance. *(From Iriyama K, Asakawa T, Koike H, et al: is extensive lymphadenectomy necessary for surgical treatment of intramucosal carcinoma of the stomach? Arch Surg 124:309, 1989. Copyright 1989, American Medical Association.)*

- The Lauren system separates gastric adenocarcinoma into intestinal or diffuse types based on histology.
- The intestinal variant typically arises in the setting of a recognizable precancerous condition such as gastric atrophy or intestinal metaplasia.
- Men more commonly affected than women.
- Incidence increases with age.
- Dominant histology in areas in which gastric cancer is epidemic.
- The diffuse form is poorly differentiated.
- Composed of signet ring cells.
- To spread submucosally.
- Metastasizes early.
- Route of spread is generally by transmural extension and through lymphatic invasion.
- Not generally arise in the setting of prior gastritis, is more common in women.
- Slightly younger age group.
- Type A.
- Familial occurrences.
- Intraperitoneal metastases are frequent.
- Clinical presentation.
  - Gastric adenocarcinoma lacks specific symptoms early in the course of the disease.
  - Early vague epigastric discomfort mistaken for gastritis, leading to symptomatic treatment for 6 to 12 months.
  - Typically, however, the pain is constant, nonradiating, and unrelieved by food ingestion.
  - Proximal tumors involving the GE junction often present with dysphagia, whereas distal antral tumors may present as gastric outlet obstruction.
  - Clinically significant GI bleeding is rare, but as many as 15% of patients may develop hematemesis and 40% of patients are anemic.
  - Patients may present with a palpable abdominal mass, a palpable supraclavicular (Virchow's) or periumbilical (Sister Mary Joseph's) lymph node, peritoneal metastasis palpable by rectal examination (Blumer's shelf), or a palpable ovarian mass (Krukenberg's tumor).
- Preoperative evaluation.
  - Flexible upper endoscopy is the diagnostic modality of choice.
  - During endoscopy, multiple biopsies (seven or more) should be obtained around the ulcer crater to facilitate histologic diagnosis.
  - If multiple biopsies are taken, the diagnostic accuracy of the procedure approaches 98%. The addition of direct

brush cytology to multiple biopsies may increase the diagnostic accuracy of the study.

- Some centers are using endoscopic ultrasonography (EUS) to assist in the staging of this disease. EUS can gauge the extent of gastric wall invasion and evaluate local nodal status.
- Once the diagnosis of gastric cancer is confirmed, further studies should include a complete blood count, serum chemistries to include liver function tests, coagulation studies, chest x-ray examination, and a CT scan of the abdomen. In women, a pelvic CT scan or ultrasound is also recommended. CT of the chest may be needed for proximal gastric cancers.
- The reported accuracy for CT staging of lymph node metastasis ranges from 25% to 86%.
- Laparoscopy can detect metastatic disease in 23% to 37% of patients judged to be eligible for potentially curative resection by current generation CT scanning.
- Laparoscopy improves palliation by avoiding nontherapeutic laparotomy in approximately one fourth of patients presumed to have localized gastric cancer.
- Cytologic analysis of peritoneal fluid or of fluid obtained by peritoneal lavage may reveal the presence of free intraperitoneal gastric cancer cells, identifying patients with otherwise occult carcinomatosis.
- Staging.
  - The pathologic staging system currently in use worldwide is the American Joint Committee on Cancer (AJCC) tumor-lymph node-metastasis (TNM) staging system.
  - Minimum of 15 nodes must be evaluated for accurate staging. Nodal staging is then determined by the number of positive nodes with pN1 reflecting 1 to 6 positive nodes, pN2 7 to 15 positive nodes, and pN3 more than 15 positive nodes.
  - The term R status was first described by Hermanek in 1994 and is used to describe the tumor status after resection.
  - The term R0 describes a microscopically margin negative.
  - R1 indicates removal of all macroscopic disease but microscopic margins are positive.
  - R2 indicates gross residual disease.
  - The Japanese Classification for Gastric Carcinoma (JCGC) staging system was designed to describe the anatomic locations of nodes removed during gastrectomy. Sixteen distinct anatomic locations of lymph nodes are described.
  - Recommendation for nodal basin dissection dependent on the location of the primary.

- Surgical treatment.
  - Location of disease. In the absence of distant metastatic spread, aggressive surgical resection of the gastric tumor is justified.
  - Because gastric tumors are characterized by extensive intramural spread, a line of resection at least 6 cm from the tumor mass is necessary to ensure a low rate of anastomotic recurrence.
  - Tumors of the cardia and proximal stomach account for 35% to 50% of all gastric adenocarcinomas.
  - For proximal lesions, either total gastrectomy or proximal gastric resection is necessary to remove the tumor.
  - Incidence of morbidity and mortality following proximal gastric resections was 52% and 16%, respectively, compared to 38% and 8% for total gastrectomy. Thus, total gastrectomy should be considered the procedure of choice for proximal gastric lesions. Distal tumors account for approximately 35% of all gastric cancers.
  - Thus, a luminal margin of 5 to 6 cm is recommended with frozen section analysis when a subtotal gastric resection is performed for adenocarcinoma.
  - JCGC D categories are used to define the extent of lymphatic dissection performed.
  - A D1 resection refers to the removal of group 1 lymph nodes, D2 to dissection of group 1 and group 2 nodes, whereas a D3 resection stands for a D2 resection plus removal of paraaortic lymph nodes. To effect complete removal of station 10 (parasplenic) and station 11 (parapancreatic) Japanese surgeons perform splenectomy and partial pancreatectomy during D2 resections for primaries whose drainage includes these echelons. Because of the increased morbidity in the patients receiving these adjunctive resections, Western surgeons do not typically resect the spleen or pancreas unless involved by direct extension from a T4 tumor.
  - It is clear that any extended resection is accompanied by an increase in morbidity and mortality without an improvement in survival. Thus, local organ resection, especially of the spleen, pancreas, or transverse colon, should be performed only when needed to accomplish an R0 resection.
  - Extended D2 lymph node dissections are routinely performed in Japan and have been demonstrated in studies performed in that country to provide a survival benefit over more limited D1 dissections.

- However, randomized controlled trials in the West of D2 versus D1 disections for gastric cancer have failed to demonstrate a survival benefit for the extended dissections.
- Extended lymph node dissections for gastric cancer remains an investigational treatment option and should be performed at specialized centers in the context of a clinical trial.
- Palliative treatment.
  - Twenty percent to 30% of gastric cancer patients present with stage IV disease.
  - The goal of palliative treatment is the relief of symptoms with minimal morbidity.
  - Complete staging is necessary to determine the appropriate method of palliation for individual patients.
  - Nonoperative therapies include laser recanalization and endoscopic dilation, with or without stent placement. Patients who undergo stent placement for gastric outlet obstruction are frequently able to tolerate solid foods and may not require additional interventions.
- Adjuvant therapy.
  - Southwest Cancer Oncology Group trial (INT-00116). This trial evaluated two cycles of 5-FU and leucovorin with subsequent concurrent chemoradiotherapy, using the same chemotherapeutic agents as adjuncts following an R0 resection of gastric adenocarcinoma.
  - Median survival for the surgery only arm was 27 months compared with 36 months ($p = .005$) for the chemoradiotherapy group.
  - Three-year survival 41% in the surgery group, compared to 50% in the chemoradiation therapy group ($p = .005$).
  - These data would support the addition of postoperative chemoradiation to the treatment of patients with resectable gastric adenocarcinoma.
- Outcomes.
  - Overall, 5-year survival after the diagnosis of gastric cancer is 10% to 21%.
  - Patients who undergo a potentially curative resection have a better prognosis with a 5-year survival rate of 24% to 57%.
  - Recurrence rates after gastrectomy remain high, ranging from 40% to 80%.
  - The most common sites of locoregional recurrence are the gastric remnant at the anastomosis, in the gastric bed, and in the regional nodes. Hematogenous spread occurs to the liver, lung, and bone.

- Surveillance.
  - Most recurrences occur within the first 3 years.
  - Follow-up should include a complete history and physical examination.
  - Laboratory: complete blood counts, liver function tests obtained as clinically indicated.
  - Chest x-rays films and CT scans of the abdomen and pelvis when clinically suspicious of a recurrence.
  - Yearly endoscopy should be considered in patients who have undergone a subtotal gastrectomy.

Gastric Lymphoma

- Epidemiology.
  - The stomach is the most common site for lymphomas in the GI system.
  - Patients often present with vague symptoms, namely epigastric pain, early satiety, and fatigue.
  - Peak incidence in the sixth and seventh decades and are more common in men (male-to-female ratio 2:1).
  - Most commonly occur in the gastric antrum.
  - Patients are considered to have gastric lymphoma if the stomach is the exclusive or predominant site of disease.
- Pathology.
  - The most common gastric lymphoma is diffuse large B-cell lymphoma (55%) followed by extranodal marginal cell lymphoma (mucosal-associated lymphoid tissue [MALT]) (40%), Burkitt's lymphoma (3%), and mantle cell and follicular lymphomas (each <1%).
  - Immunodeficiencies and *H. pylori* infection are risk factors for the development of primary diffuse large B-cell lymphoma.
  - In 1983 Isaacson and Wright noted that the histology of primary low-grade gastric B-cell lymphoma resembled that of MALT.
  - MALT lymphomas were recently reclassified as "extranodal marginal zone lymphomas of MALT-type."
  - Evidence of *H. pylori* infection can be found in almost every instance of gastric MALT lymphoma.
  - MALT lymphoma is characterized by t (1; 14)(p22; q32) and t (11; 18)(q21; q21), both of which result in impaired responsiveness to apoptotic signaling and increased nuclear factor κB (NF-κB) activity. Recent evidence suggests that the t (11; 18)(q21; q21) and B-cell lymphoma/leukemia 10 (Bcl-10) nuclear expression may predict for

nonresponsiveness to treatment by *H. pylori* eradication and lymphoma regression.

- *Burkitt's lymphomas of the stomach are associated with Epstein-Barr virus infections.*
- Very aggressive and tends to affect a younger aged population.
- *Most commonly found in the cardia or body of the stomach as opposed to the antrum.*

- Evaluation.
  - Endoscopy generally reveals nonspecific gastritis or gastric ulcerations with mass lesions being unusual. Occasionally a submucosal growth pattern will render endoscopic biopsies nondiagnostic.
  - Evidence of distant disease should be sought through upper airway examination, bone marrow biopsy, and CT of the chest and abdomen to detect lymphadenopathy. Any enlarged lymph nodes should be biopsied. *H. pylori* testing should be performed by histology and if negative confirmed by serology.
- Staging.
  - When possible, the TNM staging system should be used.
- Treatment.
  - The role of resection in gastric lymphoma remains controversial, and many patients are now being treated with chemoradiation.
  - The risk of perforation in patients treated with chemotherapy has been overstated in the past and approaches 5%. The most common chemotherapeutic combination is cyclophosphamide, doxorubicin, vincristine, and prednisone (CHOP).
  - Patients with early stage (stage IE, IIE) disease.
  - Similar disease free 5-year survival rates in patients treated with surgery, chemotherapy, and radiation therapy versus chemotherapy and radiation therapy alone (82% vs 84.4%; NS). Radiation therapy is limited in usefulness for larger tumors with local control rates dropping from 100% for tumors 3 cm or less to 60% to 70% for tumors larger than 6 cm.
  - Patients who present with late stage disease are not amenable to surgical cure and should be referred for chemotherapy.
  - Patients with disseminated lymphoma cannot be cured surgically and the operation should focus on obtaining enough tissue for diagnosis and the repair of perforations.
  - Patients with early-stage MALT lymphomas and some patients with very limited diffuse large B-cell lymphoma

may be effectively treated by *H. pylori* eradication alone. Successful eradication resulted in remission in more than 75% of cases.

- Some patients will continue to demonstrate the lymphoma clone after *H. pylori* eradication, suggesting the lymphoma became dormant rather than disappeared.
- The presence of transmural tumor extension, nodal involvement, transformation into a large cell phenotype, transformation t (11; 18), or nuclear Bcl-10 expression all predict for failure after *H. pylori* eradication alone.
- A small subset of MALT lymphoma patients will be *H. pylori*-negative. In these patients, consideration should be given to surgical resection, radiation, and chemotherapy. Five-year disease-free survival with multimodality treatment is greater than 95% is stage IE and 75% in stage IIE disease.

Gastric Sarcomas

- Epidemiology.
  - Gastric sarcomas arise from mesenchymal components of the gastric wall and compose about 3% of all gastric malignancies. Gastrointestinal stromal tumors (GISTs) are the most common mesenchymal tumor of the GI tract and are most frequently located in the stomach (60% to 70%). Patients usually present after the fourth decade, with the mean age of 60 at diagnosis.
- Pathology.
  - Histologically, originate from the cells of Cajal, autonomic nerve related GI pacemaker cells that regulate intestinal motility.
  - Cellular, spindle cell, or occasionally pleomorphic mesenchymal tumors located in the GI tract and express the Kit (CD117, stem cell factor receptor) protein. Kit is a transmembrane tyrosine kinase receptor, the ligand for which is stem cell factor.
  - Most GISTs (70% to 80%) also are positive for CD34, a hematopoietic progenitor cell antigen.
  - A subset of GISTs lack c-*kit* mutations and have intragenic activation mutations in a related tyrosine kinase receptor, platelet-derived growth factor-alpha.
- Staging.
  - Tumors that show low mitotic frequency (five or fewer mitosis per 50 high power fields [HPF]) usually have a benign behavior. Tumors with mitotic counts over 5 per 50 HPF are considered malignant, whereas tumors with more than 50 mitosis per 50 HPF are classified as high-grade

malignant. Malignancy is also associated with tumors greater than 5 cm in size, cellular atypia, necrosis, or local invasion. Mutations of c-*kit* occur predominantly in malignant GISTs and are an unfavorable prognostic marker. Most c-*kit* mutations occur in exon 11 and result in activation of c-*kit*. More than 80% of gastric GISTs are classified as benign according to the previous criteria.

- Benign gastric GISTs occur more frequently than malignant ones (3:1 to 5:1).
- Clinical manifestation and evaluation.
  - The most common presentations of gastric GISTs are GI bleeding and pain and dyspepsia.
  - Endoscopic biopsy is diagnostic in approximately 50% of the cases.
- Treatment.
  - The goal of surgery is a margin-negative resection to include *en bloc* resection of adjacent organs if involved by direct extension.
  - Rupture of the tumor should be avoided to prevent inoculation of the peritoneal cavity with tumor cells. Lymph node metastases are rare (<10%).
  - No known added benefit of extended lymphadenectomy. Most recurrences will occur in the first 2 years, presenting as local disease frequently associated with liver metastases.
  - Salvage surgery to resect recurrent disease has not been demonstrated to improve survival. Overall 5-year survival for gastric GISTs is 48% (19% to 56%) with survival after complete surgical resection ranging from 32% to 63%.
  - Radiation therapy has not been proven to be effective in their management and only 5% of tumors respond to doxorubicin-based cytotoxic chemotherapy. Imatinib mesylate (formerly ST1517, now Glivic/Gleevec [Novartis]) is a competitive inhibitor of certain tyrosine kinases, including the kinases associated with the transmembrane receptor Kit and platelet-derived growth factor receptors.
  - Fifty-four percent of patients exhibiting at least a partial response. Imatinib mesylate is approved for use in CD117-positive unresectable and/or metastatic GISTs.

OTHER GASTRIC LESIONS

Hypertrophic Gastritis (Ménétrier's Disease)

- Ménétrier's disease (hypoproteinemic hypertrophic gastropathy) is a rare, acquired, premalignant disease characterized by massive gastric folds in the fundus and corpus of the stomach, giving the mucosa a cobblestone or cerebriform appearance. Histologic examination reveals foveolar hyperplasia.

● The condition is associated with protein loss from the stomach.

● Associated with cytomegalovirus infection in children and *H. pylori* infection in adults. In addition, increased transforming growth factor α (TGF-α) has been noted in the gastric mucosa of patients with the disease.

● Twenty-four hour pH monitoring reveals hypochlorhydria or achlorhydria, and a chromium-labeled albumin test reveals increased GI protein loss.

● Some benefit has been shown through the use of anticholinergic drugs, acid suppression, octreotide, and *H. pylori* eradication. Total gastrectomy should be performed on patients who continue to have massive protein loss despite optimal medical therapy or if dysplasia or carcinoma develops.

Mallory-Weiss Tear

● Mallory-Weiss tears are related to forceful vomiting, retching, coughing, or straining that result in disruption of the gastric mucosa high on the lesser curve at the GE junction. They account for 15% of acute upper GI hemorrhages.

● Overall mortality is 3% to 4%, with the greatest risk in patients with portal hypertension.

● Portal hypertension.

● Most patients with active bleeding can be managed by endoscopic methods.

● Angiographic intra-arterial infusion of vasopressin or transcatheter embolization may be of use in very selective high-risk cases.

● If surgery is required, the lesion at the GE junction is approached through an anterior gastrotomy and the bleeding site oversewn with several deep 2-0 silk ligatures to reapproximate the gastric mucosa in an anatomic fashion.

Dieulafoy's Gastric Lesion

● Dieulafoy's lesions account for 0.3% to 7% of nonvariceal upper GI hemorrhages. Bleeding from a gastric Dieulafoy's lesion is caused by an abnormally large (1 to 3 mm), tortuous artery coursing through the submucosa.

● Generally the mucosal defect is 2 to 5 mm in size and is surrounded by normal-appearing gastric mucosa. The lesions generally occur 6 to 10 cm from the GE junction generally in the fundus near the cardia.

- Esophagogastroduodenoscopy is the diagnostic modality of choice, correctly identifying the lesion in 80% of patients.
- Repeated endoscopies may be needed to correctly identify the lesion.
- Attempts should be made to stop the bleeding using endoscopic modalities.
- Angiography can be useful in cases in which endoscopy could not definitely identify the source.
- Gelfoam embolization has been reported to successfully control bleeding in patients with Dieulafoy's, although the reported experience is limited.
- Surgery reserved for patients in whom other modalities have failed. The surgical management consists of gastric wedge resection to include the offending vessel.
- The difficulty locating the lesion unless it is actively bleeding.
- The surgical procedure can be facilitated by asking the endoscopist to tattoo the stomach when the lesion is identified.
- Surgical approach.
- Wide wedge resection.
- Can be approached laparoscopically, combined with intraoperative endoscopy.

Gastric Varices

- Gastric varices can develop secondary to portal hypertension, in conjunction with esophageal varices, or secondary to sinestral hypertension from splenic vein thrombosis.
- The incidence of bleeding from gastric varices is less than 10%.
- The incidence of bleeding can be as high as 78% in patients with splenic vein thrombosis and fundic varices.
- Gastric varices in the setting of splenic vein thrombosis are readily treated by splenectomy. Patients with bleeding gastric varices should have an abdominal ultrasound to document splenic vein thrombosis before surgical intervention, because gastric varices are most often associated with generalized portal hypertension.
- Gastric varices in the setting of portal hypertension should be managed like esophageal varices.
- Volume resuscitated correction of abnormal coagulation profiles.
- Temporary tamponade.
- Sengstaken-Blakemore.
- Successful eradication of the esophageal varices through banding or sclerotherapy often results in obliteration of

the gastric varices. Because gastric varices arise in the sub-mucosa, a common complication associated with gastric variceal sclerotherapy is ulceration.

● Endoscopic variceal band ligation can achieve hemostasis in approximately 89% of patients; however, concerns over gastric perforations with this technique have tempered its use. Transjugular intrahepatic portosystemic shunt (TIPS) can be effective in controlling gastric variceal hemorrhage, with rebleeding rates around 30%. A gastrorenal shunt between gastric varices and the left renal vein is present in 85% of patients with gastric varices.

● Balloon-occluded retrograde transvenous obliteration (BRTO) has been reported to have a high success rate (100%) with a low recurrence rate (0% to 5%). The major complication of this procedure is aggravation of esophageal varices secondary to a rise in portal pressure as a consequence of occluding the gastrorenal shunt.

Gastric Volvulus

● Gastric volvulus is an uncommon condition. Torsion occurs along the stomach's longitudinal axis (organoaxial) in approximately two thirds of cases and along the vertical axis (mesenteroaxial) in one third of cases.

● Organoaxial gastric volvulus occurs acutely and is associated with a diaphragmatic defect, whereas mesenteroaxial volvulus is partial (less than 180 degrees), recurrent, and is not associated with a diaphragmatic defect.

● The sudden onset of constant and severe upper abdominal pain, recurrent retching with production of little vomitus, and the inability to pass a nasogastric tube constitute Borchardt's triad.

● The diagnosis can be confirmed by barium contrast study or upper GI endoscopy. Acute volvulus is a surgical emergency. Through a transabdominal approach the stomach is reduced and uncoiled.

● The diaphragmatic defect is repaired.

● In the unusual case strangulation has occurred (5% to 28%), the compromised segment of stomach is resected.

Bezoars

● Bezoars are collections of nondigestible materials, usually of vegetable origin (phytobezoar) but also of hair (tricho-bezoar).

- The symptoms of gastric bezoars include early satiety, nausea, pain, vomiting, and weight loss.
- Dan et al in 1959 were the first to suggest enzymatic therapy to attempt dissolution of the bezoar. Papain, found in Adolph's meat tenderizer (AMT), is given in a dose of 1 teaspoon in 150 to 300 mL water several times daily.
- Alternative enzymes such as cellulase have been used with some success. Generally, enzymatic debridement is followed by aggressive Ewold tube lavage or endoscopic fragmentation. Failure of these therapies would necessitate surgical removal.
- Trichobezoars tend to form a cast of the stomach.
- Small trichobezoars may respond to endoscopic fragmentation, vigorous lavage, or enzymatic therapy. However, these techniques are of limited usefulness, and larger trichobezoars require surgical removal.
- The small bowel should be examined to be certain additional bezoars are not present.

CHAPTER 45

SMALL INTESTINE

ANATOMY

Neurovascular Supply

- Blood supply, except for the proximal duodenum, comes entirely from the superior mesenteric artery.
- Innervation is provided by both parasympathetic and sympathetic divisions of the autonomic nervous system.

Microscopic Anatomy

- The small bowel wall consists of four layers:
  - Serosa.
  - Muscularis propria.
  - Submucosa.
  - Mucosa.
- The epithelial layer is a continual sheet of epithelial cells covering the villi and lining the crypts.

PHYSIOLOGY

Digestion and Absorption

- Digestion and eventual absorption of nutrients, water, electrolytes, and minerals is the main role of the small intestine.

Carbohydrates

- The enzymes responsible for the final digestion of the starch molecules are concentrated in the brush border of the luminal surface.
- After dietary carbohydrate is reduced to monosaccharides by surface digestion, transport of the released hexoses is carried by specific mechanisms.
  - *Glucose* and *galactose* are absorbed by a carrier-mediated active transport.
  - *Fructose* is absorbed through a process of facilitated diffusion.

Protein

- In the small intestine, protein comes in contact with pancreatic proteases.
- The intraluminal action of the pancreatic proteases yields 70% short-chain peptides and 30% amino acids.

Fat

- Dietary fat is absorbed predominantly in the jejunum, with only approximately 500 to 600 mg lost in the stool every day; this is replaced by resynthesis from cholesterol.
- Unconjugated bile acids are absorbed in the jejunum by passive diffusion; conjugated bile acids that form micelles are absorbed in the ileum by active transport and are reabsorbed into the enterohepatic circulation from the distal ileum.

Water, Electrolytes, and Vitamins

- Approximately 8 to 10 L of water per day enter the small intestine; much of this is absorbed by simple diffusion.
- Sodium and chloride are absorbed along the small bowel by active transport.
- Calcium is absorbed, particularly in the proximal intestine (duodenum and jejunum), by a process of active transport; absorption appears to be facilitated by an acid environment and is enhanced by vitamin D and parathyroid hormone.
- Iron is absorbed as either a heme or nonheme component in the duodenum by an active process.
- Fat-soluble vitamins are carried in mixed micelles and transported to the lymph. Water-soluble vitamins are absorbed by active or passive mechanisms.

ENDOCRINE FUNCTION

Gastrointestinal Hormones

- The small bowel is the largest endocrine organ in the body.
- Gastrointestinal (GI) hormones play a major role in pancreaticobiliary and intestinal secretion and motility. In addition, certain GI hormones exert a trophic effect on both normal and neoplastic intestinal mucosa and pancreas.
- The location, major stimulants of release, primary actions, and diagnostic and therapeutic uses of the more important GI hormones are summarized in Table 45–1.

TABLE 45–1. Gastrointestinal Hormones

Hormone	Location	Major Stimulants of Peptide Secretion	Primary Effects
Gastrin	Antrum, duodenum (G cells)	Peptides, amino acids, antral distention, vagal and adrenergic stimulation, gastrin-releasing peptide (bombesin)	Stimulates gastric acid and pepsinogen secretion Stimulates gastric mucosal growth
Cholecystokinin	Duodenum, jejunum (I cells)	Fats, peptides, amino acids	Stimulates pancreatic enzyme secretion Stimulates gallbladder contraction Relaxes sphincter of Oddi Inhibits gastric emptying
Secretin	Duodenum, jejunum (S cells)	Fatty acids, luminal acidity, bile salts	Stimulates release of water and bicarbonate from pancreatic ductal cells Stimulates flow and alkalinity of bile Inhibits gastric acid secretion and motility and inhibits gastrin release
Somatostatin	Pancreatic islets (D cells), antrum, duodenum	Gut: fat, protein, acid, other hormones (e.g., gastrin, cholecystokinin) Pancreas: glucose, amino acids, cholecystokinin	Universal "off" switch: Inhibits release of gastrointestinal hormones Inhibits gastric acid secretion Inhibits small bowel water and electrolyte secretion Inhibits secretion of pancreatic hormones
Gastrin-releasing peptide (mammalian equivalent of bombesin)	Small bowel	Vagal stimulation	Universal "on" switch: Stimulates release of all gastrointestinal hormones (except secretin) Stimulates gastrointestinal secretion and motility Stimulates gastric acid secretion and release of antral gastrin Stimulates growth of intestinal mucosa and pancreas

Continued

TABLE 45–1. Gastrointestinal Hormones—cont'd

Hormone	Location	Major Stimulants of Peptide Secretion	Primary Effects
Gastric inhibitory polypeptide	Duodenum, jejunum (K cells)	Glucose, fat, protein adrenergic stimulation	Inhibits gastric acid and pepsin secretion Stimulates pancreatic insulin release in response to hyperglycemia
Motilin	Duodenum, jejunum	Gastric distention, fat	Stimulates upper gastrointestinal tract motility May initiate the migrating motor complex
Vasoactive intestinal peptide	Neurons throughout the gastrointestinal tract	Vagal stimulation	Primarily functions as a neuropeptide Potent vasodilator Stimulates pancreatic and intestinal secretion Inhibits gastric acid secretion
Neurotensin	Small bowel (N cells)	Fat	Stimulates growth of small and large bowel mucosa Glucagon-like peptide-1
Enteroglucagon	Small bowel (L cells)	Glucose, fat	Stimulates insulin release Inhibits pancreatic glucagon release Glucagon-like peptide-2 Potent enterotrophic factor
Pentide YY	Distal small bowel	Fatty acids, cholecystokinin	Inhibits gastric and pancreatic secretion Inhibits gallbladder contraction

IMMUNE FUNCTION

- Gut-associated lymphoid tissue is localized in three areas: Peyer's patches, lamina propria lymphoid cells, and intra-epithelial lymphocytes.
- One of the major protective immune mechanisms for the intestinal tract is the synthesis and secretion of IgA. Secretory IgA inhibits the adherence of bacteria to epithelial cells and prevents their colonization and multiplication.

OBSTRUCTION

Etiology

- The causes of a small bowel obstruction can be divided into three categories:
  - Extraluminal etiologies such as adhesions, hernias, carcinomas, and abscesses.
  - Processes intrinsic to the bowel wall (e.g., primary tumors).
  - Intraluminal obturator obstruction (e.g., gallstones, enteroliths, foreign bodies, and bezoars).
- Adhesions secondary to previous surgeries are, by far, the most common etiology of small bowel obstruction.
- Malignant tumors account for approximately 20% of the cases of small bowel obstruction. The majority of these tumors are metastatic lesions that obstruct the intestine secondary to peritoneal implants that have spread from an intraabdominal primary tumor.
- Hernias are the third leading cause of intestinal obstruction and account for approximately 10% of all cases.
- An important etiology of small bowel obstruction that is not routinely considered is obstruction associated with an intra-abdominal abscess.

Pathophysiology

- Early in the course of an obstruction, intestinal motility and contractile activity increase in an effort to propel luminal contents past the obstructing point.
- Later, the intestine fatigues and dilates, with contractions becoming less frequent and less intense.
- As the bowel dilates, water and electrolytes accumulate both intraluminally and in the bowel wall itself. This massive third-space fluid loss accounts for the dehydration and hypovolemia.

- Oliguria, azotemia, and hemoconcentration can accompany the dehydration. Hypotension and shock can ensue.
- Other consequences of bowel obstruction include increased intraabdominal pressure, decreased venous return, and elevation of the diaphragm, compromising ventilation.

Clinical Manifestations and Diagnosis

- In most patients, a meticulous history and physical examination complemented by plain abdominal x-rays are all that is required to establish the diagnosis.
- More sophisticated radiographic studies may be necessary in certain patients in whom the diagnosis and etiology are uncertain.

History

- The cardinal symptoms of intestinal obstruction include colicky abdominal pain, nausea, vomiting, abdominal distention, and a failure to pass flatus and feces (i.e., obstipation).

Physical Examination

- Abdominal distention.
- Early in the course of bowel obstruction, auscultation of the abdomen may demonstrate hyperactive bowel sounds with audible rushes associated with vigorous peristalsis (i.e., borborygmi).
- Late in the obstructive course, minimal or no bowel sounds are noted.
- Mild abdominal tenderness may be present with or without a palpable mass; localized tenderness, rebound, and guarding suggest peritonitis and the likelihood of strangulation.
- A careful examination must be performed to rule out incarcerated hernias.
- A rectal examination should be done to assess for intraluminal masses and to examine the stool for occult blood, which may be an indication of a malignancy, intussusception, or infarction.

Radiologic and Laboratory Examinations

- Characteristic findings on supine x-rays are dilated loops of small intestine without evidence of colonic distention.

Upright x-rays demonstrate multiple air fluid levels, which often layer in a stepwise pattern.

- Computed tomography (CT) has proven beneficial. CT is helpful if an extrinsic cause of bowel obstruction (e.g., abdominal tumors, inflammatory disease, or abscess) is suggested.
- Barium studies, in particular enterolysis, have been a useful adjunct in certain patients with a presumed obstruction.
- Laboratory examinations are not helpful in the diagnosis of patients with small bowel obstruction but are extremely important in assessing the degree of dehydration.
- Leukocytosis may be found in patients with strangulation; however, an elevated white cell count does not necessarily denote strangulation. Conversely, the absence of leukocytosis does not eliminate strangulation as a possibility.

Simple Versus Strangulating Obstruction

- Most patients with small bowel obstruction are classified as *simple* obstructions that involve mechanical blockage of the flow of luminal contents without compromising viability of the intestinal wall.
- In contrast, *strangulation* obstruction, which usually involves a closed-loop obstruction, can lead to intestinal infarction and is associated with increased morbidity and mortality.
- It is *important to remember* that bowel ischemia and strangulation cannot be reliably diagnosed or excluded preoperatively in all cases by any known clinical parameter, combination of parameters, or by current laboratory and x-ray examinations.

Treatment

Fluid Resuscitation and Antibiotics

- Patients require aggressive intravenous replacement with an isotonic saline solution such as Ringer's lactate.
- Urine output, electrolytes, hematocrit, and white cell counts should be monitored.
- Broad-spectrum antibiotics are given prophylactically by some surgeons.

Tube Decompression

- Nasogastric suction using a Levin tube is an important adjunct to the supportive care of patients with obstruction.

- Use of long intestinal tubes (such as Cantor or Baker tubes) is not indicated.

Operative Management

- The patient with a complete small bowel obstruction requires operative intervention.
- The nature of the problem dictates the approach to management.
  - Patients with an adhesive band may be treated by lysis of adhesions.
  - Incarcerated hernias can be managed by manual reduction of the herniated segment of bowel and closure of the defect.

Management of Specific Problems

Recurrent Intestinal Obstruction

- An initial nonoperative trial is usually desirable and often safe. In those patients who do not respond conservatively, reoperation is required.
- External plication procedures have been described but not routinely performed.
- Pharmacologic agents, including steroids and other anti-inflammatory agents, cytotoxic drugs, and antihistamines, have been used with limited success.

Acute Postoperative Obstruction

- Plain abdominal x-ray films are usually not helpful in distinguishing an ileus from obstruction. CT scans may be useful in this regard, and, in particular, enteroclysis studies may be quite helpful in determining if an obstruction exists.
- Conservative management should be attempted for a partial obstruction. Complete obstruction requires reoperation and correction of the underlying problem.

Ileus

- Defined as intestinal distention and the slowing or absence of passage of luminal contents without a demonstrable mechanical obstruction.
- Can result from a number of causes including drug-induced, metabolic, neurogenic, and infectious.

- Treatment is entirely supportive with nasogastric decompression and intravenous fluids.

INFLAMMATORY DISEASES

Crohn's Disease

- A chronic, transmural inflammatory disease of the GI tract of unknown cause.
- Can involve any part of the alimentary tract but most commonly affects the small intestine and colon.

Incidence and Epidemiology

- Most common primary surgical disease of the small bowel; the incidence is highest in North America and Northern Europe.
- Primarily attacks young adults in the second and third decades of life. However, a bimodal distribution is apparent with a second smaller peak occurring in the sixth decade of life.
- Strong familial association, with the risk of developing Crohn's disease increased approximately 30-fold in siblings and 13-fold for all first-degree relatives.

Etiology

- The cause of Crohn's disease remains unknown.
- A number of potential causes have been proposed, with the most likely possibilities include an infectious, immunologic, or genetic etiology.
- Individuals with allelic variants of the *NOD2* gene (IBD1 locus) have a 40-fold relative risk of Crohn's disease compared with the general population.

Pathology

- The most common sites of occurrence are the small intestine and colon.
- The disease process is discontinuous and segmental. In patients with colonic disease, rectal sparing is characteristic of Crohn's disease and helps to distinguish it from ulcerative colitis.
- Perirectal and perianal involvement occurs in about one third of patients with Crohn's disease, particularly those with colonic involvement.

Gross Pathologic Features

- Areas of diseased bowel separated by areas of grossly appearing normal bowel called *skip areas* are commonly encountered.
- A striking finding of Crohn's disease is extensive fat wrapping caused by the circumferential growth of the mesenteric fat around the bowel wall.
- As the disease progresses, the bowel wall becomes increasingly thickened, firm, rubbery, and virtually incompressible.
- On opening the bowel, the earliest gross pathologic lesion is a superficial aphthous ulcer noted in the mucosa.
- The ulcers are characteristically linear and may coalesce to produce transverse sinuses with islands of normal mucosa in between, thus giving the characteristic cobblestone appearance.

Microscopic Features

- Characteristic histologic lesions of Crohn's disease are *non-caseating granulomas* with Langhans' giant cells.
- Granulomas appear later in the course and are found in the wall of the bowel or in regional lymph nodes in 60% to 70% of patients.

Clinical Manifestations

- Typical patient is the young adult in the second or third decade of life.
- Onset of disease is often insidious, with a slow and protracted course.
- Characteristically, there are symptomatic periods of abdominal pain and diarrhea interspersed with asymptomatic periods.
- Most common symptom is intermittent and colicky abdominal pain.
- Diarrhea is the next most frequent symptom and is present, at least intermittently, in approximately 85% of patients.
- Systemic nonspecific symptoms include a low-grade fever (present in about one third of the patients), weight loss, loss of strength, and malaise.
- The main intestinal complications include obstruction and perforation.
- More commonly, fistulas occur between the sites of perforation and adjacent organs.
- Long-standing Crohn's disease predisposes to cancer of both the small intestine and colon.

- Perianal disease (fissure, fistula, stricture, or abscess) is common.
- Extraintestinal manifestations of Crohn's disease may be present in 30% of patients (Box 45–1).

Diagnosis

- Crohn's disease should be considered in patients with chronic, recurring episodes of abdominal pain, diarrhea, and weight loss.
- Barium radiographic studies of the small bowel may reveal a number of characteristic findings including the following:
  - Cobblestone appearance of the mucosa composed of linear ulcers, transverse sinuses, and clefts.
  - Long lengths of narrowed terminal ileum *(Kantor's string sign)* in long-standing disease.
  - Segmental and irregular patterns of bowel involvement.
  - Fistulas between adjacent bowel loops and organs.
- CT scanning may be useful in demonstrating the marked transmural thickening, and it can also aid in diagnosing extramural complications of Crohn's disease.
- In most instances, Crohn's disease of the colon can be readily distinguished from ulcerative colitis; however, in 5% to 10% of patients, the delineation between Crohn's and ulcerative colitis may be difficult, if not impossible, to make (Table 45–2).

Box 45–1. Extraintestinal Manifestations of Crohn's Disease

Skin
Erythema multiforme
Erythema nodosum
Pyoderma gangrenosum

Eyes
Iritis
Uveitis
Conjunctivitis

Joints
Peripheral arthritis
Ankylosing spondylitis

Blood
Anemia
Thrombocytosis

Phlebothrombosis
Arterial thrombosis

Liver
Nonspecific triaditis
Sclerosing cholangitis

Kidney
Nephrotic syndrome
Amyloidosis

Pancreas
Pancreatitis

General
Amyloidosis

TABLE 45–2. Diagnosis of Crohn's Colitis Versus Ulcerative Colitis

	Crohn's Colitis	Ulcerative Colitis
Symptoms and Signs		
Diarrhea	Common	Common
Rectal bleeding	Less common	Almost always
Abdominal pain (cramps)	Moderate to severe	Mild to moderate
Palpable mass	At times	No (unless large cancer)
Anal complaints	Frequent (>50%)	Infrequent (<20%)
Radiologic Findings		
Ileal disease	Common	Rare (backwash ileitis)
Nodularity, fuzziness	No	Yes
Distribution	Skip areas	Rectum extending upward and continuously
Ulcers	Linear, cobblestone, fissures	Collar-button
Toxic dilatation	Rare	Uncommon
Proctoscopic Findings		
Anal fissure, fistula, abscess	Common	Rare
Rectal sparing	Common (50%)	Rare (5%)
Granular mucosa	No	Yes
Ulceration	Linear, deep, scattered	Superficial, universal

Medical and Dietary Therapy

- There is no cure for Crohn's disease, so both medical and surgical therapy is mainly palliative and directed toward relieving acute exacerbations or complications of the disease.
- Sulfasalazine (Azulfidine), an aminosalicylate, has shown a clear benefit in patients with colitis and ileocolitis.
- Corticosteroids, particularly prednisone, have been beneficial in the induction of remission in active Crohn's disease.
- Other immunosuppressive agents that have been used with some effectiveness include azathioprine, 6-mercaptopurine, methotrexate, cyclosporine, and tacrolimus (FK-506).
- The most promising therapy to emerge in recent years are treatments using cytokines (e.g., interleukin [IL]-10) and anti-cytokines. Treatment with monoclonal antibody to tissue necrosis factor (TNF)-α (e.g., Infliximab) demonstrated a rapid control of active Crohn's disease, tissue healing, and potential remission.
- Certain antibiotics have also been found to be effective in the primary therapy of Crohn's disease.

● Nutritional therapy using chemically defined elemental diets and total parenteral nutrition (TPN) has been used with varying success.

Surgical Therapy

● The indications for operation are limited to complications that include the following:
  ● Intestinal obstruction.
  ● Intestinal perforation with fistula formation or abscess.
  ● Free perforation.
  ● GI bleeding.
  ● Urologic complications.
  ● Cancer.
  ● Perianal disease.
● Operative treatment of a complication should be limited to that segment of bowel involved with the complication and no attempt should be made to resect more bowel even though grossly evident disease may be apparent.
● Surgery is not curative but oftentimes can provide patients with significant symptomatic relief.

Typhoid Enteritis

● Remains a significant problem in developing countries.
● An acute systemic infection of several weeks' duration caused primarily by *Salmonella typhosa* and initiated after oral ingestion of the typhoid bacillus.
● Hyperplasia of the reticuloendothelial system, including lymph nodes, liver and spleen, is characteristic of typhoid fever.
● Peyer's patches in the small bowel become hyperplastic and may subsequently ulcerate with complications of hemorrhage or perforation.
● The diagnosis of typhoid fever is confirmed by isolating the organism from blood (positive in 90% of the patients during the first week of the illness), bone marrow, and stool cultures.
● Treatment of typhoid fever and uncomplicated typhoid enteritis is accomplished by antibiotic administration.
● Complications requiring potential surgical intervention include hemorrhage and perforation.

Enteritis in the Immunocompromised Host

● The growing acquired immunodeficiency syndrome (AIDS) epidemic and the widespread use of immunosuppressive agents after organ transplantation has resulted in a number of rare and exotic pathogens infecting the GI tract.

- The surgeon may be asked to evaluate the immunocompromised patient with abdominal pain, an obvious acute abdomen, or GI bleeding. A number of protozoal (e.g., *Cryptosporidium, Microsporium*), bacterial (e.g., *Salmonella, Shigella*), viral (e.g., cytomegalovirus), and fungal (e.g., histoplasmosis) organisms may be responsible.

Mycobacteria

- Mycobacterial infection is a frequent cause of intestinal disease in immunocompromised hosts. This can be either secondary to *Mycobacterium tuberculosis* or *Mycobacterium avium* complex (MAC).
- The usual route of infection is by swallowed organisms that directly penetrate the intestinal mucosa.
- Clinically, patients with MAC present with diarrhea, fever, anorexia, and progressive wasting.
- The most frequent site of intestinal involvement of *M. tuberculosis* is the distal ileum and cecum, with 85% to 90% of patients demonstrating disease at this site.
- The diagnosis of mycobacterial infection is made by identification of the organism in tissue, either by direct visualization with an acid-fast stain, by culture of the excised tissue, or by polymerase chain reaction (PCR) techniques.
- The treatment of *M. tuberculosis* is similar in the immunocompromised or nonimmunocompromised host. The organism is usually responsive to multidrug, antimicrobial therapy.

NEOPLASMS

General Considerations

- Small bowel neoplasms are exceedingly rare.
- Only 5% of all GI neoplasms and only 1% to 2% of all malignant tumors of the GI tract occur in the small bowel.
- The mean age of presentation is 62 years for benign tumors and approximately 57 years for malignant lesions.
- Males have a higher incidence of small bowel cancer than females.
- Highest cancer rates found among the Maori of New Zealand and ethnic Hawaiians.
- Depending on the series, either adenocarcinoma or carcinoid tumor is the most common malignant neoplasm.

Diagnosis

- High index of suspicion required.
- An upper GI tract series with small intestinal follow-through yields an accurate diagnosis in 50% to 70% of patients with malignant neoplasms of the small intestine.

Clinical Manifestations

Benign Neoplasms

- Benign GI stromal tumors (GISTs), which arise from the interstitial cell of Cajal, and adenomas are the most frequent of the benign tumors.
- Most patients with benign neoplasms remain asymptomatic, and the neoplasms are only discovered at autopsy or as incidental findings.
- Of the remainder, pain, most often related to obstruction, is the most frequent complaint.
- Hemorrhage is the next most common symptom, which is usually occult.

Malignant Neoplasms

- The most common malignant neoplasms of the small bowel in the approximate order of frequency are adenocarcinomas, carcinoid tumors, malignant GISTs, and lymphomas.
- In contrast with benign lesions, malignant neoplasms almost always produce symptoms, the most common of which include pain and weight loss.
- Diarrhea with tenesmus and passage of large amounts of mucus may occur.
- GI bleeding is manifested by anemia and guaiac-positive stools or occasionally by melena or hematochezia.
- A palpable mass may be felt in 10% to 20% of patients, and perforations develop in about 10%, usually secondary to lymphomas and sarcomas.

Treatment

- Complications of benign neoplasm that most often require treatment include bleeding and obstruction; segmental resection and primary anastomosis are most commonly performed.
- The treatment for malignant neoplasms of the small bowel is wide resection including regional lymph nodes. This may

require pancreaticoduodenectomy (Whipple operation) for duodenal lesions.

- Adjuvant radiation and chemotherapy have little role in the treatment of patients with adenocarcinomas of the small bowel. There may be some improvement in survival when radiotherapy is used in patients with sarcomas. Radiotherapy and chemotherapy combined with surgical excision provide the best survival rates for patients with lymphomas.

- Adenocarcinoma has the poorest prognosis, with an overall survival rate of 15% to 20%. Malignant GISTs and lymphomas have a 5-year survival rate of approximately 25% to 35%.

- Imatinib mesylate (Gleevec), a tyrosine kinase inhibitor which blocks the unregulated c-*kit* (CD177) tyrosine kinase, appears to be effective in the treatment of certain metastatic GISTs.

Carcinoid Tumors

- The GI tract is the most common site for carcinoid tumors. After the appendix, the small intestine is the second most frequently affected site in the GI tract.

- In the small intestine, carcinoids almost always occur within the last 2 feet of the ileum.

- Arise from enterochromaffin cells (Kulchitsky cells) found in the crypts of Lieberkuhn.

- Most patients are in the fifth decade of life.

- Carcinoid tumors may be derived from the foregut, midgut, or hindgut.

- Foregut carcinoids characteristically produce low levels of serotonin (5-hydroxytryptamine [5-HT]) but may secrete 5-hydroxytryptophan (5-HTP) or adrenocorticotrophic hormone (ACTH).

- Midgut carcinoids are characterized by having high serotonin production.

- Hindgut carcinoids rarely produce serotonin but may produce other hormones such as somatostatin and peptide YY.

- The primary importance of carcinoid tumors is the malignant potential of the tumors themselves. Although the carcinoid syndrome can occur and is quite dramatic in its most florid form, it occurs in only a small percentage of patients with malignant carcinoids.

Pathology

- Seventy percent to 80% of carcinoids are asymptomatic and found incidentally at time of operation.

- In the GI tract, more than 90% of carcinoids are found in three sites: the appendix (45%), the ileum (28%), and the rectum (16%).
- The malignant potential (ability to metastasize) is related to location, size, depth of invasion, and growth pattern.
- Small bowel carcinoids are multicentric in 20% to 30% of patients. This tendency to multicentricity exceeds that of any other malignant neoplasm of the GI tract.
- Another unusual observation is the frequent coexistence of a second primary malignant neoplasm of a different histologic type. This is usually a synchronous adenocarcinoma (most commonly in the large intestine), which can occur in 10% to 20% of patients with carcinoid tumors.

Clinical Manifestations

Carcinoid Tumors

- The most common symptoms include abdominal pain, which is variably associated with partial or complete small intestinal obstruction.
- Diarrhea and weight loss may also occur.

Malignant Carcinoid Syndrome

- The malignant carcinoid syndrome is a relatively rare disease, occurring in less than 10% of patients with carcinoid tumors.
- The syndrome is most commonly associated with carcinoid tumors of the GI tract, particularly from the small bowel.
- Common symptoms and signs include cutaneous flushing (80%); diarrhea (76%); hepatomegaly (71%); cardiac lesions, most commonly right heart valvular disease (41% to 70%); and asthma (25%).
- Malabsorption and pellagra (dementia, dermatitis, and diarrhea) are occasionally present and are thought to be caused by excessive diversion of dietary tryptophan.

Diagnosis

- Carcinoid tumors produce serotonin, which is then metabolized in the liver and the lung to the pharmacologically inactive 5-hydroxyindoleacetic acid (5-HIAA). Elevated urinary levels of 5-HIAA measured over 24 hours by high-performance liquid chromatography are highly specific.

- A novel imaging study that takes advantage of the fact that many of these tumors possess somatostatin receptors is somatostatin receptor scintigraphy using indium-111-labeled (^{111}In) pentetreotide.

Treatment

- Treatment of patients with small bowel carcinoid tumors is based on their size, site of the tumor, and the presence or absence of metastatic disease.
- For primary tumors of less than 1 cm in diameter without evidence of regional lymph node metastasis, a segmental intestinal resection is adequate. For patients with lesions more than 1 cm, with multiple tumors, or with regional lymph node metastasis, regardless of the size of the primary tumor, wide excision of bowel and mesentery are required.
- Anesthesia may precipitate a carcinoid crisis characterized by hypotension, bronchospasm, flushing, and tachycardia predisposing to arrhythmias; treatment is intravenous octreotide.
- In patients with carcinoid tumors and widespread metastatic disease, surgery is still indicated. In contrast to metastases from other tumors, there is a definite role for surgical debulking.
- In the case of widespread multiple hepatic metastases, hepatic artery ligation or percutaneous embolization has produced good results.
- Medical therapy for patients with malignant carcinoid syndrome is primarily directed toward the relief of symptoms caused by the excess production of humoral factors. Various long-acting analogues of somatostatin, such as octreotide (Sandostatin), relieve symptoms (diarrhea and flushing) of the carcinoid syndrome in most patients.
- Cytotoxic chemotherapy has only had limited success.
- In summary, treatment of carcinoid tumors requires a multidisciplinary approach and combined modalities may be the best option, including surgical debulking, hepatic artery embolization or chemoembolization, and medical therapy.

Prognosis

- Carcinoid tumors have the best prognosis of all small bowel tumors, whether the disease is localized or metastatic.
- Resection of a carcinoid tumor localized to its primary site approaches a 100% survival rate.

- Five-year survival rates are approximately 65% among patients with regional disease and 25% to 35% among those with distant metastasis.

Metastatic Neoplasm

- Metastatic tumors involving the small bowel are much more common than primary neoplasms.
- The most common metastases to the small intestine are those arising from other intra-abdominal organs.
- Metastases from extra-abdominal tumors are rare but may be found in patients with cutaneous melanoma (most common extra-abdominal source), adenocarcinoma of the breast, and carcinoma of the lung.
- Treatment is palliative resection to relieve symptoms.

DIVERTICULAR DISEASE

- Diverticular disease of the small intestine is relatively common; it may present as either true or false diverticula.
- A true diverticulum contains all layers of the intestinal wall and is usually congenital; false diverticula consist of mucosa and submucosa protruding through a defect in the muscle coat and are usually acquired defects.
- Duodenal diverticula are the most common acquired diverticula of the small bowel, and Meckel's diverticulum is the most common true congenital diverticulum of the small bowel.

Duodenal Diverticula

Incidence and Etiology

- Diverticula of the duodenum are relatively common, representing the second most common site for diverticulum formation after the colon.
- Occur twice as often in women as in men and are rare in patients younger than 40 years.
- Although the typical location is in the second portion of the duodenum, approximately 10% of duodenal diverticula develop more distally and laterally.

Clinical Manifestations

- Most duodenal diverticula are asymptomatic and are usually noted incidentally.

- Less than 5% will require surgery because of a complication of the diverticulum itself.
- Major complications include obstruction of the biliary or pancreatic ducts, hemorrhage, perforation, and, rarely, "blind loop" syndrome.

Treatment

- Most duodenal diverticula are asymptomatic and benign, and, when they are found incidentally, they should be left alone.
- The most common and most effective treatment for a symptomatic duodenal diverticulum is diverticulectomy.

Jejunal and Ileal Diverticula

Incidence and Etiology

- Diverticula of the small bowel are much less common than duodenal diverticula.
- These are false diverticula occurring mainly in an older age group.
- Multiple, usually protrude from the mesenteric border of the bowel and are embedded within the small bowel mesentery.
- Etiology is thought to be a motor dysfunction of the smooth muscle or the myenteric plexus.

Clinical Manifestations

- Usually found incidentally at laparotomy or during performance of an upper GI study; most remain asymptomatic.
- Acute complications such as intestinal obstruction, hemorrhage, or perforation can occur but are rare.
- Chronic symptomology includes vague chronic abdominal pain, malabsorption, functional pseudoobstruction, and chronic low-grade GI hemorrhage.

Treatment

- For incidentally noted, asymptomatic jejunoileal diverticula, no treatment is required.
- Treatment for complications of obstruction, bleeding, and perforation is usually by intestinal resection and end-to-end anastomosis.
- Patients presenting with malabsorption secondary to the blind loop syndrome and bacterial overgrowth within the diverticulum can usually be treated with antibiotics.

Meckel's Diverticulum

Incidence and Etiology

- Most commonly encountered congenital anomaly of the small intestine, occurring in approximately 2% of the population.
- Located on the antimesenteric border of the ileum approximately 45 to 60 cm proximal to the ileocecal valve.
- Results from incomplete closure of the omphalomesenteric duct.
- Not uncommon to find heterotopic tissue within the Meckel's diverticulum, the most common of which is gastric mucosa (present in 50% of all Meckel's diverticula), and pancreatic mucosa (present in approximately 5% of diverticula).

Clinical Manifestations

- Most are entirely benign and are incidentally discovered.
- Most common clinical presentation is GI bleeding, which occurs in 25% to 50% of patients who present with complications; hemorrhage is the most common symptomatic presentation for children aged 2 years or younger.
- Another common presenting symptom is intestinal obstruction, which may occur as a result of a volvulus, intussusception, or, rarely, incarceration of the diverticulum in an inguinal hernia (Littre's hernia).
- Diverticulitis accounts for approximately 10% to 20% of symptomatic presentations and is more common in adult patients.

Diagnostic Studies

- In children, the single most accurate diagnostic test for Meckel's diverticula is scintigraphy with sodium ^{99m}Tc-pertechnetate.
- In adults, however, ^{99m}Tc-pertechnetate scanning is less accurate. The sensitivity and specificity can be improved by the use of pharmacologic agents such as pentagastrin and glucagon or H_2-receptor antagonists (e.g., cimetidine).

Treatment

- The treatment of a symptomatic Meckel's diverticulum should be prompt surgical intervention with resection of the diverticulum or resection of the segment of ileum bearing the diverticulum.

- Controversy still exists regarding the optimal treatment of a Meckel's diverticulum noted as an incidental finding.

MISCELLANEOUS PROBLEMS

Small Bowel Ulcerations

- Relatively uncommon and may be attributed to Crohn's disease, typhoid fever, tuberculosis, lymphoma, and ulcers associated with gastrinoma.
- Drug-induced ulcerations can occur and have been attributed to enteric-coated potassium chloride tablets, corticosteroids, and nonsteroidal anti-inflammatory drugs (NSAIDs).
- Treatment of complications is segmental resection and intestinal reanastomosis.

Ingested Foreign Bodies

- Foreign bodies are swallowed, usually accidentally, by children or adults.
- Intentional ingestion is sometimes seen in the incarcerated and the mentally deranged.
- For most patients, treatment is observation; surgery is required for complications (e.g., perforation, obstruction).

Enterocutaneous Fistulas

- Most commonly iatrogenic, usually the result of a surgical misadventure.
- Less than 2% occur spontaneously and are usually the result of Crohn's disease.
- Classified according to their location and volume of daily output.
- In general, the more proximal the fistula in the intestine, the more serious the problem with greater fluid and electrolyte loss.
- Factors that prevent the spontaneous closure of fistulas are shown in Box 45–2.
- Radiographic investigation of the fistula is accomplished by injection of water-soluble contrast material through the fistula tract.
- CT scan is helpful in determining if underlying collections of fluid or pus are present.
- Major complications include sepsis, fluid and electrolyte depletion, necrosis of the skin at the site of external drainage, and malnutrition.

> **Box 45–2. Factors Preventing Spontaneous Fistula Closure**
>
> High output (>500 mL/24 hr)
> Severe disruption of intestinal continuity (>50% of bowel circumference)
> Active inflammatory bowel disease of bowel segment
> Cancer
> Radiation enteritis
> Distal obstruction
> Undrained abscess cavity
> Foreign body in the fistula tract
> Fistula tract <2.5 cm in length
> Epithelialization of fistula tract

- Mortality of patients with enterocutaneous fistulas remain high, with some series reporting a 15% to 20% mortality rate.

Treatment

- Successful management requires the following:
  - Establishment of controlled drainage.
  - Management of sepsis.
  - Prevention of fluid and electrolyte depletion.
  - Protection of the skin.
  - Provision of adequate nutrition.
  - Long-acting somatostatin analog, octreotide, has been used with successful decrease in the volume of output.
- A reasonable management plan would be to follow a conservative course for 4 to 6 weeks, at which time, if closure has not been obtained, surgical management should be considered.
- The preferred operation is fistula tract excision and segmental resection of the involved segment of intestine and reanastomosis.

Pneumatosis Intestinalis

- Uncommon condition presenting as multiple gas-filled cysts of the GI tract.
- Most common in the jejunum, followed by the ileocecal region and the colon.

- Most commonly occurs in the fourth to seventh decades of life.
- Most cases are associated with chronic obstructive pulmonary disease or the immunocompromised state.
- Diagnosis is usually made radiographically by plain abdominal or barium studies.
- No treatment is necessary unless one of the very rare complications supervenes such as rectal bleeding, cyst-induced volvulus, or tension pneumoperitoneum.

Blind Loop Syndrome

- Rare condition manifested by diarrhea, steatorrhea, megaloblastic anemia, weight loss, abdominal pain, deficiencies of the fat-soluble vitamins (A, D, E, and K), and neurologic disorders.
- Etiology is bacterial overgrowth in stagnant areas of the small bowel produced by stricture, stenosis, fistulas, or diverticula.
- Treatment is parenteral vitamin B_{12} therapy and a broad-spectrum antibiotic.
- Surgical correction produces a permanent cure and is indicated in those patients who require multiple rounds of antibiotics.

Radiation Enteritis

- Small intestinal epithelium may sustain severe, acute, and chronic deleterious effects from radiation therapy used for abdominal or pelvic cancer.
- Serious late complications are unusual if the total radiation dosage is less than 4000 cGy; morbidity risk increases with dosages exceeding 5000 cGy.
- Radiation damage tends to be acute and self-limiting, with symptoms consisting of mainly diarrhea, abdominal pain, and malabsorption.
- The late effects of radiation injury are the result of damage to the small submucosal blood vessels with a progressive obliterative arteritis and submucosal fibrosis, resulting eventually in thrombosis and vascular insufficiency. This leads eventually to stricture formation with symptoms of obstruction or small bowel fistulas.
- Indications for operative intervention include obstruction, fistula formation, perforation, and bleeding.
- Operative procedures include a bypass or resection with reanastomosis.

Short Bowel Syndrome

- Results from a total small bowel length that is inadequate to support nutrition.
- Most cases occur from massive intestinal resection.
- Multiple sequential resections, most commonly associated with recurrent Crohn's disease, account for 25% of patients.
- In neonates, the most common cause of short bowel syndrome is bowel resection secondary to necrotizing enterocolitis.
- Clinical hallmarks include diarrhea, fluid and electrolyte deficiency, and malnutrition.
- The likelihood that a patient will be permanently dependent on TPN is thought to be primarily influenced by the length, location, and the health of the remaining intestine.
- Although there is considerable individual variation, resection of up to 70% of the small bowel usually can be tolerated if the terminal ileum and ileocecal valve are preserved.
- Proximal bowel resection is tolerated much better than distal resection because the ileum can adapt and increase its absorptive capacity more efficiently than the jejunum.

Treatment

- After massive small bowel resection, the treatment course may be divided into early and late phases.
- In its early phase, treatment is primarily directed at the control of diarrhea, replacement of fluid and electrolytes, and the prompt institution of TPN.
- As soon as the patient has recovered from the acute phase, enteral nutrition should begin so that intestinal adaptation may be started early and proceed successfully.
- The role of hormones administered systemically and glutamine administered enterally are being evaluated.
- A number of surgical strategies have been attempted in patients who are chronically TPN dependent with limited success; these include procedures to delay intestinal transit time, methods to increase absorptive area, and small bowel transplantation.

Vascular Compression of the Duodenum

- Vascular compression of the duodenum, also known as superior mesenteric artery syndrome or Wilkie's syndrome, is a rare condition characterized by compression of the third portion of the duodenum by the superior mesenteric artery as it passes over this portion of the duodenum.

- Symptoms include profound nausea and vomiting, abdominal distention, weight loss, and postprandial epigastric pain, which varies from intermittent to constant depending on the severity of the duodenal obstruction.
- Diagnosis is by barium upper GI series or hypotonic duodenography.
- Conservative measures are tried initially and have been increasingly successful as definitive treatment.
- The operative treatment of choice is duodenojejunostomy.

CHAPTER 46

APPENDIX

ANATOMY AND EMBRYOLOGY

- The appendix is a derivative of the midgut along with the ileum and ascending colon.
- The appendiceal artery, a branch of the ileocolic artery, supplies the appendix.
- The normal location of the appendix is retrocecal but within the peritoneal cavity, because the most inferior portion of the cecum is within the peritoneal cavity. This situation occurs approximately 65% of the time.

APPENDICITIS

Pathophysiology

- It is widely accepted that the inciting event in most instances of appendicitis is obstruction of the appendiceal lumen.

Bacteriology

- Peritoneal cultures will be positive in more than 85% of patients with gangrenous or perforated appendicitis.

Diagnosis

Clinical

- The diagnosis of acute appendicitis is made primarily on the basis of the history and the physical findings. Laboratory and radiographic examinations may provide assistance.
- The appendix is often situated at or around McBurney's point. However, it must be emphasized that the exact anatomic location of the appendix can be at any point on a 360-degree circle surrounding the base of the cecum.

Radiographic

- Abdominal radiographs.

- Ultrasound.
  - Most studies of graded compression ultrasound demonstrate a sensitivity of more than 85% and a specificity of more than 90%.
- Computed tomography (CT).
  - CT is especially useful in distinguishing those patients presenting late in their clinical course (48 to 72 hours) who may have developed a phlegmon or abscess, thus altering potential therapy.
  - A reasonable estimate is that CT is 90% sensitive to the detection of intra-abdominal inflammation, with an 80% to 90% positive predictive value.

Laboratory

- A completely normal leukocyte count and differential is uncommon in patients with appendicitis but can be seen.

Types of Treatment

- The treatment of appendicitis varies somewhat depending on the stage of the disease. In general, patients should receive fluid resuscitation before surgery. Appendectomy is required.

Acute Appendicitis

- Patients with acute, nonperforated appendicitis should undergo urgent appendectomy.
- There are a number of antibiotics that can be used as long as they provide activity against enteric anaerobic and gram-negative bacteria.
- An overall negative exploration rate of 20% should not be viewed as a gold standard with the availability of ultrasound- and CT-assisted diagnosis.

Perforated Appendicitis with Peritonitis

- It is important to ensure that the patient has been adequately resuscitated before undertaking an operation. Patients with perforated disease have established peritonitis and should receive appropriate broad-spectrum intravenous antibiotic therapy targeted against gram-negative aerobes and anaerobes prior to appendectomy.

Late Presentation with or without a Mass

● The preferred approach to the management of the appendiceal mass is percutaneous drainage, which is performed under image guidance (ultrasound or CT) and intravenous antibiotics directed against aerobic gram-negative and anaerobic organisms.

Interval Appendectomy

● Controversy exists, however, as to whether *interval appendectomy* (performing an elective appendectomy in the interval between bouts of appendicitis) is necessary to prevent recurrent bouts of appendicitis.

Chronic or Recurrent Appendicitis

● May occur, but is uncommon.

Appendicitis during Pregnancy

● Suspicion of appendicitis should lead to early surgical intervention in all trimesters. Negative laparotomy results in minimal fetal loss.

Special Considerations

● Intraoperative management of the noninflamed appendix.
● Crohn's disease.
  • Patients who undergo exploration for presumed appendicitis and have evidence of Crohn's disease should undergo appendectomy.
● Meckel's diverticulum.

Postoperative Complications

Infection

  • Infection remains the most common complication after the operative treatment of appendicitis. Although infection can occur in a number of locations, surgical site infection predominates.
  • The treatment of intra-abdominal abscess is usually percutaneous drainage and intravenous antibiotics with good results.

Bowel Obstruction

Infertility

- The risk of tubal infertility in female patients after appendicitis is unclear.

Miscellaneous

- Elderly patients have a higher rate of complications.

NEOPLASMS

Adenocarcinoma

- Carcinoids are the most common appendiceal neoplasm.
- The 5-year survival rate for appendiceal carcinoma is 55% and varies with the stage of the tumor.
- In general, mucinous carcinoma or adenocarcinoma of the appendix is seen in older patients thought to have acute appendicitis.

Carcinoid Tumors

- They are derived from midgut argentaffin cells, possibly of neural crest origin. The appendix or the small bowel has been reported to be the most frequent site for carcinoid tumors.
- Most appendiceal carcinoid tumors are asymptomatic or found incidentally and are less than 1 cm. Simple appendectomy is adequate treatment.
- Lesions greater than 2 cm have a higher incidence of distant metastases and should be treated by right hemicolectomy with the hope of decreasing local-regional recurrence.

CHAPTER 47

COLON AND RECTUM

ANATOMY

- The colon, or large intestine, extends from the ileocecal valve to the anus and is divided into five main segments:
  - Right colon.
  - Transverse colon.
  - Left colon.
  - Sigmoid colon.
  - Rectum.
- The colon contains the same circular muscular layer underneath the serosa as does the small intestine, but its outer longitudinal muscle layer is quite distinct.
- The outer longitudinal muscular coat is concentrated into three separate longitudinal strips the taeniae coli.

Cecum

- The ileocecal valve serves as a sphincter that prevents the reflux of luminal contents from the cecum into the terminal ileum.
- The cecum, which is isolated between two sphincters, becomes a hindgut fermentation chamber; it is the widest part of the colon (7.5—8.5 cm).
- The cecum is completely enveloped by peritoneum and usually has a certain degree of mobility.

Ascending Colon and Hepatic Flexure

- The ascending colon courses upward from the right lower quadrant to the infrahepatic space, at which point it turns right and downward to become the transverse colon.

Transverse Colon

- The transverse colon is the most mobile portion of the colon and may be found in either the upper abdomen or as far down as the pelvis.

Splenic Flexure

- The angle between the transverse colon and the descending colon is designated the *splenic flexure.*

Descending Colon and Sigmoid Colon

- The descending colon courses from the splenic flexure down to the sigmoid colon at the level of the pelvic brim.
- The sigmoid colon is the S-shaped segment of the colon that extends from the pelvic brim to the peritoneal reflection; this is the narrowest portion of the colon (2.5 cm).

Rectum

- The rectum is pulled forward by the puborectalis muscle, forming the anorectal angle.
- Much of the rectum can be considered extraperitoneal, or more precisely, infraperitoneal.
- Denonvilliers fascia separates the mesorectum from the presacral fascia.

Blood Supply to the Colon

- The cecum, ascending colon, hepatic flexure, and proximal portion of the transverse colon receive arterial blood supply from the superior mesenteric artery (SMA) via the ileocolic, right colic, and middle colic arteries.
- The inferior mesenteric artery supplies blood to the distal transverse colon, splenic flexure, descending colon, and sigmoid via the left colic artery and branches of the sigmoid and superior hemorrhoidal vessels.
- A rich network of vessels that originate in both the middle and the inferior hemorrhoidal arteries supplies the rectum.
- The anastomosis or linking of arcades between the superior and inferior mesenteric vessels is known as the *long anastomosis of Riolan.*

PHYSIOLOGY

- The function of the colon is the recycling of nutrients, whereas the function of the rectum is the elimination of stool.

Recycling of Nutrients

- The ileal effluent is rich in water, electrolytes, and nutrients that resist digestion.

- The colon absorbs these substances to avoid unnecessary losses of fluids, electrolytes, nitrogen, and energy.

Colonic Flora

- This complex population of microorganisms confers great metabolic potential on the colon, primarily through its degradative abilities.
- Numbers of aerobic bacteria range from 2.4×10^3 to 1.3×10^6 cfu/sample biopsy and total anaerobic bacteria from 1.4×10^5 to $\times 10^7$ cfu/sample.
- Bacteroides species predominate throughout the colon.

Fermentation

- Bacteria supply the host with butyrate, a bacterial fermentation product that has become the main fuel for colonic epithelial cells.
- The main sources of energy for intestinal bacteria are complex carbohydrates, also known as dietary fiber.

Short Chain Fatty Acids

- Short Chain Fatty Acids (SCFAs) constitute approximately two thirds of the colonic anion concentration, mainly as acetate, propionate, and butyrate.
- SCFAs are involved in the so-called ileocolonic brake (i.e., the inhibition of gastric emptying by nutrients reaching the ileocolonic junction).

Urea Recycling

- Humans, and mammals in general, do not produce urease; however, colonic bacteria are rich in urease.
- Bacteria firmly adherent to the colonic epithelium mediate the process of urea recycling.

Absorption

- The total absorptive area is estimated to be approximately 900 cm^2.
- Between 1000 and 1500 ml of fluid is poured into the cecum by the daily ileal effluent.
- The volume of water in stool is only 100 to 150 ml per day; this 10-fold reduction represents the most efficient site of absorption in the GI tract per surface area.

- The net absorption of sodium is even higher.
- Although water is absorbed passively, sodium requires active transport.
- The colonic mucosa absorbs bile acids, thus making the colon part of the enterohepatic circulation.

Secretion

- Potassium secretion requires both Na^+, K^+-ATPase and Na^+, K^+-2Cl cotransport on the basolateral membrane and an apical potassium channel.
- Chloride is secreted by colonic epithelium at a basal rate, which is increased in pathologic conditions such as cystic fibrosis and secretory diarrhea.
- Secretion of chloride also requires the coupling of Na^+, K^+-ATPase and Na^+, K^+-2Cl cotransport to exit passively through the apical membrane.
- Colonic secretion of H^+ and bicarbonate is coupled to the absorption of Na^+ and Cl^-, respectively.

Motility

- Transit through the colon is controlled by the autonomic nervous system.
- Parasympathetic nervous fibers supply the colon via the vagi and the pelvic nerves.
- Nerve fibers reaching the colon arrange themselves in several plexuses: subserosal, myenteric (Auerbach), submucosal (Meissner), and mucosal plexuses.
- Sympathetic nerve fibers originate in the superior and inferior mesenteric ganglia.
- The effects of a meal on colonic motility are commonly called the *gastrocolic reflex.*

Formation of Stool

- An individual who passes more than three loose stools per day is considered as having diarrhea, whereas fewer than three weekly stools is considered constipation.

Defecation

- Normal defecation requires adequate colonic transit time, stool consistency, and fecal continence.
- Fecal continence implies deferment of stool elimination; discrimination among gas, liquid, and solid stool; and selective elimination of gas without stool.

DIAGNOSTIC STUDIES

- The typical signs of colorectal pathology are rectal bleeding, changes in bowel pattern, and abdominal pain.
- Plain radiography is particularly useful in patients who present with acute abdominal complaints.

Plain Radiography

- The presence, distribution, and volume of air in the colon and rectum provide useful information.

Stool Guaiac Examination

- Examination of stool for the presence of blood is essential in evaluation of patients for colonic disease.

Barium Enema

- The sensitivity of barium enema (BE) is such that even diminutive polyps can be detected; it may provide a full assessment of the colon even when distal pathology prevents retrograde advancement of a colonoscope.

Endoscopy

Rigid Proctosigmoidoscopy

- It establishes with precision the distance between a rectal lesion and the anus, a critical measurement when deciding whether to remove or preserve the anal sphincter in conjunction with a proctectomy; limited exam of distal 25 cm.

Flexible Sigmoidoscopy

- The main advantage of flexible sigmoidoscopy is that it can be performed without sedation and can be used to examine 45 cm of distal bowel.

Colonoscopy

- Colonoscopy requires sedation.
- The main advantage of colonoscopy is that it allows for examination of the entire colon and intervention.
- If a tumor is found, a biopsy is obtained, and if a pedunculated polyp is found, it is removed at the same setting.

- Colonoscopy is technically more difficult than sigmoidoscopy.
- Colonoscopy has replaced BE as the initial colorectal screening method.

Colonic Transit Study

- A colonic transit study provides information about the motility of the colon.
- The subject is given a number of radiopaque markers to swallow.
- A normal colonic transit should carry the markers throughout the colon in 5 days.
- The diagnosis of constipation can be established and then classified as either *global inertia*, when markers are dispersed throughout the colon, or *segmental dysmotility*, if they pool in a certain area.

Scintigraphy

- The tracing of tagged red cells, or bleeding scans, may be used to study lower GI hemorrhage.
- The use of scintigraphy to study colonic transit time is a logical extension of the already well-established testing of gastric emptying by scintigraphy.
- When combined into a single test of gastric emptying, small-bowel and colon transit, the study is called whole-gut transit scintigraphy, a noninvasive tool to document dysmotility of any segment of the GI tract.

Defecography

- Cinedefecography consists of recording the act of defecation with videofluoroscopy.
- Static radiographs are also taken to study the relationship between the rectum and anus and bony structures of the pelvis.
- Abnormalities of the pelvic floor are highly prevalent, particularly in females and in the elderly.

Computed Tomography

- Computed tomography (CT) is an important method for staging of colonic and rectal tumors.
- CT allows diagnosis and treatment of abscesses through the percutaneous placement of drainage catheters.

Abdominal Ultrasonography

- Advantages of ultrasonography (US) include its use in pregnant women and its portability; abdominal US is used in colorectal disease to identify and possibly treat pericolic fluid collections.

Endorectal Ultrasonography

- Transrectal ultrasound (TRUS) or endoscopic ultrasound (EUS) can easily discern the level of penetration of a rectal tumor.
- These methods can also detect perirectal lymph node enlargement and invasion of other structures, such as the levator ani and the bony pelvis.

Stool Analysis

- In all surgical patients with diarrhea, a stool sample should be examined for enteropathogens and assay of *Clostridium difficile* toxin.
- The differentiation between malabsorptive and secretory diarrhea can be made by measurement of electrolytes and osmolality in stool.
- Stool can be used to study colonic inflammation and tumor development.

PREPARATION FOR OPERATION

- The rate of wound infection in patients undergoing colonic procedures who have not received prophylactic antibiotics may be as high as 75%.
- Methods used in preparing the bowel for both endoscopic and surgical procedures have evolved since the 1960s.

Mechanical

- Much of the dry weight of feces is bacteria.
- To reduce the bulk of feces and bacteria within the colon, mechanical cleansing of the colon is the integral feature of intestinal antisepsis and colon preparation.
- Cathartics (e.g., castor oil, citrate of magnesia, sodium phosphate, polyethylene glycol) are used for mechanical cleaning.

Antibiotics

- Antibiotics are employed, in conjunction with mechanical cleansing, preoperatively to further reduce the number of bacteria within the colon.
- The regimen selected should provide broad suppression of fecal flora with high activity against aerobic and anaerobic organisms.
- The most common agents used for oral antibiotic preparation are orally administered neomycin and erythromycin base or metronidazole; these agents are generally administered at 1:00, 2:00, and 10:00 PM the day before operation.
- Appropriate regimens for parenteral antibiotics should include agents that have considerable activity against aerobes and anaerobes such as second-generation cephalosporins.

OPERATIVE PROCEDURES

Colectomy

- The excision of the colon can be performed in segments (i.e., partial colectomies) or as a whole (i.e., total abdominal colectomy).
- The most important steps in performing colectomies are identifying and preserving structures surrounding the colon and gaining control of the blood vessels that supply the colon.
- Among the structures to be identified are the right ureter and duodenum, when mobilizing the right colon, and the splenic capsule and left ureter, when mobilizing the left colon.

Proctectomy

- Excision of the rectum can be performed with inclusion of the anus and the sphincter mechanism (i.e., abdominoperineal resection [APR]) or by a transabdominal approach while preserving the anus and sphincteric mechanism (i.e., low anterior resection [LAR]).
- The difficulties in performing proctectomies are dependent of the preservation of surrounding structures and the control of blood vessels.
- The main structure to preserve while excising the rectum is the pelvic nerve plexus.
- Two major complications of APR are neurogenic bladder and sexual dysfunction.

DIVERTICULAR DISEASE

Etiology and Pathogenesis

- Diverticular disease is more prevalent in countries with a low intake of dietary fiber or non-starch polysaccharides (NSPs).
- The colon depends on the presence of a minimum amount of luminal bulk to effectively propel its contents toward the rectum.
- When the amount of bulk reaching the colon is suboptimal, the segmental contractions generate excessive pressure and lead to herniations of the mucosa through the points of least resistance of the colonic wall; these are the points of entrance of the arteriae rectae into the colonic wall.
- Acquired colonic diverticula (false) differ from congenital diverticula (true), in which all layers of the wall protrude outside of the colonic lumen.
- The incidence increases with age; 20% at age 40, 40% at age 60, and 60% at age 80 have diverticula.

Pathology

- Diverticula are usually multiple and scattered through variable lengths of colon; they are more common in the left side than the right side of the colon and typically more common in the sigmoid colon; they do not occur in the rectum.

Clinical Presentation

- Diverticular disease remains asymptomatic unless a complication develops.
- Potential complications are inflammation (diverticulitis), stricture, bleeding, and perforation.
- Contained perforations become abscesses, whereas free perforations lead to diffuse peritonitis.
- With recurrent episodes of diverticulitis, the colonic wall can become scarred and cause obstruction of the lumen (i.e., stricturing).
- Patients with abdominal complaints are often found to have diverticular disease by either BE or colonoscopy.
- Often, diverticular disease coexists in a patient with colon cancer, irritable bowel syndrome, and even inflammatory bowel disease (IBD), especially Crohn s disease.

Diverticulitis

- The typical presentation is of left lower quadrant pain, fever, and chills.
- This symptomatology has led to the naming of *left-sided appendicitis* for acute diverticulitis.

Differential Diagnosis

- Differential diagnosis includes extracolonic pathology such as appendicitis, salpingitis, pelvic inflammatory disease, perforated gastric and duodenal ulcer, and pancreatitis, as well as colonic pathology such as perforated colon cancer, IBD, colonic infarction, and infectious colitis.
- The tests of choice to assist the clinician in the diagnosis and management of diverticulitis are blood analyses, including a complete blood cell count, and imaging studies such as transabdominal US and CT scanning.
- CT scanning not only is a very useful diagnostic tool but also has therapeutic value.
- BE and endoscopy are not advisable in the acute stage of diverticulitis owing to the possible disruption of the seal created around the diverticulum.
- Antibiotic agents with bactericidal capacity over gram-negative and anaerobic bacteria should be chosen.
- If CT scanning or US confirms the presence of an abscess, the next step is percutaneous drainage under the guidance of either imaging modality.
- The most common internal fistulas caused by diverticulitis are colovesical, colovaginal, colocutaneous, colotubal, and coloenteric.
- Colovesical fistulas are easily diagnosed in male patients who promptly report pneumaturia.
- CT scanning is very sensitive for the detection of air in the bladder; a cystogram can also demonstrate the fistulous tract.

Indications for Operation

- The majority of patients with acute diverticulitis will respond to intravenous antibiotic therapy and bowel rest within 48 hours.
- Patients who require immediate operation are those with signs of either peritonitis or closed loop obstruction.
- The classic dictum in the treatment of recurrent but uncomplicated acute diverticulitis is that by the third episode, the patient should be considered for operation.

- Patients who present with abscesses should first have percutaneous drainage of the abscess.
- Clearing of infection and preparation of the bowel before resection are the primary goals in deferring operation for complicated diverticulitis.
- If these goals are achieved, the patient may have a single operation without the need for a colostomy.
- If a patient requires operation when there still is active infection in the peritoneal cavity or while the colon is filled with stool, resection with proximal diversion is required.

Surgical Options for Complications of Diverticular Disease

- Patients who require immediate operation for peritonitis or closed loop obstruction are treated by resection of the diseased segment, usually sigmoid colon, and exteriorization of the colon (colostomy) immediately proximal to the point of resection.
- The rectum is usually closed with a stapler.
- This combination of sigmoidectomy, end colostomy, and closure of the rectal stump is called the *Hartmann procedure.*
- After a period of 8 to 12 weeks, reoperation with restoration of colonic continuity is performed.
- Some surgeons prefer to perform a sigmoidectomy and coloproctostomy at the initial operation and add a loop colostomy to divert the fecal stream if anastomotic dehiscence occurs; the colostomy is closed later.

VOLVULUS

- The mobile segments of the colon are the sigmoid colon, the cecum, and the transverse colon.
- Each of these segments has the potential of twisting around the mesocolon and creating a volvulus.
- The main predisposing factor for the development of volvuli is colonic stasis with chronic distention.
- The major risk of volvulus is infarction of the segment involved.

Cecal Volvulus

- Dilatation of the cecum can precipitate the rotation of the cecum in individuals who have a mobile cecum.
- The typical presentation of patients with cecal volvulus is the sudden onset of abdominal pain and distention.

- A mass is usually palpable in either the left upper quadrant or midabdomen.
- Appendicitis, distal small bowel obstruction, pelvic inflammatory disease, and renal colic are among the most common conditions presenting with similar symptoms.
- Plain radiographs of the abdomen, both supine and erect, demonstrate a dilated and displaced cecum, usually in the left side of the abdomen; there may be a bird s beak image representing the point of torsion.
- If plain films are not helpful, the diagnosis of volvulus can be made by barium enema, which may even reduce the volvulus.

Sigmoid Volvulus

- >90% of colonic volvulus.
- Patients with chronic constipation and, often, concomitant laxative abuse, may develop a megacolon with maximal dilatation at the sigmoid.
- Typically, patients with sigmoid volvulus are elderly and debilitated.
- Some diseases predispose to sigmoid volvulus, e.g., Ogilvie s syndrome or Chagas disease.
- Patients with other conditions associated with megacolon can present with sigmoid volvulus; these include hypothyroidism, Parkinson s disease, the use of drugs with anticholinergic activity, multiple sclerosis, scleroderma, amyloidosis, and visceral neuropathies and myopathies.
- Diagnosis of sigmoid volvulus may be suspected by plain abdominal x-ray film and confirmed with water soluble contrast enema, which shows the typical bird s beak deformity.

Nonoperative Management

- There is no role for nonoperative management of patients with cecal volvulus.
- Nonoperative measures to reduce a sigmoid volvulus are usually attempted in all patients, with the exception of those with signs of ischemia.
- Sigmoid volvulus is often reduced by sigmoidoscopic or colonoscopic techniques.

Operative Management

- Operation for cecal volvulus is urgent.
- If the cecum or ileum show signs of irreversible ischemic damage, resection is required.

- The dilemma arises when the cecum and ileum are viable after the volvulus is reduced; most surgeons agree that definitive therapy in these patients is an ileocolonic resection rather than cecopexy or cecostomy.
- Operation for sigmoid volvulus can be urgent or elective (for recurrent episodes).
- Urgent surgical intervention is required when ischemia is suspected or nonoperative reduction fails.
- Sigmoid resection is indicated for both emergency and elective cases.

INFLAMMATORY BOWEL DISEASE, ULCERATIVE COLITIS, AND CROHN'S DISEASE

Etiology and Pathogenesis

- About 25% of patients with either form of IBD develop extraintestinal manifestations.
- The exact cause of IBD is still unknown; increasing evidence supports the theory that IBD is the result of dysfunctional immunoregulation in the intestinal wall.
- Epidemiologic studies suggest the presence of a genetic component in the cause of both Crohn s disease (CD) and ulcerative colitis (UC).
- Two genetic abnormalities prevalent in UC are variations in DNA repair genes and class II MHC genes.

Pathology

- The major difference between UC and CD is that in UC, the inflammatory process is limited to the colon.
- The inflammatory process in the colon is limited to the mucosa in UC; whereas, transmural inflammation is present in CD.
- Other typical pathologic findings in UC are the distribution from distal to proximal and the continuity of involvement.
- UC begins as proctitis and extends proximally without sparing any intervening mucosa.
- The involvement of the entire colon is called *universal colitis* or *pancolitis*; the terminal ileum may even become inflamed, a phenomenon called back-wash ileitis.
- In CD, the inflammatory process can involve any segment of the GI tract, including the colon and, in some cases (about 30—40%) exclusively the colon.
- Perianal involvement is relatively uncommon in UC, whereas it is quite common in CD.

Clinical Presentation

- UC has an insidious presentation with diarrhea and hematochezia.
- Once specific pharmacotherapy is initiated, most patients achieve remission within a few weeks.
- The interval of time between remission and return of symptoms is highly variable, as are the severity and frequency of relapses.
- When the symptoms of severe acute colitis are associated with radiologic evidence of colonic dilatation, the syndrome is called *toxic megacolon*.
- Extraintestinal manifestations include:
  - Peripheral arthritis.
  - Ankylosing spondylitis.
  - Primary sclerosing cholangitis.

Diagnosis

- The central diagnostic dilemma in UC is differentiation from CD, since the surgical options for each form of IBD are different.
- When still in doubt, a small bowel series should be obtained to assess the remainder of the intestine for lesions consistent with CD.
- Testing for antineutrophil cytoplasmic antibodies (ANCA) and anti-*S. cerevisiae* antibodies (ASCA) may aid in the differentiation of UC from CD.

Nonoperative Management

- The first line of pharmacotherapy for UC is the 5-ASA derivatives, of which the oldest is azulfidine.
- The second line of pharmacotherapy consists of immunomodulatory agents: corticosteroids, 6-mercaptopurine, methotrexate, cyclosporine, mycophenolate-mofetil, and tacrolimus.
- A standardized management approach advocated for patients presenting with a severe attack of UC consists of high-dose intravenous hydrocortisone, aggressive use of topical steroids, and oral 5-ASA agents.
- For patients whose disease proves to be refractory to intravenous steroids, intravenous cyclosporine has become an essential component in the management.

Operative Management

- Patients who require emergency operation are those with toxic megacolon, colonic perforation, or massive bleeding.
- Colonic obstruction is rare in UC and, when present, is usually due to cancer.
- Indications for elective operation in patients with UC are persistence of disabling symptoms despite drug therapy, intolerance to and side effects from drug therapy, and the finding of dysplasia in colonoscopic biopsies.
- Universal colonic involvement for longer than 10 years is an indication for prophylactic colectomy.
- The surgical options for UC range from the standard procto-colectomy, including an APR, to restorative proctocolec-tomy, in which the anus is preserved and the continuity of the GI tract is reconstructed by means of an ileal pouch anal anastomosis (IPAA).
- Another alternative to a permanent ileostomy is the intra-abdominal reservoir, or Kock pouch; this procedure has become a second choice to the IPAA.
- Pouches should not be used for Crohn s disease.

NEOPLASMS

- Colorectal cancer (CRC) is the second leading cause of cancer deaths in the United States for both men and women.
- Two groups of hereditary CRC are the FAP syndromes and the hereditary nonpolyposis colorectal cancer (HNPCC) syndromes (10—15% of all causes of CRC).

Adenoma-Carcinoma Sequence

- The development of CRC is a process that takes years (10—15) and evolves from initiation through well-defined phases of progression.
- At the histologic level, the earliest expression of neoplastic change is the aberrant crypt foci.
- When raised lesions become visible, they are called *adeno-matous polyps*.
- Eventually, cell differentiation is lost and polyps become dysplastic.

Genetic Mutations in Colorectal Carcinogenesis

- The various genes linked to colorectal carcinogenesis can be classified in four categories:
  - The proto-oncogenes include the K-*ras, src,* and c-*myc* genes.

- The tumor suppressor genes are the *APC* gene, *p53*, the *MCC* gene, and the *DPC4* gene.
- DNA mismatch repair genes are *hMSH2*, *MLH1*, *PMS1*, *PMS2*, and *GTBP*.
- The modifier genes include the *COX2* and the CD44*v* gene.

- The development of CRC is associated with one or more of the following genetic changes: overexpression of proto-oncogenes or risk modifier genes or underexpression of tumor suppressor genes or mismatch repair genes.
- The K-*ras* gene is the most commonly mutated oncogene.

Colorectal Polyps

- A colorectal polyp is any projecting mass that produces an elevation of the mucosa.
- Any colonic polyp should be either completely excised or undergo biopsy to assess the malignant potential.

Adenomatous Polyps

- The adenomatous polyp is the most common form of colonic polyp (67%) found in initial colonoscopy in the United States.
- Adenomas may be sessile, broad based, or pedunculated and vary in size.
- Histologically, there are three types of adenomatous polyps: tubular, villous, and tubulovillous; all possess malignant potential.
- Small pedunculated polyps are easily with a polypectomy snare.
- The excision of large and sessile lesions is much more difficult and often requires a piecemeal resection, endoscopic or bowel resection.

Hyperplastic Polyps

- This type of polyp is found in 11% of patients undergoing initial colonoscopy.
- Hyperplastic polyps are small, sessile, flat, and tank-pink and have a papillary surface.
- Pure hyperplastic polyps are not premalignant.
- All require excision for histologic confirmation.

Juvenile Polyps

- Juvenile, or retention, polyps are relatively uncommon.
- Patients with juvenile polyps usually present with bleeding and less often with intussusception at an average age of younger than 20.
- These polyps are usually pedunculated and spherical.
- Solitary juvenile polyps are not premalignant.

Familial Adenomatous Polyposis

- The modifications of the *APC* gene that result in familial adenomatous polyposis (FAP) are germline mutations caused by point mutations, deletions, or insertions in the nucleotide sequence.
- Several functions have been ascribed to *APC*, including the regulation of cell proliferation and the control of programmed cell death, or *apoptosis*.
- The inheritance pattern of FAP is autosomal dominant.

Clinical Presentation

- CRC arises early in individuals with *APC* gene mutations.
- In the typical family with FAP, 80% of individuals with *APC* gene mutation will develop polyps before the age of 20.
- Most FAP patients will die of CRC before the age of 40 if left untreated.
- Polyps are usually evenly distributed throughout the colon.
- Adenomatous polyps may occur throughout the GI tract.
- Most gastric polyps are not adenomatous polyps but rather fundic gland hyperplasia without malignant potential.
- Patients with FAP have an increased risk of ampullary cancer.
- Rare locations of extraintestinal adenomas and carcinomas include extrahepatic bile ducts, gallbladder, pancreas, adrenals, thyroid, and liver.
- Islet cell tumors have been described in individuals with the *APC* gene mutation.
- Other manifestations of FAP are congenital hypertrophy of the retinal pigment epithelium, osteomas, and fibromatosis.
- The association of FAP with brain tumors is known as Turcot s syndrome; tumors found in these patients include glioblastomas and medulloblastomas.

Surgical Options in Familial Adenomatous Polyposis

- Patients who have the *APC* gene mutation must have their colons and rectums removed.
- The advent of IPAA has solved the issue of rectal preservation by removing the mucosa at risk for cancer but maintaining the anal sphincter mechanism.

Hereditary Nonpolyposis Colorectal Cancer

- The two forms of HNPCC are known as Lynch syndrome I and II.
- HNPCC accounts for up to 6% of all forms of CRC.
- HNPCC is transmitted by an autosomal dominant inheritance.
- Peculiar features include onset at a young age (mean of 44 years), proximal distribution, predominance of the mucinous type of adenocarcinoma, and synchronous and metachronous cancers.
- Although families with Lynch syndrome I are only prone to CRC, families with Lynch syndrome II usually have both colorectal and extracolonic cancer.
- Extracolonic cancer seen in Lynch syndrome II includes carcinoma of the endometrium and ovary, transitional cell carcinoma of the ureter and renal pelvis, and, with less frequency, carcinoma of the stomach, small bowel, and pancreas.

Diagnostic Criteria

- At least 3 relatives with CRC, 2 of which are first degree.
- Involvement of at least 2 generations.
- One patient with diagnosis before age 50.

Surveillance and Management

- Surveillance colonoscopy is begun at age 25; colonoscopies are repeated every 2 years until age 35.
- When colon cancer is detected, an abdominal colectomy and ileorectal anastomosis is the procedure of choice.

Colorectal Cancer

- Prognosis is related to stage; the preferred staging system was developed by the American Joint Committee for Cancer and is known as the TNM (Tumor, Node, Metastasis) system.

- In Stage I, there is no lymph node metastasis and the tumor is either T_1 or T_2; 5-year survival, 88%.
- Stage II is defined by larger tumors, T_3 or T_4 (local invasion), with no lymph node metastasis; 5-year survival, 73%.
- Stage III is characterized by lymph node metastasis; 5-year survival, 45%.
- Stage IV includes the presence of distant metastasis; 5-year survival, less than 5%.
- The sigmoid colon (25%) and rectum (43%) are the most common sites for CRC, followed by the ascending colon (18%), transverse colon (9%), and descending colon (5%).

Colon Cancer

- The clinical presentation of colonic adenocarcinoma varies according to the location along the colon; tumors in the right side tend to grow larger than those in the left side before producing clinical manifestations.
- The size difference and the consistency of luminal contents make tumors produce obstruction in the left side more often than in the right side.
- Tumors in the right side become so large that patients develop superficial necrosis from ischemia and then chronic bleeding and anemia occurs.
- Presenting signs include a change in bowel habits, unexplained anemia and/or weight loss, dark stools, or rectal bleeding.
- Colonoscopic examination is the gold standard for the diagnosis of colon cancer; definitive diagnosis of a colonic adenocarcinoma is made by biopsy.
- Patients with CRC should undergo a metastatic work-up, including liver function tests and CEA levels.
- If any abnormality in liver function is detected, the liver must be imaged by one of many possible modalities: hepatic scintigraphy, MRI, or CT scanning.
- The presence of metastatic disease in the liver does not preclude the surgical excision of the primary tumor.

Treatment of Primary Colon Cancer

- The goals of curative surgery for CRC include removal of the primary tumor with adequate margins, regional lymphadenectomy, and restoration of colonic continuity.
- The extent of resection is determined by the location of the tumor, its blood supply and draining lymphatic vessels, and the presence or absence of direct extension into adjacent organs.

- For lesions involving the cecum, ascending colon, and hepatic flexure, right hemicolectomy is the procedure of choice.
- Left hemicolectomy is the procedure of choice for cancers of the descending colon; sigmoidectomy for cancers of the sigmoid colon.
- Total abdominal colectomy is indicated for patients with multiple primary tumors and HNPCC.

Rectal Cancer

- The most common presentation of rectal cancer is hematochezia.
- The delay in diagnosis is often because both patient and physician mistake bleeding due to rectal cancer as bleeding due to hemorrhoids.
- Other symptoms of presentation are mucus discharge, rectal pain, tenesmus, and urgency.
- The most useful diagnostic modalities used to assess extent of primary rectal cancer are endorectal ultrasound (EUS) and CT scan.

Treatment of Rectal Cancer

Low Anterior Resection (LAR)

- LAR is performed for cancer of the proximal third to two thirds of the rectum.
- LAR consists of removal of the sigmoid colon, proximal rectum, and mesorectum, with an anastomosis in the pelvis below the peritoneal reflection.

Abdominoperineal Resection (APR)

- The complete excision of the rectum, mesorectum, and anus, by concomitant dissection through the abdomen and perineum, with closure of the perineum and creation of an end colostomy.
- An APR is indicated when the cancer involves the anal sphincters, when it penetrates into the rectovaginal septum, and in patients in whom sphincter-preserving surgery is not possible.

Local Excision

- Local excision involves removal of the primary cancer by a full-thickness excision followed by reapproximation of the rectal wall.

- Patients must be carefully selected for these procedures to ensure that the risk of local recurrence is low.
- Local excisions with curative intent are indicated for mobile cancers that are less than 4 cm in diameter, that involve less than 40% of the rectal wall circumference, located within 6 cm of the anal verge, well or moderately differentiated, and exhibit no vascular or lymphatic invasion.
- There should be no evidence of nodal disease on preoperative EUS or CT scan.
- Local excisions are also used for palliation of more advanced cancers.
- Local excision can be accomplished by a transanal, transsacral, or transsphincteric approach.

RESECTION OF STRUCTURES ADJACENT TO COLORECTAL TUMORS

- Colorectal tumors often adhere to contiguous structures.
- The abdominal wall, small bowel, and bladder are most commonly involved with colon tumors.
- The uterus, adnexae, posterior vaginal wall, and bladder can be invaded by rectal carcinoma.
- Pelvic exenteration is rarely indicated for rectal cancer.

LAPAROSCOPIC SURGERY FOR COLORECTAL CANCER

- The use of laparoscopy for the surgical cure of CRC is still a controversial subject.
- The advantages are an earlier return of bowel function, decreased postoperative pain, shorter hospital stay, and earlier return to full activities.
- Some of the concerns regarding this approach are the potential inadequacy of margins of resection and of lymphadenectomy.

COMPLICATIONS OF SURGERY FOR COLORECTAL CANCER

- The most common complications are anastomotic leakage, obstruction, and infection.
- Wide pelvic dissection can result in urinary and sexual dysfunction.
- Fecal incontinence is another well-recognized complication after sphincter-saving procedures for low-lying rectal cancer.
- The most devastating complication of rectal surgery is locoregional recurrence.

ADJUVANT THERAPY

- Postoperative chemotherapy is a consideration in patients with invasive tumors and those with metastatic disease in lymph nodes.
- The standard chemotherapy is 5-fluorouracil and leucovorin.
- Radiation therapy has proved effective in patients with rectal tumors; overall survival is less than 50%; 20 to 30% pelvic recurrence.
- There are at least two advantages of postoperative over preoperative radiation therapy:
  - Staging is well established, thereby sparing the 10 to 15% of patients with stages $T_{1-2}N_0M_0$ disease unnecessary treatment.
  - Operation allows for accurate delineation of the tumor bed to be radiated.
- Conversely, there are potential disadvantages:
  - Postoperatively, there is an increased amount of small bowel in the radiation field.
  - Excisional surgery creates a hypoxic field, which is less sensitive to the effect of radiation.
  - Anal sphincter dysfunction and fecal incontinence.

CHAPTER 48

ANUS

DISORDERS OF THE ANAL CANAL

Anatomy

Anal Canal Lining

- The mucosa of the upper anal canal, like that of the rectum, is pinkish and is lined by columnar epithelium, whereas the mucosa distal to the dentate line is paler and lined by squamous epithelium devoid of hair and glands.
- Differences between the rectal columnar mucosal lining and anal squamous lining have several important clinical implications. For example, diseases affecting the rectal mucosa, such as ulcerative colitis, can extend within the transitional zone area but not distal to the dentate. Cancers proximal to the dentate are typically adenocarcinomas, and those distal are squamous or cloacogenic. At the anal verge, the lining acquires the characteristics of normal skin with its apocrine glands, and this is where infectious complications of the apocrine glands, hidradenitis suppurativa, present. Furthermore, this differentiation also demarcates differences in sensory perception, which influences the surgical approaches to anorectal conditions.

Anal Canal Musculature

- The internal sphincter, which is innervated by the autonomic nervous system, is independent of voluntary control, whereas the external sphincter, which is supplied by the inferior rectal branch of the internal pudendal nerve and the perineal branch of the fourth sacral nerve, is under voluntary control.

Physiology

- The principal function of the anal canal is the regulation of defecation and maintenance of continence. The ability to control defecation depends on the coordinated functions of the sensory and muscular activities of the anus; the

689

compliance, tone, and evacuability of the rectum; the muscular activities of the pelvic floor; and the consistency, volume, and timing of the colonic fecal movements. Perturbations of any of the critical functions can result in fecal incontinence (Table 48–1).

- The principal mechanism that provides continence is the pressure differential between the rectum (6 cm H_2O) and the anal canal (90 cm H_2O).

Diagnostic Evaluation of the Anus

History

- Bleeding is a common presenting symptom of both benign and malignant conditions of the anus and large bowel.
- Although a careful bleeding history may suggest a specific etiology, consideration must always be given to proximal bowel evaluation to exclude the possibility of more serious conditions, such as cancer.

Physical Examination

- A careful and systematic digital examination with a well-lubricated index finger gradually inserted into the anal canal helps the examiner to appreciate any mass, induration, or stricturing and to assess the resting tone and strength of the squeeze pressure of the anal sphincter.
- Any suspicious area or mass should be sampled for biopsy, with the patient's permission, so that a precise histopathologic diagnosis can be established.
- The anoscope can also be used for the same purpose; it optimizes the evaluation of lesions confined to the anus.

PELVIC FLOOR DISORDERS

Incontinence

Clinical Evaluation

- Determining the extent and nature of the problem should start by distinguishing true incontinence, that is, complete loss of solid stools, from minor incontinence, that is, occasional staining from seepage or urgency. Seepage of mucus from prolapsing hemorrhoids or from a large secretory villous polyp, urgency from colitis or proctitis, and overflow

TABLE 48–1. Common Causes for Fecal Incontinence

Category	Mechanism	Common Causes
Functional	Fecal impaction; dilated internal anal sphincter	Pelvic floor dyssynergia (difficulty relaxing sphincter when defecating); drug side effect, idiopathic, spinal cord injury
	Diarrhea rapid transit and/or large volume	Irritable bowel syndrome; infectious and metabolic causes of diarrhea
	Cognitive/psychological; social indifference	Dementia, psychosis, willful soiling
Sphincter weakness	Sphincter muscle injury	Obstetric trauma, motor vehicle accident, foreign body trauma
	Pudendal nerve injury	Obstetric trauma, diabetic peripheral neuropathy, multiple sclerosis, idiopathic
	CNS injury	Spina bifida, traumatic spinal cord injury, cerebrovascular accident, multiple sclerosis
Sensory loss	Afferent nerve injury unable to detect rectal filling	Diabetic neuropathy, spinal cord injury, multiple sclerosis

CNS, central nervous system.
Adapted from Whitehead WE, Wald A, Norton NJ: Treatment options for fecal incontinence. Dis Colon Rectum 44:134, 2001.

incontinence from fecal impaction may be confused with true incontinence.

- Fecal incontinence may be multifactorial; hence, details regarding possible causes and associated gastrointestinal disorders should be sought in the patient's history (see Table 48–1).

Medical Management

- Biofeedback training for strengthening of the anal musculature and improvement of anorectal sensation has been widely applied, particularly in cases of generalized weakness in which repairable anatomic defects are not identified.

Surgical Repair

- An expanding number of surgical options are available for correction of fecal incontinence, including everything from direct sphincter repair to artificial sphincter implantation and colostomy diversion. For discrete anatomic defects, the most common surgical approach is the direct overlapping sphincteroplasty, in which the separated muscular ends are dissected, reapproximated, and sutured (Fig. 48–1).

Prolapse of the Rectum

Pathogenesis and Clinical Presentation

- Prolapse of the rectum, or procidentia, is an uncommon problem of obscure etiology characterized by full-thickness eversion of the rectal wall through the anus. The exact cause is unclear, but the disorder tends to predominate in women, in those that strain excessively, and in those with chronic mental disorders.

Preoperative Evaluation

- The preoperative assessment of the patient should focus on establishing the extent of the prolapse; the patient's overall health status; the presence of associated bowel conditions, such as constipation; and complications, such as incontinence. All of these factors influence the operative strategy.
- Frail elderly patients and those with high-risk comorbid conditions or limited life expectancy are ideally suited for perineal procedures. Young patients, particularly those with constipation or evidence of defecating disorders, are

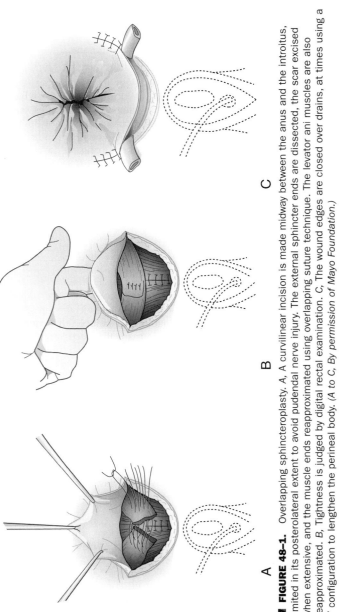

A   B   C

FIGURE 48-1. Overlapping sphincteroplasty. *A,* A curvilinear incision is made midway between the anus and the introitus, limited in its posterolateral extent to avoid pudendal nerve injury. The external sphincter ends are dissected, and the scar excised when extensive, and the muscle ends reapproximated using overlapping suture technique. The levator ani muscles are also reapproximated. *B,* Tightness is judged by digital rectal examination. *C,* The wound edges are closed over drains, at times using a Y configuration to lengthen the perineal body. *(A to C, By permission of Mayo Foundation.)*

best served with resection and fixation, using open or laparoscopic approaches.

Surgical Correction

● Two general approaches are used to achieve surgical correction of rectal prolapse: the perineal approach, which includes the Delorme and the Altemeier procedures, and the abdominal approach, which includes but is not limited to anterior resection with or without rectopexy and mesh fixation. The perineal approach is less taxing on the patient and yet has a higher recurrence rate; thus, it is ideally suited for patients with high operative risk and a limited life expectancy. An abdominal approach is preferred for young healthy patients because they can tolerate the procedure with low risk and are less likely to suffer a recurrence requiring reoperation.

RECTOCELE

Clinical Evaluation

● Symptoms attributable to a rectocele include the presentation of a vaginal bulge, inability to completely evacuate during defecation, and in most cases the necessity to digitally evacuate through the vagina or through the rectum or perineum. The etiology of rectoceles remains unclear and is probably multifactorial because it is associated with a constellation of a number of pelvic floor disorders including constipation, paradoxical muscular contraction, and neuropathies or anatomic disorders from childbirth. Rectocele may coexist with other defecation disorders such as slow-transit constipation or pelvic floor dysfunction, including pelvic organ prolapse in which factors such as age, parity, obesity, constipation, pelvic surgery, and a number of pulmonary and medical conditions may play a role. Associated disorders must be addressed to achieve resolution of all symptoms.

Treatment

Surgical Treatment

● Patients with rectoceles should be considered for surgical correction if the rectocele is greater than 2 cm and the patient has to perform digital-assisted defecation.

COMMON BENIGN ANAL DISORDERS

Hemorrhoids

Clinical Presentation and Diagnostic Evaluations

- Within the normal anal canal exist specialized, highly vascularized "cushions" forming discrete masses of thick submucosa containing blood vessels, smooth muscle, and elastic and connective tissue. They are located in the left lateral, right anterior, and right posterior quadrants of the canal to aid in anal continence. The term *hemorrhoids* should be restricted to clinical situations in which these cushions are abnormal and cause symptoms.

- Hemorrhoids can be considered external or internal; the diagnosis is based on the history, physical examination, and endoscopy. External hemorrhoids are covered with anoderm and are distal to the dentate line; they may swell, causing discomfort and difficult hygiene, but cause severe pain only if actually thrombosed. Internal hemorrhoids cause painless, bright red bleeding or prolapse associated with defecation. Internal hemorrhoids are classified according to the extent of prolapse, which influences treatment options (Table 48–2).

- Pain is not usually associated with uncomplicated hemorrhoids but more often with fissure, abscess, or external hemorrhoidal thrombosis.

TABLE 48–2. Internal Hemorrhoids: Grading and Management

Grade	Symptoms and Signs	Management
First degree	Bleeding; no prolapse	Dietary modifications*
Second degree	Prolapse with spontaneous reduction	Rubber band ligation
		Coagulation
	Bleeding; seepage	Dietary modifications
Third degree	Prolapse requiring digital reduction; bleeding	Surgical hemorrhoidectomy
	seepage	Rubber band ligation
	Bleeding; seepage	Dietary modifications
Fourth degree	Prolapsed, cannot be reduced; strangulated	Surgical hemorrhoidectomy
		Urgent hemorrhoidectomy
		Dietary modifications

*Dietary modifications include increasing consumption of fiber, bran, or psyllium and water. Dietary modifications are always appropriate for the management of hemorrhoids, if not for the acute care then for the chronic management and for prevention of recurrence after banding and/or surgery.

- Because virtually all anorectal symptoms are ascribed to hemorrhoids by patients, it is essential that other anorectal pathologies be considered and excluded.
- Colonoscopy or barium enema should be added if the hemorrhoidal disease is unimpressive; the history is somewhat uncharacteristic; or the patient is older than 40 years or has risk factors for colon cancer, such as a family history.

Nonoperative Management

- In many patients, hemorrhoidal symptoms can be ameliorated or relieved by simple measures, such as better local hygiene; avoidance of excessive straining; and better dietary habits supplemented by medication to keep stools soft, formed, and regular (see Table 48–2).
- In the absence of symptomatic external hemorrhoids, second- and some third-degree internal hemorrhoids can be treated with office procedures that produce mucosal fixation.
- Because severe perineal sepsis and even deaths have been reported after rubber band ligation, patients should be instructed to return to the emergency room if delayed or undue pain, inability to void, or a fever develops.

Surgical Treatment

- Hemorrhoidectomy is the best means of curing hemorrhoidal disease and should be considered whenever patients fail to respond satisfactorily to repeated attempts at conservative measures; hemorrhoids are severely prolapsed and require manual reduction; hemorrhoids are complicated by strangulation or associated pathology, such as ulceration, fissure, or fistula; or hemorrhoids are associated with symptomatic external hemorrhoids or large anal tags.

Anal Fissures

Clinical Presentation and Diagnostic Evaluations

- An anal fissure is a linear ulcer of the lower half of the anal canal, usually located in the posterior commissure in the midline (Fig. 48–2). Often misnamed as "rectal fissures," in fact, these lesions are truly involving just the anal tissues and are typically best seen by visually inspecting the anal verge with gentle separation of the gluteal cleft.

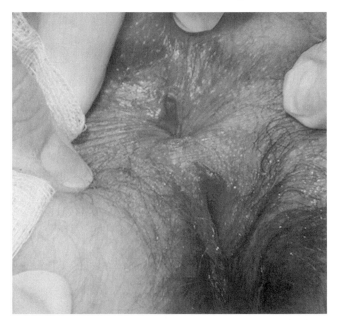

■ FIGURE 48–2. Posterior anal fissure. *(By permission of Mayo Foundation.)*

- Fissures away from these two locations should raise the possibility of associated diseases, especially Crohn's disease, hidradenitis suppurativa, or sexually transmitted disease (STD).

Pathogenesis

- It is believed that anal fissures are the result of anal sphincter hypertonia and subsequent mucosal ischemia. New information regarding the pathogenesis of anal fissures has led to the introduction of several new medical approaches, including the application of nitric oxide donors, calcium channel blockers, and botulinum injections, all of which allow for internal sphincter relaxation.

Medical Management

- Medical therapies for anal fissures are gaining in popularity, particularly for acute fissures, that is, those presenting within 3 to 6 weeks of symptom onset.

Surgical Treatment

- Patients with chronic fissures who fail medical therapy either for persistent or recurrent disease and those who develop complications can benefit from surgical therapy.
- Partial lateral internal sphincterotomy can be performed using the closed or open technique, depending on surgeon preference, training, and experience.

Anorectal Suppuration

- Although anorectal suppuration may have several causes, by far the most common is a nonspecific infection of cryptoglandular origin. Other causes are rare, except for Crohn's disease and hidradenitis suppurativa. The pathogenesis of abscesses and fistulas is usually the same, with the abscess representing the acute phase and the fistula the chronic sequela.

Abscess

- Infection originates in the intersphincteric plane, most likely in one of the anal glands. This may result in a simple intersphincteric abscess, or it may extend vertically either upward or downward, horizontally, or circumferentially, resulting in a number of clinical presentations.
- Clinical presentation: types of abscesses.

Treatment

- Abscesses should be drained when diagnosed. Simple and superficial abscesses can most often be drained under local anesthesia in the office setting in patients who are otherwise healthy. Patients who manifest systemic symptoms; those who are immunocompromised for any reason, including acquired immunodeficiency syndrome (AIDS), diabetes, cancer therapies, or chronic medical immunosuppression; and those with complex, complicated abscesses are best treated in a hospital setting.
- At times, these abscesses are sufficiently deep that needle localization of the purulent material may be required to guide the surgeon for optimizing the skin incision site. The cavity should be gently digitalized to break down loculations. Neglected abscesses can lead to devastating, necrotizing infections of the perineum that can spread and become lethal. Failure of response to local treatment or recurrent abscesses

may suggest inadequate drainage with residual pus, the presence of a fistula, or immunoincompetence. Under these circumstances, antibiotics may be useful, together with examination under anesthesia after preliminary evaluation by computed tomography of the pelvis and perineum.

Fistula in Ano

- Anorectal sepsis can be complicated by a fistula in ano in about 25% of patients during the acute phase of sepsis or within 6 months thereafter. Most fistulas derive from sepsis originating in the anal canal glands at the dentate line.
- Clinical presentation: types of fistulas.

Treatment

- A fistula may first present as an acute abscess or, at times, simply as a draining sinus that may irritate the perineal skin. On examination, subcutaneous induration may be traced from the external opening to the anal canal. Digital examination may reveal a palpable nodule in the wall of the anal canal, an indication of the primary opening. A probe can be eased gently (not forcefully) from the external skin opening to the internal, anal canal opening.
- Difficult and persistent high fistulas can be treated by sliding flap advancement made of mucosa, submucosa, and circular muscle to cover the internal opening. The Goodsall rule (Fig. 48–3) is of little help in defining the anatomy of complex and recurrent fistulas. Diagnostic tests such as pelvic magnetic resonance imaging (MRI) or endorectal ultrasound and treatment by a specialist may be helpful here.

PILONIDAL INFECTIONS

- Pilonidal infections and chronic pilonidal sinuses typically occur in the midline of the sacrococcygeal skin of young males. Although the exact pathogenesis of pilonidal disease remains elusive and controversial, hair seems to play a central role in the process of infection and in the perpetuation of granulation tissue in sinuses.

Acute Management

- Patients presenting acutely with new onset disease may have a painful fluctuant abscess or a draining infected sinus. Both can be managed with simple office therapies with

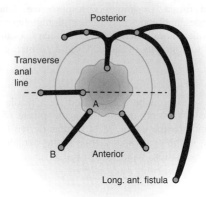

■ FIGURE 48–3. The Goodsall rule. The usual relationship of primary and secondary fistula orifices is diagrammed. The internal (primary orifice) is marked A. The rule predicts that if a line is drawn transversely across the anus, an external opening (B) anterior to this line will lead to a straight radial tract, whereas an external opening that lies posterior to the line will lead to a curved tract and an internal opening in the posterior commissure. The long anterior fistula is an exception to the rule. *(From Schrock TR: Benign and malignant disease of the anorectum. In Fromm O (ed): Gastrointestinal Surgery. New York, Churchill Livingstone, 1985, p. 612.)*

more definitive procedures reserved for patients who suffer from a recurrence.

Operative Management

- For those patients who have recurring infections, more definitive operative management is warranted. Incision and curettage is the simplest form of treatment.

LESS COMMON BENIGN ANAL DISORDERS

Rectovaginal Fistula

- A rectovaginal fistula is a communication between the epithelial-lined surfaces of the rectum and the vagina. Patients usually complain that they pass gas, mucus, blood, and/or stool through the vagina. Rectovaginal fistulas may be congenital or acquired through either trauma, inflammatory bowel disease, irradiation, neoplasia, infection, or other rare causes.

- Rectovaginal fistulas are classified as high or low depending on whether they can be corrected transabdominally or transperineally, respectively.

Surgical Repair

- In the setting of Crohn's disease, the low anovaginal fistula represents a unique challenge. Primary repair avoiding the need for a permanent stoma can be accomplished in up to 68% of patients using a variety of horizontal, linear, and sleeve advancement flaps.

Condyloma Acuminata

- Condyloma acuminata are a perineal wart disease caused by the human papillomavirus (HPV); some types are transmitted through sexual contact. Certain types, such as HPV-6 and HPV-11, are found in benign warts, whereas others, such as HPV-16 and HPV-18, are more aggressive and more commonly associated with dysplasia and malignancies.

Clinical Presentation

- Anoscopy may reveal extension in the anal canal. A giant form of the disease has been observed rarely (Buschke-Löwenstein disease). Such lesions can invade, fistulize, and be associated with verrucous carcinoma and squamous cell carcinomas.

Treatment

- Podophyllin.
- Dichloroacetic acid (bichloracetic acid).
- Intramuscular or intralesional interferon-β.
- Electrocauterization.
- Carbon dioxide laser.
- Excision with small scissors.

Sexually Transmitted Diseases and Acquired Immunodeficiency Syndrome

Clinical Presentation

- Patients with bacterial STDs may have no symptoms or may have symptoms of pruritus, bloody or mucopurulent rectal discharge, tenesmus, perineal or rectal pain, diarrhea, and fever.
- Patients with *viral* STDs may complain of anorectal pain, discharge, bleeding, and pruritus.

- Patients with *parasitic* STDs have more systemic symptoms, such as fever, abdominal cramping, and bloody diarrhea.

Acquired Immunodeficiency Syndrome

- Anorectal pathology is common in patients who are human immunodeficiency virus (HIV)-positive; affecting about one third of patients at some point in their disease. Anorectal pain, the presence of a mass, and bleeding per rectum are the most frequent presenting complaints.
- For benign noninfectious disorders, fissures and ulcers are the most common presenting problem.
- Neoplastics disorders in HIV-positive patients include condyloma, anal intraepithelial neoplasia (AIN), epidermoid carcinoma, and Kaposi's sarcoma; the incidence of each of these being higher in HIV-positive than HIV-negative patients.

Hidradenitis Suppurativa

- Hidradenitis suppurativa is a chronic inflammatory process affecting the apocrine glands of the perianal region characterized by abscesses and sinuses formation. Although recent dermatologic investigations call into question the site of origin of hidradenitis, implicating occluding spongiform infundibulofolliculitis (a follicular disease), hidradenitis has traditionally been considered the result of keratotic debris plugging the apocrine gland.
- A number of factors have been implicated in the development and perpetuation of hidradenitis, including the use of depilatories, close shaving, poor personal hygiene, tight-fitting and synthetic clothing, and antiperspirants.

Clinical Presentation

Treatment

- When hidradenitis sinus tracks are well established but relatively superficial, they can be unroofed or laid open.

Crohn's Disease of the Anorectum

Clinical Presentation

- Anal manifestations of Crohn's disease can be most devastating because of their painful nature and their threat to the patient's continence, and they occur in nearly 20% of patients with Crohn's disease. Patients may suffer from fissure, fistulas, and abscesses.

Evaluation and Treatment

- It is now increasingly recognized that patients with Crohn's disease can also present with common anorectal conditions such as fissures, abscesses, and fistulas. In the absence of evidence of rectal or perianal Crohn's, these conditions may be best treated using standard approaches. Although caution is advised against aggressive approaches when treating a Crohn's patient with anorectal problems, undertreatment of symptomatic conditions is also discouraged.

NEOPLASTIC DISORDERS

- Neoplasms of the anal area are rare and represent a wide spectrum of benign and malignant tumors. Benign lesions may range from innocuous *in situ* Bowen's disease to clinically aggressive verrucous lesions; malignant lesions range from favorable early-stage squamous cell cancers of the anal margin to anal canal adenocarcinoma and melanoma. In all instances, it is essential for clinicians to consider tumor location with reference to clear landmarks, such as anal verge, dentate line, and anorectal ring. For a number of reasons, the anatomy of the anus should be differentiated into two parts: the *anal margin* and the *anal canal.*
- Clinical evaluations.

Anal Margin Tumors

Bowen's Disease

- *Bowen's disease* is an *in situ* intraepithelial squamous cell carcinoma that rarely (5%) invades or metastasizes.
- The concept that Bowen's disease is frequently associated with internal malignancies justifying extensive diagnostic investigations has been challenged and refuted.
- In the absence of an underlying invasive component, the disease can be cured by wide and full-thickness excision of all the affected skin.

Paget's Disease

- Extramammary Paget's disease of the anus is a rare intraepithelial adenocarcinoma. The presence of intraepithelial adenocarcinoma in an area of squamous epithelium has led to speculation about the origin of Paget's cells. A number of concepts have been proposed, including the possibility that they are derived from pluripotent epidermal stem cells, arise from apocrine or sweat glands, or are metastatic from underlying adenocarcinomas.

● Patients with underlying rectal adenocarcinoma should undergo abdominal perineal resection (APR) while those with epidermoid anal canal cancer can be treated with combined radiation and chemotherapy. For patients with an invasive component, treated with radical therapy, the 5-year crude survival rate is only 54%.

Basal Cell Carcinoma

● Basal cell carcinoma is a rare type of anal canal tumor.
● On occasion, it may be difficult to differentiate a cloacogenic (or basaloid) carcinoma arising in the transitional zone from a basal cell cancer arising in the anal skin. The distinction is crucial because of the dramatic behavioral difference and is based on location and histologic features.

Squamous Cell Carcinoma

● Wide local excision is recommended for early anal margin squamous cell carcinoma; results are excellent.

Verrucous Carcinoma

● Verrucous carcinoma, also referred to as *giant condyloma acuminatum* or *Buschke-Löwenstein tumors* are poorly defined and best considered as intermediate lesions between condyloma acuminatum and invasive squamous cell carcinomas based on their common HPV etiology.

Anal Canal Neoplasms

Epidermoid Carcinoma

● Tumors arising in the anal canal or in the transitional zone that have a squamous, basaloid, cloacogenic, or mucoepidermoid epithelium share a similar behavior in clinical presentation, response to treatment, and prognosis and are considered collectively.
● The introduction of multimodality therapy combining irradiation and chemotherapy promised to preserve continence, avoid colostomy, and offer similar survival advantage. In keeping with this concept, local excision alone remains an option for superficial, early-stage lesions, which have been associated with variable survivorship (61% to 87%; 100% in

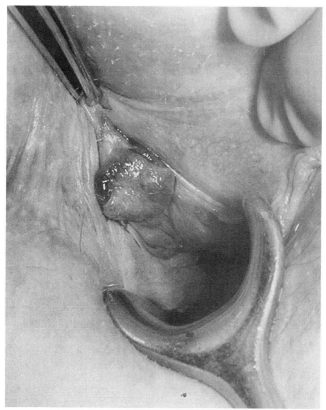

■ FIGURE 48–4. Anal canal amelanotic melanoma. *(By permission of Mayo Foundation.)*

at least one study) if the lesion was smaller than 2 cm. Although some small superficial lesions can be treated with local excision, most patients are best treated with combined chemotherapy and irradiation.

Melanoma

● Melanoma involving the anal canal can produce a mass, pain, or bleeding and is not infrequently amelanotic (Fig. 48–4). Overall, the outlook of patients with such tumors is poor, with a 5-year survival rate hovering around 10% to, at most, 26%.

CHAPTER 49

THE LIVER

- The liver is invested in peritoneum except for the gallbladder bed, the porta hepatis, and posteriorly on either side of the inferior vena cava (IVC) in two wedge-shaped areas (called the bare area of the liver to the right of the IVC).
- The primitive liver plays a central role in the fetal circulation.
- In the adult liver, the remnant of the left umbilical vein becomes the ligamentum teres, which runs in the falciform ligament into the umbilical fissure, and the remnant of the ductus venosus becomes the ligamentum venosum at the termination of the lesser omentum under the left liver.
- The functional anatomy (Figs. 49–1 and 49–2) of the liver is composed of eight segments, which are each supplied by a single portal triad (pedicle) composed of a portal vein, hepatic artery, and a bile duct.
- The main scissura contains the middle hepatic vein that runs in an anterior-posterior direction from the gallbladder fossa to the left side of the vena cava and divides the liver into right and left hemilivers.
- The umbilical fissure is *not* a scissura, does not contain a hepatic vein, and contains the left portal pedicle (triad containing the left portal vein, hepatic artery, and bile duct), which runs in this fissure branching to feed the left liver.
- However, the left portal triad has a long extrahepatic course of up to 3 or 4 cm and runs transversely along the base of segment 4 in a peritoneal sheath that is the upper end of the lesser omentum.
- The caudate lobe (segment 1) is the dorsal portion of the liver and embraces the IVC on its posterior surface and lies posterior to the left portal triad inferiorly and the left and middle hepatic veins superiorly.
- The vascular inflow and biliary drainage to the caudate lobe comes from both the right and left systems.
- The portal vein provides about 75% of hepatic blood flow, and, although it is postcapillary and largely deoxygenated, its large volume flow rate provides 50% to 70% of the liver's oxygenation.
- Cephalad to its formation behind the neck of the pancreas, the portal vein runs behind the first portion of the duodenum

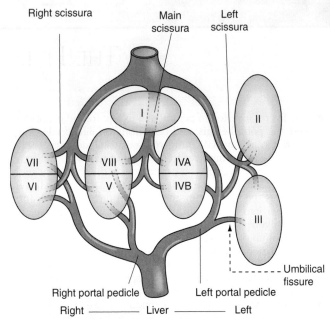

■ FIGURE 49–1. A schematic demonstrating the segmental anatomy of the liver. Each segment receives its own portal pedicle (triad of portal vein, hepatic artery, and bile duct). The eight segments are illustrated and the four sectors, divided by the three main hepatic veins running in scissurae are shown. The umbilical fissure (not a scissura) is shown to contain the left portal pedicle. *(From Blumgart LH, Hann LE: Surgical and radiologic anatomy of the liver and biliary tract. In Blumgart LH, Fong Y (eds): Surgery of the Liver and Biliary Tract. London, WB Saunders, 2000, pp 3–34.)*

and into the hepatoduodenal ligament where it runs along the right border of the lesser omentum usually posterior to the bile duct and hepatic artery.
- There are a number of connections between the portal venous system and the systemic venous system.
- The anatomy of the portal vein and its branches is relatively constant and has much less variation than the ductal and hepatic arterial system.
- The hepatic artery, representing high flow oxygenated systemic arterial flow, provides approximately 25% of the hepatic blood flow and 30% to 50% of its oxygenation.

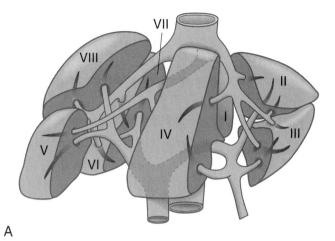

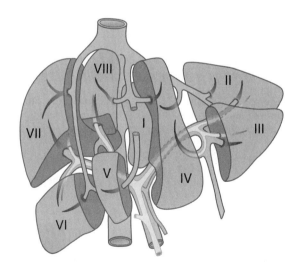

FIGURE 49–2. Segmental anatomy of the liver. *A,* As seen at laparotomy in the anatomic position. *B,* In the ex-vivo position. *(From Blumgart LH, Hann LE: Surgical and radiologic anatomy of the liver and biliary tract. In Blumgart LH, Fong Y (eds): Surgery of the Liver and Biliary Tract. London, WB Saunders, 2000, pp 3–34.)*

- The common description of the arterial supply to the liver and biliary tree is only present approximately 60% of the time.
- An accessory vessel is described as an aberrant origin of a branch that is in addition to the normal branching pattern. A replaced vessel is described as an aberrant origin of a branch that substitutes for the lack of the normal branch.
- The intrahepatic bile ducts are terminal branches of the main right and left hepatic ductal branches that invaginate Glisson's capsule at the hilum along with corresponding portal vein and hepatic artery branches forming the peritoneal covered portal triads.
- The short right hepatic duct meets the longer left hepatic duct forming the confluence anterior to the right portal vein, constituting the common hepatic duct.
- The common bile/hepatic duct runs along the right side of the hepatoduodenal ligament (free edge of the lesser omentum) to the right of the hepatic artery and anterior to the portal vein.
- At the choledochoduodenal junction a complex muscular complex known as the sphincter of Oddi regulates bile flow and prevents reflux of duodenal contents into the biliary tree.
- A peritoneal layer covers the majority of the gallbladder except for the portion adherent to the liver.
- The cystic duct is variable in its length, its course, and its insertion into the main biliary tree.
- Anomalies of the hepatic ductal confluence are common; the normal anatomy described previously is present about two thirds of the time.
- The supraduodenal and infrahilar bile duct are predominantly supplied by two axial vessels that run in a 3-o'clock and 9-o'clock position.
- A lobule is made up of a central terminal hepatic venule surrounded by four to six terminal portal triads forming a polygonal unit.
- This functional hepatic unit provides a structural basis for the many metabolic and secretory functions of the liver.
- A one-way reciprocal relationship between hepatic artery and portal vein flow has been demonstrated.
- The physiologic role of bile is twofold: first to dispose of certain substances secreted into bile and second to provide enteric bile salts to aid in the digestion of fats.
- Thus, the liver, in part, serves as an epithelial structure that moves solutes from blood to bile and provides a route of secretion of bile into the intestines.
- Canalicular bile flow is largely due to water flow in response to active solute transport.

- Thus, the active secretion of bile salts from hepatocyte to bile and from ileal enterocytes to the portal vein are the engine behind the enterohepatic circulation.
- Albumin is made exclusively in the liver and is the predominant serum binding protein.
- The liver is also responsible for the so-called acute phase response, a protein synthetic response by the liver to trauma or infection.
- Along with the intestine, the liver is responsible for the metabolism of the fat-soluble vitamins A, D, E, and K.
- The liver is responsible for synthesizing almost all of the identified coagulation factors and many of the fibrinolytic system components and several plasma regulatory proteins of coagulation and fibrinolysis.
- For the surgeon, assessment of hepatic function and estimation of the ability of a hepatic remnant to be sufficient after liver resection is also of obvious importance.

HEPATIC ABSCESS

Pyogenic Abscess

- The incidence of pyogenic liver abscess has remained similar over 60 years.
- The development of a hepatic abscess occurs when the inoculum of bacteria, regardless of the route of exposure, exceeds the liver's ability to clear it.
- Hepatic infections from the biliary tree are presently the most common identifiable cause of hepatic abscess.
- The portal venous system drains the gastrointestinal tract; therefore, any infectious disorder of the gastrointestinal tract can result in an ascending portal vein infection (pyelophlebitis) with exposure of the liver to large amounts of bacteria.
- Any systemic infection (endocarditis, pneumonia, osteomyelitis, etc.) can result in bacteremia and infection of the liver via the hepatic artery.
- Possible explanations for cryptogenic hepatic abscess are undiagnosed abdominal pathology, resolved infective process at the time of presentation, or host factors such as diabetes or malignancy rendering the liver more susceptible to transient hepatic artery or portal vein bacteremias.
- In series that evaluated colonoscopy and endoscopic retrograde cholangiopancreatography (ERCP) in patients with cryptogenic abscess, the yield has been low and often is only fruitful in patients with some objective finding that

might have suggested a subclinical abnormality (e.g., mildly elevated bilirubin).

- Abscesses from pyelophlebitis or cholangitis tend to be polymicrobial with a high preponderance of gram-negative rods. Systemic infections, on the other hand, usually cause infection with a single organism.
- The most common organisms cultured are *Escherichia coli* and *Klebsiella pneumoniae.*
- The classic description of the presenting symptoms of hepatic abscess are fever, jaundice, and right upper quadrant pain and tenderness. Unfortunately, this presentation is present only 10% of the time.
- The most essential element to making the diagnosis of hepatic abscess is radiographic imaging studies.
- Ultrasound (US) and computed tomography (CT) are the mainstays in diagnostic modalities for hepatic abscess.
- Differentiating pyogenic abscess from other cystic infective diseases of the liver such as amebic abscess or echinococcal cyst is important because of differences in treatment.
- Over the last 20 years, percutaneous catheter drainage has become the treatment of choice for most patients.
- Surgery should be reserved for patients who require surgical treatment of the primary pathology (e.g., appendicitis) or for those who have failed percutaneous techniques.

Amebic Abscess

- Amebiasis is largely a disease of tropical and developing countries but is also a significant problem in developed countries because of immigration and travel between countries.
- In contrast to pyogenic hepatic abscesses, patients with amebic liver abscesses tend to be Hispanic males, aged 20 to 40 with a history of travel to (or origination from) an endemic area. A male preponderance of greater than 10:1 has been reported in almost all studies.
- It is felt that the trophozoites reach the liver through the portal venous system.
- Amebic liver abscesses are thus formed by progressing, localized hepatic necrosis resulting in a cavity containing acellular proteinaceous debris surrounded by a rim of invasive amebic trophozoites.
- Approximately 80% of patients with amebic liver abscess present with symptoms lasting from a few days to 4 weeks.
- Greater than 70% of patients with amebic liver abscess do not have detectable amebae in their stool, the most useful laboratory evaluation is the measurement of circulating

antiamebic antibodies, which are present in 90% to 95% of patients.

- Typical findings on abdominal US are a rounded lesion abutting the liver capsule (see previous discussion) without significant rim echoes interpreted as an abscess wall.
- In situations in which amebic serology is inconclusive and therapeutic trial of antibiotics is either deemed inappropriate or has failed to improve symptoms, consideration should be given to diagnostic aspiration.
- The mainstay of treatment for amebic abscesses is metronidazole (750 mg orally three times per day for 10 days), which is curative in more than 90% of patients.
- In general, aspiration is recommended for diagnostic uncertainty (see previous discussion), for failure to respond to metronidazole therapy in 3 to 5 days, or in abscesses felt to be at high risk for rupture.
- Although amebic liver abscess usually has a benign course, there are uncommon complications that the practitioner must be aware of.

Hydatid Disease

- Hydatid disease or echinococcosis is a zoonosis that occurs primarily in sheep grazing areas of the world but is common worldwide because the dog is a definitive host.
- In a definitive host, the scoleces would develop into an adult tapeworm, but in the intermediate host they can only differentiate into a new hydatid cyst.
- The clinical presentation of a hydatid cyst is largely asymptomatic until complications occur.
- Rupture of the cyst into the biliary tree or bronchial tree or free rupture into the peritoneal, pleural, or pericardial cavities can occur. Free ruptures can result in disseminated echinococcosis and/or a potentially fatal anaphylactic reaction.
- A number of findings on US can be diagnostic and depend on the stage of the cyst at the time of the examination.
- In patients with suspected biliary involvement, ERCP or percutaneous transhepatic cholangiography (PTC) may be necessary.
- The treatment of hepatic hydatid cysts is primarily surgical. In general, most cysts should be treated, but in elderly patients with small, asymptomatic, calcified cysts, conservative management is appropriate.
- When bile duct communication is diagnosed at operation or preoperatively, it must be meticulously searched for.

- In recent years, however, a number of authors have reported percutaneous aspiration and injection of scolecoidal agents with early success rates on the order of 70%. This technique has significant limitations and should only be used in very well selected cases.

Cholangitis

- Recurrent pyogenic cholangitis (RPC) is a syndrome of repeated attacks of cholangitis secondary to biliary stones and strictures that involve the extra- and intrahepatic ducts.
- Strictures can be found anywhere in the biliary tree but more commonly involve the intrahepatic main hepatic ducts and most often involve the left hepatic duct.
- The typical patient with RPC is young, Asian, and of a lower-socioeconomic background and presents with repeated bouts of cholangitis.
- Evaluation of the anatomic distribution of disease is critical to formulating a sound therapeutic plan.
- At the definitive operation the goal is to clear the biliary tree of stones and to bypass or enlarge strictures.

BENIGN NEOPLASMS

Adenoma

- Liver cell adenoma (LCA) is a relatively rare benign proliferation of hepatocytes in the context of a normal liver.
- The normal architecture of the liver is not present in these lesions.
- Although in the past, imaging studies lacked the accuracy to diagnose LCA, modern day imaging techniques can identify the majority of these tumors.
- The two major risks of LCA are rupture (with potentially life-threatening intraperitoneal hemorrhage) and malignant transformation.
- Most authorities recommend resection because of a very low mortality in experienced hands and the previously mentioned risks of observation.
- The mass is characterized by a central fibrous scar with radiating septae, although no central scar is seen in about 15% of cases.

Focal Nodular Hyperplasia (FNH)

- Most patients with FNH present as an incidental finding at laparotomy or more commonly on imaging studies.

- With advances in hepatobiliary imaging, most cases of FNH can be diagnosed radiologically with reasonable certainty.
- Fine needle aspiration for the diagnosis of FNH is often unrevealing.
- The treatment of FNH, therefore, depends on diagnostic certainty and symptoms.

HEMANGIOMA

- Hemangioma is the most common benign tumor of the liver.
- Enlargement of hemangiomata are by ectasia rather than neoplasia.
- Most commonly, hemangiomata are asymptomatic and incidentally found.
- Radiologic investigation can reliably make the diagnosis in most cases.
- Percutaneous biopsy of a suspected hemangioma is potentially dangerous and inaccurate and is therefore contraindicated.
- Although the natural history of liver hemangioma has not been well documented, it appears that most remain stable over time with a very low risk of rupture or hemorrhage.

MALIGNANT NEOPLASMS

Hepatoma

- Hepatocellular carcinoma (HCC) is the most common primary malignancy of the liver and one of the most common malignancies worldwide accounting for more than 1 million deaths annually.
- Many years of research have documented a clear association between persistent hepatitis B virus (HBV) infection and the development of HCC.
- Hepatitis C virus (HCV) has recently been discovered to be a major cause of chronic liver disease in Japan, Europe, and the United States where there is a relatively low rate of HBV infection.
- HCV is an RNA virus that does not integrate into the host genome; therefore, the pathogenesis of HCV-related HCC may be more related to chronic inflammation and cirrhosis rather than direct carcinogenesis.
- Cirrhosis is not required for the development of HCC, and HCC is not an inevitable result of cirrhosis.
- Chronic alcohol abuse and smoking are both associated with an increased risk of HCC, and there may be a synergistic effect between the two as well as with HBV and HCV infection.

- Unfortunately, in unscreened populations, HCC tends to present at a late stage because of the lack of symptoms in early stages.
- Small, incidentally noted tumors are becoming a more common presentation because of the knowledge of specific risk factors, screening programs, and the increasing use of high-quality abdominal imaging.
- In the past, liver radioisotope scans and angiography were common methods of diagnosis, but US, CT, and magnetic resonance imaging (MRI) have largely replaced these studies.
- Alpha fetoprotein (AFP) measurements can be very helpful in the diagnosis of HCC.
- Patients with appropriate risk factors and suggestive radiology (with or without an elevated AFP) who are candidates for potentially curative surgical therapy do not require preoperative biopsy.
- Most patients with HCC have two diseases, and survival is as much related to the tumor as it is to cirrhosis.
- HCC largely metastasizes to the lung, bone, and peritoneum, and preoperative history should focus on symptoms referable to these areas.
- Assessment of liver function is absolutely critical in considering treatment options for a patient with HCC.
- The tumor-node-metastasis (TNM) staging system is not routinely used for HCC because it does not accurately predict survival because it does not take liver function into account.
- Most HCC probably starts as a single tumor, but ultimately multiple satellite lesions can develop secondary to portal vein invasion and metastases.
- Complete excision of HCC either by partial hepatectomy or by total hepatectomy and transplant is the only treatment modality with curative potential.
- The most commonly cited negative prognostic factors are tumor size, cirrhosis, infiltrative growth pattern, vascular invasion, intrahepatic metastases, multifocal tumors, lymph node metastases, margin less than 1 cm, and lack of a capsule.
- Comparing results of resection to transplantation is difficult and the two should be viewed as complimentary rather than competitive.
- Percutaneous ethanol injection (PEI) is a useful technique for ablating small tumors.
- Transarterial therapy for HCC is based on the fact that the majority of the tumor's blood supply is from the hepatic artery.

- Percutaneous transarterial embolization can induce ischemic necrosis in HCC resulting in response rates as high as 50%.
- Transarterial radiotherapy is potentially promising therapy for HCC as primary therapy or as adjuvant therapy.
- Systemic chemotherapy with a variety of agents has been ineffective for the treatment of HCC and has a minimal role in the treatment of HCC.

Distinct Variations of HCC

- Fibrolamellar HCC (FHCC) is a variant of HCC with remarkably different clinical features that are summarized in Table 49–1.

Intrahepatic Cholangiocarcinoma (IHC)

- The majority (40% to 60%) of these tumors involve the biliary confluence (Klatskin's tumor), but approximately 10% emanate from intrahepatic ducts, presenting as a liver mass.
- Complete resection is the treatment of choice for IHC.

Hepatoblastoma

- Hepatoblastoma is the most common primary hepatic tumor of childhood.
- A variety of sarcomas can rarely present as primary liver tumors but must always be considered metastatic lesions until proven otherwise.

METASTATIC TUMORS

- The most common malignant tumors of the liver are metastatic lesions.

TABLE 49–1. Comparison of Standard Hepatocellular Carcinoma (HCC) and Fibrolamellar Hepatocellular Carcinoma (FHCC)

Characteristic	HCC	FHCC
Male female ratio	2:1–8:1	1:1
Median age	55	25
Tumor	Invasive	Well circumscribed
Resectability	<25%	50–75%
Cirrhosis	90%	5%
α-Fetoprotein positive	80%	5%
Hepatitis B positive	65%	5%

- Although an elevated carcinoembryonic antigen (CEA) is not specific for recurrent colorectal cancer, a rising CEA on serial examinations and a new solid mass on imaging studies are diagnostic of metastatic disease.
- The majority of these cases are associated with widespread disease and/or unresectable hepatic disease, and it is estimated that about 5% to 10% of these cases are candidates for a potentially curative liver resection.
- The presence of extrahepatic disease and the inability to resect all disease in the liver are absolute contraindications for liver resection.
- Although long-term survival after liver resection for hepatic colorectal metastases is clearly possible, recurrence of disease is quite common.
- Adjuvant systemic chemotherapy after liver resection for metastatic colorectal cancer is not supported by prospective trials.
- Thus, the goal of treatment is often more focused on quality of life rather than prolongation of life.
- A number of effective nonsurgical therapies exist for neuroendocrine liver metastases.
- Liver resection can play a role in patients whose tumor can be completely encompassed.
- The other role surgery plays is in those patients who have failed medical therapy and have recalcitrant symptoms of hormonal excess.
- Formal resections with wide margins are not necessary for neuroendocrine tumors and techniques such as enucleations or wedge resections are good options.
- Prognosis tends to be dismal if there is extrahepatic disease, multiple tumors, large tumors, or a short disease-free interval.
- In most series, liver resection for genitourinary tumors has the best prognosis, and in well-selected patients liver resection should be considered.

CYSTIC LESIONS

- Simple cysts of the liver contain serous fluid, do not communicate with the biliary tree, and do not have septations.
- Treatment of simple hepatic cysts is only indicated if they are symptomatic or if there is diagnostic uncertainty.
- Surgical therapy is achieved by fenestration or unroofing the portion of the cyst that is extrahepatic.
- Cystadenoma of the liver is a rare neoplasm that usually presents as a large cystic mass (usually 10 to 20 cm).

Polycystic Liver Disease

- Liver cysts are commonly seen in patients with the autosomal dominant inherited adult polycystic kidney disease.
- Treatment of polycystic liver disease is reserved for severe symptoms related to large cysts and complications.
- Because of the risk of malignancy and recurrent cholangitis treatment is excision with re-establishment of bilioenteric continuity.
- When intrahepatic bile duct cysts are localized, hepatic resection with or without biliary reconstruction is the treatment of choice.
- Series from the 1970s and 1980s often reported mortality rates in excess of 10% and were often as high as 20%, especially for major resections.
- In experienced centers, perioperative mortality is routinely 5% or less.
- Because many resections encompass tumors and normal liver, the concept of "functional liver parenchyma" is important because there is often compensatory hypertrophy of normal liver when tumors occupy a significant amount of the liver volume.
- In general, one should always revert back to the segmental anatomy of the liver if there is any confusion about the description of a liver resection.

HEMOBILIA

- Hemobilia is defined as bleeding into the biliary tree from an abnormal communication between a blood vessel and bile duct.
- The most common cause of hemobilia is iatrogenic trauma to the liver and biliary tree.
- Clinical sequelae of hemobilia are related to blood loss and the formation of potentially occlusive blood clots in the biliary tree.
- Upper gastrointestinal bleeding seen in conjunction with biliary symptoms must always raise the suspicion of hemobilia.
- Once hemobilia is suspected, the first evaluation should be upper gastrointestinal endoscopy, which rules out other sources of hemorrhage and may visualize bleeding from the ampulla of Vater.
- Arterial angiography is now recognized as the test of choice when hemobilia is suspected and will reveal the source of bleeding in about 90% of cases.

- The first line of therapy for major hemobilia is transarterial embolization (TAE) and success rates of 80% to 100% are reported.
- Surgery is indicated when conservative therapy and TAE have failed.
- Bilhemia is an extremely rare condition in which bile flows into the bloodstream either through the hepatic veins or portal vein branches.

CHAPTER 50

SURGICAL COMPLICATIONS OF CIRRHOSIS AND PORTAL HYPERTENSION

- Cirrhosis is the end result of a variety of mechanisms causing hepatocellular injury, including toxins (alcohol), viruses (hepatitis B and hepatitis C), prolonged cholestasis (extrahepatic and intrahepatic), autoimmunity (lupoid hepatitis), and metabolic disorders (hemochromatosis, Wilson's disease, alpha$_1$-antitrypsin deficiency). Although the mechanisms are diverse, the pathologic response is uniform: hepatocellular necrosis followed by fibrosis and nodular regeneration.
- Cirrhosis causes two major phenomena: hepatocellular failure and portal hypertension.
- Only 10% to 15% of heavy drinkers develop alcoholic cirrhosis.
- Hepatic failure and variceal hemorrhage are the first and second most common causes of death, respectively, in patients with cirrhosis.
- In contrast, since 1980, the surgical management of chronic liver disease with hepatic transplantation has been highly successful, with long-term survival rates generally greater than 70%.

ANATOMY, PHYSIOLOGY, AND PATHOPHYSIOLOGY OF PORTAL HYPERTENSION

- Because increased portal venous resistance is usually the initiator of portal hypertension, classifications of this disorder are generally based on the site of elevated resistance.
- The most common cause of prehepatic portal hypertension is portal vein thrombosis, which accounts for about half of cases of portal hypertension in children.
- Isolated splenic vein thrombosis (left-sided portal hypertension) is usually secondary to pancreatic inflammation or neoplasm. This variant of portal hypertension is important to recognize because it is easily reversed by splenectomy alone.

721

- Alcoholic cirrhosis, the most common cause of portal hypertension in the United States, usually causes increased resistance to portal flow at the sinusoidal (secondary to deposition of collagen in Disse space) and postsinusoidal (secondary to regenerating nodules distorting small hepatic veins) levels.
- Portal hypertension is defined by a portal pressure above 5 mm Hg.
- The collateral network through the coronary and short gastric veins to the azygos vein is the most important one clinically because it results in formation of esophagogastric varices.

EVALUATION OF THE PATIENT WITH CIRRHOSIS

- Key aspects of the assessment of a patient with suspected chronic liver disease or one of the complications of portal hypertension are the following: (1) diagnosis of the underlying liver disease, (2) estimation of functional hepatic reserve, (3) definition of portal venous anatomy and hepatic hemodynamic evaluation, and (4) identification of the site of upper gastrointestinal hemorrhage, if present.
- Precise identification of the site of bleeding is essential because hemorrhage secondary to portal hypertension may be from esophageal varices, gastric varices, ectopic varices, portal hypertensive gastropathy (PHG), or portal colopathy and because a significant fraction of patients with portal hypertension bleed from other lesions.

History and Physical Examination

- Subtle clues to the presence of underlying chronic liver disease on physical examination are spider angiomas, palmar erythema, testicular atrophy, and gynecomastia.

Laboratory Tests

- Cirrhosis is often accompanied by anemia, leukopenia, and thrombocytopenia.
- Although many patients with portal hypertension have some degree of hypersplenism, it is unusual to find a platelet count of less than 50,000 per mm^3 or a white blood cell count of less than 2000 per mm^3.
- Hypoalbuminemia and/or a prolonged international normalized ratio (INR) are usually reliable indices of chronic rather than acute liver disease.

- Increased disease activity may be an important risk factor in patients who undergo surgery.
- In the absence of prior blood transfusions, a total bilirubin level of greater than 3 mg per 100 mL is indicative of severe hepatic decompensation and a high operative risk status.
- Hepatitis serology should be obtained in most patients with cirrhosis.
- Unexpected hepatic functional deterioration in a patient with cirrhosis is often a result of the development of hepatocellular carcinoma, which can be diagnosed in about 60% of patients by an elevated alpha-fetoprotein level. All newly diagnosed cirrhotic patients should be screened for hepatocellular carcinoma by determining alpha-fetoprotein level and by obtaining a computed tomography (CT) scan of the liver.

Liver Biopsy

- Percutaneous liver biopsy is a useful technique for establishing the cause of cirrhosis and for assessing activity of the liver disease.

Measurement of Hepatic Functional Reserve

- The time-honored method of assessing hepatic functional reserve is Child's classification or one of its modifications. The most commonly used scheme is the Child-Pugh classification (Table 50–1), which includes two clinical variables in addition to three biochemical indices. Although not a direct measure of hepatic functional reserve, no other test has

TABLE 50–1. Child-Pugh Criteria for Hepatic Functional Reserve

Clinical and Laboratory Measurement	Patient Score for Increasing Abnormality		
	1	2	3
Encephalopathy (grade)	None	1 or 2	3 or 4
Ascites	None	Mild	Moderate
Bilirubin (mg/dL)	1–2	2.1–3	≥3.1
Albumin (g/dL)	≥3.5	2.8–3.4	≥2.7
Prothrombin time (increase, sec)	1–4	4.1–6	≥6.1

Grade A, 5 and 6; grade B, 7–9; grade C, 10–15.

surpassed it with respect to predicting operative outcome or assessing long-term prognosis in the unoperated patient.

- The Model for End-Stage Liver Disease (MELD) scale that consists of serum bilirubin and creatinine levels, INR, and etiology of liver disease has recently been found to be as predictive of mortality as the Child-Pugh score.
- Now that hepatic transplantation has become a realistic option for many patients with cirrhosis, accurate quantitation of hepatocellular function to determine which patients are transplantation candidates has become even more important.

Hepatic Hemodynamic Assessment

- In patients with alcoholic cirrhosis and many varieties of nonalcoholic cirrhosis, portal pressure can be indirectly estimated by measurement of hepatic venous wedge pressure.
- The portal pressure should be expressed as the portal pressure gradient, which is the difference between the portal pressure and the inferior vena cava pressure. It is an important measurement because a gradient in excess of 10 mm Hg is necessary for varices to form and a pressure higher than 12 mm Hg is required for varices to bleed.
- Because splanchnic venous thrombosis may be the cause of portal hypertension or develop as a result of cirrhosis, portal venous anatomy should be defined before performing a portosystemic shunt operation. Although selective visceral angiography has been the most frequently used method for visualization of the portal venous system and for qualitative estimation of hepatic portal perfusion, this relatively invasive approach is presently being replaced in many institutions by less invasive methods such as CT angiography, Doppler ultrasonography, and magnetic resonance imaging.
- Doppler ultrasonography is a noninvasive technique for assessment of portal venous patency, direction of portal flow, and shunt patency status.

Diagnosis of Bleeding

- The key procedure for diagnosing the site of upper gastrointestinal hemorrhage in a patient with portal hypertension is endoscopy. Before endoscopy, the patient should be hemodynamically stabilized and the stomach evacuated of blood clots with a large-bore lavage tube.
- Upper gastrointestinal tract bleeding in patients with portal hypertension is caused by the portal hypertension in about 90% of instances.

- Portal hypertensive bleeding is most commonly from esophagogastric varices (esophageal varices, 80%; gastric varices, 20%).
- Isolated gastric varices should raise the suspicion of splenic vein thrombosis. Hemorrhage from gastric fundal varices can be especially severe and is associated with a higher likelihood of recurrent bleeding and mortality than bleeding from esophageal varices. The endoscopic diagnosis of variceal hemorrhage can be established by either observing a bleeding varix (about 25% of patients) or by observation of moderate-to large-sized varices and no other lesions in a patient who has recently experienced a major upper gastrointestinal tract hemorrhage (loss of more than 2 units of blood).
- The only nonvariceal cause of portal hypertensive bleeding is PHG and much less commonly, portal colopathy.
- Endoscopic ultrasound is a more sensitive diagnostic test than endoscopy alone for detection of gastric varices.

VARICEAL HEMORRHAGE

- Bleeding from esophagogastric varices is the single most life-threatening complication of portal hypertension, responsible for about one third of all deaths in patients with cirrhosis. Overall, acute variceal bleeding is associated with a mortality rate of about 25% to 30%.
- The risk for death from bleeding is mainly related to the underlying hepatic functional reserve.
- The greatest risk for rebleeding from varices is within the first few days after the onset of hemorrhage; the risk declines rapidly between then and 6 weeks after hemorrhage onset, when it returns to the prehemorrhage risk level.

Pathogenesis

- Esophagogastric varices do not bleed until portal pressure exceeds 12 mm Hg, and then they bleed in only one third to one half of patients.
- The three key variables that are predictive of variceal bleeding are Child-Pugh class, variceal size, and the presence and severity of red wale markings (indicative of epithelial thickness).

Treatment

- The many treatment modalities available suggest that no single therapy is entirely satisfactory for all patients or for all clinical situations. Sequential therapies are often necessary. Nonoperative treatments are generally preferred for acutely bleeding patients because they are often high operative risks because of decompensated hepatic function.

Treatment of the Acute Bleeding Episode

- Endoscopic treatment (sclerosis or ligation), which has become the mainstay of nonoperative treatment of acute hemorrhage in most centers, controls bleeding in more than 85% of patients, allowing an interval of medical management for improvement of hepatic function, resolution of ascites and encephalopathy, and enhancement of nutrition before definitive treatment for prevention of recurrent bleeding. Pharmacotherapy can be initiated in any hospital and some trials suggest that it is just as effective as endoscopic treatment.
- TIPS has replaced operative shunts for managing acute variceal bleeding when pharmacotherapy and endoscopic treatment fail to control bleeding.
- Endoscopy to determine the cause of bleeding should be performed as soon as the patient is stabilized. If a bleeding esophageal varix is observed or suspected because of an overlying clot, sclerotherapy or variceal ligation should be performed during the initial endoscopy if the expertise is available.
- Because infections are common in patients with bleeding varices, prophylactic antibiotics should be initiated.
- Randomized trials have shown that somatostatin and its longer acting analogue octreotide are as efficacious as endoscopic treatment for control of acute variceal bleeding. These agents are also associated with fewer adverse side effects than vasopressin.
- Because of the minimal adverse effects and ease of administration, octreotide is now commonly used as an adjunct to endoscopic therapy.
- The major advantages of variceal tamponade with the Sengstaken-Blakemore tube are immediate cessation of bleeding in more than 85% of patients and widespread availability of this device, including small community hospitals (Fig. 50–1). Endotrachial intubation is required for airway protection.
- Because of the effectiveness of endoscopic treatment and pharmacotherapy for acute variceal bleeding, balloon tamponade is infrequently required. It may be lifesaving, however, when exsanguinating hemorrhage prevents acute endoscopic treatment and in patients in whom

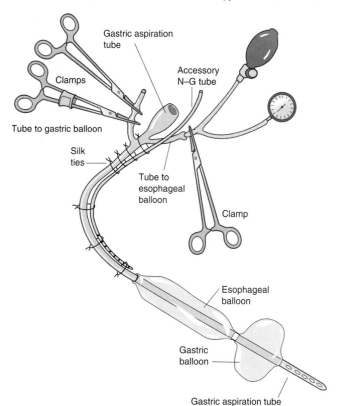

■ FIGURE 50–1. The modified Sengstaken-Blakemore tube. Note the accessory nasogastric tube for suctioning of secretions above the esophageal balloon and the two clamps, one secured with tape, to prevent inadvertent decompression of the gastric balloon. *(From Rikkers LF: Portal hypertension. In Goldsmith H (ed): Practice of Surgery. Philadelphia, Harper & Row, 1981, pp 1–37.)*

sclerotherapy has failed and who do not respond to pharmacotherapy.

- Endoscopic treatment (variceal sclerosis or ligation) is the most commonly used therapy for both management of the acute bleeding episode and prevention of recurrent hemorrhage. In the acute setting, sclerotherapy and band ligation have been shown to be equally efficacious.

- Failure of endoscopic treatment should be declared when two sessions fail to control hemorrhage.
- TIPS is a technique that accomplishes portal decompression without an operation.
- At present, TIPS should not be recommended as initial therapy for acute variceal hemorrhage but should be used only after less invasive treatments, such as endoscopic therapy and pharmacotherapy, have failed to control bleeding.
- One clear indication for TIPS is a short-term bridge to liver transplantation for patients in whom endoscopic treatment has failed.
- Patients with advanced hepatic functional decompensation (Child's Class C), even those who are not transplantation candidates, may be better served by TIPS than by an emergency operation when less invasive approaches fail to control bleeding.
- Hemodynamic studies suggest that TIPS is a nonselective shunt, and several investigations have demonstrated a similar frequency of encephalopathy after TIPS has been previously reported after nonselective shunts. Another disadvantage of the procedure is that shunt stenosis or occlusion develops in as many as half of patients within 1 year of TIPS insertion.
- The most common situations requiring either urgent or emergency surgery are failure of acute endoscopic treatment, failure of long-term endoscopic therapy, hemorrhage from gastric varices or PHG, and failure of TIPS placement.
- Selection of the appropriate emergency operation should mainly be guided by the experience of the surgeon.
- A commonly performed shunt operation in the emergency setting is the portacaval shunt because it rapidly and effectively decompresses the portal venous circulation.
- The major disadvantage of emergency surgery is that operative mortality rates exceed 25% in most reported series.

Prevention of Recurrent Hemorrhage

- Seventy percent of patients who have bled from varices will rebleed.
- In most institutions, initial treatment consists of pharmacotherapy or endoscopic therapy with portal decompression by means of TIPS or an operative shunt reserved for failures of first-line treatment. Hepatic transplantation is used for patients with end-stage liver disease.
- The objective of pharmacotherapy is to reduce the hepatic vein wedge pressure (HVWP) below 12 mm Hg, a level at which variceal bleeding does not occur.

- Thus, two obstacles to effective treatment with drugs are variability of response to the drug and lack of an easily measured hemodynamic index to monitor therapy.
- A meta-analysis of 11 controlled trials of nonselective beta-adrenergic blockade has shown that this treatment significantly decreases the likelihood of recurrent hemorrhage and demonstrates a trend toward decreased mortality.
- Long-term pharmacotherapy should be used only in compliant patients who are observed closely by their physicians. Although an attractive approach because of its noninvasiveness, pharmacotherapy, like endoscopic therapy, is associated with a high incidence of rebleeding.
- Since the late 1970s, chronic endoscopic therapy has become the most common treatment for prevention of recurrent variceal hemorrhage.
- The objective of chronic endoscopic therapy is to eradicate esophageal varices.
- Several controlled trials and a meta-analysis comparing endoscopic sclerotherapy to variceal ligation have shown a significant advantage to the latter technique.
- Although fewer patients receiving endoscopic treatment than medical treatment experienced rebleeding in all of the investigations, recurrent bleeding still occurred in about half of endoscopic therapy patients.
- Thus, chronic endoscopic therapy is a rational initial treatment for many patients who bleed from esophageal varices, but subsequent treatment with TIPS, a shunt procedure, a nonshunt operation, or hepatic transplantation should be anticipated for a significant percentage of patients. Because of its relatively high failure rate, a course of chronic endoscopic therapy should not be undertaken for noncompliant patients and those living a long distance from advanced medical care.
- A major limitation of TIPS, however, is a high incidence (up to 50%) of shunt stenosis or shunt thrombosis within the first year.
- Until TIPS technology improves, an operative shunt is probably preferable in patients who require long-term portal decompression.
- Clinical evidence of the nonselectivity of TIPS is its effectiveness in resolving medically intractable ascites and a fairly high frequency of post-TIPS encephalopathy (about 30%).
- Fewer patients rebled after TIPS (19%) than following endoscopic treatment (47%), but encephalopathy was significantly more common in TIPS patients (34%). TIPS dysfunction developed in 50% of patients.

- Thus, liver transplantation candidates who fail endoscopic and/or pharmacotherapy are well suited for TIPS followed by transplantation when a donor organ becomes available.
- Another group of patients in whom TIPS may be advantageous includes those with advanced hepatic functional decompensation who are unlikely to survive long enough for the TIPS to malfunction. Because it functions as a side-to-side portosystemic shunt, TIPS is also effective in the treatment of medically intractable ascites.
- Portosystemic shunts are clearly the most effective means of preventing recurrent hemorrhage in patients with portal hypertension.
- Diversion of portal blood, however, which contains hepatotropic hormones, nutrients, and cerebral toxins, is also responsible for the adverse consequences of shunt operations, namely portosystemic encephalopathy and accelerated hepatic failure. Depending on whether they completely decompress, compartmentalize, or partially decompress the portal venous circulation, portosystemic shunts can be classified as nonselective, selective, or partial.

Nonselective Shunts

- The end-to-side portacaval shunt is the prototype of nonselective shunts and is the only shunt procedure that has been compared to conventional medical management in randomized, controlled trials.
- Although no survival advantage could be demonstrated for shunt patients, all of these studies had a crossover bias in favor of medically treated patients, several of whom received a shunt when they developed intractable recurrent variceal hemorrhage.
- Other important findings of these randomized trials include reliable control of bleeding in shunted patients; variceal rebleeding in more than 70% of medically treated patients; and spontaneous, often severe, encephalopathy in 20% to 40% of shunted patients.
- Because the liver and intestines are both important contributors to ascites formation, side-to-side portosystemic shunts are the most effective shunt procedures for relieving ascites and preventing recurrent variceal bleeding.
- A major disadvantage of prosthetic interposition shunts is a high graft thrombosis rate that approaches 35% during the late postoperative interval. This problem can be avoided by using autogenous vein (internal jugular vein) rather than a prosthetic graft.

- A conventional splenorenal shunt that is of sufficient caliber to remain patent gradually dilates and eventually causes complete portal decompression and portal flow diversion.
- In summary, nonselective shunts effectively decompress varices. Because of complete portal flow diversion, however, they are complicated by frequent postoperative encephalopathy and accelerated hepatic failure. Side-to-side nonselective shunts effectively relieve ascites and prevent variceal hemorrhage.

Selective Shunts

- The distal splenorenal shunt consists of anastomosis of the distal end of the splenic vein to the left renal vein and interruption of all collateral vessels, such as the coronary and gastroepiploic veins, connecting the superior mesenteric and gastrosplenic components of the splanchnic venous circulation. This results in separation of the portal venous circulation into a decompressed gastrosplenic venous circuit and a high-pressure superior mesenteric venous system that continues to perfuse the liver.
- Because sinusoidal and mesenteric hypertension is maintained and important lymphatic pathways are transected during dissection of the left renal vein, the distal splenorenal shunt tends to aggravate rather than relieve ascites. Thus, patients with medically intractable ascites should not undergo this procedure.
- A splenic vein diameter of less than 7 mm is a relative contraindication to the procedure because the incidence of shunt thrombosis is high when using a small-diameter vein.
- Although the distal splenorenal shunt results in portal flow preservation in more than 85% of patients during the early postoperative interval, the high-pressure mesenteric venous system gradually collateralizes to the low-pressure shunt, resulting in loss of portal flow in about half of patients by 1 year.
- Henderson and coworkers have shown that portal flow is maintained in most patients with nonalcoholic cirrhosis and noncirrhotic portal hypertension (e.g., portal vein thrombosis).
- Six of the seven controlled comparisons of the distal splenorenal shunt to nonselective shunts have included predominantly alcoholic cirrhotic patients. None of these trials has demonstrated an advantage to either procedure with respect to long-term survival. Three of the studies have found a lower frequency of encephalopathy after the distal splenorenal shunt, whereas the other trials have shown no difference in the incidence of this postoperative complication.

- Mainly because of these inconsistent results of the controlled trials, there is no consensus as to which shunting procedure is superior in patients with alcoholic cirrhosis. Because the quality of life (encephalopathy rate) was significantly better in the distal splenorenal shunt group in three of the trials, however, there appears to be an advantage to selective variceal decompression even in this population.
- Considerably fewer data are available regarding selective shunting in nonalcoholic cirrhosis and in noncirrhotic portal hypertension.
- Several controlled trials have also compared the distal splenorenal shunt with chronic endoscopic therapy. In these investigations, recurrent hemorrhage was more effectively prevented by selective shunting than by sclerotherapy, but hepatic portal perfusion was maintained in a significantly higher fraction of patients undergoing sclerotherapy. Despite this hemodynamic advantage, encephalopathy rates have been similar after both therapies.
- The survival results of these two studies suggest that endoscopic therapy is a rational, initial treatment for patients who bleed from varices if sclerotherapy failure is recognized and such patients promptly undergo surgery or TIPS. However, patients living in remote areas are less likely to be salvaged by shunt surgery when endoscopic treatment fails, and a selective shunt may be preferable initial treatment for such patients.
- In a nonrandomized comparison to TIPS, the distal splenorenal shunt had lower rates of recurrent bleeding, encephalopathy, and shunt thrombosis.
- Partial shunts.
    - The objectives of partial and selective shunts are the same: (1) effective decompression of varices, (2) preservation of hepatic portal perfusion, and (3) maintenance of some residual portal hypertension.
- More recently, a small-diameter interposition portacaval shunt using a polytetrafluoroethylene graft, combined with ligation of the coronary vein and other collateral vessels, has been described. When the prosthetic graft is 10 mm or less in diameter, hepatic portal perfusion is preserved in most patients.
- The objectives of these procedures are either ablation of varices or, more commonly, extensive interruption of collateral vessels connecting the high-pressure portal venous system with the varices.
- The most effective nonshunt operation is extensive esophagogastric devascularization combined with esophageal transection and splenectomy.

- In Japan, the results with this operation have been excellent, with rebleeding rates of less than 10%. Extensive devascularization procedures, however, have generally been less successful in North American patients with alcoholic cirrhosis.
- Liver transplantation is not a treatment for variceal bleeding per se but rather must be considered for all patients who present with end-stage hepatic failure whether or not it is accompanied by bleeding.
- There is accumulating evidence that variceal bleeders with well-compensated hepatic functional reserve (Child's Class A and B) are better served by nontransplantation strategies initially.
- Patients with variceal bleeding who are transplantation candidates include nonalcoholic cirrhotic patients and abstinent alcoholic cirrhotic patients with either limited hepatic functional reserve (Child's Class B and C) or a poor quality of life secondary to their disease (e.g., encephalopathy, fatigue, or bone pain).
- An algorithm for definitive management of variceal hemorrhage is shown in Figure 50–2. Patients are first grouped according to their transplantation candidacy.
- Transplantation candidates with either decompensated hepatic function or a poor quality of life secondary to their liver disease should undergo transplantation as soon as possible. Most future transplantation and nontransplantation candidates should undergo initial endoscopic treatment and/or pharmacotherapy unless they bleed from gastric varices or PHG or live in remote geographic locations and have limited access to emergency tertiary care. Patients who live in remote locations and those who fail endoscopic and drug therapy should receive a selective shunt if they meet the criteria for this operation.
- TIPS is clearly indicated for patients with endoscopic treatment failure who may require transplantation in the near future and for nontransplantation candidates with advanced hepatic functional deterioration.
- Nontransplantation operations are now necessary less frequently, the survival results are better because high operative risk patients are managed by other means, and emergency surgery has nearly been eliminated.

Prevention of Initial Variceal Hemorrhage (Prophylactic Therapy)

- In these investigations, survival of shunted patients was actually less than that of medically treated patients because

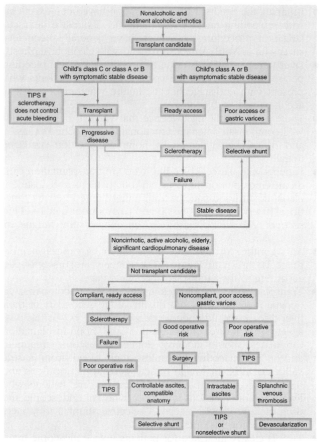

■ FIGURE 50–2. Algorithm for definitive therapy of variceal hemorrhage (see text). *(Modified from Rikkers LF: Portal hypertension. In Levine BA, Copeland E, Howard R, et al (eds): Current Practice of Surgery, Vol. 3. New York, Churchill Livingstone, 1995.)*

of accelerated hepatic failure secondary to complete portal diversion.

● Endoscopic treatment, however, cannot be advocated for prophylaxis because controlled trials have shown no consistent benefit, and some have demonstrated a higher rebleeding rate and a lower survival rate in the sclerotherapy group than in medically treated controls. In contrast, most trials of beta-blockade as prophylactic therapy have found a reduced incidence of initial variceal hemorrhage in treated patients.

- Because beta-blockade has been associated with few adverse side effects, it can be recommended for reliable patients with varices that have never bled.

ASCITES AND THE HEPATORENAL SYNDROME

- Ascites is usually an indicator of advanced cirrhosis and is associated with a 1-year survival rate of approximately 50% compared with a 1-year survival rate of greater than 90% for patients with cirrhosis but without ascites.
- Portal hypertensive ascites is initiated by altered hepatic and splanchnic hemodynamics, which cause transudation of fluid into the interstitial space.
- Both the liver and intestines are important sites of ascites formation, and clinically significant ascites is rare in patients with extrahepatic portal hypertension.
- Because avid sodium retention by the kidneys is one of the key mechanisms in the development of ascites, a central goal of treatment is to achieve a negative sodium balance.
- More commonly, diuretic therapy is required and will resolve this complication of portal hypertension in greater than 90% of patients. Because secondary hyperaldosteronism is a key pathogenetic mechanism in the formation of ascites, a rational first-line diuretic is spironolactone.
- Diuretic therapy can be associated with significant complications because it can lead to a reduction in intravascular volume and, potentially, renal dysfunction.
- As a general guideline, patients with new onset ascites that is barely detectable on physical examination should be placed on salt restriction alone. However, patients with more advanced or tense ascites will usually require the combination of sodium restriction and diuretic therapy.
- Five percent to 10% of patients with ascites are refractory to medical treatment and require more invasive measures. The two mainstays of therapy in this group of patients are large volume paracentesis combined with intravenous albumin administration and TIPS.
- Although initially effective in most patients, a surgically placed peritoneovenous shunt is seldom used in the management of medically refractory ascites because of its associated complications such as occlusion, infection, and disseminated intravascular coagulation.
- Cirrhotic patients with ascites who develop fever, abdominal tenderness, or worsening hepatic and/or renal function should

undergo a diagnostic paracentesis to rule out spontaneous bacterial peritonitis.

- Before culture results are available, antibiotic therapy should be initiated when spontaneous bacterial peritonitis is suspected.
- Another life-threatening complication of portal hypertension is the hepatorenal syndrome that develops almost exclusively in patients with tense ascites and declining hepatic function.
- The only reliable treatment for the hepatorenal syndrome is liver transplantation.

ENCEPHALOPATHY

- The most common setting for the development of encephalopathy is in patients with cirrhosis who undergo a procedural shunt.
- Almost certainly the syndrome is multifactorial with the bulk of evidence supporting ammonia as the main cerebral toxin.
- Encephalopathy develops spontaneously in less than 10% of patients, and this form of the syndrome is almost entirely confined to those patients who undergo a procedural shunt. More commonly, one or more of the following precipitating factors induce the syndrome: gastrointestinal hemorrhage, excessive diuresis, azotemia, constipation, sedatives, infection, and excess dietary protein.
- Key to the management of encephalopathy is identifying and then eliminating whatever precipitating factors are responsible.
- The only drugs with proven effectiveness are neomycin, a poorly absorbed antibiotic that suppresses urease-containing bacteria, and lactulose, a nonabsorbable disaccharide that acidifies colonic contents and also has a cathartic effect.
- Lactulose is the mainstay of therapy for chronic encephalopathy as long-term use of neomycin may cause nephrotoxicity or ototoxicity in some patients.

CHAPTER 51

BILIARY TRACT

NORMAL ANATOMY

- The extrahepatic biliary tract consists of the bifurcation of the left and right hepatic ducts, the common hepatic duct and common bile duct, and the cystic duct and gallbladder.
- The right hepatic duct.
- The common hepatic duct.
- The common bile duct.
- The distal common bile duct and pancreatic duct may join outside the duodenal wall to form a long common channel or within the duodenal wall to form a short common channel or they may enter the duodenum through two distinct ostia.
- The gallbladder is a pear-shaped reservoir in continuity with the common hepatic and common bile ducts via the cystic duct.

COMMON ANOMALIES AND VARIATIONS

- Anatomic variations in the cystic duct and hepatic ducts are common.
- The cystic duct usually enters the common bile duct at an acute angle.
- An accessory hepatic duct or cholecystohepatic duct may also enter the gallbladder.
- Anomalies of the gallbladder are much less frequent than variations in ductal anatomy. Agenesis of the gallbladder.

NORMAL ANATOMY AND VARIATIONS

- The gallbladder is supplied by the cystic artery, which most commonly is a single branch of the right hepatic artery.
- The blood supply to the extrahepatic biliary tree.

BILE DUCTS

- The bile ducts, gallbladder, and sphincter of Oddi act in concert to modify, store, and regulate the flow of bile.

- Secretin increases bile flow.
- The bile duct epithelium is also capable of water and electrolyte absorption.

GALLBLADDER

- The main functions of the gallbladder are to concentrate and store hepatic bile during the fasting state and deliver bile into the duodenum in response to a meal.
- The gallbladder mucosa has the greatest absorptive capacity per unit area of any structure in the body. Bile is usually concentrated 5- to 10-fold.
- Active NaCl transport by the gallbladder epithelium.
- Water is passively absorbed.
- As the gallbladder bile becomes concentrated, several changes occur in the capacity of bile to solubilize cholesterol.
- The gallbladder epithelial cell secretes at least two important products into the gallbladder lumen: glycoproteins and hydrogen ions.
- Mucin gel.
- Decrease in gallbladder bile pH through a sodium-exchange mechanism.
- The gallbladder s normal acidification process lowers the pH of entering hepatic bile from 7.5 to 7.8 down to 7.1 to 7.3.

GALLBLADDER

- Gallbladder filling is facilitated by tonic contraction of the ampullary sphincter, which maintains a constant pressure in the common bile duct (10 to 15 mm Hg).
- Periods of filling are punctuated by brief periods of partial emptying (10% to 15% of its volume).
- Hormone motilin.
- One of the main stimuli to gallbladder emptying is the hormone cholecystokinin (CCK).
- When stimulated by eating, the gallbladder empties 50% to 70% of its contents within 30 to 40 minutes. Gallbladder refilling.

SPHINCTER OF ODDI

- The human sphincter of Oddi is a complex structure that is functionally independent from the duodenal musculature.
- High-pressure zone between the bile duct and the duodenum. The sphincter regulates the flow of bile and pancreatic juice into the duodenum, prevents the regurgitation of duodenal

contents into the biliary tract, and also diverts bile into the gallbladder.

- High-pressure phasic contractions.
- Both neural and hormonal factors influence the sphincter of Oddi.
- Pressure and phasic wave activity diminish in response to CCK.
- Neurally mediated reflexes link the sphincter of Oddi with the gallbladder and stomach.
- Bile in the gallbladder or bile ducts in the absence of gallstones or any other biliary tract disease is normally sterile. In the presence of gallstones or biliary obstruction the prevalence of bactibilia increases. The presence of positive bile cultures is influenced by several factors including the severity or type of biliary disease and the patient s age.
- Chronic cholecystitis.
- Acute cholecystitis.
- Common bile duct stones.
- Cholangitis.
- Gram-negative aerobes are the organisms most frequently isolated from bile in patients with symptomatic gallstones, acute cholecystitis, or cholangitis. *Escherichia coli.*
- *Klebsiella* species.
- *Pseudomonas.*
- *Enterobacter.*
- Other common isolates include the gram-positive aerobes, enterococcus, and *Streptococcus viridans.*
- Anaerobes.
- *Bacteroides* species.
- *Clostridium.*
- Small but significant role in biliary infections.
- *Candida* species are also being increasingly recognized particularly in critically ill patients.
- Polymicrobial infections are more common in patients with cholangitis.
- The source of bacteria in patients with biliary tract infections is controversial. Most evidence favors an ascending route via the duodenum.
- Antibiotics should be used prophylactically in most patients undergoing elective biliary tract surgery or other biliary tract manipulations.
- The risk of postoperative infectious complications corresponds to the presence of bactibilia.
- In low-risk patients undergoing laparoscopic cholecystectomy for chronic cholecystitis.
- In high-risk patients a single dose of the first-generation cephalosporin cefazolin provides good coverage.

- Therapeutic antibiotics are used in patients with acute cholecystitis and acute cholangitis.
- Second- or third-generation cephalosporins, aminoglycosides, ureidopenicillins, carbapenems, and the fluoroquinolones.
- Ureidopenicillins offer the advantage of gram-positive coverage, including the enterococci and of anaerobic coverage.
- Jaundice is a frequent manifestation of biliary tract disorders.
- Normal serum bilirubin ranges from 0.5 to 1.3 mg/dL.
- The presence of conjugated bilirubin in the urine is one of the first changes noted by patients.
- Bilirubin is the normal breakdown product of hemoglobin produced from senescent red blood cells.
- Insoluble unconjugated bilirubin.
- Uridine diphosphate (UDP)-glucuronyl transferase.
- Bilirubin monoglucuronide and bilirubin diglucuronide.
- Conjugated bilirubin.
- In the terminal ileum and colon, bilirubin is converted to urobilinogen.
- Urobilinogen is either re-excreted into the bile or excreted by the kidneys into the urine.

DIAGNOSTIC EVALUATION

- The differential diagnosis of jaundice parallels the metabolism of bilirubin.
- Common causes of increased bilirubin production include the hemolytic anemias and acquired causes of hemolysis.
- Bilirubin uptake.
- Impaired excretion of bilirubin.
- Extrahepatic biliary obstruction.
- The physician must be able to distinguish among defects in bilirubin uptake, conjugation, or excretion from extrahepatic biliary obstruction.
- A careful history, physical examination, routine laboratory tests, and noninvasive radiologic imaging will differentiate.
- Jaundice from common bile duct stones is usually transient.
- The gradual onset of painless jaundice with associated weight loss is suggestive of a malignancy. If jaundice occurs after cholecystectomy, retained bile duct stones or an injury to the bile duct should be suspected.
- Laboratory tests that should be performed in all jaundiced patients include serum direct and indirect bilirubin, alkaline phosphatase, transaminases, amylase, and a complete blood cell count.
- Unconjugated (indirect) hyperbilirubinemia.
- Conjugated (direct) hyperbilirubinemia.

- The highest elevations in serum bilirubin are usually found in patients with malignant obstruction.
- Common bile duct stones are usually associated with a more moderate increase in serum bilirubin.
- Alkaline phosphatase.
- The goals of radiologic evaluation of the jaundiced patient include confirmation of biliary obstruction, identification of the site and cause, and selection of the appropriate treatment modality.
- Ultrasound is often the initial screening test.
- Computed tomography (CT) scanning is also very sensitive at identifying biliary dilation.
- Spiral CT scanning provides additional staging information.
- Cholangiography is often necessary to delineate the site and cause of biliary obstruction.
- Magnetic resonance cholangiography (MRC).
- Both endoscopic retrograde cholangiography (ERC) and percutaneous transhepatic cholangiography (PTC) are invasive procedures.
- ERC is most useful in imaging patients with periampullary tumors and choledocholithiasis.
- PTC is the preferred technique in patients with proximal biliary obstruction.

ENDOSCOPIC MANAGEMENT

- Several conditions causing jaundice can also be treated at the time of endoscopic cholangiography. The common bile duct can be cleared of stones.
- Malignant biliary strictures involving the mid or distal common bile duct are also amenable to endoscopically placed stents.

PERCUTANEOUS MANAGEMENT

- The percutaneous route is favored in patients with more proximal bile duct obstruction.
- A careful evaluation of the overall general medical condition of the patient and accurate staging are necessary for the patient with obstructive jaundice.
- Preoperative assessment.
- Cardiac risk factors.
- Respiratory status.
- Renal function.
- Overall performance status.
- Alterations in hepatic and pancreatic function, the gastrointestinal barrier, immune function, hemostatic mechanisms, and wound healing.

- Endotoxemia may contribute to renal, cardiac, and pulmonary insufficiency.
- Altered cell-mediated immunity increases the risk of infection, whereas coagulation disorders make these patients prone to bleeding problems.
- Preoperative risk factors.
- Presence of sepsis (cholangitis).
- Renal insufficiency.
- Control of sepsis and intensive nutritional support.
- Preoperative relief of jaundice has been proposed as a method to decrease the risk of surgery.
- Several prospective randomized studies have shown that the routine use of preoperative biliary drainage does not reduce operative morbidity or mortality.
- A recent meta-analysis also concluded that preoperative biliary drainage increased rather than decreased overall complications.
- Several studies have documented a higher incidence of infectious complications.
- Preoperative biliary drainage.
- It may be useful in carefully selected patients with advanced malnutrition or biliary sepsis.
- Bile facilitates the intestinal absorption of lipids and fat-soluble vitamins and represents the route of excretion for certain organic solids, such as bilirubin and cholesterol.
- The major organic solutes are bilirubin, bile salts, phospholipids, and cholesterol.
- Bilirubin.
- Bile salts.
- Phospholipids.
- Cholesterol.
- Gallstones represent a failure to maintain certain biliary solutes, primarily cholesterol and calcium salts, in a solubilized state. Gallstones are classified by their cholesterol content as either cholesterol or pigment stones. Pigment stones are further classified as either black or brown.
- In most American populations, 70% to 80% of gallstones are cholesterol.
- Biliary sludge, a mixture of cholesterol crystals, calcium bilirubinate granules, and a mucin gel matrix.

CHOLESTEROL GALLSTONES

- The pathogenesis of cholesterol gallstones is clearly multifactorial but essentially involves three stages: (1) cholesterol supersaturation in bile, (2) crystal nucleation, and (3) stone growth.

- The key to maintaining cholesterol in solution is the formation of both micelles and cholesterol-phospholipid vesicles.
- Cholesterol solubility depends on the relative concentration of cholesterol, bile salts, and phospholipid.
- Triangular coordinates.
- Cholesterol supersaturation is present in many normal humans.
- Nucleation refers to the process in which solid cholesterol monohydrate crystals form and conglomerate. Nucleation occurs more rapidly in gallbladder bile of patients with cholesterol stones.
- For gallstones to cause clinical symptoms, they must obtain a size sufficient to produce mechanical injury to the gallbladder or obstruction of the biliary tree.
- Defects in gallbladder motility increase the residence time of bile in the gallbladder thereby playing a role in stone formation.
- Gallstone formation occurs after use of long-term parenteral nutrition, after vagotomy, and in patients with somatostatin-producing tumors or in those receiving long-term somatostatin therapy.

PIGMENT GALLSTONES

- Calcium bilirubinate and calcium palmitate also form major components of pigment gallstones.
- Pigment gallstones are classified as either black or brown pigment stones. Black pigment stones are typically tarry and are associated frequently with hemolytic conditions or cirrhosis.
- Brown pigment stones are earthy in texture and are typically found in the bile ducts.
- Once gallstones develop, they remain silent (asymptomatic) or they can produce biliary pain by obstructing the cystic duct.
- Additional complications include acute cholecystitis, choledocholithiasis, gallstone pancreatitis, gallstone ileus, and gallbladder carcinoma. The prevalence of gallstones is related to a number of factors including age, gender, weight, family history, and ethnic background.
- Common dietary factors and medications can also influence the risk of developing symptomatic gallstones.
- Gallstones are common.
- Approximately 1% to 2% of asymptomatic individuals with gallstones will develop serious symptoms or complications related to their gallstones per year.
- Over a 20-year period, two thirds of asymptomatic patients with gallstones will remain symptom-free.

- Patients with mild symptoms have a higher risk of developing gallstone-related complications or requiring cholecystectomy.
- At least 6% to 8% per year will require a cholecystectomy to manage their gallbladder symptoms.
- Delay in managing symptomatic gallstones with laparoscopic cholecystectomy may contribute to the high prevalence of gallstone-related complications.

ABDOMINAL RADIOGRAPH

- Abdominal plain films have a low yield in diagnosing biliary tract problems.
- Only 10% to 15% of gallstones will contain sufficient calcium to be radiopaque on abdominal radiographs.

ULTRASOUND

- Ultrasound has become the procedure of choice for documenting gallstones and is also extremely useful at identifying biliary dilation.
- An acoustic shadow.
- Gravity-dependent movement.
- The accuracy of ultrasound at diagnosing gallstones approaches 100%.
- Overall, the false-negative rate for ultrasound in detecting gallstones is approximately 5%.

CHOLESCINTIGRAPHY

- Cholescintigraphy provides a noninvasive evaluation of the liver, gallbladder, bile duct, and duodenum with both anatomic and functional information.
- Nonvisualization of the gallbladder with prompt filling of the common bile duct and small intestine is consistent with cystic duct obstruction.
- The primary use of cholescintigraphy is in the diagnosis of acute cholecystitis.
- The sensitivity and specificity of cholescintigraphy for diagnosing acute cholecystitis are each about 95%. False-positive results are increased in the setting of gallbladder stasis.

MISCELLANEOUS

- Abdominal CT scans are more useful in the evaluation of gallbladder cancer than calculous disease.

PATHOGENESIS

- The term chronic cholecystitis implies an ongoing or recurrent inflammatory process involving the gallbladder. In most patients (more than 90%), gallstones are the causative factor.

CLINICAL PRESENTATION

- The primary symptom associated with chronic cholecystitis or symptomatic cholelithiasis is pain often labeled biliary colic. The term biliary colic is inaccurate.
- Constant pain in most patients. The pain is usually located in the right upper quadrant.
- Classically, the pain of biliary colic occurs following a greasy meal, the pain often begins at night-time waking the patient from sleep.
- The duration of pain is typically 1 to 5 hours.
- Pain lasting beyond 24 hours suggests acute inflammation or cholecystitis.
- Nausea and vomiting often accompany each episode.
- Bloating and belching are also present in 50% of patients.
- The physical examination is usually completely normal in patients with chronic cholecystitis.
- Laboratory values are also usually normal in patients with uncomplicated gallstones.

DIAGNOSIS

- The diagnosis requires two things: (1) abdominal pain consistent with biliary colic and (2) the presence of gallstones.
- In most cases treatment is not necessary in asymptomatic patients.
- The differential diagnosis should include gastroesophageal reflux disease, acute pancreatitis, peptic ulcer disease, or irritable bowel syndrome.
- The presence of gallstones should also be documented. Ultrasound is quite sensitive (95% to 98%).

MANAGEMENT

- The treatment of choice for patients with symptomatic gallstones is elective laparoscopic cholecystectomy.
- The mortality rate is approximately 0.1% with cardiovascular complications being the most frequent cause of death. The most significant complication following laparoscopic cholecystectomy is injury to the biliary tract.

- Conversion to an open cholecystectomy is necessary in less than 5% of patients.
- Conversion rates are increased in elderly, obese, and male patients.
- The long-term results of laparoscopic cholecystectomy in appropriately selected patients with chronic cholecystitis are excellent.
- More than 90% of patients rendered symptom-free following cholecystectomy.

PATHOPHYSIOLOGY

- In 90% to 95% of cases, acute cholecystitis is related to gallstones.
- In the most severe cases (5% to 18%), this process can lead to ischemia and necrosis of the gallbladder wall.
- Initially, acute cholecystitis is an inflammatory process.
- In the most severe cases, generalized sepsis may be present.

CLINICAL PRESENTATION

- Right upper quadrant abdominal pain is the most common complaint in patients with acute cholecystitis.
- The pain of acute cholecystitis persists for longer than an uncomplicated episode of biliary colic.
- On physical examination, focal tenderness and guarding are usually present.
- A mass may be present in the right upper quadrant and a Murphy s sign may also be elicited.
- A mild leukocytosis is usually present; mild elevations in serum bilirubin, alkaline phosphatase, the transaminases, and amylase may be present.

DIAGNOSIS

- Ultrasound is the most useful radiologic examination in the patient with suspected cholecystitis.
- Focal tenderness directly over the gallbladder (sonographic Murphy s sign) is also suggestive of acute cholecystitis. Ultrasound has a sensitivity and specificity of 85% and 95%, respectively, for diagnosing acute cholecystitis.
- Radionuclide scanning is used less frequently; in the right clinical setting, it is highly sensitive (95%) and specific (95%) for acute cholecystitis.

MANAGEMENT

- Once the diagnosis of acute cholecystitis is made, the patient should have oral intake limited and be started on intravenous antibiotics.
- Parenteral analgesia should also be administered.
- Nonsteroidal analgesics, which inhibit prostaglandin synthesis, reduce gallbladder mucin production and, therefore, reduce pressure and pain.
- Open cholecystectomy has been the standard treatment for acute cholecystitis for many years.
- Laparoscopic cholecystectomy has become the preferred approach for most patients with acute cholecystitis.
- The conversion rate in the setting of acute cholecystitis (4% to 35%) is higher than with chronic cholecystitis.
- The timing of cholecystectomy for acute cholecystitis has been studied for several decades.
- Twenty percent of patients in the delayed surgery arm failed initial medical therapy.
- No significant differences were observed in the conversion rate.
- No significant differences in the complication rate were observed.
- However, hospital stay and, therefore, cost was significantly reduced in both trials in the early laparoscopic cholecystectomy group.
- Several retrospective series have demonstrated advantages to proceeding with laparoscopic cholecystectomy soon after the diagnosis of acute cholecystitis is made.
- In most patients with acute cholecystitis, laparoscopic cholecystectomy should be attempted soon (24 to 48 hours) after the diagnosis is made.

COMPLICATIONS

- Acute cholecystitis may progress to empyema of the gallbladder, emphysematous cholecystitis, or perforation of the gallbladder.
- In each case, emergency cholecystectomy is warranted.
- Empyema occurs with bacterial proliferation in an obstructed gallbladder.
- Emphysematous cholecystitis develops more commonly in males and patients with diabetes mellitus.
- Perforation of the gallbladder occurs in up to 10% of cases of acute cholecystitis.

- Perforation is most frequently (50% of cases) contained within the subhepatic space.
- Rarely, the gallbladder perforates freely into the peritoneal cavity.
- In most patients, cholecystectomy can be performed and is the best treatment of complicated acute cholecystitis. Occasionally, the inflammatory process obscures the structures in the triangle of Calot.
- In these patients, partial cholecystectomy and drainage avoids injury to the common bile duct.
- Percutaneous transhepatic cholecystostomy can drain the gallbladder.
- Interval laparoscopic cholecystectomy should then be performed after a delay of 3 to 4 months.
- Acute acalculous cholecystitis accounts for 5% to 10% of all patients with acute cholecystitis and is the diagnosis in approximately 1% to 2% of patients undergoing cholecystectomy. The disease often has a more fulminant course than acute calculous cholecystitis.
- Acute acalculous cholecystitis usually occurs in the critically ill patient.
- The etiology of acute acalculous cholecystitis remains unclear.
- Stasis is common.
- Visceral ischemia is also a common denominator.
- The symptoms and signs of acute acalculous cholecystitis are similar to acute calculous cholecystitis.
- CT scan and ultrasound findings are similar.
- Cholescintigraphy will demonstrate absent gallbladder filling.
- The false-positive rate may be as high as 40%.
- Emergency cholecystectomy is the appropriate treatment.
- Open cholecystectomy will usually be required.
- Mortality rate remains high (40%) in large part because of the concomitant illnesses.
- A subgroup of patients presenting with typical symptoms of biliary colic will not have any evidence of gallstones on ultrasound examination.
- Further investigations: esophagogastroduodenoscopy or even an endoscopic retrograde cholangiogram.
- The CCK-Tc-hepatobiliary iminodiacetic acid (HIDA) scan has been useful in identifying patients with this disorder. CCK is infused intravenously.
- An ejection fraction less than 35% at 20 minutes is considered abnormal.
- Patients with symptoms of biliary colic and an abnormal gallbladder ejection fraction should be managed with a laparoscopic cholecystectomy.

- Between 85% and 94% of patients will be asymptomatic or improved by cholecystectomy.
- Cholecystectomy is the most common gastrointestinal operation performed in the United States.
- The number of cholecystectomies performed in the United States has increased to 700,000 per year.
- The majority of these procedures can be safely completed using the laparoscopic technique.
- Uncontrolled coagulopathy is one of the few current contraindications to laparoscopic cholecystectomy.
- Patients with severe chronic obstructive pulmonary disease or congestive heart failure may not tolerate the pneumoperitoneum.
- The major contraindication to completing a laparoscopic cholecystectomy is an inability to clearly identify all of the anatomic structures.
- A liberal policy of converting represents good surgical judgment.
- The conversion rate for elective laparoscopic cholecystectomy ranges up to 5%.
- The technical difficulty of laparoscopic cholecystectomy is increased in several clinical settings.
- Morbid obesity.
- Prior upper abdominal surgery.
- Well-compensated cirrhosis.

LAPAROSCOPIC CHOLECYSTECTOMY

- Conversion to an open operation should be discussed with the patient.
- A Foley catheter and orogastric tube are inserted.
- Both open and closed methods have been used to establish a pneumoperitoneum.
- Open technique.
- Special blunt-tipped cannula (Hasson).
- Once an adequate pneumoperitoneum has been established, an 11-mm trocar is inserted through the supraumbilical incision. The laparoscope with attached video camera is then inserted.
- Additional trocars are inserted under direct vision.
- The two smaller ports are used for grasping the gallbladder and placing it in the ideal position for an antegrade cholecystectomy.
- Lateral port.
- Medial 5-mm cannula.
- The junction of the gallbladder and cystic duct is identified.

- The triangle of Calot is cleared of all fatty and lymphatic tissue.
- Once the cystic duct is identified, an intraoperative cholangiogram may be performed.
- Once the cholangiogram is completed, two clips are placed distally on the cystic duct.
- Alternatively, the common bile duct may be evaluated for stones using laparoscopic ultrasound. The sensitivity of laparoscopic ultrasound for detecting common bile duct stones is comparable to intraoperative cholangiography.
- The next step is the division of the cystic artery.
- Clips are placed proximally and distally on the artery.
- The gallbladder is dissected out of the gallbladder fossa.
- Just before removing the gallbladder from the liver, the operative field is carefully searched for hemostasis.
- The gallbladder.
- Is usually removed through the umbilical port.
- Many centers have demonstrated that elective laparoscopic cholecystectomy can be safely performed as an outpatient procedure.

OPEN CHOLECYSTECTOMY

- Open cholecystectomy can be performed through either an upper midline or right subcostal (Kocher) incision.
- The cystic duct is identified and ligated distally.
- A cholangiogram is performed.
- The cystic artery is ligated and divided.
- The gallbladder is dissected out of the gallbladder bed.
- A cystic duct cholangiogram is performed.
- A closed suction drain is placed if there is concern about the security of the cystic duct closure.
- Common bile duct stones are classified both by their point of origin and the time at which they are discovered relative to cholecystectomy.
- Most common bile duct calculi form initially in the gallbladder and migrate through the cystic duct into the common bile duct.
- From primary common bile duct calculi.
- Form within the biliary tract.
- Retained.
- Recurrent.
- Primary common duct stones are associated with biliary stasis and infection. Primary stones are usually of the brown pigment type.
- Biliary cultures are positive in most patients with common duct stones.

- The underlying abnormality leading to biliary stasis usually must be identified.

PRESENTATION

- Approximately 7% to 15% of patients undergoing cholecystectomy will have common bile duct stones.
- Biliary obstruction from stones is often transient.
- Clinical features suspicious for biliary obstruction resulting from common bile duct stones include biliary colic, jaundice, lightening of the stools, and darkening of the urine.
- Fever and chills.
- Elevated serum bilirubin (>3.0 mg/dL), serum aminotransferases, and alkaline phosphatase.
- Serum bilirubin has the highest positive predictive value.
- However, laboratory values may be normal in up to one third of patients with choledocholithiasis.
- Standard ultrasound examination can provide additional information.
- The prevalence of choledocholithiasis is significantly higher in the setting of a dilated common bile duct.
- Echogenic shadows consistent with calculi are only visible in 60% to 70% of patients.
- MRC.
- Has a sensitivity and specificity of 95% and 89% at detecting choledocholithiasis.
- Endoscopic cholangiography has been the gold standard for diagnosing common bile duct calculi preoperatively.
- The advantage of providing a therapeutic option at the time common duct stones are identified.
- Complications of diagnostic cholangiography include pancreatitis and cholangitis.
- Endoscopic ultrasound (EUS) has also been used to identify bile duct stones.
- The choice of radiologic studies to evaluate a patient with suspected choledocholithiasis should be based on the probability of this diagnosis. Patients at highest risk for choledocholithiasis should undergo endoscopic cholangiography.
- MRC.
- Intraoperative cholangiography.

ENDOSCOPIC MANAGEMENT

- Endoscopic sphincterotomy and stone extraction.
- Permits common bile duct stones to be removed without the need for conventional surgery.

- Particularly useful for patients before cholecystectomy.
- Endoscopic clearance can avoid the need for an open operation.
- Common bile duct calculi not suspected preoperatively but detected on intraoperative cholangiography may also be suitable for endoscopic management.
- Endoscopic sphincterotomy and stone extraction is also the procedure of choice for patients with retained common bile duct stones after cholecystectomy.
- Endoscopic sphincterotomy and stone extraction is well tolerated in most patients. Complications occur in 5% to 8% of patients: cholangitis, pancreatitis, perforation, bleeding.
- The overall mortality rate is 0.2% to 0.5%.
- Following endoscopic sphincterotomy and stone extraction, patients with a stone-filled gallbladder remain at high risk of developing future biliary symptoms.

LAPAROSCOPIC COMMON BILE DUCT EXPLORATION

- Laparoscopic exploration of the common bile duct for choledocholithiasis enables appropriate patients to undergo complete management of their calculous biliary tract disease with one invasive procedure.
- Once the presence of stones is confirmed, balloon-tipped Fogarty catheters are inserted through the cystic ductotomy.
- A small flexible choledochoscope is next introduced.
- Occasionally, the cystic duct will need to be dilated.
- Clearance of all common bile duct stones is achieved in 75% to 95% of patients with laparoscopic common bile duct exploration.

OPEN COMMON BILE DUCT EXPLORATION

- Open common bile duct exploration is performed much less frequently now than 15 years ago.
- After mobilizing the duodenum, a longitudinal choledochotomy is made.
- A combination of techniques are all used to remove stones from the bile duct.
- The flexible and rigid choledochoscope are both useful.
- A T-tube is placed in the common bile duct.
- A completion cholangiogram is performed.
- The common bile duct may be explored through a large cystic duct.
- In patients with a nondilated common bile duct (<4 mm), a transduodenal sphincteroplasty should be performed.

- In patients with definite sphincter stenosis, multiple common bile duct stones, primary common bile duct stones, or intrahepatic stones, a drainage procedure (Roux-en-Y choledochojejunostomy, transduodenal sphincteroplasty, or choledochoduodenostomy) should be performed.
- Open common bile duct exploration is associated with low operative mortality and operative morbidity; the rate of retained common bile duct stones is less than 5%.
- Abdominal pain or other symptoms originally attributed to the gallbladder may persist or recur months or years following cholecystectomy.
- A retained common bile duct stone or bile duct injury or leak.
- Pancreatitis, peptic ulcer disease, gastroesophageal reflux, wound neuroma, or even irritable bowel syndrome.
- A long cystic duct stump.
- Abnormalities in the sphincter of Oddi.

SPHINCTER OF ODDI DYSFUNCTION

- Pain characteristic of biliary colic and episodes of recurrent acute pancreatitis have been attributed to a poorly defined clinical syndrome described as dysfunction of the sphincter of Oddi.
- A structural or functional abnormality.
- Fibrosis of the sphincter.
- Sphincter of Oddi dyskinesia or spasm.
- Sphincter of Oddi dysfunction should be suspected in patients with typical episodic biliary-type pain without an obvious organic cause. Approximately 1% of patients undergoing cholecystectomy are estimated to have sphincter of Oddi dysfunction.
- Numerous diagnostic tests have been used but none are sensitive or specific.
- Elevated serum amylase or transaminases.
- Ultrasound evidence of sphincter of Oddi dysfunction.
- Delayed emptying of contrast from the common bile duct.
- Endoscopic manometry has also been used and an elevated basal sphincter pressure (>40 mm Hg) has been correlated with successful response to sphincter ablation.
- Both endoscopic sphincterotomy and transduodenal sphincteroplasty with transampullary septectomy have been used to manage patients with sphincter of Oddi dysfunction.
- Results dependent on the presence of objective signs of sphincter dysfunction.
- When objective evidence of sphincter dysfunction is present.

- Sixty percent to 80% of patients will be pain-free or improved following sphincterotomy or sphincteroplasty.
- Gallstone ileus is mechanical obstruction of the gastrointestinal tract from a large gallstone, most commonly following passage of the stone through a spontaneous biliary-enteric fistula.
- Seventy-five percent of these fistulas develop between the gallbladder and duodenum.
- Biliary enteric fistulas usually follow an episode of acute cholecystitis.
- Gallstone ileus occurs most commonly in the elderly.
- Patients with gallstone ileus present with signs and symptoms of intestinal obstruction.
- Abdominal films will demonstrate small bowel distension and air-fluid levels.
- The site of obstruction is most frequently in the narrowest part of the small intestine (ileum).
- The initial management of gallstone ileus includes relieving the obstruction.
- By removing the gallstone through an enterotomy.
- In patients with a significant inflammatory process in the right upper quadrant.
- The fistula can be addressed at a second laparotomy.
- Intrahepatic stones or hepatolithiasis is endemic in East Asia. In the United States, hepatolithiasis is associated with more common biliary tract conditions such as benign biliary strictures, primary sclerosing cholangitis, choledochal cyst, and biliary tract tumors.
- Factors important in the pathogenesis of intrahepatic stones include bile stasis, bacterial infection, and biliary mucin.
- Most intrahepatic stones are brown pigment stones.

CLINICAL PRESENTATION

- Most patients with hepatolithiasis experience cholangitis (67%) and right upper quadrant pain (63%), jaundice (39%), and pruritus (6%).

MANAGEMENT

- The goal of therapy is correction of the underlying biliary disorder and clearance of all stones from the intrahepatic biliary tree.
- Long-term biliary access is critical.
- The surgical approach includes cholecystectomy, resection of the extrahepatic biliary tree.

- Choledochoscopy and extraction of any intrahepatic stones.
- Roux-en-Y hepaticojejunostomy either over transhepatic stents.
- A partial hepatic resection may be required. Approximately 50% of patients will require further procedures.
- Clearance rates of 94% have been reported.
- Polypoid lesions of the gallbladder (PLG) are being identified more frequently.
- PLGs are present in 3% to 7% of normal subjects and in 2% to 12% of cholecystectomy specimens.
- Lesions include benign pseudotumors (cholesterol polyps, adenomyomatosis) and benign (adenoma) and malignant (adenocarcinoma) neoplasms.
- Cholesterol polyps are the most common PLG.
- Adenomyomatosis appears as a sessile polyp.
- Adenoma and adenocarcinoma may be sessile or pedunculated.
- Factors associated with malignancy include age older than 60 years, coexistence of gallstones, a documented increase in size, and size greater than 10 mm.
- All patients with symptomatic PLGs should undergo laparoscopic cholecystectomy.
- Asymptomatic PLGs less than 10 mm without ultrasound features of neoplasia may be safely observed.
- Benign biliary strictures occur in association with a wide variety of conditions including chronic pancreatitis, primary sclerosing cholangitis, acute cholangitis, and several autoimmune diseases or following either blunt or penetrating abdominal trauma.
- Most benign strictures follow iatrogenic bile duct injury, most commonly during laparoscopic cholecystectomy. Most injuries are recognized intraoperatively or during the early postoperative period.
- With unrecognized or inappropriately managed biliary strictures, recurrent cholangitis, secondary biliary cirrhosis, and portal hypertension may eventually develop.

PATHOGENESIS

- Most bile duct injuries occur during cholecystectomy.
- The overall rate of bile duct problems at 0.85% or 1 in every 120 laparoscopic cholecystectomies. The incidence of major bile duct injuries is about 0.55%, and the incidence of bile leaks or minor injuries is 0.3%.
- Several factors have been implicated.

- Surgeon training and experience.
- Local operative factors can also increase the difficulty of the procedure and, therefore, the risk of injury.
- Increased in patients with complications of gallstones including acute cholecystitis, pancreatitis, cholangitis, and obstructive jaundice.
- Additional factors include chronic inflammation, obesity, fat in the periportal area, poor exposure, and bleeding obscuring the operative field.
- Increased patient age, male gender, a long period of symptoms, number of attacks.
- Aberrant biliary anatomy is often cited as a factor in biliary injuries.
- Intraoperatively, several factors have been implicated in biliary injuries. The classic laparoscopic injury occurs when the cystic duct and common bile duct are brought into alignment and the common bile duct is mistaken for the cystic duct.
- Often the right hepatic artery is injured as well.
- Other intraoperative factors include excessive traction on the cystic duct, dissecting too deep in the liver parenchyma, poor clip placement on the cystic duct, or injudicious use of cautery.
- Routine operative cholangiography has been recommended to decrease or prevent biliary injuries.
- Biliary injuries and stricture also occur following other abdominal operations.
- Following common bile duct exploration.
- Gastrectomy.

PRESENTATION

- Patients with bile duct injuries can present intraoperatively, in the early postoperative period, or months or years after the initial injury.
- Approximately, 25% of major ductal injuries will be recognized intraoperatively.
- Patients with a bile leak from the cystic duct stump will usually present within 1 week of cholecystectomy.
- Occasionally, bile will begin leaking externally through a drain or surgical incision.
- With injuries involving occlusion of the common hepatic or bile duct, jaundice with or without abdominal pain is the common mode of presentation. Less commonly, patients will present months or years after biliary surgery with cholangitis or cirrhosis.

DIAGNOSIS

- An orderly sequence of diagnostic tests will usually establish the diagnosis.
- An abdominal CT scan or ultrasound will identify peritoneal fluid or an abscess or biloma. Perihepatic or other intra-abdominal fluid collections should be percutaneously drained.
- Tc-IDA scan. In patients with a surgical drain and an external bile leak, the biliary anatomy can often be determined with a sinogram through the drain.
- In the absence of an external bile leak, the biliary anatomy can be defined with an endoscopic retrograde cholangiogram.
- The diagnostic evaluation is slightly different in the jaundiced patient.
- A CT scan or ultrasound, percutaneous transhepatic cholangiography and placement of a transhepatic stent will decompress the biliary tree.

MANAGEMENT

- The appropriate management of biliary tract injuries depends on the time of diagnosis after the initial injury and the type, extent, and level of the injury. Cystic duct bile leaks can usually be managed with percutaneous drainage of any intra-abdominal fluid collections, followed by placement of a biliary endoprosthesis.
- Lateral bile duct should be managed with placement of a T-tube.
- Isolated hepatic ducts smaller than 3 mm or those draining a single hepatic segment can be safely ligated. Ducts larger than 3 mm are more likely to drain several segments or an entire lobe and need to be reimplanted.
- Major bile duct injuries including transections of the common bile or common hepatic duct should be repaired if recognized at the time of cholecystectomy.
- Injuries diagnosed after the early postoperative period should be repaired in 6 to 8 weeks when the acute inflammation has resolved. The goal of surgical repair is a tension-free, mucosa-to-mucosa duct enteric anastomosis.
- In most cases either an end-to-side Roux-en-Y choledochojejunostomy or, more commonly, a Roux-en-Y hepaticojejunostomy should be performed.
- Bilateral hepaticojejunostomies may be necessary. Transhepatic stents placed preoperatively are useful technical aids.

- Biliary strictures in which the duct remains intact or postoperative anastomotic strictures are also amenable to either percutaneous or endoscopic dilation and/or stenting.

RESULTS

- Acceptable results are achieved in most patients undergoing operative repair of bile duct stricture or injury.
- The operative mortality has been less than 1% in several large series.
- Long-term follow-up is necessary.
- Two thirds of recurrences will become symptomatic within 2 years after repair.
- In one large series, 91% of patients were free of jaundice and cholangitis after undergoing operative repair of a laparoscopic bile duct injury.
- More proximal strictures have a lower success rate. Percutaneous balloon dilation and stenting also has a significantly lower success rate (64%) than operative repair.
- The impact of the injury on quality of life may persist.
- Acute cholangitis is a bacterial infection of the biliary ductal system, which varies in severity from mild and self-limited to severe and life-threatening. The clinical triad of fever, jaundice, and pain was first described in 1877 by Charcot.

PATHOPHYSIOLOGY

- Clinical cholangitis results from a combination of two factors: significant bacterial concentrations in the bile and biliary obstruction.
- The most common organisms recovered include *E. coli, Klebsiella pneumonia,* the enterococci, and *Bacteroides fragilis.*
- Normal biliary pressures range from 7 to 14 cm H_2O.
- With partial or complete biliary obstruction, intrabiliary pressures rise to 18 to 29 cm H_2O, and organisms rapidly appear in both the blood and lymph. The fever and chills are the result of systemic bacteremia.

ETIOLOGY

- The most common causes of biliary obstruction are choledocholithiasis, benign strictures, biliary enteric anastomotic strictures, and cholangiocarcinoma or periampullary cancer.
- In recent years, malignant strictures have become a frequent cause of cholangitis.

CLINICAL PRESENTATION

- Cholangitis may present with a wide spectrum of disease.
- Self-limited illness, toxic cholangitis, a severe illness, including jaundice, fever, abdominal pain, mental obtundation, and hypotension (Reynold s pentad). Fever is the most common presenting symptom.
- Jaundice as a frequent physical finding is also commonly present.

DIAGNOSIS

- Laboratory tests can support evidence of biliary obstruction. Leukocytosis, hyperbilirubinemia, and elevations of alkaline phosphatase and transaminases.
- Radiologic studies are also helpful in confirming the diagnosis.
- Cholangiography is usually required.

MANAGEMENT

- The initial treatment of the patient with cholangitis includes antibiotics. Some patients can be managed as outpatients with oral antibiotics. Patients with toxic cholangitis may require intensive care unit monitoring.
- Most patients will require intravenous fluids and antibiotics.
- Most patients with cholangitis respond to antibiotic therapy alone. In the 15% of patients who do not respond to antibiotics within 12 to 24 hours or in patients with toxic cholangitis, emergency biliary decompression may be necessary.
- Endoscopically.
- Percutaneous transhepatic route.
- Proximal perihilar obstruction or a biliary-enteric anastomotic stricture, percutaneous drainage may be the preferred route.
- Choledocholithiasis and cholangitis associated with peri-ampullary malignancies are best approached endoscopically.
- Successful endoscopic common bile duct stone clearance can be achieved in more than 90% of patients.
- The mortality for patients treated surgically is considerably higher than for patients successfully managed endoscopically.
- The mortality rate associated with an episode of gallstone cholangitis is approximately 2% but is higher in patients with toxic cholangitis (5%). Renal failure, hepatic abscess, and malignancy are all associated with higher morbidity and mortality.

- Hepatic abscesses should be considered in patients who do not respond to therapy.
- Primary sclerosing cholangitis is a cholestatic liver disease characterized by fibrotic strictures involving the intrahepatic and extrahepatic biliary tree.
- The clinical course of patients with sclerosing cholangitis is highly variable.
- Recent studies suggest that genetic and immunologic factors are important in the pathogenesis.

ASSOCIATED DISEASES

- Several diseases have been associated with primary sclerosing cholangitis. The strongest association exists between inflammatory bowel disease, primarily ulcerative colitis, and sclerosing cholangitis. The incidence of ulcerative colitis in patients with sclerosing cholangitis ranges from 60% to 72%. Patients with sclerosing cholangitis are also at increased risk of developing cholangiocarcinoma.

CLINICAL PRESENTATION

- The natural history of patients with primary sclerosing cholangitis is highly variable.
- The mean age at presentation for patients with primary sclerosing cholangitis ranges from 40 to 45 years, and two thirds of patients with primary sclerosing cholangitis are male.
- Patients present with signs and symptoms of cholestatic liver disease or with abnormal serum liver function tests.
- Approximately 75% of patients will be symptomatic at presentation.
- Symptoms of bacterial cholangitis are uncommon.
- The median survival for patients with primary sclerosing cholangitis from the time of diagnosis ranges from 10 to 12 years.

DIAGNOSIS

- The diagnosis of primary sclerosing cholangitis is usually made by endoscopic retrograde cholangiopancreatography. Diffuse multifocal strictures are most commonly found.
- Involvement of the extrahepatic ducts alone without intrahepatic duct involvement occurs in 5% to 10% of patients.
- The hepatic duct bifurcation is often the most severely strictured segment of the biliary tree.

MANAGEMENT

- Medical therapy for primary sclerosing cholangitis has been disappointing to date. Ursodeoxycholate lowers serum bilirubin and transaminases but has not improved symptoms or delayed disease progression. Biliary strictures in patients with primary sclerosing cholangitis have been dilated or stented.
- Symptomatic patients with persistent jaundice are also candidates for surgical therapy. Resection of the extrahepatic biliary tree with bilateral hepaticojejunostomies has yielded reasonable short-term results in patients with significant extrahepatic or bifurcation strictures. Surgical resection should only be performed in patients without cirrhosis.
- Patients in whom a cholangiocarcinoma cannot be excluded should also be explored.
- Ahrendt et al reported 146 patients.
- Survival was significantly longer in the noncirrhotic patients with primary sclerosing cholangitis managed with surgical resection than in the group of patients managed nonoperatively.
- Primary sclerosing cholangitis is a progressive disease that eventually results in biliary cirrhosis. Liver transplantation has produced excellent results.
- Overall 5-year actuarial patient survival is as high as 85%, and 5-year graft survival of 72% has been reported.
- Choledochal cyst is a rare congenital dilation of the extrahepatic and/or intrahepatic biliary tract.
- Incidence of choledochal cyst is only between 1 in 100,000 and 1 in 150,000 people in Western countries but is much more common in Japan. Choledochal cysts are three to eight times more common in women than men.

ETIOLOGY AND CLASSIFICATION

- The frequent presentation of choledochal cysts in infancy supports a congenital origin. An anomalous pancreatobiliary duct junction (APBDJ) has also been documented in between 90% and 100% of patients.
- Long common channel.
- Reflux of pancreatic juice into the biliary tract results in increased biliary pressures and inflammatory changes.
- The current classification of choledochal cysts was initially proposed by Alonso-Lej and was subsequently modified by Todani.
- Type I cysts are the most common and compose 50%.

- Type IV cysts also occur frequently.
- Type II.
- Type III.
- Type V cysts are much less common.

CLINICAL PRESENTATION

- The classic clinical triad includes right upper quadrant pain, jaundice, and an abdominal mass.
- The clinical presentation differs between children and adults. In adults, abdominal pain and jaundice are present frequently.
- Laboratory evaluation may demonstrate mild liver function abnormalities.
- The diagnosis can be established with ultrasound or CT scanning is required to determine the type of choledochal cyst.

MANAGEMENT

- Appropriate management of type I and type II choledochal cysts should include cholecystectomy, resection of the extra-hepatic biliary tract including the choledochal cyst, and Roux-en-Y hepaticojejunostomy.
- Cholangiocarcinoma is uncommon in children with chole-dochal cysts, but the risk of cholangiocarcinoma may be as high as 30% in adults and supports the role of resection in the management. Resection of the extrahepatic biliary tract is also recommended for type IV cysts.
- Cancer of the gallbladder is an aggressive malignancy that occurs predominantly in the elderly.
- The prognosis for most patients is poor.
- An aggressive surgical approach for patients with localized gallbladder cancer has produced encouraging results.

INCIDENCE

- Gallbladder cancer is the fifth most common gastrointestinal malignancy. Cancer of the gallbladder is two to three times more common in females than males.
- Approximately 5,000 new cases are diagnosed annually in the United States, and the overall incidence of gallbladder cancer is 2.5 cases per 100,000.
- Gallbladder cancer is more common in Native Americans.

ETIOLOGY

- Several factors have been associated with an increased risk of developing gallbladder cancer.
- Gallstones, an APBDJ, porcelain gallbladder, choledochal cysts, and primary sclerosing cholangitis.
- Cholelithiasis is present in 75% to 90% of cases.
- Approximately 1% of all elective cholecystectomies performed for cholelithiasis will harbor an occult gallbladder cancer.

PATHOLOGY AND STAGING

- Ninety percent of cancers of the gallbladder are classified as adenocarcinoma. Squamous cell, oat cell, undifferentiated, and adenosquamous cancers and carcinoid tumors are much less frequent.
- At diagnosis, 25% of cancers are localized to the gallbladder wall, 35% have associated metastases to regional lymph nodes or extension into adjacent organs, and 40% have already metastasized to distant sites.
- Hepatic involvement with gallbladder cancer can occur by direct invasion through the gallbladder bed, angiolymphatic portal tract invasion, or distant hematogenous spread.
- The appropriate management and overall prognosis are strongly dependent on tumor stage.

CLINICAL PRESENTATION

- Gallbladder cancer most often presents with right upper quadrant abdominal pain.
- Weight loss, jaundice, and an abdominal mass are less common.
- The largest group of patients present with symptoms of chronic cholecystitis.
- Another common presentation is similar to acute cholecystitis.
- Signs and symptoms of malignant biliary obstruction with jaundice are also common. Patients can also present with symptoms of a nonbiliary malignancy.
- Gallbladder cancer is often misdiagnosed.

DIAGNOSIS

- Ultrasonography is often the first diagnostic modality.
- The sensitivity of ultrasound in the detection of gallbladder cancer ranges from 70% to 100%. CT usually demonstrates a mass replacing the gallbladder.

- Spiral CT also demonstrates the adjacent vascular anatomy. With newer magnetic resonance (MR) techniques, gallbladder cancers may also be easily visualized.
- Cholangiography also may be helpful in diagnosing jaundiced patients with gallbladder cancer. The typical cholangiographic finding in gallbladder cancer is a long stricture of the common hepatic duct.

MANAGEMENT

- The appropriate operative procedure for the patient with localized gallbladder cancer is determined by the pathologic stage.
- Cholecystectomy is adequate therapy for patients with T1 tumors.
- Bile spillage is associated with poor survival even in early stage (T1 and T2) gallbladder cancer. Thus, patients with preoperatively suspected gallbladder cancer should undergo open cholecystectomy.
- Cancer of the gallbladder with invasion beyond (Stages II to III) the gallbladder muscularis is associated with an increasing incidence of regional lymph node metastases and should be managed with an extended cholecystectomy including lymphadenectomy.
- Resection of the common bile duct.
- A 2-cm margin beyond the palpable or sonographic extent of the tumor.
- A wedge resection of the liver.
- An anatomic liver resection.
- Staging laparoscopy should be performed before attempted resection.
- In most cases, therapy for gallbladder cancer is palliative.
- The results of chemotherapy in the treatment of patients with gallbladder cancer have been quite poor.
- Gemcitabine.
- Trials of chemoradiation in patients with stage II and III disease need to be performed.

SURVIVAL

- Survival in patients with gallbladder cancer is strongly influenced by the pathologic stage.
- T1a have a uniformly excellent prognosis. Invasion into the muscular wall (T1b) of the gallbladder increases the risk of recurrent cancer after curative resection.
- Invasion into the subserosa (T2) increases the risk of regional lymph node metastases to 33% to 50%. Five-year

survival in patients with T2 tumors is improved following extended cholecystectomy.

- Five-year overall survival for resected patients with stage IIA and stage IIB gallbladder cancer of 28% to 63% and 19% to 25%, respectively.
- Most patients with gallbladder cancer have advanced, unresectable disease.
- Fewer than 15% of all patients with gallbladder cancer are alive after 5 years.
- Cholangiocarcinoma is an uncommon tumor, which may occur anywhere along the intrahepatic or extrahepatic biliary tree. These tumors are located most commonly at the hepatic duct bifurcation.
- Most patients with cholangiocarcinomas present with jaundice.
- When possible, surgical resection does offer a chance for long-term disease-free survival.

INCIDENCE

- Between 2500 and 3000 new cases of cholangiocarcinoma are diagnosed annually in the United States.
- The incidence of cholangiocarcinoma in the United States is approximately 1.0 per 100,000 people per year.

RISK FACTORS

- A number of diseases have been linked to cholangiocarcinoma including primary sclerosing cholangitis, choledochal cysts, and hepatolithiasis.
- Primary sclerosing cholangitis.
- Choledochal cysts.
- Hepatolithiasis.
- Prior biliary-enteric anastomosis may also increase the future risk of cholangiocarcinoma.
- The risk of bile duct cancer was higher following transduodenal sphincteroplasty and choledochoduodenostomy than hepaticojejunostomy and was most strongly associated with recurrent episodes of cholangitis.

STAGING AND CLASSIFICATION

- Cholangiocarcinoma is best classified anatomically into three broad groups: (1) intrahepatic, (2) perihilar, and (3) distal.
- Cancers of the hepatic duct bifurcation have also been classified according to their anatomic location.

- Type I tumors are confined to the common hepatic duct, and type II tumors involve the bifurcation.
- Type IIIa and IIIb tumors extend into either the right or left secondary intrahepatic ducts.
- Type IV tumors involve the secondary intrahepatic ducts on both sides.
- Cholangiocarcinoma is also staged according to the tumor-node-metastasis (TNM) classification.
- Stage IA.
- Stage IIA.
- Stage IIA.

CLINICAL PRESENTATION

- More than 90% of patients with perihilar or distal tumors present with jaundice.
- Except for jaundice, the physical examination is usually normal.

DIAGNOSIS

- At the time of presentation, most patients with perihilar and distal cholangiocarcinoma will have a total serum bilirubin level greater than 10 mg/dL.
- Serum CA 19-9 may also be elevated.
- The radiologic evaluation of patients with cholangiocarcinoma should delineate the overall extent of the tumor.
- Abdominal ultrasound or CT scanning.
- After documentation of bile duct dilation, biliary anatomy has been traditionally defined cholangiographically.
- The percutaneous route is favored in these patients.
- MRC has documented diagnostic accuracy comparable to percutaneous and endoscopic cholangiography.
- Prolonged efforts to establish a tissue diagnosis are not indicated.

MANAGEMENT

- Curative treatment of patients with cholangiocarcinoma is only possible with complete resection. The operative approach depends on the site and extent of the tumor.
- For patients with intrahepatic cholangiocarcinoma, partial hepatectomy is the procedure of choice.
- Patients with perihilar tumors (Bismuth type I or II) are candidates for local tumor excision.

- If preoperative evaluation suggests involvement of the right or left hepatic duct (Bismuth type IIIa or IIIb), right or left hepatic lobectomy, respectively, should be planned.
- To achieve negative margins, resection of the adjacent caudate lobe may be required.
- For patients with resectable distal cholangiocarcinoma, pancreatoduodenectomy is the optimal procedure.
- Surgical exploration should be undertaken in good risk patients.
- Selective use of laparoscopy.
- In patients with extensive metastatic disease, preoperative biliary stents may be left in place.
- In patients with locally advanced unresectable perihilar tumors, several operative approaches are available.
- Most distal bile duct tumors are respectable.
- Patients with unequivocal evidence of unresectable cholangiocarcinoma at initial evaluation are palliated nonoperatively.
- Endoscopically and percutaneously.
- Metallic stents.
- No prospective, randomized trials have been reported, and a well-controlled, but not randomized, trial reported no benefit for postoperative adjuvant radiation.
- Chemotherapy has also not been shown to improve survival.
- The combination of radiation and chemotherapy may be more effective than either agent alone.
- The role of adjuvant chemoradiation must be tested in patients with cholangiocarcinoma.
- Long-term survival in patients with cholangiocarcinoma is highly dependent on the stage of disease.
- For resectable intrahepatic cholangiocarcinoma, overall 5-year survival ranges from 30% to 40%.
- Overall 5-year survival for patients with resectable perihilar tumors has been only 10% to 20%.
- Patients with resectable distal bile duct cancer have the highest rate of resection.
- The 5-year survival rate of 28% to 45%.
- Hepatocellular carcinoma and liver metastases can cause obstructive jaundice.
- Hepatic cystadenomas and cystadenocarcinomas arise from the biliary epithelium may also cause bile duct obstruction.
- Primary and secondary hepatic tumors can also produce biliary obstruction by metastasizing to hilar or pericholedochal lymph nodes.
- Lymphoma can also result in biliary obstruction.
- Lymphomas usually respond to chemotherapy.

CHAPTER 52

EXOCRINE PANCREAS

ANATOMY

Location

- The pancreas lies posterior to the stomach and lesser omentum in the retroperitoneum of the upper abdomen. It extends obliquely, rising slightly as it passes from the medial edge of the duodenal C-loop to the hilum of the spleen. It lies anterior to the inferior vena cava, aorta, splenic vein, and left adrenal gland.

Regions

- The pancreas is divided into four regions: the head and uncinate process, neck, body, and tail. The head lies within the duodenal C-loop and its uncinate process extends posteriorly and medially to lie behind the portal and superior mesenteric veins and superior mesenteric artery.

Blood Supply and Lymph Nodes

- Both the celiac trunk and the superior mesenteric artery provide the arterial supply to the pancreas.

Innervation

- The principal, and possibly only, pathway for pancreatic pain involves nociceptive fibers arising in the pancreas. They pass through the celiac ganglia to form the greater, lesser, and least splanchnic nerves that pass to cell bodies in the thoracic sympathetic chain.

Ducts

- The main pancreatic duct, or duct of Wirsung, arises in the tail of the pancreas and terminates at the papilla of Vater in the duodenum.
- The duct of Santorini (i.e., the minor, or accessory, pancreatic duct) is smaller than the main duct. It extends from the main

duct to enter the duodenum at the lesser papilla. That papilla lies approximately 2 cm proximal and slightly anterior to the major papilla.

EMBRYOLOGY AND HISTOLOGY

Organogenesis

Histology

- The mature pancreas is an endocrine organ made up of the islets of Langerhans and an exocrine organ consisting of acinar and ductal cells.

Cell Differentiation

CONGENITAL ANOMALIES

Pancreas Divisum

- Failure of the dorsal and ventral pancreatic duct systems to join during embryogenesis is referred to as pancreas divisum. It results in a pancreas with divided drainage because the dorsal pancreas drains, via the duct of Santorini, to empty at the lesser papilla, and the ventral pancreas, composed of the head and uncinate process, drains via Vater's papilla. Pancreas divisum has been noted in up to 11% of autopsy cases.
- On the other hand, the presence of pancreas divisum and the development of pancreatitis are, in most patients, not related to each other in a cause-effect manner and the corollary of this may also be true (i.e., that attempts to widen the orifice of the dorsal duct at the lesser papilla in patients with pancreas divisum and pancreatitis are unlikely to be of benefit).

Ectopic and Accessory Pancreas

Annular Pancreas

- Annular pancreas refers to the presence of a band of normal pancreatic tissue that partially or completely encircles the second portion of the duodenum and extends into the head of the pancreas. It usually contains a duct that joins the main pancreatic duct.

- Treatment usually involves bypass, via duodenojejunostomy, rather than resection.

Developmental Pancreatic Cysts

PHYSIOLOGY

Protein Secretion

- With the possible exception of the lactating mammary gland, the exocrine pancreas synthesizes protein at a greater rate, per gram of tissue, than any other organ. More than 90% of that protein consists of digestive enzymes. Most of the digestive enzymes are synthesized and secreted by acinar cells as inactive proenzymes or zymogens that, in health, are activated only after they reach the duodenum where enterokinase activates trypsinogen and the trypsin catalyses the activation of the other zymogens.

Electrolyte Secretion

- Although stimulation of acinar cells results in the secretion of a small amount of serum-like fluid, most of the fluid and electrolytes secreted from the pancreas arises from duct cells.
- Taken together, the result of these events is the secretion of a bicarbonate-rich fluid into the duct and the discharge, into the circulation, of protons. In the absence of secretin stimulation, pancreatic juice has a more plasma-like composition because it is composed primarily of acinar cell secretions and there is little duct cell secretion of chloride to permit exchange with bicarbonate. With secretin stimulation, chloride secretion is increased, flow rates rise, and chloride-bicarbonate exchange results in juice that is rich in bicarbonate and poor in chloride.

Integrated Physiology

- Acidification of the duodenum and the presence of bile in the duodenum promote secretin release. In addition, in the duodenum and proximal small intestine, the presence of fat and protein and their partial breakdown products stimulates the release of cholecystokinin, and this cholecystokinin stimulates enzyme secretion from acinar cells. The intestinal phase of pancreatic secretion accounts for 70% to 75% of meal-stimulated pancreatic secretion.

Feedback Loop

PANCREATITIS

Definition and Classification

- Pancreatitis can be classified as either *acute* or *chronic* based on its clinical characteristics, pathologic changes, and natural history. Clinically, acute pancreatitis is usually characterized by the acute onset of symptoms in a previously healthy individual and the disappearance of those symptoms as the attack resolves. In contrast, patients with chronic pancreatitis may have had prior attacks or symptoms of either exocrine or endocrine insufficiency before the current attack and their symptoms may persist even after resolution of the current attack. From a clinical standpoint, however, attacks of *either* acute or chronic pancreatitis can be characterized by the abrupt onset of symptoms that are often similar. Thus, without the test of time or a tissue sample, it may be difficult or impossible to determine if a first attack is one of acute or chronic pancreatitis.

Pathology

- The pathologic changes of acute pancreatitis include parenchymal and peripancreatic fat necrosis and an associated inflammatory reaction. The extent of these changes is directly related to the severity of an attack. In mild pancreatitis, changes frequently include interstitial edema and infiltration of inflammatory cells with relatively little necrosis, whereas, in severe pancreatitis, extensive necrosis, thrombosis of intrapancreatic vessels, vascular disruption, and intraparenchymal hemorrhage can be seen. With infection, intrapancreatic or peripancreatic abscesses involving areas of necrosis can also develop. The major changes of chronic pancreatitis include fibrosis and loss of both endocrine and exocrine elements. In addition, an acute inflammatory reaction may be superimposed on a background of chronic inflammation.

Etiology

- Both acute and chronic pancreatitis are frequently associated with other disease entities collectively referred to as the etiologies of pancreatitis (Box 52–1). In developed countries, roughly 70% to 80% of patients with pancreatitis have their pancreatitis in association with either biliary tract stone disease or

---

Box 52–1. Etiologies of Pancreatitis

Acute Pancreatitis
Biliary tract stones
Drugs
ERCP
Ethanol abuse
Hypercalcemia
Hyperlipidemia
Idiopathic
Infections
Ischemia
Parasites
Postoperative
Scorpion sting
Trauma

Chronic Pancreatitis
Autoimmune
Duct obstruction
Ethanol abuse
Hereditary
Hypercalcemia
Hyperlipidemia
Idiopathic

ERCP, endoscopic retrograde cholangiopancreatography.

ethanol abuse. For the most part, biliary tract stone disease is associated with acute pancreatitis, whereas chronic pancreatitis is associated with the intake of large amounts of ethanol over protracted periods. In 10% to 15% of pancreatitis cases, no etiology can be identified and those individuals are said to have idiopathic pancreatitis.

Biliary Tract Stones

- The onset of acute pancreatitis is frequently associated with the passage of biliary tract stones through the terminal biliopancreatic duct into the duodenum. Stones can be retrieved from the stools of roughly 90% of patients with stone-induced pancreatitis.
- Although the bile reflux theory, often referred to as the "common channel theory," was originally favored, subsequent studies have cast doubt on its validity and most observers now believe that it is stone-induced pancreatic duct obstruction

and ductal hypertension, rather than bile reflux, that triggers acute pancreatitis.

Abuse of Ethanol

● The most frequent cause of morphologically defined chronic pancreatitis is ethanol abuse, but, occasionally, ethanol can also induce acute pancreatitis. There is no threshold rate of consumption below which ethanol consumption is not associated with an increased incidence of pancreatitis.

Drugs (Box 52-2)

● Exposure to certain drugs is, perhaps, the third most frequent cause of pancreatitis, but the mechanisms by which those drugs cause pancreatitis is not known.

Box 52–2. Drugs Associated with Pancreatitis

Definite Cause
5-Aminosalicylate
6-Mercaptopurine
Azathioprine
Cytosine arabinoside
Dideoxyinosine
Diuretics
Estrogens
Furosemide
Metronidazole
Pentamidine
Tetracycline
Thiazide
Trimethoprim-sulfamethoxide
Valproic acid

Probable Cause
Acetaminophen
α-Methyl-DOPA
Isoniazid
L-Asparaginase
Phenformin
Procainamide
Sulindac

DOPA, dihydroxyphenylalanine.

Obstruction

● Even in the absence of biliary tract stones, pancreatic duct obstruction can cause pancreatitis. Thus, pancreatitis has been associated with duodenal lesions such as duodenal ulcers, duodenal Crohn's disease, and periampullary tumors. It can also be triggered by a periampullary diverticulum, particularly if that diverticulum is filled with debris or food particles. Pancreatitis can also be the result of a pancreatic duct stricture or disruption following blunt pancreatic trauma or duct obstruction caused by a pancreatic tumor. Most patients with obstruction-induced pancreatitis have chronic, rather than acute, pancreatitis. This type of chronic pancreatitis affects only the obstructed portion of the pancreas, and it can be cured by removing the obstructed part of the pancreas.

Hereditary and Autoimmune Pancreatitis

● There has been considerable recent interest in the few patients who develop pancreatitis on a hereditary basis. It is generally believed that spontaneous trypsinogen activation normally occurs to a slight degree within the pancreas but that, in health, the pancreas is protected from injury by the presence of trypsin inhibitors. In hereditary pancreatitis, genetic mutations are believed to cause this protective process to fail either because a trypsin that is resistant to inhibition is synthesized or because the trypsin inhibitors themselves are defective. In either case, the result could be expected to be further intra-pancreatic activation of trypsin and, possibly, other digestive enzymes, eventually leading to repeated episodes of pancreatitis. In hereditary pancreatitis, those attacks begin at a young age and lead to chronic changes including fibrosis, calcifications, and loss of both exocrine and endocrine function. The incidence of pancreatic cancer is also markedly increased in patients with hereditary pancreatitis. Hereditary pancreatitis is an autosomal dominant disease with incomplete penetrance. Pancreatic cancer most frequently develops in those with a paternal pattern of inheritance.

● Pancreatitis can be the result of an autoimmune process, and, in those patients, it is frequently associated with other autoimmune diseases such as primary sclerosing cholangitis, Sjögren's syndrome, and primary biliary cirrhosis. Recently, a distinct form of autoimmune pancreatitis has been described in which there is a severe, sclerosing process characterized by intense lymphocyte and plasmacyte infiltration.

Other Miscellaneous Causes of Pancreatitis

- Pancreatitis can result from pancreatic trauma even without major duct disruption or stricture. In those cases, the inflammatory process is usually related to contusion or laceration of the gland and possibly disruption of small ducts. Pancreatitis can occur during the postoperative period in patients undergoing procedures on or near the pancreas or procedures associated with either hypoperfusion or atheroembolism (cardiopulmonary bypass, cardiac transplantation, and renal transplantation). The injection of the pancreatic duct that occurs during endoscopic retrograde pancreatography or during sphincter of Oddi manometry can also cause pancreatitis. Both acute and chronic pancreatitis can be caused by metabolic abnormalities, especially those leading to hypercalcemia (i.e., hyperparathyroidism) and those leading to hyperlipidemia (Types I, IV, or V hyperlipoproteinemias).
- In places such as Trinidad, scorpion stings are a frequent cause of pancreatitis. Scorpion toxin contains a potent pancreatic secretagogue, and, presumably, the excessive pancreatic stimulation that follows exposure to this toxin leads to pancreatic injury.

Idiopathic Pancreatitis

- In most series, roughly 20% of patients have pancreatitis without an identifiable etiology. Some of those individuals have gallbladder sludge or microcrystals, and further attacks can be prevented by either cholecystectomy or biliary sphincterotomy.

Pathophysiology of Acute and Chronic Pancreatitis

- It is generally believed that acute pancreatitis is triggered by obstruction of the pancreatic duct and that the injury begins within pancreatic acinar cells. That injury is believed to include, and possibly be the result of, intra-acinar cell activation of digestive enzyme zymogens including trypsinogen. Chronic pancreatitis is believed to reflect repeated episodes of subclinical acute pancreatitis with unrecognized pancreatic necrosis evolving into pancreatic fibrosis.

Presentation of an Acute Attack

- The clinical presentation, diagnosis, and management of an acute attack of pancreatitis are similar regardless of whether that attack is *acute* or *chronic* pancreatitis. In fact, many describe patients with chronic pancreatitis who present with acute symptoms as having *acute on chronic* pancreatitis. On the other hand, the long-term management of patients with acute and chronic pancreatitis may differ considerably. The former primarily involves elimination of the inciting cause, whereas, for chronic pancreatitis, irreversible changes have usually occurred before diagnosis and long-term management primarily involves treatment of pain and pancreatic exocrine and endocrine insufficiency. For these reasons, this discussion of clinical presentation focuses on issues relevant to an acute attack and does not make distinctions based on whether that is an attack of acute or chronic pancreatitis.

Symptoms

- Abdominal pain, nausea, and vomiting are the dominant symptoms of pancreatitis. Typically, the pain is located in the epigastrium, but it may also involve both upper quadrants, the lower abdomen, or the lower chest. It may have a pleuritic component and be felt in one or both shoulders. Most patients describe the pain as being knife-like and radiating straight through to the mid-central back. It is usually abrupt in onset and slowly increases in magnitude to reach a maximal level. The pain is usually constant, although it may be somewhat relieved by leaning forward or lying on the side with the knees drawn upward. Patients with chronic pancreatitis frequently describe similar prior attacks that are often noted to occur within 12 to 24 hours of ethanol consumption. The nausea and vomiting of pancreatitis usually persists even after the stomach has been emptied.
- Although vomiting and retching may be relieved by passage of a nasogastric tube, the pain usually persists even after gastric decompression.

Physical Findings

- Pancreatitis patients are frequently noted to be rolling or moving around in search of a more comfortable position and, in this sense, they are unlike patients with a perforated viscus who often remain motionless because movement worsens their pain. Patients with severe pancreatitis usually appear ill and anxious. Hyperthermia, tachycardia, tachypnea, and hypotension caused by hypovolemia are common. Hypovolemia can also result in collapsed neck veins, dry skin, dry mucous membranes, and diminished subcutaneous elasticity. Because pleuritic and abdominal pain may make breathing difficult, breath sounds in the lower lung fields are usually diminished and atelectasis may be present. A pleural effusion can often be detected on either side although it is more commonly found on the left. Patients with severe pancreatitis frequently develop an acute lung injury that can clinically present as the acute respiratory distress syndrome (ARDS). Occasionally, patients with pancreatitis have alterations in their mental status because of drug or ethanol exposure, hypotension, hypoxemia, or release of circulating toxic agents from the inflamed pancreas. Some degree of jaundice is common. In gallstone-induced acute pancreatitis, the jaundice may reflect distal bile duct obstruction, but jaundice can also occur in nonbiliary pancreatitis either as a result of duct obstruction caused by the inflamed pancreas or as a result of cholestasis induced by the severe illness itself. Because of ileus, bowel sounds are usually diminished during an attack of pancreatitis and the abdomen may become distended and tympanitic. Direct, percussion, and rebound abdominal tenderness and both voluntary and involuntary guarding are common. These findings may be localized to the epigastrium, or they may be diffusely present throughout the abdomen. An epigastric mass, reflecting the inflamed pancreas and surrounding tissues, may be felt in the upper abdomen or left upper quadrant. On rare occasions, flank ecchymoses (Grey Turner's sign) or periumbilical ecchymoses (Cullen's sign), which result from retroperitoneal hemorrhage, can be seen during severe pancreatitis. Occasionally, patients develop areas of tender subcutaneous induration and erythema that resemble erythema nodosum but that, in the case of pancreatitis, are caused by subcutaneous fat necrosis.

Diagnosis

Routine Blood Tests

- Pancreatitis can induce a diffuse capillary leak syndrome that, when combined with vomiting, can result in significant fluid losses. The resulting hypovolemia can be marked. It usually leads to an increased hematocrit, hemoglobin, blood urea nitrogen, and creatinine. Serum albumin levels may be markedly depressed, particularly if fluid losses are corrected by administration of albumin-free crystalloid solutions. The serum electrolytes may be normal, but, with significant vomiting, a hypochloremic metabolic alkalosis can develop. The white blood cell count is usually elevated with an associated left shift in the differential count. Blood glucose may be elevated either because of associated diabetes mellitus or because of increased glucagon and catecholamine release combined with diminished insulin release. Hyperbilirubinemia is relatively common during the early stages of pancreatitis.

● Hypertriglyceridemia is routinely noted in patients who have hyperlipidemia-induced pancreatitis. Hypertriglyceridemia can also be induced by exposure to ethanol; therefore, the diagnosis of pancreatitis should always be suspected when lactescent serum is found when evaluating an alcoholic patient with abdominal pain. Many patients with pancreatitis appear to have hypocalcemia, but, for the most part, that hypocalcemia can be explained by the hypoalbuminemia that accompanies pancreatitis. Occasionally however, patients with severe pancreatitis have a reduction in their free, ionized, calcium that is not a reflection of hypoalbuminemia. This type of hypocalcemia is associated with a poor prognosis. Some of these patients manifest tetany and carpopedal spasm, making treatment with calcium mandatory.

● Patients with severe pancreatitis can also develop disseminated intravascular coagulation. In those cases, thrombocytopenia, elevated levels of fibrin degradation products, a decreased fibrinogen level, prolonged partial thromboplastin time, and a prolonged prothrombin time can be observed.

Amylase Measurement

● Serum amylase activity is usually, but not always, elevated during pancreatitis, but the magnitude of that elevation does not parallel the severity of the attack. In fact, as many as 10% of patients with lethal pancreatitis may have near-normal or normal amylase levels.

● Elevations that persist beyond a week suggest either ongoing inflammation or the development of a complication such as pseudocyst, abscess, or pancreatic ascites.

● In most cases, patients with hyperamylasemia that is not due to pancreatitis have only mild elevations in the circulating amylase level (i.e., two- to threefold elevations from the normal value), whereas those with pancreatitis usually have greater elevations.

Other Blood Tests

- Circulating lipase levels usually increase during pancreatitis. That increase usually parallels the rise in amylase activity, but the elevations of lipase activity may persist even after amylase activity has returned to normal. Thus, serum lipase measurement may be particularly helpful when patients are first seen several days after the onset of symptoms.

Imaging Studies

- In general, the plain chest and abdominal x-ray films are not particularly helpful in the diagnosis of pancreatitis, although they may be useful in patient management by revealing other causes for the patient's symptoms (e.g., pneumonia, perforated hollow viscus, mechanical bowel obstruction). In patients with pancreatitis, radiographs of the chest frequently reveal basal atelectasis and elevation of the diaphragm caused by splinting of respiration. Pleural effusions, most common on the left, can also be seen. Plain abdominal films usually show the gas pattern of a paralytic ileus, but, occasionally, retroperitoneal gas bubbles indicating infection with gas-forming organisms can be seen. Pancreatic calcifications that are pathognomonic of chronic pancreatitis and are caused by the formation of calcified intraductal protein plugs may be seen on the routine abdominal films. Transcutaneous ultrasound (US) may be useful in demonstrating the presence of gallbladder stones and/or dilated bile ducts, but US examination has limited value because of the presence of intestinal gas in the upper abdomen.
- Computed tomography (CT) has been shown to be particularly helpful in the diagnosis and management of patients with pancreatitis. During the early stages of an attack, CT can image the upper abdomen and pancreas without being obscured by overlying or surrounding intestinal gas. When combined with bolus administration of intravenous contrast material, helical CT can detect the subtle changes of mild pancreatitis (i.e., pancreatic swelling and edema) and the changes of more severe pancreatitis (i.e., varying degrees of pancreatic necrosis and the presence of peripancreatic or intrapancreatic fluid collections). Both clinical and experimental studies have demonstrated the close parallel that exists between nonperfused pancreas seen on CT examination and necrosis seen on morphologic examination of the pancreas. Later during the evolution of an attack, CT can be used to detect and follow pseudocysts and to permit fine needle aspiration of areas

suspected of harboring pancreatic infection. The timing of CT during an attack of pancreatitis is a matter of considerable controversy. One study, using an experimental model of pancreatitis in rodents, suggested that early CT with administration of intravenous contrast material could adversely effect the course of pancreatitis and worsen outcome, but this conclusion has not been borne out by other studies, and, at present, it is generally believed that early performance of contrast-enhanced CT does not worsen pancreatitis. On the other hand, there may be little or no value in obtaining a CT in patients with obvious pancreatitis because early CT is unlikely to alter treatment. Early CT may be particularly helpful when the diagnosis of pancreatitis is in doubt.

Differential Diagnosis

● The differential diagnosis of pancreatitis includes any process that can cause upper abdominal pain and tenderness, nausea, and vomiting (Box 52–3).

Prognosis of an Acute Attack

● The ultimate severity of an attack appears to be determined by events that occur within the first 24 to 48 hours. Most patients experience only a mild self-limited illness, which can be expected to resolve with only supportive care, but approximately 10% of patients experience a severe attack. Severe attacks are more common in acute pancreatitis, but they can also occur when an acute attack is superimposed on chronic pancreatitis (i.e., so-called acute on chronic pancreatitis). Severe attacks are also more common in patients older than age 60; those experiencing a first attack; those with postoperative pancreatitis; and those with methemalbuminemia, hypocalcemia, Grey Turner's sign, or Cullen's sign.

● Among the clinical scoring systems, the most widely used are those developed in New York by Ranson's group (Table 52–1)

Box 52–3. Differential Diagnosis of Acute Pancreatitis

Bowel obstruction
Cholecystitis/cholangitis
Mesenteric ischemia/infarction
Perforated hollow viscus

TABLE 52–1. Ranson's Prognostic Signs

Admission	Initial 48 Hours
Gallstone Pancreatitis	
Age >70 yr	Hct fall >10
WBC >18,000/mm³	BUN elevation >2 mg/100 mL
Glucose >220 mg/100 ML	Ca²⁺ >8 mg/100 mL
LDH >40 IU/L	Base deficit >5 mEq/L
AST >250 U/100 mL	Fluid sequestration >4 L
Non-Gallstone Pancreatitis	
Age >55 yr	Hct fall >10
WBC >16,000/mm³	BUN elevation >5 mg/100 mL
Glucose >200 mg/100 mL	Ca²⁺ >8 mg/100 mL
LDH >350 IU/L	Pao₂ >55 mm Hg
AST >250 U/100 mL	Base deficit >4 mEq/L
	Fluid sequestration >6 L

AST, aspartate transaminase; BUN, blood urea nitrogen; Ca²⁺, calcium; Hct, hematocrit; LDH, lactate dehydrogenase; Pao₂, arterial oxygen; WBC, white blood count.
Adapted from Ranson JHC, Rifkind KM, Roses DF, et al: Prognostic signs and the role of operative management in acute pancreatitis. Surg Gynecol Obstet 139:69–81, 1974 and Ranson JHC. Etiological and prognostic factors in human acute pancreatitis: A review. Am J Gastroenterol 77–633, 1982.

and in Glasgow by Imrie's group. Patients with fewer than three of the prognostic criteria can be expected to have a mild attack with little morbidity and a mortality rate of less than 1%. On the other hand, with the presence of more prognostic factors, increased morbidity and mortality can be expected; thus, with three or four of Ranson's criteria, the mortality rate may reach 15%, and 50% of patients may need to be treated in an intensive care unit. Most patients with five or six signs will require intensive care, and, with seven or eight of Ranson's signs, the mortality rate may reach 90%.

- The second version of the Acute Physiology and Chronic Health Evaluation (APACHE II) scoring system has also been used to predict the severity of a pancreatitis attack. An APACHE II score of 8 or more is generally indicative of a severe attack. The APACHE II scoring system has the advantage of continually quantifying disease severity. Although the APACHE II system can be used at the time of admission, recent studies have suggested that an admission score that worsens over the initial 48 hours of hospitalization despite aggressive treatment or the score itself 48 hours after admission may be particularly accurate in predicting the severity of the attack and a poor outcome.

Treatment of an Acute Attack

- An acute attack of pancreatitis evolves in two, somewhat overlapping, phases. The initial phase, which lasts for 1 to 2 weeks, involves an acute inflammatory and autodigestive process that takes place within and around the pancreas. It may have systemic effects as well. In patients with severe pancreatitis, this initial phase of pancreatitis seamlessly evolves into a later phase that may last for weeks or months. This later phase of pancreatitis is primarily characterized by the development of local complications that are, themselves, the result of necrosis, infection, and pancreatic duct rupture.

Initial Treatment

- The initial management of patients with pancreatitis should focus on establishing the diagnosis, estimating its severity, addressing the major symptoms (i.e., pain, nausea, vomiting, and hypovolemia), and limiting its progression. On occasion, however, exploration may be required to establish the diagnosis with certainty, especially when the diagnosis is uncertain and the patient has not responded favorably to aggressive nonoperative treatment. Patients with predicted severe pancreatitis should be treated in an intensive care unit because it is in this group that fluid and respiratory management may be particularly challenging and both morbidity and mortality are, essentially, confined to this group.

Management of Pain

- The pain of pancreatitis may be severe and difficult to control. Most patients require narcotic medications. Meperidine or its analogues are probably preferable to morphine in this setting because morphine can induce spasm of the sphincter of Oddi and that could at least theoretically worsen biliary pancreatitis.

Fluid and Electrolyte Management

- Aggressive fluid and electrolyte repletion is the most important element in the initial management of pancreatitis. Fluid losses can be enormous and can lead to marked hemoconcentration and hypovolemia. Inadequate fluid resuscitation during the early stages of pancreatitis can worsen the severity of an attack and lead to subsequent complications. The fluid depletion that occurs in pancreatitis results from the additive effects of losing fluid both externally and internally. The external fluid losses are caused by repeated episodes of vomiting and worsen by nausea, which limits fluid intake.

- Internal fluid losses, which are usually even greater than the external losses, are caused by fluid sequestration into areas of inflammation (i.e., the peripancreatic retroperitoneum) and into the pulmonary parenchyma and soft tissues elsewhere in the body. These latter losses result from the diffuse capillary leak phenomenon that is triggered by proinflammatory factors released during pancreatitis.

- Many of the patients with chronic pancreatitis are alcoholics who, even before the onset of pancreatitis, had hypoalbuminemia and hypomagnesemia. Those problems are exacerbated by the losses of pancreatitis.

- Although hypocalcemia is common particularly during a severe attack, the low total serum calcium is usually attributable to the low levels of circulating albumin and no treatment is needed when ionized calcium is normal. Occasionally, however, ionized calcium levels may also be depressed and tetany and carpopedal spasm can occur. Under those circumstances, aggressive calcium repletion is indicated.

- During the first several days of a severe attack, circulating levels of many proinflammatory factors, including cytokines and chemokines, are elevated. This "cytokine storm," in many cases, triggers the systemic immune response syndrome (SIRS), and, consequently, the hemodynamic parameters of these patients may resemble those of sepsis associated with other disease states.

Role of Nasogastric Decompression

- The nausea and vomiting of pancreatitis can result in significant fluid and electrolyte losses. Furthermore, retching can lead to gastroesophageal mucosal tears and result in upper gastrointestinal bleeding (i.e., the Mallory-Weiss syndrome). To increase patient comfort, nasogastric decompression may be needed, although the institution of nasogastric drainage has not been shown to alter the eventual outcome of an attack.

Role of Prophylactic Antibiotics

- Over the past decade, three separate studies have indicated that prophylactic antibiotics are useful in the management of patients with severe pancreatitis, but no benefit was observed when prophylactic antibiotics were given to patients with mild pancreatitis.

● In patients with severe pancreatitis, benefit was observed with regimens that included imipenem alone, imipenem with cilastatin, and cefuroxime.

● Although these recent studies argue strongly for administration of prophylactic antibiotics to patients with severe pancreatitis, there is an opposing view that is becoming increasingly widespread. According to that school of thought, administration of prophylactic antibiotics favors emergence of resistant organisms in the area of pancreatic injury. That may be particularly true for fungal strains such as *Candida*.

Nutritional Support

● Patients with severe pancreatitis may be unable to eat for prolonged periods, and an alternative route for providing nutrition is required. Traditionally, these patients have been given parenteral nutrition administered via a central venous catheter. Widely differing opinions exist regarding the time that total parenteral nutrition should be started. Some advocate starting within the first day or two, whereas others delay starting total parenteral nutrition until the early phase of pancreatitis, characterized by extensive fluid shifts and high fluid requirements, has been completed. I favor the latter approach.

● Several investigative groups have recently demonstrated that most patients with pancreatitis, including those with severe pancreatitis, can actually tolerate small amounts of enterally administered nutrients. They have shown that those nutrients can be tolerated if given either into the stomach (via a naso-gastric tube) or into the small intestine (via a nasojejunal tube). Pancreatic infections are believed to occur because gut bacteria are translocated across the injured bowel wall adjacent to areas of pancreatic injury. Theoretically, enteral nutrition exerts a trophic effect on the injured bowel wall that could reduce this translocation and, thus, reduce the incidence of pancreatic infections.

Treatments of Limited or Unproved Value

● Peritoneal dialysis, designed to eliminate the proinflammatory factors released into the abdomen during pancreatitis, might theoretically be expected to reduce the severity of pancreatitis. Indeed, early anecdotal studies did support the use of peritoneal dialysis in patients with severe pancreatitis, but a more recent, prospective, randomized multi-institutional study showed that peritoneal dialysis was of no benefit.

- Other attempts to reduce gastrointestinal and/or pancreatic secretion (i.e., histamine-2 blockers, proton pump inhibitors, antacids, atropine, somatostatin, glucagon, and calcitonin) have not been shown to be beneficial in the treatment of pancreatitis. Similarly, the use of anti-inflammatory agents (i.e., steroids, prostaglandins, and indomethacin) have not been helpful, although recent experimental studies have suggested that specific inhibition of cyclooxygenase-2 might be beneficial.

Treatment of Early Systemic Complications of Pancreatitis

- Cardiovascular collapse is largely caused by hypovolemia, and its management requires aggressive fluid and electrolyte repletion. This may necessitate placement of a central venous or Swan-Ganz monitoring catheter. Changes in hematocrit, filling pressures, and cardiac output can be used to monitor the adequacy of treatment, but changes in blood pressure, pulse, and urine output do not accurately and reliably reflect the adequacy of fluid replacement.
- The pulmonary manifestations of pancreatitis include atelectasis and acute lung injury.
- Management includes good pulmonary toilet combined with close monitoring of pulmonary function. For many patients, intubation and respiratory support may be required. Renal failure in pancreatitis is usually prerenal and is associated with a poor prognosis.
- Stress-induced gastroduodenal erosions account for most of the gastrointestinal bleeding in pancreatitis, and prophylaxis with antacids, histamine-2 receptor antagonists, or proton pump inhibitors may be appropriate. Very rarely, massive bleeding can result from injury to peripancreatic vascular structures leading to hemorrhage into the retroperitoneum.
- Some patients with severe pancreatitis develop disseminated intravascular coagulation, but it rarely causes bleeding and prophylactic heparinization is usually not indicated.

Role of Early Endoscopy and Stone Extraction

- Patients with mild pancreatitis may ultimately require endoscopic duct clearance to prevent recurrent attacks, but they rarely benefit from early endoscopy because their pancreatitis generally resolves spontaneously within several days. On the other hand, the role of early endoscopic duct clearance in the initial management of patients with severe biliary pancreatitis is more controversial. Three randomized, controlled, prospective studies have differing results. One study indicated that early stone clearance reduced the severity and mortality of biliary pancreatitis, whereas a second study indicated that early duct clearance reduced the incidence of infectious complications. The third study concluded that early endoscopy and duct clearance actually adversely affected the course of pancreatitis because it was associated with a high incidence of complications. At present, most experts would favor early (i.e., <48 hours after the onset of symptoms) endoscopic intervention in severe biliary pancreatitis, but further studies are needed.

Role and Timing of Cholecystectomy in Patients with Gallstone Pancreatitis

- In general, patients with gallstone pancreatitis should undergo some form of definitive treatment before discharge from the hospital, but that intervention should take place as soon as possible after resolution of their attack. Further delaying the intervention would increase the chances that additional stones might be passed and another attack of pancreatitis might be triggered.
- Thus, good surgical risk patients are better managed by cholecystectomy.

Treatment of Later Complications

Definitions

- In 1992, an international symposium was held to resolve the confusion that had arisen concerning the terminology used to describe the local complications of pancreatitis and the value of specific treatments for those complications. The following definitions were agreed on at that conference.
    - *Acute fluid collections.* These occur during the early stages of severe pancreatitis in 30% to 50% of patients and lack a wall of granulation or fibrous tissue, and more than half regress spontaneously.
    - *Pancreatic and peripancreatic necrosis.* These are areas of nonviable pancreatic or peripancreatic tissue that may

be either sterile or infected. They typically include areas of fat necrosis, and the necrotic tissue has a putty-like or paste-like consistency.

- *Pancreatic pseudocyst.* These are collections of pancreatic juice, usually rich in digestive enzymes, that are enclosed by a nonepithelialized wall composed of fibrous and granulation tissue.
- When pus is present, the infected pseudocyst is referred to as a *pancreatic abscess.* Leakage or rupture of a pseudocyst into the peritoneal cavity results in *pancreatic ascites.* A *pancreaticopleural fistula* results from erosion of a pseudocyst into the pleural space.
- *Pancreatic abscess.* These are circumscribed intra-abdominal collections of pus, usually in proximity to the pancreas, that contain little or no necrotic tissue but arise as a consequence of pancreatitis. An infected pseudocyst should be considered a pancreatic abscess. Pancreatic abscess and infected pancreatic necrosis represent the extremes of a spectrum that include lesions with varying amounts of necrosis.
- The material has a liquid consistency whereas, in infected pancreatic necrosis, necrosis predominates and the material is paste or putty-like.

Diagnosis

- Contrast-enhanced CT is particularly valuable as a means of quantifying the extent of pancreatic necrosis (i.e., non-enhancement). The maturation of a pseudocyst can be followed by both contrast-enhanced CT and endoscopic ultrasound (EUS).
- When the clinical suspicion of infection is high, fine needle aspiration of peripancreatic or intrapancreatic fluid for culture and Gram stain analysis may be particularly helpful. The procedure is most frequently done with CT guidance, and it is safe when performed by experienced radiologists.

Management of Sterile and Infected Acute Fluid Collections

- Sterile acute fluid collections usually resolve spontaneously, and no specific treatment is indicated. Attempts to drain acute fluid collections, either by using percutaneously placed drains or by intervening surgically, should be discouraged because they are usually unnecessary, and, furthermore, they are likely to lead to infection.

Management of Sterile and Infected Necrosis

- The role of surgical intervention in the management of patients with *sterile* pancreatic or peripancreatic necrosis has been the subject of considerable controversy.

- There is, however, a consensus that patients with *infected* necrosis require some form of intervention. Prospective studies have indicated that infection of areas of necrosis can occur at any time but that it usually occurs during the initial 3 to 4 weeks of an attack.

- The conventional approach to managing infected necrosis involves laparotomy and surgical débridement of the infected, devitalized tissue. Repeated operations and débridements may be needed. The timing of the initial débridement appears to be closely related to the outcome (i.e., those undergoing later operations do better and require fewer repeat operations than those undergoing early operation).

- The goal of operation, in patients with infected necrosis, is to remove as much as possible of the infected, necrotic tissue and to provide drainage for the remaining viable exocrine tissue. Many different ways of achieving these goals have been described (Box 52–4), and, although each has its advocates, none has been proven to be superior to the others.

Box 52–4. Management Options for Infected Pancreatic Necrosis

Conventional Approach
Débridement with reoperation when clinically indicated or at planned intervals
Débridement with open or closed packing and reoperation when clinically indicated or at planned intervals
Débridement with continuous lavage

Unconventional Approach
Antibiotics alone
Antibiotics with percutaneous drainage
Antibiotics with endoscopic drainage
Antibiotics with surgical drainage but not débridement
Antibiotics with débridement via minimally invasive surgery

Management of Pancreatic Pseudocysts

- Recent reports have shown that many pseudocysts eventually resolve without complications and that intervention is not mandatory in all cases unless the pseudocysts are symptomatic, enlarging, or associated with complications. The likelihood that a pseudocyst will resolve spontaneously, however, is dependent on its size. Large pseudocysts (i.e., greater than 6 cm in diameter) are more likely to become symptomatic either because they are tender or because of their mass effect on adjacent organs.

- Pancreatic pseudocysts that erode into a neighboring vessel can result in formation of a pseudoaneurysm with *hemosuccus pancreaticus* and upper gastrointestinal bleeding.

- Most patients who develop symptomatic pseudocysts are best managed by pseudocyst drainage. In poor surgical risk patients, percutaneous catheter drainage can be considered, but, in my experience, that approach leads to considerable morbidity because of catheter-induced infection and the development of a prolonged external pancreatic fistula. Internal drainage can avoid these problems and seems preferable.

- Surgical internal drainage of pseudocysts is usually accomplished by creating either a Roux-en-Y cyst-jejunostomy, a side-to-side cyst-gastrostomy, or a side-to-side cyst duodenostomy.

Management of Pancreatic Ascites and Pancreatico-pleural Fistulas

- Pancreatic ascites occurs when pancreatic juice gains entry into the peritoneal cavity either from a pancreatic duct disruption or from a leaking pseudocyst. The diagnosis can usually be made when high amylase levels are found in the ascitic fluid. The initial treatment usually is nonoperative and involves attempts to decrease pancreatic secretion by elimination of enteral feeding, institution of nasogastric drainage, and administration of the antisecretory hormone somatostatin. Repeated paracentesis may also be helpful. Roughly 50% to 60% of patients can be expected to respond to this treatment with resolution of pancreatic ascites within 2 to 3 weeks. Persistent or recurrent ascites can be treated either endoscopically or surgically. Endoscopic treatment involves endoscopic pancreatic sphincterotomy with or without placement of a transpapillary pancreatic duct stent.

- This approach is designed to allow the site of leakage to seal. Surgical treatment of pancreatic ascites, usually preceded by

performance of an endoscopic retrograde cholangiopancreatography (ERCP) to identify the site of duct disruption,
involves either resection (for leaks in the pancreatic tail)
or internal Roux-Y drainage.

Management of Pancreatitis-Induced False Aneurysms

- Rarely, pancreatic pseudocysts or areas of pancreatic
  necrosis can erode into pancreatic or peripancreatic vascular
  structures.
- Therapeutic angiographic embolization is most appropriate
  for the unstable patient, and this approach may also provide
  definitive treatment, particularly for those patients whose
  false aneurysm is in the pancreatic head. For those whose
  false aneurysm is in the tail of the pancreas, subsequent
  distal pancreatectomy, once the patient is stabilized, may
  provide more secure hemostasis.

CHRONIC PANCREATITIS

Pathology and Etiology of Chronic Pancreatitis

- Chronic pancreatitis is characterized by irreversible changes
  including pancreatic fibrosis and the loss of functional
  pancreatic exocrine and/or endocrine tissue.

Diagnosis of Chronic Pancreatitis

- There has been considerable confusion concerning the clinical distinction between chronic and acute pancreatitis.
  Largely, this confusion results from the fact that, from a
  clinical standpoint, attacks of chronic pancreatitis may be
  indistinguishable from those of acute pancreatitis. Fortunately,
  the initial management of acute or chronic pancreatitis
  attacks is identical as is the management of complications
  such as infection, necrosis, and pseudocyst (see the section
  on treatment). On the other hand, the two forms of pancreatitis have natural histories that differ considerably, and the
  long-term management of chronic pancreatitis presents
  challenges that are not inherent to the management of acute
  pancreatitis.

History

- Patients with chronic pancreatitis may describe prior
  episodes of pancreatic-type abdominal pain, and 60% to

80% of patients have a long history of ethanol abuse. There may be a family history of pancreatitis suggestive of the presence of hereditary pancreatitis or a history of autoimmune diseases including primary sclerosing cholangitis and Sjögren's syndrome that should raise suspicion of pancreatitis on an autoimmune basis. Diabetes mellitus and/or a history suggestive of malabsorption (i.e., steatorrhea) indicate that significant pancreatic endocrine and/or exocrine function has been lost, and this is most compatible with the diagnosis of chronic pancreatitis.

● Repeated use of heating pads or hot water bottles to treat the chronic pain may result in skin lesions (erythema *ab igne*) that define the distribution of the pain (Fig. 52–1). Some patients experience no pain.

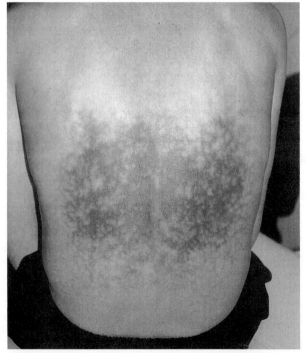

■ **FIGURE 52–1.** Erythema *ab igne*. Skin injury, characterized by keratinocyte injury and melanocyte activation, is induced by mild and repeated exposure to infrared sources. This patient with chronic pancreatitis repeatedly applied a heating pad to the painful area on his back.

Imaging Studies

- Radiographs or CT scans showing pancreatic calcifications are diagnostic of chronic pancreatitis.
- The absence of pancreatic calcifications does not rule out a diagnosis of chronic pancreatitis. Perhaps the most sensitive methods for diagnosing chronic pancreatitis are those that provide images of the pancreatic ductal system—ERCP, CT cholangiopancreatography (CTCP), or magnetic resonance cholangiopancreatography (MRCP).
- Chronic pancreatitis is characterized by irregularities of the pancreatic ducts, ductal strictures, and areas of duct dilation.
- Some patients with chronic pancreatitis develop dilated main pancreatic ducts (large duct disease), whereas others retain ducts of normal or even smaller than normal caliber (small duct disease).

Pancreatic Function Tests

- Tubeless tests involve measuring the stool content of fat, measuring stool content of digestive enzymes, or orally administering a pancreatic digestive enzyme substrate and quantitating enzyme activity in the gut by measuring metabolic product in either the urine or exhaled gases. These tests, although nonintrusive, are notoriously insensitive; therefore, normal results are not very helpful. The more invasive tube tests involve placement of a collecting tube in the duodenum and measuring pancreatic bicarbonate or enzyme output after meal or hormone stimulation of the pancreas.

Natural History

- More often, the disease remains painful; addicting doses of narcotics are required; and loss of function results in diabetes, steatorrhea, and profound weight loss.

Treatment of Pancreatic Malabsorption

- Theoretically, pancreatic malabsorption of fat should be corrected by oral administration of exogenous lipase. Unfortunately, most orally administered lipase is inactivated as it traverses the acidic environment of the stomach allowing only 8% to 15% of ingested lipase activity to reach the duodenum. Some of that lipase may be ineffective, because of low duodenal pH.

- The use of acid-inhibiting agents (e.g., proton pump inhibitors) and enterically coated microsphere delivery systems can partially compensate for these problems.

Treatment of Pain in Chronic Pancreatitis

Medical Management

- Complete abstinence from ethanol is advised for patients with alcohol-induced pancreatitis, but symptoms may persist even after complete abstinence. Attacks of hyperlipidemia-induced pancreatitis can be prevented by normalizing lipid levels with medication and/or dietary changes. Some patients with autoimmune pancreatitis are cured by administration of steroids.
- Toskes and coworkers have noted that some of their patients with painful chronic pancreatitis have diminished pain if pancreatic secretion is reduced either by oral administration of pancreatic enzymes or by administration of the inhibitory hormone somatostatin.

Endoscopic Management

- Endoscopic pancreatic sphincterotomy has been reported to benefit some patients with elevated sphincter of Oddi pressures. Endoscopic minor pancreatic sphincterotomy has been used to treat patients with pancreatitis and pancreas divisum.

Neuroablative Procedures

- Pain from the pancreas is carried in sympathetic fibers that traverse the celiac ganglia, reach the sympathetic chain through the splanchnic nerves, and then ascend to the cortex. Celiac plexus nerve blocks performed either percutaneously or endoscopically have been used to abolish this pain with inconsistent results. Recently, splanchnicectomy performed in the chest via a thoracoscopic approach has been used with reports of transient improvement in 70% of patients and long-lasting pain control in 50%.

Surgical Treatment of Chronic Pancreatitis

- The two indications for surgical intervention are pain and concern over the possible presence of cancer. After the diagnosis of chronic pancreatitis has been established, surgical intervention should be considered when (1) the pain is severe enough to limit the patient's lifestyle and/or reduce productivity and (2) the pain persists despite complete abstinence from alcohol and administration of non-narcotic analgesics.

Drainage Procedures for Patients with Small Ducts

● Patients with small (i.e., <4 to 5 mm) pancreatic ducts, particularly those whose pancreatitis is caused by obstruction at the ampullary level, may benefit from transduodenal sphincteroplasty of the common bile duct with division of the septum that lies between the pancreatic duct and bile duct (pancreatic septotomy). Sphincteroplasty of the lesser papilla might be appropriate for patients with pancreas divisum. On the other hand, most patients with chronic pancreatitis have multiple areas of duct stricture throughout the pancreas and are unlikely to benefit from these transduodenal procedures.

Drainage Procedures for Patients with Dilated Ducts

● The ideal treatment for these patients involves creating an anastomotic connection between the dilated duct and the intestinal lumen. There is little agreement concerning the minimum duct size needed to perform these anastomoses. Ducts larger than 1 cm in diameter are clearly large enough, but many surgeons perform duct-to-intestine drainage procedures with ducts as small as 5 mm.
● In appropriately selected patients (i.e., those with large ducts and those with intraductal stones), longitudinal pancreaticojejunostomy, performed according to the Partington and Rochelle modification of the Puestow procedure, has been reported to result in immediate pain relief in more than 80% of patients and long-term pain relief in roughly 60% of patients. More recently, Frey further modified the procedure by including removal of part of the pancreatic head, thereby marsupializing the duct as it dives deeply in the pancreas to reach the ampulla of Vater.

Resective Procedures

● Painful chronic pancreatitis can be treated with resection the body and tail of the pancreas (distal pancreatectomy), with resection of the head and uncinate process of the pancreas (Whipple procedure), with subtotal pancreatectomy that spares a rim of pancreas along the inner curve of the duodenum, and with total pancreatectomy.

- Most experts believe that it is the inflammatory process in the pancreatic head that controls both the severity of symptoms and the further progression of the disease in the remainder of the gland. Perhaps because of this, resection of the pancreatic head has been shown to completely relieve the pain of chronic pancreatitis in 70% to 80% of patients. Resection of the pancreatic head can be accomplished by a standard pancreaticoduodenectomy (Whipple procedure) or by its pylorus-preserving modification (pylorus-preserving Whipple procedure). Relief of symptoms by either procedure is comparable, but some claim that the quality of life and gastrointestinal function is better after the pylorus-preserving operation. Beger and colleagues have modified the Whipple procedure even further by coring out the head of the pancreas and preserving the duodenum and distal bile duct. They claim that this "duodenum-preserving pancreatic head resection" yields results that are as good as or better than those achieved with the standard Whipple procedure.

BENIGN EXOCRINE TUMORS

- Most benign pancreatic exocrine tumors are cystic but not all cystic tumors are benign. Benign cystic tumors, which account for 10% to 15% of pancreatic tumors, are usually asymptomatic, but, when symptoms develop, they are usually related to pressure or obstruction of an adjacent organ.

Serous Cystadenoma

- These tumors account for 20% to 40% of cystic pancreatic neoplasms.
- Rare cases of malignant serous cystic lesions have been reported but most are benign and have no malignant potential. Typically, they are large, spherical masses that contain a watery fluid and have a central, calcified stellate scar.
- Resection is indicated when the diagnosis is in doubt or when they become symptomatic.

Mucinous Tumors

- These tumors account for 20% to 40% of cystic tumors. Even if benign at the time of diagnosis, they are usually considered to have malignant potential. Two types have been described but neither type usually communicates with the pancreatic duct. One form contains areas of ovarian-like stroma, is almost always found in women, and is almost always found in the pancreatic tail. The more common type, however, lacks ovarian stroma and it can be found anywhere in the pancreas. It occurs equally in both sexes. For both types, imaging studies usually indicate that the lesion is composed of one or more very large cysts (i.e., macrocystic) although microcystic mucinous tumors can also occur.

- Prolonged survival (i.e., >5 years) can be anticipated in more than 50% of patients if these tumors are resected before the development of invasive malignancy, but, even after the development of malignant changes and invasion, long-term survival is still better than for ductal adenocarcinoma.

Intraductal Papillary Mucinous Neoplasm (IPMN)

- Intraductal papillary mucinous tumor (IPMT), also known as IPMN is another type of cystic pancreatic neoplasm. Although first described in Japan in the 1980s, it is now being recognized worldwide, and its incidence appears to be rapidly increasing.
- IPMT patients can experience pancreatitis when mucus, secreted by the tumor, transiently obstructs the orifice of the pancreatic duct. The diagnosis of IPMT can be made with near certainty if mucus is seen extruding through a large, fish-mouth like papillary orifice at the time of endoscopy.
- IPMT is believed to follow an adenoma-carcinoma sequence, and it can be classified according to the Pan-IN classification scheme that categorizes tumors as having minimal or no dysplasia (PanIN-1), moderate dysplasia (PanIN-2), or severe dysplasia/carcinoma *in situ* (PanIN-3). The natural history of tumors with only mild or no dysplasia is not known, but those with severe dysplasia and/or carcinoma *in situ* are very likely to become locally invasive and metastasize if left unresected. Resection with, at worst, PanIN-1 changes at the margin, before development of invasive malignancy, is usually curative. This may mandate total pancreatectomy. When resection is performed after development of invasive malignancy, cure rates are relatively low.

Management of Cystic Pancreatic Neoplasms

- A recent history of pancreatitis, enzyme-rich fluid in the cyst, and communication between the cyst and the pancreatic duct suggests that the cystic lesion is a postpancreatic (i.e., inflammatory) pseudocyst. Patients with asymptomatic pseudocysts can be left untreated. It should be recognized, however, that occasionally these features can also be associated with neoplastic cystic lesions; therefore, these patients should be closely followed. Serous cystadenomas, diagnosed by finding glycogen-rich cells on fine needle aspiration biopsy, can also be followed without resection if they are not symptomatic.

- The finding of mucin in the cyst, mucin-secreting cells on biopsy, a high cyst fluid viscosity, or a high cyst fluid carcinoembryonic antigen (CEA) is suggestive, but not diagnostic, of a potentially malignant tumor.
- Because of these uncertainties, all neoplastic cysts should be resected.

Solid-Pseudopapillary Tumor of the Pancreas

- This relatively uncommon tumor often occurs in young women and follows a benign course. Local resection is usually curative, although incomplete removal can result in local recurrence and malignant varieties have been described.
- In suitable operative candidates, solid-pseudopapillary tumors of the pancreas should be resected.

MALIGNANT PANCREATIC TUMORS

Incidence and Epidemiology

- Pancreatic cancer affects 25,000 to 30,000 people in the United States each year and is the fourth or fifth leading cause of cancer-related death in this country. It occurs more frequently in men than in women, and it is more common among blacks than whites. Roughly 80% of cases occur between the ages of 60 and 80, and less than 2% occur in people younger than 40. Other risk factors include a history of hereditary or chronic pancreatitis, cigarette smoking, and occupational exposure to carcinogens. The incidence of diabetes mellitus is increased in patients with pancreatic cancer, but the relationship of diabetes to pancreas cancer is controversial.

Pathology

- Ductal adenocarcinoma and its variants account for 80% to 90% of all pancreatic neoplasms and for an even greater fraction of the malignant tumors. Roughly 70% of ductal cancers arise in the pancreatic head or uncinate process.

- They are usually larger than 3 cm in diameter, and both nodal and distant metastases are also frequently present. Those originating in the body or tail of the pancreas are often larger and more likely to have spread before their presence is known.
- In addition, perineural growth of the tumor is highly characteristic of this cancer and may account for the propensity of pancreatic cancer to extend into neighboring neural plexuses causing both upper abdominal and back pain.
- Cancers such as mucinous noncystic carcinoma (colloid carcinoma), signet-ring-cell carcinoma, adenosquamous carcinoma, anaplastic carcinoma, giant-cell carcinoma, and sarcomatoid carcinoma are considered to be variants of ductal adenocarcinoma that differ primarily in their degree of differentiation and their morphologic appearance.
- Other forms of pancreas cancer include acinar-cell carcinomas, which are most common in the fifth to seventh decade of life and most frequently present as large masses in the body or tail of the pancreas. Pancreatoblastoma is a very rare form of pancreas cancer that usually presents in young children. Nonepithelial cancers of all types, including leiomyosarcomas, liposarcomas, plasmacytomas, and lymphomas can also develop within the pancreas, but these tumors are quite rare. Lymphomas of the pancreas, if diagnosed before resection, are usually best treated with chemoradiation.

Development and Molecular Biology

- Almost all pancreatic cancers and most of the precursor lesions, demonstrate codon 12 mutations of the *K-ras* oncogene.
- Mutation of the p53 tumor suppressor gene is the most common genetic event in all human cancers, and it is observed in 75% of pancreatic cancers.
- Mutations resulting in the functional loss of other tumor suppressor genes, including *p16, SMAD 4, DPC,* and *DCC* are also commonly observed in pancreatic cancer. Other much less frequent tumor suppressor gene deletions that have been observed in pancreatic cancers result in the loss of the retinoblastoma gene and the adenomatous polyposis coli *(APC)* gene.
- Several growth factor systems are commonly upregulated in pancreatic cancer either by increased expression of their

receptors or by increases in the relevant ligands. The most commonly observed changes involve the epidermal growth factor (EGF) receptor family that includes the EGF receptor (which responds to EGF and to transforming growth factor-α) and the HER 2, 3, and 4 receptors. Overexpression of EGF receptors or its ligands is correlated with tumor invasiveness, enhanced potential for metastasis, and a poorer prognosis.

- Precursor ductal lesions have been identified and the step-wise progression toward invasive cancer and metastasis has been related to the accumulated presence of multiple genetic abnormalities.

Hereditary Pancreatic Cancer Syndromes

- Pancreatic cancer has been observed to be increased in families with hereditary nonpolyposis colon cancer (HNPCC), those with familial breast cancer (associated with the *BRCA2* mutation), those with Peutz-Jeghers syndrome, those with ataxia-telangiectasia, and those with the familial atypical multiple mole melanoma (FAMMM) syndrome. Patients with hereditary pancreatitis are also at increased risk of developing pancreatic cancer. This is particularly true in those with a paternal pattern of inheritance who may have a 75% risk of developing pancreatic cancer. Even in the absence of one of these familial cancer syndromes or hereditary pancreatitis, individuals with a family history of pancreatic cancer, especially those with two or more pancreatic cancer-affected first-degree relatives, have an increased risk of developing pancreatic cancer.

Symptoms and Signs

- The symptoms, once they develop, are determined by the location of the tumor in the pancreas (Table 52–2). Those in the head or uncinate process of the pancreas make their presence known by causing bile duct, duodenal, or pancreatic duct obstruction. Symptoms include unexplained episodes of pancreatitis, painless jaundice, nausea, vomiting, steatorrhea, and unexplained weight loss. With further spread beyond the pancreas, these patients may note upper abdominal and/or back pain when peripancreatic nerve plexuses are involved and ascites when peritoneal carcinomatosis or portal vein occlusion develops. Patients with tumors arising in the neck, body, or tail of the pancreas usually do not develop jaundice or gastric outlet obstruction. Their symptoms may be limited to unexplained weight loss and vague upper

TABLE 52–2.   Signs and Symptoms of Pancreatic Cancer

Frequent	Infrequent
Pancreatic Head Cancers	
Weight loss (92%)	Nausea (37%)
Pain (72%)	Weakness (35%)
Jaundice (82%)	Pruritus (24%)
Dark Urine (63%)	Vomiting (37%)
Light stools (62%)	
Anorexia (64%)	
Pancreatic Body/Tail Cancers	
Weight loss (100%)	Jaundice (7%)
Pain (87%)	Dark Urine (5%)
Weakness (43%)	Light stools (6%)
Nausea (45%)	Pruritus (4%)
Anorexia (33%)	
Vomiting (37%)	

abdominal pain until the tumor has grown extensively and spread beyond the pancreas. New onset diabetes mellitus is occasionally the first symptom of an otherwise occult pancreatic cancer. Recent studies have suggested that this form of diabetes may be mediated by a factor released from the tumor that either inhibits insulin release from islets or induces peripheral insulin resistance. Unexplained migratory thrombophlebitis (Trousseau's syndrome) may be associated with pancreatic and other types of malignancy. It is probably a paraneoplastic phenomenon that results from a tumor-induced hypercoagulable state.

- Liver nodules indicative of metastases can sometimes be felt. Metastatic subumbilical (Sister Mary Joseph node) and pelvic peritoneal (Blummer's shelf) deposits and left supraclavicular lymphadenopathy (Virchow's node) indicate the presence of distant metastases. Malignant ascites, caused by peritoneal carcinomatosis, may also be present. With portal, splenic, or superior mesenteric vein occlusion, mesenteric venous pressures may be increased and collateral channels, including gastroesophageal varices and a caput medusae, may develop. Distal common bile duct obstruction caused by the tumor often leads to bile duct and gallbladder distention. Thus, a palpable gallbladder in a patient with painless jaundice (i.e., Courvoisier's sign) should suggest the presence of a periampullary neoplasm.

Blood Tests

- The two most widely used pancreatic cancer serum markers are the CEA and the Lewis blood-group carbohydrate antigen CA 19-9. Both are frequently elevated in patients with advanced disease, but, unfortunately, the circulating levels of these tumor markers are often normal in patients with early, potentially curable, tumors. Thus, using these tumor markers to screen patients with vague symptoms or those in high-risk groups has not been shown to be useful in detecting early disease. With a cutoff value of 37 U/mL, CA 19-9 has been reported to have a sensitivity of 86% and a specificity of 87%. CA 19-9 can also be elevated in patients with cholangitis and jaundice not caused by pancreatic cancer. Extremely high levels of either the CA 19-9 or CEA usually indicate unresectable and/or metastatic disease.

Imaging Studies

- For most patients, the initial imaging study is a transcutaneous US examination. It may reveal a pancreatic mass and indicate whether that mass is solid or cystic. It can also aid in the diagnosis of jaundiced patients by revealing the presence of extrahepatic ductal dilation in the absence of demonstrable biliary tract stones. Transcutaneous US, regardless of its findings, is usually followed by helical contrast-enhanced CT, performed in conjunction with intravenous infusion of contrast material.
- Pancreatic cancer usually appears as a hypodense mass with poorly demarcated edges.
- When performed and interpreted by experienced radiologists, CT has a specificity for diagnosing pancreatic tumors of 95% or better. Its sensitivity depends on the size of the tumor, exceeding 95% for tumors larger than 2 cm in diameter.
- Positron emission tomography (PET) may be of value in diagnosing small pancreatic tumors that escape CT or magnetic resonance imaging (MRI) detection, but the sensitivity and specificity of PET scanning remains to be established.
- ERCP may be particularly helpful in evaluating patients with obstructive jaundice without a detectable mass on CT or MRI.
- The "double duct sign" on ERCP is highly suggestive of a pancreatic head cancer but benign processes, such as chronic pancreatitis or autoimmune pancreatitis, can also produce a double duct sign.
- Resection will be indicated regardless of the ERCP findings.

The Role of Biopsy

- Biopsy to confirm the presence and identify the type of cancer is usually required before chemoradiation therapy of unresectable pancreatic tumors or neoadjuvant treatment of resectable tumors. Percutaneous biopsy, performed with either CT or US guidance, or transduodenal biopsy, performed with EUS guidance, are routinely used in these situations.

- For these reasons, most surgeons would not recommend routine preoperative biopsy for confirmation of the diagnosis in the management of patients with potentially resectable lesions. It should be recognized, however, that if this policy of not performing preoperative biopsy is followed, 5% to 10% of patients undergoing resection for suspected cancer will be found to have benign lesions.

Staging of Pancreatic Cancer

- The American Joint Commission on Cancer (AJCC) staging system is widely used to stage pancreatic cancer (Table 52–3). This system uses the tumor-lymph node-metastasis (TNM) classification to define the tumor extent, nodal metastases, and distant metastases. T*is*, which denotes *in situ* cancer, corresponds to PanIN-3 (i.e., the most advanced of the ductal cancer precursor lesions). T1 and T2 cancers are confined to the pancreas and either less than 2 cm or greater than 2 cm in diameter. T3 and T4 lesions extend beyond the pancreas. T3 lesions are considered to be potentially resectable

TABLE 52–3. American Joint Committee on Cancer: TNM System for Staging of Pancreatic Cancer

Stage	T Status	N Status	M Status
Stage 0	Tis	N0	M0
Stage IA	T1	N0	M0
Stage IB	T2	N0	M0
Stage IIA	T3	N0	M0
Stage IIB	T1	N1	M0
	T2	N1	M0
	T3	N1	M0
Stage III	T4	Any N	M0
Stage IV	Any T	Any N	M1

Adapted from AJCC Cancer Staging Handbook, 6th ed. New York, Springer, 2002, pp 179–188.

because they do not involve the celiac axis or superior mesenteric artery.

- T4 lesions are considered to be unresectable because they involve the critical peripancreatic arteries. N1 lesions have positive regional nodes and M1 lesions have distant metastases, whereas N0 and M0 lesions lack both of these features. Distant metastases are common, and they are most frequently located in the liver, lung, or on the peritoneal surfaces of the abdomen.

- Stage 1 and stage 2 cancers are amenable to resection. Poor prognostic signs include aneuploidy, large tumor size (T2), the presence of positive regional nodes (N1), and an incomplete resection at the pancreatic or retroperitoneal margin.

- Stage 3 and stage 4 cancers are considered to be unresectable, either because of distant metastases (stage 4) or because of major arterial involvement (stage 3). Mean survival for patients with stage 3 tumors ranges from 8 to 12 months, whereas survival for patients with stage 4 tumors is only 3 to 6 months.

- Circumferential encasement, invasion, or occlusion of the portal vein and superior mesenteric vein and/or the superior mesenteric artery is generally considered to be a sign of unresectability, although, strictly speaking, resection is still technically possible if only the venous structures are involved. Partial encasement (i.e., involvement of 30% to 60% of the circumference of the vein) may result in distortion of the vein and the appearance of a tear drop shaped rather than a round structure.

- Other CT changes suggestive of unresectability include extension beyond the pancreatic capsule and into the retroperitoneum, involvement of neural or nodal structures surrounding the origin of either the celiac axis or superior mesenteric artery, and extension of the tumor along the hepatoduodenal ligament.

The Role of Laparoscopy in Staging

- The role of staging laparoscopy in the management of pancreatic cancer is controversial. Proponents claim that 20% to 40% of patients believed to have stage 1 or 2 disease have unrecognized small metastases to peritoneal surfaces (diaphragm, liver, etc.) and that those metastases can be laparoscopically detected, thus preventing a needless laparotomy. Our own experience indicates that, with high-quality modern imaging techniques, very few patients with pancreatic head tumors are deemed unresectable at operation merely because they are found to have metastases that might have been found by laparoscopy.

- For these reasons, it is my practice to perform staging laparoscopy for potentially resectable body or tail lesions. For pancreatic head lesions that are deemed respectable by preoperative routine staging, laparoscopy is not advocated.

Resectional Surgery for Pancreatic Head and Uncinate Process Tumors

- Tumors of the head, neck, and uncinate process of the pancreas account for approximately 70% of pancreatic tumors. They are generally resected by pancreaticoduodenectomy, with or without preservation of the pylorus and proximal duodenum.
- The pylorus-preserving operation is technically easier and faster, but it may be associated with a higher incidence and more prolonged delayed gastric emptying.

Complications of Pancreaticoduodenectomy

- When performed by experienced surgeons in high-volume centers, the operative mortality of pancreaticoduodenectomy is 2% to 4%. Anastomotic leaks, intra-abdominal abscesses, and delayed gastric emptying account for most perioperative complications after pancreaticoduodenectomy. Leakage from the pancreatic anastomosis, resulting in a pancreatic fistula, occurs in 15% to 20% of patients. With adequate drainage, these fistulas usually heal within several weeks.
- A recent randomized trial addressing this subject concluded that prophylactic administration of a somatostatin analogue in this setting is not beneficial. Biliary fistulas are much less common than pancreatic fistulas after pancreaticoduodenectomy but they also usually heal if adequate drainage is achieved. Delayed gastric emptying occurs in 15% to 40% of patients and almost always resolves with time.
- Erythromycin, which has a structure that resembles motilin, acts as an agonist at motilin receptors and has been used to treat these patients. Success has been reported using this approach, but my experience with this use of erythromycin has been disappointing.
- The endocrine pancreas has considerable functional reserve and, for that reason, most patients do not develop diabetes after resection of the pancreatic head. In fact, some patients with tumor-induced diabetes may have resolution of their diabetes after resection. In contrast, pancreatic malabsorption

and steatorrhea are relatively common long-term problems. It may reflect exocrine secretory insufficiency, an obstruction at the pancreatic-jejunal anastomosis, or poor postoperative mixing of secreted enzymes with food.

Results of Pancreaticoduodenectomy for Pancreatic Cancer

- Five-year survival rates of 15% to 20% have been reported from some centers but rates of 10% to 15% are more common, and the vast majority of those patients who survive for 5 years succumb over the subsequent 5 years.
- Negative margins, in one study, were associated with a 26% 5-year survival, whereas positive margins were associated with an 8% 5-year survival.
- The 5-year survival of node-positive patients, in one series, was reported to be 14%, whereas 5-year survival of node-negative patients was 36%.

Resectional Surgery for Pancreatic Body and Tail Tumors

- Most body and tail cancers have already metastasized to distant sites or extended locally to involve nodes, nerves, or major vessels by the time of diagnosis. Splenic vein involvement and/or occlusion is not uncommon and, by itself, is not a sign of nonresectability.
- Splenectomy should be performed for malignant tumors, but splenic preservation is not contraindicated when benign tumors are being removed.
- Complications of distal pancreatectomy include subphrenic abscess, which may occur in 5% to 10% of patients, and pancreatic duct leak, which has been reported to occur in up to 20% of patients.
- Somatostatin administration frequently reduces the output of these pancreatic fistulas, but it does not appear to alter the time of fistula closure.
- Only 10% of cancers involving the tail or body of the pancreas are resectable at the time of diagnosis. The 5-year survival of patients who are deemed resectable is somewhat lower than that of patients with resectable cancer of the pancreatic head.

Palliative Nonsurgical Treatment for Pancreatic Cancers

- Establishing the diagnosis and relieving symptoms of jaundice, gastric outlet obstruction, and pain are the goals of palliative nonsurgical treatment.

- Decompression of the obstructed biliary tract can be achieved using either an endoscopic or a percutaneous-transhepatic approach. The former has been shown, in randomized trials, to yield better results with fewer associated complications. At the time of ERCP, a transpapillary stent is placed across the obstructed segment of bile duct. Either plastic or expandable metal stents can be used, but metal stents give more complete and more long-lasting relief of jaundice.
- Pancreatic tumors can extend into and obstruct the duodenum leading to gastric outlet obstruction.
- Pancreatic body tumors can invade the third or fourth portion of the duodenum and also cause obstruction.
- For lesions that are not amenable to stents, surgical intervention gastrojejunostomy may be required.
- Most patients can be adequately treated with orally or transcutaneously administered analgesics. Narcotic medications may be required. When and if this fails, percutaneous CT guided or endoscopic US guided celiac plexus block may be helpful.

Palliative Surgical Management of Pancreatic Cancer

- Surgical palliation is, for the most part, used for patients who are undergoing laparotomy for anticipated respectable disease and found to be unresectable at the time of surgery. In that situation, biliary tract decompression can be achieved by creating either a cholecystojejunostomy or a choledochojejunostomy.
- Duodenal obstruction can be managed by creation of a side-to-side gastrojejunostomy in which an antecolic jejunal loop is anastomosed to the posterior wall of the gastric antrum. Duodenal obstruction, even in advanced pancreatic cancer, occurs in less than 25% of patients; therefore, considerable controversy surrounds whether a prophylactic gastrojejunostomy should be performed before the development of gastric outlet obstruction.
- Palliation of pain can be achieved, intraoperatively, by injecting alcohol into the celiac plexus, and some surgeons routinely perform operative celiac plexus block at the time of surgical palliation. This is usually accomplished by injecting 15 to 20 mL of 50% ethanol into the celiac plexus on either side of the aorta, and, in one randomized prospective trial, this treatment has been reported to reduce postoperative pain and the need for postoperative analgesics in patients with unresectable pancreatic cancers.

Chemoradiation Therapy

- For the most part, the best results have been achieved using radiotherapy combined with either 5-fluorouricil or gemcitabine.

PANCREATIC AND PANCREATICODUODENAL TRAUMA

- Three percent to 12% of patients with severe abdominal trauma have pancreatic injury. On average, these patients have 3.5 other organs injured and isolated pancreatic injury is uncommon. Roughly two thirds of pancreatic injuries are the result of penetrating trauma and the remaining one third are due to blunt trauma.
- The mortality rate for pancreatic trauma is closely related to the nature of the injury. Thus, the mortality rate associated with blunt trauma is 17% to 19%, whereas, with stab wounds, it is 3% to 5%, with gunshot wounds 15% to 22%, and with shotgun wounds 46% to 56%.

Diagnosis

- Serum amylase levels are elevated in most patients with significant pancreatic trauma, but they are also increased in up to 90% of severe abdominal trauma patients who do not have pancreatic injury.
- On the other hand, a progressive rise in serum amylase activity is a more specific indicator of pancreatic injury. Contrast-enhanced CT, which is increasingly being used as a screening test of patients with major abdominal trauma, is the most useful noninvasive method of evaluating patients with suspected pancreatic injury, but even high-quality CT examinations may be either falsely negative or falsely positive.
- The management of pancreatic injuries will depend on the presence of pancreatic duct disruption, major associated vascular injury, and/or significant injury to peripancreatic organs especially the duodenum. Vascular and duodenal injury can be evaluated at the time of exploratory laparotomy, but the integrity of the pancreatic duct may be difficult to determine at the time of operation unless the pancreas is transected or pancreatic juice is seen to be extravasating from the region of the duct. In the absence of these findings, pancreatography is required to localize or exclude a duct injury.

Management

- The Pancreas Organ Injury Scale developed by the American Association for the Surgery of Trauma can be used to grade pancreatic injuries (Box 52–5). Management of pancreatic injuries is determined by the site and grade of that injury. Grade I injuries that involve minor contusions or lacerations of the gland without duct injury should be treated expectantly. Drainage is usually not needed. On the other hand, grade II injuries, which involve major contusions or lacerations of the gland without duct injury, are traditionally treated by débridement, adequate hemostasis, and placement of sump drains.
- Transection of the neck, body, or tail of the pancreas or parenchymal injury to those areas accompanied by duct injury is considered a grade III injury.

The Classical Treatment of Grade III Injuries Involves Resection of the Pancreas to the Left of the Injury along with Splenectomy

- Because of overwhelming postsplenectomy sepsis, splenic conservation might be considered for children with grade III injuries. When the location of a grade III injury is to the right of the pancreatic neck, the surgeon should consider débriding the site of injury and conserving, rather than resecting, the uninjured body and tail by anastomosing it to a Roux-en-Y jejunal limb.

Box 52–5. Grading and Treatment of Pancreatic Injuries

Grade I: Minor contusion or laceration without duct injury
  Treatment: Observation alone
Grade II: Major contusion or laceration without duct injury
  Treatment: Débridement, drainage, possible repair
Grade III: Distal transection or injury with duct injury
  Treatment: Distal resection, possible Roux-en-Y drainage
Grade IV: Proximal transection or injury involving ampulla

or

Grade V: Massive disruption of the pancreatic head
  Treatment: Damage control, hemostasis/drainage; resection and possible Roux-en-Y drainage; triple-tube decompression; duodenal diverticularization; pancreaticoduodenectomy

---

Adapted from Moore EE, Cogbill TH, Malangoni MA, et al: Organ injury scaling: II. Pancreas, duodenum, small bowel, colon, and rectum. J Trauma 30:1427–1429, 1990.

- Grade IV and grade V injuries present the greatest surgical challenge because they involve the head of the pancreas and, in addition, they also usually involve the adjacent duodenum and/or papilla of Vater. Because of their location, grade IV and grade V injuries are also the ones that are most likely to involve major adjacent vascular structures.
- In unstable patients or in those with major associated injuries, this "damage control" approach may be all that is done at the initial operation and definitive repair may be postponed until the patient's condition has improved.
- Short of radical resection, however, other options designed to divert gastric, pancreatic, and biliary secretions away from the duodenum should be considered for the management of patients with grade IV and V injuries. These include duodenal diverticularization, pyloric exclusion/gastrojejunostomy, and triple-tube decompression. Duodenal diverticularization is accomplished by performing antrectomy and gastrojejunostomy to achieve gastric diversion; choledochostomy to divert bile if the ampulla is injured; tube duodenostomy for decompression of the duodenum; suture repair of any duodenal injuries and extensive periduodenal and peripancreatic drainage. Pyloric exclusion with gastrojejunostomy is a simpler method of protecting the injured duodenum, and it does not permanently alter function.

CHAPTER 53

SPLEEN

SPLENIC ANATOMY

- The visceral relationships of the spleen are with the proximal greater curvature of the stomach, the tail of the pancreas, the left kidney, and the splenic flexure of the colon. The parietal peritoneum adheres firmly to the splenic capsule, except at the splenic hilum. The peritoneum extends superiorly, laterally, and inferiorly, creating folds, which form the suspensory ligaments of the spleen. The splenophrenic and splenocolic ligaments are usually relatively avascular. The splenorenal ligament extends from the anterior left kidney to the hilum of the spleen as a two-layered fold in which the splenic vessels and the tail of the pancreas are invested. These two layers continue anteriorly and superiorly to the greater curvature of the stomach to form the two leaves of the gastrosplenic ligament through which the short gastric arteries and veins course.
- The splenic artery is a tortuous vessel that arises from the celiac trunk; it courses along the superior border of the pancreas. The branches of the splenic artery include the numerous pancreatic branches, the short gastric arteries, the left gastroepiploic artery, and the terminal splenic branches.
- The splenic vein runs inferior to the artery and posterior to the pancreatic tail and body. It receives several short tributaries from the pancreas. The splenic vein joins the superior mesenteric vein at a right angle behind the neck of the pancreas to form the portal vein. The inferior mesenteric vein often empties into the splenic vein; it may also empty into the superior mesenteric vein at or near the confluence of the splenic vein and superior mesenteric vein.

SPLENIC FUNCTION

- The spleen has important hematopoietic functions during early fetal development, with both red and white blood cell production.
- Although the hematopoietic function is usually lost during fetal development, the spleen continues to function as a

sophisticated filter because of the unique circulatory system and lymphoid organization, and it has both blood cell monitoring and management functions and important immune functions throughout life.

- The formed blood elements must pass through slits in the lining of the venous sinuses; if they cannot pass, they are trapped in the spleen and ingested by splenic phagocytes. Experimental animal studies have demonstrated that an intact splenic arterial system is necessary for optimal control of infection. Removal of the spleen results in loss of both the immunologic and filtering functions.

- The most important function of the spleen is probably its mechanical filtration, which removes senescent erythrocytes and likely contributes to control of infection. The spleen is important in clearing circulating pathogens that reside within erythrocytes, for example, malarial parasites, or bacteria such as *Bartonella* species. Mechanical filtration by the spleen may also be important for removal of unopsonized, noningested bacteria from the circulation. It may be particularly important for clearing microorganisms for which the host has no specific antibody.

- Splenic filtering function is important for maintaining normal erythrocyte morphology and function. Normal red blood cells are biconcave and deform relatively easily to facilitate both passages through the microvasculature and optimal oxygen and carbon dioxide exchange. The spleen is an important site for the processing of immature erythrocytes and for repair or destruction of deformed or aged erythrocytes.

- In the asplenic condition, there are several characteristic alterations in the morphologic appearance of the peripheral red blood cells, with the presence of target cells (immature cells), Howell-Jolly bodies (nuclear remnant), Heinz bodies (denatured hemoglobin), Pappenheimer bodies (iron granules), stippling, and spur cells. Aged red blood cells (120 days) that have lost enzymatic activity and membrane plasticity are trapped and destroyed in the spleen (Box 53–1).

- Another major function of the spleen is the maintenance of normal immune function and host defenses against certain types of infectious agents. It is well established that people lacking a spleen are at a significantly higher risk for overwhelming postsplenectomy infection (OPSI) with fulminant bacteremia, pneumonia, or meningitis, as compared with those with normal splenic function. Major pathogens in OPSI are organisms such as *Streptococcus pneumoniae,* in which polysaccharide capsules requiring both antibody and complement are important in host defense against these organisms.

> ## Box 53–1. Biologic Substances Removed by the Spleen
>
> **In Normal Subjects**
> Red blood cell membrane
> Red blood cell surface pits and craters
> Howell-Jolly bodies
> Heinz bodies
> Pappenheimer bodies
> Acanthocytes
> Senescent red blood cells
> Particulate antigen
>
> **In Patients with Disease**
> Spherocytes (hereditary spherocytosis)
> Sickle cells, hemoglobin C cells
> Antibody-coated red blood cells
> Antibody-coated platelets
> Antibody-coated white blood cells

Modified from Eichner ER: Splenic function: Normal, too much and too little.
Am J Med 66:311, 1979.

Asplenic subjects have defective activation of complement by the alternative pathway, leaving them more susceptible to infection.

- The spleen is a major site of production for the opsonins properdin and tuftsin, and removal of the spleen results in decreased serum levels of these factors. Properdin can initiate the alternative pathway of complement activation to produce destruction of bacteria and foreign and abnormal cells. Tuftsin is a tetrapeptide that enhances the phagocytic activity of both polymorphonuclear leukocytes and mononuclear phagocytes.

SPLENECTOMY FOR BENIGN HEMATOLOGIC CONDITIONS

Immune Thrombocytopenic Purpura

- *Immune* thrombocytopenic purpura (ITP) is also referred to as *idiopathic* thrombocytopenic purpura. A low platelet count, a normal bone marrow, and the absence of other causes of thrombocytopenia characterize this disease. ITP is principally a disorder of increased platelet destruction mediated by autoantibodies to platelet membrane antigens that results in platelet phagocytosis by the reticuloendothelial system. Bone marrow megakaryocytes are present in normal or sometimes increased numbers; however, there is relative marrow failure in that the marrow does not increase production sufficiently to compensate for platelet destruction in the spleen. In adults, ITP is more common in young women than men. Seventy-two percent of patients older than 10 years are women, and 70% of affected women are younger than 40 years. In children, ITP is manifested somewhat differently. It affects both sexes equally, and its onset is typically abrupt, with severe thrombocytopenia; however, spontaneous permanent remissions are the rule, occurring in about 80% of affected children. Children who develop the chronic thrombocytopenia are usually girls older than 10 years and present with a longer history of purpura.

● Patients with ITP often present with a history of purpura, epistaxis, and gingival bleeding. Hematuria and gastrointestinal bleeding occur less commonly, and intracerebral hemorrhage is a rare but sometimes fatal event. The diagnosis of ITP requires exclusion of other causes of thrombocytopenia (Box 53–2). Apparent thrombocytopenia may be an artifactual report on a complete blood count because of *in vitro* platelet clumping or the presence of giant platelets. Mild thrombocytopenia may occur in 6% to 8% of otherwise normal pregnant women and in up to one fourth of women with pre-eclampsia. Several drugs are known to induce thrombocytopenia, including heparin, quinidine, quinine, and sulfonamides. Human immunodeficiency virus (HIV) infection and other viral infections may cause thrombocytopenia that may be mistaken for ITP. Other conditions that may be associated with thrombocytopenia include myelodysplasia, congenital thrombocytopenia, thrombotic thrombocytopenic purpura, chronic disseminated intravascular coagulation, autoimmune diseases such as systemic lupus erythematosus, and lymphoproliferative disorders such as chronic lymphocytic leukemia (CLL) and non-Hodgkin's lymphoma (NHL).

● Management of patients with ITP varies according to the severity of the thrombocytopenia. Patients with asymptomatic disease and platelet counts greater than 50,000/mm^3 may simply be followed with no specific treatment. Platelet counts greater than 50,000/mm^3 are seldom associated with spontaneous clinically important bleeding, even with invasive procedures. Patients with platelet counts between 30,000 and 50,000/mm^3 who do not have symptoms may also be observed without treatment; however, careful follow-up is

---

Box 53–2. **Differential Diagnosis of Immune Thrombocytopenic Purpura**

Falsely Low Platelet Count
In vitro platelet clumping caused by ethylenediamine tetra-acetic acid (EDTA)-dependent or cold-dependent agglutinins
Giant platelets

Common Causes of Thrombocytopenia
Pregnancy (gestational thrombocytopenia, preeclampsia)
Drug-induced thrombocytopenia (common drugs include heparin, quinidine, quinine, and sulfonamides)
Viral infections, such as human immunodeficiency virus, rubella, infectious mononucleosis
Hypersplenism due to chronic liver disease

Other Causes of Thrombocytopenia That Have Been Mistaken for Immune Thrombocytopenic Purpura
Myelodysplasia
Congenital thrombocytopenias
Thrombotic thrombocytopenic purpura and hemolytic-uremic syndrome
Chronic disseminated intravascular coagulation

Thrombocytopenia Associated With Other Disorders
Autoimmune diseases, such as systemic lupus erythematosus
Lymphoproliferative disorders (chronic lymphocytic leukemia, non-Hodgkin's lymphoma)

From George JN, El-Harake MA, Raskob GE: Chronic idiopathic thrombocytopenic purpura. N Engl J Med 331:1207–1211, 1994.

essential in these patients because they are at risk for more severe thrombocytopenia. The initial medical treatment is with glucocorticoids, usually prednisone (1 mg/kg body weight per day). About two thirds of patients treated in this manner experience an increase in their platelet count to more than 50,000/mm^3, usually within 1 week of treatment, although it sometimes requires up to 3 weeks. Up to 26% of patients may have a complete response with glucocorticoid therapy. Patients with platelet counts greater than 20,000/mm^3 who are symptom-free, or who have only minor purpura, do not require hospitalization. Treatment of ITP is indicated in patients with platelet counts of less than

20,000 to 30,000/mm^3 or for those with platelet counts of less than 50,000/mm^3 and significant mucus membrane bleeding or risk factors for bleeding, such as hypertension, peptic ulcer disease, or a vigorous lifestyle.

● Although platelet transfusions are necessary for controlling severe hemorrhage, they are seldom indicated in patients with ITP in the absence of severe hemorrhage. Intravenous immunoglobulin is important in the management of acute bleeding and for preparing patients for operation or delivery in the case of pregnancy. The usual dose is 1 g/kg per day for 2 days. This dose increases the platelet count in most patients within 3 days. It also increases the efficacy of transfused platelets. Administration of intravenous immunoglobulin is also appropriate in patients with platelet counts of less than 20,000/mm^3 who are being prepared for splenectomy.

● Splenectomy was the first effective treatment described for ITP and was an established therapeutic modality long before glucocorticoid therapy was introduced in 1950. About two thirds of patients achieve a complete response with normalization of platelet counts after splenectomy and require no further therapy. Splenectomy is indicated in patients with refractory severe symptomatic thrombocytopenia, in patients requiring toxic doses of steroids to achieve remission, and in patients with a relapse of thrombocytopenia after initial glucocorticoid treatment. Splenectomy is an appropriate consideration for patients who have had the diagnosis of ITP for 6 weeks and continue to have a platelet count of less than 10,000/mm^3 whether or not bleeding symptoms are present. Splenectomy is also indicated for patients who have had the diagnosis of ITP for up to 3 months and have experienced a transient or incomplete response to primary therapy and have a platelet count of less than 30,000/mm^3. Splenectomy should be considered for women in the second trimester of pregnancy who have failed glucocorticoid and intravenous immunoglobulin therapy and have platelet counts of less than 10,000/mm^3 or who have platelet counts of less than 30,000/mm^3 and bleeding problems. Splenectomy is probably not indicated in nonbleeding patients who have had a diagnosis of ITP for 6 months, have platelet counts of greater than 50,000/mm^3, and are not engaged in high-risk activities.

● Most patients who respond to splenectomy with increased platelet counts do so within the first 10 days after their operation. Durable platelet responses have been correlated with platelet counts greater than 150,000/mm^3 by the 3rd postoperative day or greater than 500,000/mm^3 on the 10th postoperative day. The immediate response rates among series collected between 1980 and 1998 range from 71% to 95%, with relapse rates of 4% to 12% (Tables 53–1 and 53–2).

- For patients with chronic ITP who fail to achieve complete response after splenectomy, the options range from simple observation in patients with no bleeding symptoms and platelet counts of more than 30,000/mm³ to continued long-term prednisone therapy (Table 53–3). Single-agent treatment with azathioprine or cyclophosphamide may be considered, but response to these agents may require up to 4 months of treatment. Patients who fail to respond to splenectomy or have relapsing disease after an initial response should be investigated for the presence of accessory spleen. Accessory spleen may be found in as many as 10% of these patients.

- About 10% to 20% of otherwise symptom-free patients infected with HIV develop ITP. Splenectomy may be performed safely in this cohort of patients and produces sustained increases in platelet levels in more than 80%. Splenectomy does not increase the risk of progression to acquired immunodeficiency syndrome (AIDS), and a recent cohort study suggested that the absence of a spleen during the asymptomatic phase of HIV infection may delay disease progression.

Hereditary Spherocytosis

- Hereditary spherocytosis is an autosomal dominant disease that results from a deficiency of spectrin, a red blood cell cytoskeletal protein. This protein defect causes a membrane abnormality in the red blood cells resulting in small, spherical, and rigid erythrocytes. These cells have increased osmotic fragility. These spherocytes are more susceptible to becoming trapped in the spleen and destroyed. The clinical features of this disease include anemia, occasionally with jaundice, and splenomegaly. The diagnosis is made by identification of spherocytes on the peripheral blood smear, an increased reticulocyte count, increased osmotic fragility, and a negative Coombs test.

- Splenectomy decreases the rate of hemolysis and usually leads to resolution of the anemia. Splenectomy is usually performed in childhood shortly after diagnosis.

- It is generally recommended that the operation be delayed until after the fourth year of life to preserve immunologic function of the spleen in young children who are most at risk for OPSI. There is a high incidence of pigmented gallstones among patients with spherocytosis, similar to other hemolytic anemias, and ultrasound should be performed before

TABLE 53–1. Hematologic Response after Laparoscopic Treatment of Immune Thrombocytopenia Purpura

Study	Patients (n)	ITP (n)	AS (n [%])	IR (n [%])	RR (n [%])
Cadiere et al, 1994	17	8	2 (11.8)	NA	NA
Emmermann et al, 1995	27	20	2 (7.4)	19 (95.0)	0 at 14 mo
Poulin et al, 1995	22	22	6 (27.2)	NA	NA
Yee and Akpata, 1995	25	14	2 (8.0)	11 (76.0)	NA
Brunt et al, 1996	26	17	3 (11.5)	13 (76.0)	NA
Flowers et al, 1996	43	22	4 (9.3)	18 (82.0)	0 at 21 mo
Gigot et al, 1996	18	16	7 (39.0)	NA	2 (12.5) at 14 mo
Smith et al, 1996	10	8	2 (20.0)	NA	0
Friedman et al, 1997	63	28	11 (17.5)	NA	NA
Park et al, 1997	22	8	2 (9.0)	NA	NA
Tsiotos and Schlinkert, 1997	18	18	1 (5.6)	17 (94.0)	0
Katkhouda et al, 1998	103	67	17 (16.5)	56 (83.6)	4 (6.0) at 38 mo
Total	394	237	59/394 (15.0)	134/158 (85.0)	6/151 (4.0)

AS, total number of patients with accessory spleens; IR, immediate response to immune thrombocytopenic purpura (ITP); NA, data not available; RR, relapse rate in ITP.
From Katkhouda N, Hurwitz MB, Rivera RT, et al: Laparoscopic splenectomy: Outcome and efficacy in 103 consecutive patients. Ann Surg 228:568–578, 1998.

TABLE 53-2. Results in 749 Collected Cases of Open Splenectomy

Study	Patients (n)	Morbidity (n [%])	Mortality (n [%])	ITP (n)	AS (n [%])	IR (n [%])	RR (n [%])
DiFino et al, 1980	37	9 (24.3)	0	37	2 (5.4)	27 (73.0)	9 (24.3)
Mintz et al, 1981	66	13 (14.1)	1 (1.4)	66	20 (28.2)	56 (84.8)	6 (9.0)
Musser et al, 1984	306	118 (24.0)	18 (6.0)	65	58 (19.0)	50 (77.0)	NA
Jacobs et al, 1986	102	15 (14.7)	0	102	NA	95 (93.1)	11 (10.7)
Akwari et al, 1987	100	8 (8.0)	0	100	18 (18.0)	71 (71.0)	4 (4.0)
Julia et al, 1990	138	NA	NA	138	NA	114 (83.0)	23 (17.0)
Total	749	163/611 (26.7)	19/611 (3.1)	508	98/611 (16.0)	413/508 (81.3)	53/443 (12.0)

AS, total number of patients with accessory spleens; ITP, immune thrombocytopenic purpura; IR, immediate response in ITP; NA, data not available; RR, relapse rate in ITP.

From Katkhouda N, Hurwitz MB, Rivera RT, et al: Laparoscopic splenectomy: Outcome and efficacy in 103 consecutive patients. Ann Surg 228:568–578, 1998.

TABLE 53–3. Treatment Options for Patients with Chronic Immune Thrombocytopenic Purpura Unresponsive to Initial Glucocorticoid Therapy and Splenectomy

Intervention	Indication	Outcome
Observation	No bleeding symptoms; platelet count of ≥30,000–50,000/mm³	Platelet count may remain stable, but the risk for more severe thrombocytopenia with serious bleeding is unknown
Prednisone	Symptomatic thrombocytopenia, with bleeding symptoms; platelet count of ≤30,000–50,000/mm³	Goal is a safe platelet count with a minimal dose, such as 10 mg every other day; steroid toxicity is the limiting factor
Azathioprine or cyclophosphamide	Symptomatic thrombocytopenia, with bleeding symptoms; platelet count of ≤30,000–50,000/mm³	Response may require 4 months of treatment; complete recovery may occur in 10%–40% of patients
Other regimens	Symptomatic thrombocytopenia, with bleeding symptoms; platelet count of ≤30,000–50,000/mm³	Some regimens promising in small, preliminary studies; in others, few patients recover completely
Resection of accessory spleen or spleens	Symptomatic thrombocytopenia in a patient who is a good candidate for surgery	Complete recoveries reported in a few patients; symptomatic improvement in some others
Observation (with glucocorticoid of intravenous immune globulin as needed to treat or prevent bleeding)	Unresponsive to treatment	Some patients require frequent supportive therapy; others have minimal symptoms despite severe thrombocytopenia; spontaneous remissions may occur

From George JN, El-Harake MA, Raskob GE: Chronic idiopathic thrombocytopenic purpura. N Engl J Med 331:1207–1211, 1994.

splenectomy. If gallstones are present, it is appropriate to perform cholecystectomy at the time of the splenectomy.

Hemolytic Anemia Resulting from Erythrocyte Enzyme Deficiency

- Glucose-6-phosphate dehydrogenase deficiency and pyruvate kinase deficiency are the two predominant hereditary conditions associated with hemolytic anemia. These deficiencies result in abnormal glucose use and metabolism, leading to increased hemolysis. Pyruvate kinase deficiency is an autosomal recessive condition in which there is decreased red blood cell deformability resulting in increased hemolysis. The spleen is the site of erythrocyte entrapment and destruction in patients with deficiency of pyruvate kinase. These patients often have splenomegaly, and splenectomy has been shown to decrease their transfusion requirements. For the previously mentioned reasons of preserving immunologic function, splenectomy is usually delayed until after 4 years of age in patients with this condition.
- Glucose-6-phosphate dehydrogenase deficiency is an X-linked hereditary condition that is most frequently seen in people of African, Middle Eastern, or Mediterranean ancestry. Hemolytic anemia occurs in most patients after exposure to certain drugs or chemicals. Splenectomy is rarely indicated in patients with glucose-6-phosphate dehydrogenase.

Hemoglobinopathies

- Thalassemia and sickle cell disease are hereditary hemolytic anemias that result from abnormal hemoglobin molecules. This results in abnormal shape of the erythrocyte, which may be subject to splenic sequestration and destruction. Sickle cell anemia is the result of the homozygous inheritance of hemoglobin S.
- Under conditions of reduced oxygen tension, hemoglobin S molecules crystallize within the cell, which results in an elongated, distorted cell with a crescent shape. These altered erythrocytes are rigid and incapable of deforming in microvasculature. This lack of deformation results in capillary occlusion and thrombosis, ultimately leading to microinfarction. This occurs with particular frequency in the spleen. The spleen is enlarged during the first decade of life in most patients with sickle cell disease and then with progressive infarction caused by repeated attacks of vaso-occlusion and infarction, resulting in autosplenectomy. The spleen in patients

with sickle cell disease usually atrophies by adulthood, although splenomegaly may occasionally persist into adult life.

- Thalassemias constitute a group of hemoglobin disorders that also result in hemolytic anemia. Thalassemias are inherited as autosomal dominant traits and occur as a result of a defect in hemoglobin synthesis. This results in variable degrees of hemolytic anemia. Splenic infarction, splenomegaly, and hypersplenism may be predominant features of either sickle cell disease or thalassemia.

- Hypersplenism and acute splenic sequestration are life-threatening disorders in children with sickle cell anemia and thalassemia. In these conditions, there may be rapid splenic enlargement, resulting in severe pain and requiring multiple blood transfusions. In addition to acute splenic sequestration crisis, these patients may suffer from symptomatic massive splenomegaly causing discomfort and interfering with daily activities. Indications for splenectomy in patients with sickle cell disease include acute splenic sequestration crisis, hypersplenism, and splenic abscess.

SPLENECTOMY FOR MALIGNANCY

Lymphomas

Hodgkin's Disease

- Hodgkin's disease is a malignant lymphoma that typically affects young adults in their 20s and 30s. Most patients have asymptomatic lymphadenopathy at the time of diagnosis, and most present with cervical node enlargement.

- The disease is pathologically staged according to the Ann Arbor classification. Stage I represents disease in a single lymphatic site, whereas stage II indicates the presence of disease in two or more lymphatic sites on the same side of the diaphragm. Stage III indicates the presence of lymphatic disease (includes splenic involvement) on both sides of the diaphragm. Stage IV disease is disseminated into extralymphatic sites such as liver, lung, or bone marrow. Subscript E indicates single or contiguous extralymphatic involvement in stages I to III, and subscript S represents splenic involvement. Patients with constitutional symptoms are classified as B (presence) or A (absence), for example, stage IIA or IIB.

- Historically, staging laparotomy including splenectomy provided essential pathologic staging information that was necessary to select appropriate therapy for Hodgkin's disease. The purpose of staging laparotomy is to pathologically stage the presence and extent of disease below the diaphragm.

- Advances in imaging techniques, with widespread availability of dynamic helical computed tomography (CT) scan and lymphangiography and increasing availability of fluorodeoxyglucose positron-emission tomography imaging, have improved nonoperative staging of Hodgkin's disease. The improved nonoperative staging, along with the use of less toxic systemic chemotherapeutics for earlier stages of Hodgkin's disease, has led to a dramatic decrease in the numbers of patients requiring staging laparotomy. Patients at high risk for relapse, especially those with B symptoms and those with evidence of intra-abdominal involvement on one or more of the diagnostic imaging studies, require systemic chemotherapy and should not undergo a staging laparotomy. Staging laparotomy and splenectomy are appropriate for selected patients with an early clinical stage of disease (stage IA or IIA) in whom pathologic staging of the abdomen will significantly influence the therapeutic management.

Non-Hodgkin's Lymphomas

- Splenomegaly or hypersplenism is a common occurrence during the course of NHL. Splenectomy is indicated for patients with NHL for treatment of massive splenomegaly when the bulk of the spleen contributes to abdominal pain, fullness, and early satiety. Splenectomy may also be effective in the treatment of patients who develop hypersplenism with associated anemia, thrombocytopenia, and neutropenia.
- Splenectomy occasionally plays an important role in the diagnosis and staging of patients who present with isolated splenic disease. The most common primary splenic neoplasm is NHL. The spleen is involved in 50% to 80% of NHL patients, but fewer than 1% of patients present with splenomegaly without peripheral lymphadenopathy.
- For those patients with low-grade NHL who had spleen-predominant features, survival was significantly improved after splenectomy (median, 108 months) as compared with patients receiving similar treatment without splenectomy (median, 24 months).

Leukemia

Hairy Cell Leukemia

- Hairy cell leukemia is a rare disease that represents about 2% of adult leukemias. Splenomegaly, pancytopenia, and neoplastic mononuclear cells in the peripheral blood and bone marrow characterize the disease. The hairy cells are usually B lymphocytes that have cell membrane ruffling, which appears as cytoplasmic projections under the light microscope. The patients are usually elderly men with palpable splenomegaly. About 10% of cases have an indolent course requiring no specific therapy, but most require therapy for cytopenias such as symptomatic anemia, infectious complications from neutropenia, or hemorrhage from thrombocytopenia.

- Splenectomy and alpha$_2$ interferon have been the standard treatment of hairy cell leukemia until recently; this approach is being replaced with systemic administration of purine analogues, such as 2-chlorodeoxyadenosine and deoxycoformycin, as initial treatment. Splenectomy is still indicated for some patients with massive enlargement of the spleen or with evidence of hypersplenism that is refractory to medical therapy. Splenectomy provides a highly effective and sustained palliation of these problems, and most patients show definite hematologic improvement after the procedure. About 40% of patients experience normalization of their blood counts after splenectomy. The responses to splenectomy usually last for 10 or more years, and about half of patients will require no further therapy. Patients with diffusely involved bone marrow who do not have significant splenomegaly are far less likely to achieve a significant benefit from splenectomy. The current 4-year survival rate after diagnosis of hairy cell leukemia is about 80%, as compared with 60% for patients diagnosed in the 1970s.

Chronic Lymphocytic Leukemia

- CLL is a B-cell leukemia that is characterized by the progressive accumulation of relatively mature, but functionally incompetent, lymphocytes. CLL occurs more frequently in men and usually occurs after 50 years of age. Staging of CLL is according to the Rai staging system, which correlates well with prognosis. Stage 0 includes bone marrow and blood lymphocytosis only; stage I includes lymphocytosis and enlarged lymph nodes; stage II includes lymphocytosis and enlarged spleen, liver, or both; stage III includes lymphocytosis and anemia; and stage IV includes lymphocytosis with thrombocytopenia. Chlorambucil has long been the mainstay of medical therapy and was useful for the palliation of symptoms; however, there is increasing interest in using purine analogues, such as fludarabine, as first-line therapy, with some studies showing improved rates of remission. Bone marrow transplantation has also become increasingly used in the treatment of CLL, and both allotransplantation and autotransplantation approaches are being investigated.

● The role of splenectomy in the treatment of CLL continues to be for palliation of symptomatic splenomegaly and for treatment of cytopenia related to hypersplenism. Relief of bulk symptoms from splenomegaly is virtually always successful, whereas the hematologic response rates for correction of anemia and thrombocytopenia are between 60% and 70%.

Chronic Myelogenous Leukemia

● Chronic myelogenous leukemia (CML) is a myeloproliferative disorder that results from neoplastic transformation of myeloid elements.

● CML may occur from childhood to old age. CML usually presents with an indolent or chronic phase that is asymptomatic. Progression to the accelerated phase is marked by the onset of symptoms such as fever, night sweats, and progressive splenomegaly; however, this phase may also be asymptomatic and detectable only from changes in the peripheral blood or bone marrow. The accelerated phase may give rise to the blastic phase, which is characterized by the previously listed symptoms as well as anemia, infectious complications, and bleeding. Splenomegaly with splenic sequestration of blood elements often contributes to these symptoms.

● Treatment of CML is primarily medical and may include hydroxyurea, interferon-alfa, and high-dose chemotherapy with bone marrow transplantation. Symptomatic splenomegaly and hypersplenism in patients with CML may be effectively palliated by splenectomy. Otherwise, the role of splenectomy in the treatment of CML has been controversial. Randomized studies of patients with CML have demonstrated no survival benefit when splenectomy is performed during the early chronic phase. Splenectomy has also not resulted in a survival benefit when performed before allogeneic bone marrow transplantation. Thus, splenectomy before allogeneic bone marrow transplantation is recommended only for patients with significant splenomegaly.

Nonhematologic Tumors of the Spleen

● The spleen is a site of metastatic tumor in up to 7% of autopsies of cancer patients. The primary solid tumors that most frequently metastasize to the spleen are carcinomas of the breast, lung, and melanoma; however, virtually any primary malignancy may metastasize to the spleen. Metastases to the spleen are often asymptomatic but may be associated with symptomatic splenomegaly or even spontaneous splenic rupture. Splenectomy may provide effective palliation in carefully selected symptomatic patients with splenic metastasis.

- Vascular neoplasms are the most common primary splenic tumors that include both benign and malignant variants. Hemangiomas are usually incidental findings identified in spleens removed for other reasons. Angiosarcomas (or hemangiosarcomas) of the spleen have been associated with environmental exposure to thorium dioxide or monomeric vinyl chloride, but they most often occur spontaneously. Patients with these tumors may present with splenomegaly, hemolytic anemia, ascites, and pleural effusions or spontaneous splenic rupture. These are highly aggressive tumors that have a poor prognosis.

- Lymphangiomas are usually benign endothelium-lined cysts that may become symptomatic by causing splenomegaly. Lymphangiosarcoma within a cystic lymphangioma has been reported. Splenectomy is appropriate for diagnosis, treatment, or palliation of the conditions cited previously.

SPLENECTOMY FOR MISCELLANEOUS BENIGN CONDITIONS

Splenic Cysts

- Cystic lesions of the spleen have been recognized with increasing frequency since the advent of CT scanning and ultrasound imaging. Splenic cysts are classified as true cysts, which may be either nonparasitic or parasitic, and pseudocysts. Cystic-appearing tumors of the spleen include cystic lymphangiomas and cavernous hemangiomas, as discussed previously. Primary true cysts of the spleen account for about 10% of all nonparasitic cysts of the spleen. Most nonparasitic cysts are pseudocysts and are secondary to trauma. The diagnosis of true splenic cysts is commonly made in the second and third decades of life. True cysts are characterized by a squamous epithelial lining, and many are considered congenital. These epithelial cells are often positive for CA 19-9 and carcinoembryonic antigen by immunohistochemistry, and patients with epidermoid cysts of the spleen may have elevated serum levels of one or both of these tumor-associated antigens. Despite the presence of these tumor markers, these cysts are benign and apparently do not have malignant potential greater than any other native tissue.

- Often, true splenic cysts are asymptomatic and found incidentally. When symptomatic, patients may complain of vague upper abdominal fullness and discomfort, early satiety, pleuritic chest pain, shortness of breath, left back or shoulder pain, or renal symptoms from compression of the left kidney. A palpable abdominal mass may be present. The presence of symptoms is often related to the size of the cysts, and cysts smaller than 8 cm are rarely symptomatic. Rarely, these cysts may present with acute symptoms related to rupture, hemorrhage, or infection. The diagnosis of splenic cysts is best made with CT imaging. Operative intervention is indicated for symptomatic cysts and for large cysts. Either total or partial splenectomy may provide successful treatment. The clear advantage of partial splenectomy is the preservation of splenic function. Preservation of at least 25% of the spleen appears sufficient to protect against pneumococcal pneumonia.

- Most true splenic cysts are parasitic cysts in areas of endemic hydatid disease (*Echinococcus* species). Radiographic imaging may reveal cyst wall calcifications or daughter cysts.

- Splenectomy is the treatment of choice, and great care should be taken to avoid rupture of the cysts intraoperatively. The cysts may be sterilized by injection of a 3% sodium chloride solution, alcohol, or 0.5% silver nitrate, as has been recommended for hydatid cysts of the liver.

- Pseudocysts account for 70% to 80% of all nonparasitic cysts of the spleen. A history of prior trauma can usually be elicited. Splenic pseudocysts are not epithelial lined. Radiographic imaging may demonstrate focal calcifications in up to half of cases. Most splenic pseudocysts are unilocular, and the cysts are smooth and thick-walled. Small asymptomatic splenic pseudocysts (less than 4 cm) do not require treatment and may undergo involution over time. When the pseudocysts are symptomatic, patients often present with left upper quadrant and referred left shoulder pain. Symptomatic pseudocysts should be treated surgically. If the spleen can be safely and completely mobilized and partial splenectomy accomplished to include the cystic portion of the spleen, this technique offers effective therapy that preserves splenic function. Presented with less favorable conditions, the surgeon should not hesitate to perform total splenectomy. Successful percutaneous drainage has also been reported for splenic pseudocysts although the success rate with this approach as compared with surgical intervention has not been determined. The 90% success rate of image-guided percutaneous drainage of unilocular splenic abscesses suggests that this may be a reasonable initial approach for the management of symptomatic splenic pseudocysts.

Splenic Abscess

- Splenic abscess is an uncommon and potentially fatal illness. The incidence in autopsy series approximates 0.7%. The mortality for splenic abscess ranges from about 80% for multiple abscesses in immunocompromised patients to about 15% to 20% in previously healthy patients with solitary unilocular lesions. Predisposing illnesses include malignancies, polycythemia vera, endocarditis, previous trauma, hemoglobinopathy (e.g., sickle cell disease), urinary tract infection, intravenous drug abuse, and AIDS. About 70% of splenic abscesses result from hematogenous spread of the infecting organism from another location, as occurs with endocarditis, osteomyelitis, and intravenous drug abuse.
- The clinical presentation of splenic abscess is often nonspecific and insidious, including abdominal pain, fever, peritonitis, and pleuritic chest pain. The abdominal pain is localized in the left upper quadrant less than half the time and is more often vague abdominal pain. Splenomegaly is present in a minority of patients. The diagnosis is made most accurately by CT; however, it may also be made with ultrasonography. Two thirds of splenic abscesses in adults are solitary, and the remaining one third are multiple. These ratios are reversed in children.
- Unilocular abscesses are amenable to CT-guided drainage, and this approach, along with systemic antibiotic administration, has a success rate that is in excess of 75% (and the success rate may be as high as 90% when only patients with unilocular collections are considered). Failure of a prompt clinical response to percutaneous drainage should lead to splenectomy without delay. Multilocular abscesses should usually be treated by splenectomy, with drainage of the left upper quadrant and antibiotic administration.

The Wandering Spleen

- Wandering spleen is a rare finding, accounting for only a fraction of a percent of all splenectomies.
- Wandering spleen is most often diagnosed in children or women between the ages of 20 and 40 years.
- Most patients with wandering spleen are asymptomatic. Symptomatic patients often present with recurrent episodes

of abdominal pain. This is likely related to tension on the vascular pedicle or intermittent torsion. Torsion of the splenic vessels may lead to venous congestion and splenomegaly. Severe and persistent pain is suggestive of splenic torsion and ischemia. On examination, a mobile abdominal mass may be present along with abdominal tenderness. The diagnosis may be most readily confirmed with a CT scan of the abdomen. The typical finding is the absence of a spleen in its normal position and the presence of a spleen in an ectopic location. Intravenous contrast injection during the CT scan provides valuable information. Lack of contrast enhancement of the spleen suggests splenic torsion, as does a whorled appearance to the splenic pedicle. Lack of splenic perfusion on the CT scan may be helpful in guiding the operative decision for splenectomy versus splenopexy.

SPLENIC TRAUMA

General Considerations

- Injury to the spleen is the most common indication for laparotomy after blunt mechanisms of injury. Motor vehicular crashes continue to be the major source of injury in industrialized nations.
- Splenic injuries are produced by rapid deceleration, compression, energy transmission through the posterolateral chest wall over the spleen, or puncture from an adjacent rib fracture. Rapid deceleration results in the spleen continuing in a forward motion while being tethered at the point of attachment. Injuries produced by deceleration forces result in capsular avulsion along the various ligamentous attachments and linear or stellate fractures of varying depths. Because of its solid structural characteristics and density, energy transfer to the spleen is relatively efficient. Injuries caused by assaults or falls are usually a result of direct blows over the lower chest wall, with transmission of energy resulting in splenic lacerations and fractures.

Diagnosis

- The history and physical examination continue to be the basis from which splenic injury should be diagnosed.
- On physical examination, evidence of peritoneal irritation (tenderness, guarding, rebound) is sometimes apparent. Recently extravasated blood, however, is a fairly benign

peritoneal irritant, and large amounts of blood may be contained in the free peritoneal cavity with minimal physical findings.

● Significant injury producing hemorrhage is indicated by the hemodynamic status of the patient. Hypotension or tachycardia should alert the clinician to the potential for splenic injury. At the initial trauma assessment, apparent injuries that may yield enough blood loss individually or in aggregate to produce physiologic changes in hemodynamics should be noted. If blood loss from long bone or pelvic fractures or from external losses from lacerations cannot be attributed, an intra-abdominal source must be assumed, and the spleen is the most common source.

Diagnostic Peritoneal Lavage (DPL)

● DPL was introduced by Root and colleagues in 1965. That modality remained the standard diagnostic procedure for blunt abdominal trauma evaluations for the subsequent 20 years. Initially, results were interpreted from a grossly positive examination or from quantification of red and white blood cells in the large effluent. A positive DPL consisted of either 10 mL of gross blood aspirated with catheter insertion or a microscopically positive examination. For microscopic examination in adults, 1 L of crystalloid solution is instilled through a periumbilical catheter inserted by either open or closed technique. Assuming complete instillation of the liter, positive examinations consisted of a red blood cell count higher than $100,000/mm^3$ or a white blood cell count higher than $500/mm^3$ in the completely mixed effluent. The dilution factor that produces a red blood cell count of more than $100,000/mm^3$ accounts for about 30 to 40 mL of blood in the peritoneal cavity. A microscopically positive examination by white blood cell count criteria is indicative of peritoneal inflammation generally produced by hollow viscus injury.

● After the introduction of DPL, multiple investigators demonstrated sensitivities approaching 99% and specificities in the range of 95% to 98%.

● As CT began to be applied for trauma diagnostics, it was observed that small splenic injuries had occurred and that the patient remained hemodynamically stable. It was further noted that enough blood was present to have caused a positive lavage. Coincident with that development was the observation by surgeons that many of the positive DPL procedures led to laparotomies in which there was indeed a splenic injury but often of a relatively trivial nature without active bleeding. Based on these parallel observations, the term *nontherapeutic laparotomy* began surfacing in the splenic injury literature, and it began to be appreciated that DPL was perhaps too sensitive.

Computed Tomography

- The early incidental CT observations of damaged spleens in stable patients ushered in the era of nonoperative management.
- The anatomic definition of injury provided objective criteria for classification of degrees of splenic injury. The American Association for the Surgery of Trauma developed a splenic injury grading scale through a consensus methodology (Table 53–4).

Ultrasound

- During the 1990s, ultrasound was introduced and firmly established as an important diagnostic tool for evaluating blunt abdominal trauma.
- The acronym FAST (focused abdominal sonogram for trauma) has been applied to this quick survey, which takes about 3 minutes to complete in experienced hands. Significant bowel distention, obesity, and subcutaneous emphysema compromise the examination. Initial concerns were with the sensitivity and reproducibility of FAST.
- Tso and colleagues reported in 1992 on 163 stable patients evaluated by ultrasound before either DPL or CT and found a 91% sensitivity, with all cases of clinically significant hemoperitoneum being identified.
- The reported data would suggest that with a structured training format, FAST can be expeditiously taught to practicing surgeons.
- Ultrasound has emerged as a replacement for DPL. It appears to be as sensitive in detecting free intraperitoneal blood and is less invasive and quicker. The most important application is in evaluating the hemodynamically unstable patient with multiple injuries. A positive ultrasound would generally mandate expeditious exploratory laparotomy. The place for ultrasound use in the stable patient has been less clear. As nonoperative management has become so prominent, CT has become indispensable in defining the location and degree of organ injury. Ultrasound is not capable of accurately defining those anatomic characteristics.

TABLE 53–4. American Association for the Surgery of Trauma Splenic Injury Scale (1994 Revision)

Grade	Type	Injury Description
I	Hematoma	Subcapsular, <10% surface area
	Laceration	Capsular tear, <1-cm parenchymal depth
II	Hematoma	Subcapsular, 10%–50% surface area; intraparenchymal, <5 cm in diameter
	Laceration	1–3 cm parenchymal depth, which does not involve a trabecular vessel
III	Hematoma	Subcapsular, >50% surface area or expanding; ruptured subcapsular or parenchymal hematoma
		Intraparenchymal hematoma >5 cm or expanding
	Laceration	>3 cm parenchymal depth or involving trabecular vessels
IV	Laceration	Laceration involving segmental or hilar vessels producing major devascularization (>25% of spleen)
	Vascular	Hilar vascular injury that devascularizes spleen

Adapted from Moore EE, Cogbill TH, Jurkovich GJ, et al: Organ injury scaling: Spleen and liver (1994 revision). J Trauma 38:323, 1995.

Issues Concerning Operation

Indications for Exploration

- The clearest indication for urgent operation is hemodynamic instability.
- Because there can be no *standard* criteria for hemodynamic instability, a general guideline is to operate for a systolic blood pressure below 90 mm Hg or a pulse of more than 120 beats/minute if there is not immediate response to 1 to 2 L of crystalloid resuscitation and when physical examination, ultrasound, or DPL indicates intra-abdominal blood loss. Indications for operation based on CT findings are delineated in a subsequent section of this chapter on nonoperative management.

Technical Issues

- A midline incision is usually preferred for trauma exploration. This approach is expeditious and provides access to all areas of the abdominal cavity, including the retroperitoneum. A left subcostal approach may be preferred when laparotomy is directed by CT findings. The small bowel and lesser sac are easily evaluated from this incision.
- After rapid evacuation of free blood and clots to assess other sources of injury, including the liver and mesentery, the spleen should be mobilized into the wound. Splenic mobilization should be accomplished by the fundamental operative principle of traction and countertraction. In the case of splenic mobilization, traction and countertraction are based on the spleen and its suspensory ligaments.
- The incision begins at the phrenocolic ligament, continuing through the ligaments to the stomach near the highest short gastric vessels. Division should occur 1 to 2 cm from the spleen to avoid injury to both spleen and diaphragmatic muscle. Continued tension on the tissues allows gradual mobilization anterior to the spleen as deeper layers of filmy connective tissue planes are placed under tension and easily visualized and divided. The dissection should progress such that the left adrenal gland is visualized and left undisturbed in its posterior location. As this dissection progresses through these thin connective tissue planes, the posterior surface of the pancreas and the splenic vein densely adherent to the pancreas are visualized.
- Laparotomy pads are placed in the left upper quadrant to maintain the spleen in the wound.

- Splenectomy is usually indicated under the following circumstances: (1) the patient is unstable, (2) other injuries require prompt attention, (3) the spleen is extensively injured with continuous bleeding, and (4) bleeding is associated with hilar injury.

- As noted earlier in this chapter, thrombocytosis occurs in about half of postoperative patients in the initial weeks after splenectomy. The thrombocytosis may increase the risk for deep vein thrombosis. When the platelet count rises above $750,000/mm^3$, many surgeons treat the patient with antiplatelet therapy, low-dose heparin, or low-molecular-weight heparin. Pimpl and colleagues reviewed 37,000 autopsies over 20 years of adults who died after splenectomy and compared them with a deceased population of 403 who did not have splenectomy. These investigators found higher incidence rates of lethal pneumonia, sepsis with multiple organ failure, purulent pyelonephritis, and pulmonary embolism in the splenectomy group. They concluded that splenectomy carries a considerable lifelong risk for severe infection and thromboembolism.

Splenorrhaphy

- Splenorrhaphy was applied to nearly half of splenic injuries at the height of its use. A general rule is that if more than one unit of blood is required for salvage, splenectomy should be performed. Beyond that, the risks associated with transfusion generally outweigh the risks of OPSI. Four types of splenorrhaphy have been used: (1) superficial hemostatic agents (cautery, oxidized cellulose, absorbable gelatin sponge, topical thrombin), (2) suture repair, (3) absorbable mesh wrap, and (4) resectional débridement.

- Superficial hemostatic approaches are useful for American Association for the Surgery of Trauma grades I and II injuries (see Table 53–4). They may also be adjunctive in higher grades of injury. The argon-beam coagulator has received some support, but there is no clinical evidence that it is superior to other approaches.

- Suture repair of lacerations in grades II and III injuries has become common. When feasible, temporary occlusion of the splenic artery may reduce blood loss and facilitate repair. A problem with suture repair is the tendency for the sutures to tear the spleen further when tied. Pledgeted repairs reduce that occurrence. Many surgeons have used Teflon pledgets. The use of pledgets constructed of 2- to 3-cm absorbable gelatin sponge wrapped in oxidized cellulose and secured with suture ties to resemble a cigarette has been commonly applied.

- Mesh wrapping has been effectively used for grade III and some grade IV injuries. Investigators from Cook County Hospital provided some of the earliest data and description of this technique. Disposable mesh, composed of either polyglycolic acid or polyglactin, has been used. If knitted mesh is used, a keyhole about 1 to 2 cm in diameter is cut in the middle of the mesh and is stretched, so that the spleen can be delivered through it, resulting in the keyhole around the splenic hilum. The edges of the mesh are then approximated with a running suture over the top, so that the spleen is effectively enclosed in a mesh sac. If woven mesh is used, it will not stretch; thus, the keyhole for surrounding the hilum is designed by dividing one side of a square piece of mesh to the center and constructing an appropriately sized circular hole. The mesh is tightened around the hilum by reapproximating the severed mesh. The mesh is secured over the top of the spleen as described previously.
- Resectional débridement has been applied for major fractures, usually involving the upper or lower pole (grade II or IV). The raw surfaces are approximated. Pledgeted materials are of considerable benefit for reapproximating those edges. At least one third of the splenic mass is necessary to maintain immunocompetence.
- Most patients who currently undergo operation for splenic injury have active bleeding or destructive injuries requiring splenectomy. Heightened awareness of risk for transmission of viral disease, especially hepatitis, with blood transfusion has also dampened enthusiasm for splenic repair.

Nonoperative Management

- Currently, 70% to 90% of children with splenic injury are successfully treated without operation, and 40% to 50% of adult patients with splenic injury are managed nonoperatively in large-volume trauma centers. The lower percentage of nonoperatively managed splenic injury in adults than in children has been a source of speculation. It has been suggested that anatomic differences between adults and children are responsible, including a more elastic, cartilaginous rib cage providing protection and more elastin in the spleen producing contraction and some degree of hemostasis in children. Powell and colleagues, however, have produced data demonstrating that the differences in management of splenic injury between adults and children are most likely related to mechanisms of injury.

- A fundamental rule for consideration of nonoperative management is the requirement that the patient be hemodynamically stable. In addition, institutional resources should be such that the patient can be monitored in a critical care environment and that operating room facilities and personnel are available in the event of sudden bleeding that requires splenectomy. Most grade I and grade II injuries can be managed nonoperatively; these account for about 60% to 70% of cases of nonoperative management.

- Analysis of failure rates is important in evaluating criteria for selecting appropriate patients for nonoperative management. Although age greater than 55 years has been reported to be associated with high failure rates, others have refuted that observation. Nonoperative management failure rates from recent series are shown in Table 53–5.

- An important finding that has been correlated with failed nonoperative management is the presence of a vascular blush on CT examination. Schurr and associates reported on 309 blunt splenic injuries, of which 29% were managed nonoperatively. They noted a 13% failure rate; two thirds of the failures were associated with a vascular blush. Those vascular blushes were proved to represent false aneurysms of intraparenchymal branches of the splenic artery. The cause of failure from false aneurysms is gradual enlargement of the aneurysm, with rupture of the aneurysm and spleen. This pathophysiology most likely accounts for many of the instances of "delayed splenic rupture" noted from the past.

- Controversy exists concerning the need for follow-up CT evaluations. Some institutions have suggested that follow-up scans are unnecessary. Davis and colleagues, however, noted that 74% of vascular blushes were seen only in follow-up studies. Because a high rate of failure was noted with the finding, these investigators recommend follow-up scans within 2 to 3 days for all but the most trivial lesions. The reasons for absence of vascular blush on initial scans include missed 1-cm cut protocol and lysis of initial clot.

Evidence-Based Medicine Evaluation

- The Agency for Health Care Policy and Research has also developed a system of assessing confidence levels for recommendations based on that data classification system, which is presented in Box 53–3.

TABLE 53–5. Comparison of Results of Nonoperative Management of Blunt Splenic Injuries from Published Series

Study	Splenic Injuries (n)	Cases Planned		
		Nonoperatively Managed (%)	Nonoperative Success (%)	Failure (%)
Shackford and Molin, 1990	1866	13	69	31
Schurr et al, 1995	309	25	87	13
Smith et al, 1996	166	47	97	3
Morrell et al, 1996	135	18	52	48
Davis et al, 1998	524	61	94	6
Myers et al, 1999	204	68	93	7
Cocanour et al, 1999	368	57	86	14
Bee et al, 2001	558	77	92	8

*Excluded grade IV and V injuries.

**Box 53–3. Categorization of Strengths of
Recommendations Based on a Medical
Literature Review of a Specified Topic***
**According to Methodologies Derived
from the Agency for Health Care Policy
and Research**

Level 1
This recommendation is convincingly justifiable based on the
available scientific information alone. It is usually based on
class I data; however, strong class II evidence may from
the basis for a level 1 recommendation, especially if the
issue does not lend itself to testing in a randomized
format. Conversely, weak or contradictory class I data may
not be able to support a level 1 recommendation.

Level 2
This recommendation is reasonably justifiable by available
scientific evidence and strongly supported by expert
critical care opinion. It is usually supported by class II data
or a preponderance of class III evidence.

Level 3
This recommendation is supported by available data, but
adequate scientific evidence is lacking. It is generally
supported by class III data. This type of recommendation
is useful for educational purposes and in guiding future
studies.

*See Table 54–1.

- To develop the guidelines for splenic injury, a study group
  consisting of seven surgeons identified 50 English-language
  clinical articles published between 1976 and 1996 addressing
  pertinent questions about blunt splenic injury management.
  The recommendations based on the classification and assessment of those published data are listed in Box 53–4.

ELECTIVE LAPAROSCOPIC SPLENECTOMY

- The technique of laparoscopic splenectomy was first described
  in 1992. In experienced hands, laparoscopic splenectomy can
  be performed as safely and effectively as open splenectomy,
  particularly for hematologic diseases in which the spleen
  size is normal or only slightly enlarged.

> **Box 53–4. Eastern Association for the Surgery of Trauma* Recommended Patient Management Guidelines for the Nonoperative Management (NOM) of Blunt Injuries to the Liver and the Spleen**
>
> **Level I**
> There are insufficient data to suggest NOM as a level I recommendation for the initial management of blunt injuries to the liver and/or spleen in the hemodynamically stable patient.
>
> **Level II**
> 1. There are class II and mostly class III data to suggest that NOM of blunt hepatic and/or splenic injuries in a hemodynamically stable patient is reasonable.
> 2. Severity of hepatic or splenic injury (as suggested by CT grade or degree of hemoperitoneum), neurologic status, and/or the presence of associated injuries are not contraindications to NOM.
> 3. Abdominal CT is the most reliable method to identify and assess the severity of the injury to the spleen or liver.
>
> **Level III**
> 1. The clinical status of the patient should dictate the frequency of follow-up scans.
> 2. Initial CT of the abdomen should be performed with oral and intravenous contrast agents to facilitate the diagnosis of hollow-viscus injuries.
> 3. Medical clearance to resume normal activity status should be based on evidence of healing.
> 4. Angiographic embolization is an adjunct in the NOM of the hemodynamically stable patient with hepatic and splenic injuries and evidence of ongoing bleeding.

*See their website at *www.east.org*.
CT, computed tomography.

● Results of laparoscopic splenectomy for benign hematologic diseases, such as ITP, should be compared with the standard of open splenectomy, which is technically feasible in 100% of patients and is associated with a hospital mortality rate of less than 1% and a morbidity rate of 10% to 20%. In a retrospective literature review of 1358 patients who underwent open splenectomy, the rate of wound-related complications was estimated to be 3%. The mean postoperative hospital stay ranged from 7.5 to 11 days. In patients with splenomegaly secondary to malignant hematologic disorders, however, the operative mortality rates are increased in the range of 0% to 18% and morbidity rates are increased in the range of 19% to 56%, respectively.

- In comparison, laparoscopic splenectomy can be completed in about 90% of properly selected patients. The incidence of conversion to open splenectomy is between 0% and 20%. Most of the conversions are caused by intraoperative bleeding, but lack of surgical experience, extensive adhesions, large splenomegaly, and obesity are also involved.

- Yee and colleagues' and Glasgow and associates' experience reported a conversion rate of 36% during the initial 11 laparoscopic splenectomies; during the subsequent operations, the conversion rate dropped to 0% to 5%.

- In two reviews of laparoscopic series that included 418 and 948 patients, respectively, the mean operative time for laparoscopic splenectomy ranged from 88 to 261 minutes, with an open conversion rate ranging from 0% to 30% (Table 53–6). In a multivariate analysis by Friedman and coworkers, operative time was significantly related to patient age, hematologic diagnosis, operative technique, and splenic weight. The perioperative morbidity rates averaged 8% and 12%, respectively (range 0% to 30%), and the mortality rate was 0.7% (0% to 6%). Most deaths were attributable to the patient's underlying diseases or hematologic disorder. In the review by Gigot and associates of 984 patients, 119 had reported complications. Bleeding was the most frequent perioperative complication and has been significantly linked to the surgeon's learning curve. The mean number of patients requiring intraoperative or postoperative transfusions was 13%, ranging from 0% to 40%. Local complications, including wound-related complication (seroma, hematoma, infection, evisceration, or incisional hernia) occurred in 1.5%. Postoperative bleeding occurred in 1% of patients, and 73% of these cases required re-exploration. Pancreatic complications (pancreatitis or pancreatic fistula) occurred in 0.6% and subphrenic abscess in 0.5%. General postoperative complications occurred in 7.4%; most (3.2%) were pleuropulmonary.

- Postoperative recovery after laparoscopic splenectomy is surprisingly fast, as has previously been observed with laparoscopic cholecystectomy. The length of stay ranged from 1.8 to 6 days after laparoscopic splenectomy. Most patients are able to return to full activities within 1 week if their underlying hematologic disorder allows. In Flowers'

TABLE 53–6. Retrospective Case-Control Series Comparing Open and Laparoscopic Splenectomies in Adults

	Yee et al, 1995		Rhodes et al, 1995		Brunt et al, 1996		Watson et al, 1997		Diaz et al, 1997		Friedman et al, 1997		Delaitre & Pitre, 1997		Smith et al, 1996		Glasgow et al, 1997		Hashizume et al, 1996	
	OS	LS	OS	LS	OS	LS	OS	LS	OS	LS	OS	LS	OS	LS	OS	LS	OS	LS	OS	LS
Patients	25	25	11	24	20	26	47	13	15	15	74	63	28	28	10	10	28	52	41	10
Operative time (min)	156	198†	75	120	134	202‡	84	88	116	196‡	121	153	127	183*	131	261*	156	196‡	249	100‡
Delay before regular diet (days)	4.3	2.1†	—	—	4.1	1.4‡	—	—	—	—	3.2	1.5*	—	—	4.4	1.9*	4.3	2	—	—
Blood loss (mL)	273	319	—	—	222	376	—	—	359	385	437	259	—	—	—	—	274	320	512	176*
Transfusion rate	12	16	—	—	15	10	13	0	—	—	27	3.5	36	29	20	40	18	27	—	—
Complications (%)	12	8	8	27	23	23	19	0	13	6.7	22	12	32	11	20	20	14	10	46	0
POHS	6.7	5.1*	7	3‡	5.8	2.5‡	10	2‡	8.8	2.3‡	6.7	3.5*	8.6	5.1*	5.8	3*	6.7	4.8*	20	8.2
Total hospital costs USD × 10³	13,433	9207	—	—	—	—	4224	2238	16,362	18,015	10,900	9700*	—	—	13,196	17,071	17,876	20,295	9264	6438‡
Cure rate at FU in ITP (%)	76	81	—	—	75	75	83	92	75	80	—	—	86	93	—	81	81	74	63	80
Mean FU (mo)	24	8	—	—	6.5	6.5	60	14	20	29	13.5	19	—	—	30	21	21	16	—	—
As detected (%)	—	—	—	—	5	5	6	15	23	12*	—	—	18	11	—	—	—	—	—	—
Return to full activity (days)	—	—	—	—	—	—	—	—	—	—	—	—	—	—	6 wk	1–2 wk	—	—	—	—

FU, follow-up; ITP, immune thrombocytopenic purpura; LS, laparoscopic splenectomy; OS, open splenectomy; POHS, postoperative hospital stay; USD, U.S. dollars.

*p < .05.
†p < .001.
‡p = .0005.

From Gigot JF, Lengele B, Gianello P, et al: Present status of laparoscopic splenectomy for hematologic diseases: Certitudes and unresolved issues. Semin Laparosc Surg 5:159, 1998.

study, 9% of patients returned to work in 7 days, and all patients with uncomplicated laparoscopic splenectomy were fully recovered by 21 days regardless of profession. Although a prospective, randomized comparison has not been conducted, several retrospective case-control series have compared the laparoscopic approach to an open splenectomy (see Table 53–6).

- Open splenectomy for the treatment of ITP achieves a long-term cure rate of 65% to 90%. In clinical series of laparoscopic splenectomy, the mean follow-up is usually limited to 1 to 2 years. During this short follow-up, reports of 76% to 100% success rates have been published. Similarly, Katkhouda and associates reported that the treatment of ITP appears to be at least as good after laparoscopic surgery as after the open technique in comparisons of separate series (see Tables 53–1 and 53–2). Gigot and colleagues reported on 279 patients with ITP in which an absence of initial response and/or recurrent thrombocytopenia occurred in approximately 15% (Table 53–7).

- The causes of recurrence in patients with ITP are multifactorial, but residual accessory spleens are well known to be one of the factors of recurrence. There have been several reported cases of recurrent thrombocytopenia secondary to retained accessory spleens (see Table 53–7). This issue of accessory spleens has been prominent in the discussion of the role of laparoscopic splenectomy. Autopsy studies have demonstrated that the incidence of accessory spleens in the normal population is about 10%. In clinical series, however, accessory spleens have been reported in 15% to 30% of patients. The incidence of accessory spleen in recently reviewed splenectomy series since 1980 is 15% to 16%.

- Although the indications for a laparoscopic splenectomy remain the same as open splenectomy, some cases require caution in performing laparoscopically. Absolute contraindications to the laparoscopic approach include severe cardiopulmonary disease, cirrhosis, and pregnancy. Variceal short gastric vessels compounded by the coagulopathy of liver disease present an unacceptable risk of operative hemorrhage and temper enthusiasm for the laparoscopic approach in patients with portal hypertension. Thrombocytopenia in pregnancy is frequently gestational. Surgery is reserved for the failure of medical management and associated with a fetal mortality of 31%. Although laparoscopic cholecystectomy has been shown to be safe in the second trimester of pregnancy, results of laparoscopic splenectomy in this rare patient population have not been reported.

TABLE 53–7. Long-Term Hematologic Cure Rate after Laparoscopic Treatment of Immune Thrombocytopenic Purpura Patients

Study	Patients (n)	Mean Follow-Up (mo [range])	Absence of Initial Response and/or Recurrent Thrombocytopenia	Residual Accessory Spleen Detected
Emmermann et al, 1995	20	14 (1–28)	1	?
Yee et al, 1995	14	At discharge	4	1
Liew and Storey, 1995	6	?	1	1
Legrand et al, 1996	9	12 (1–26)	1	?, ?
Parent et al, 1995	11	— (6–9)	1	?, ?
Flowers et al, 1996	22	21 (3–36)	4	?
Dexter et al, 1996	6	24 (17–33)	0	—
Zamir et al, 1996	15	— (2–36)	0	—
Katkhouda et al, 1996	20	20 (1–46)	0	—
Watson et al, 1997	13	14 (5–21)	1	1
Tsiotos and Schinkert, 1997	18	15 (1–30)	1	?, ?
Lee and Kim, 1997	15	?	3	?, ?
Glasgow et al, 1997	16	?	4	1
Delaitre and Pitre, 1997	26	— (3–48)	2	?, ?
Decker et al, 1998	17	12.5 (1–28)	4	?, ?
Trias et al, 1998	32	12 (1–50)	9	3
Gigot, 1998*	19	45 (22–63)	6	3

*Unpublished data.
?, data not given despite treatment failures—not assessed; —, no treatment failures, therefore not assessed.

- Initially, splenomegaly was felt to be an absolute contraindication to the laparoscopic approach. Increasing experience and improvement of surgical devices have made this a relative contraindication. Splenic size and surgeon experience are the determining factors. Although technically feasible, laparoscopic splenectomy in the patient with splenomegaly can be a challenge. The introduction of hand-assisted laparoscopic surgery (HALS) has led some surgeons to approach these larger spleens with outcomes similar to the totally laparoscopic approach.
- Our preference has been to use the lateral decubitus approach. The initial dissection is begun by mobilization of the splenic flexure of the colon. The splenocolic ligament is divided using sharp dissection. This mobilizes the inferior pole of the spleen and allows the spleen to be retracted cephalad. Great care is taken to avoid rupture of the splenic capsule during retraction.
- The lateral peritoneal attachments of the spleen are then incised using either sharp dissection or ultrasonic shears. A 1-cm cuff of peritoneum is left along the lateral aspect of the spleen to be grasped if the spleen must be drawn medially. The lesser sac is entered along the medial border of the spleen. With the spleen elevated, the short gastric vessels and main vascular pedicle are visualized. The tail of the pancreas is also visualized and avoided at this point as it approaches the splenic hilum. The short gastric vessels are divided.
- The use of hemoclips should be minimized throughout the procedure and especially around the hilum because the clips may interfere with future applications of a stapling device. The stapler will not function if a clip is caught within its jaws, and this can result in significant bleeding from hilar vessels.
- After the short gastric vessels have been divided, the splenic pedicle may be carefully dissected from both the medial and lateral aspects (an advantage over the anterior approach). After the artery and vein are dissected, the vessels are divided by application of endoscopic vascular staplers or suture ligatures.
- The surgeon should be acutely aware of the position of the tail of the pancreas during the hilar division. The pancreatic tail lies within 1 cm of the splenic hilum in 75% of patients and touches the splenic hilum in 30%.
- To remove the detached spleen, a puncture-resistant nylon extraction bag is introduced through one of the trocar sites, typically the left lateral site. The bag is opened within the abdominal cavity, and the spleen is placed into the bag.

The drawstring is grasped and the bag is closed, leaving only the superior pole attachments to be divided at this stage. The open end of the closed bag is brought outside the abdomen through the supraumbilical or epigastric trocar site. The spleen is then morcellated with ring forceps and with finger fracture and is removed in fragments.

- Postsplenectomy thrombocytosis may be associated with both hemorrhagic and thromboembolic phenomena. This occurs particularly in patients with myeloproliferative disorders such as CML, agnogenic myeloid dysplasia, essential thrombocytosis, and polycythemia vera. Thrombosis of the mesenteric, portal, and renal veins may be a life-threatening sequela of postsplenectomy thrombocytosis. The lifelong risk of deep venous thrombosis and pulmonary embolism has not been well defined but may be significant. In review of 37,012 autopsies over a 20-year period, Pimpl and colleagues identified 202 deceased adults who had a history of splenectomy and matched them with a cohort of 403 deceased patients who had not undergone splenectomy. Pulmonary embolism was the major or contributory cause of death more often in the splenectomy group (35.6%) than in the control group (9.7%).

- OPSI is among the more devastating sequelae of asplenia and is the most common fatal late complication of splenectomy. Hyposplenism in the neonatal period has been suggested to contribute to the poor outcomes from neonatal sepsis. The exact incidence of OPSI has been difficult to determine. The incidence of infection in postsplenectomy patients is likely to be under-reported. In the same autopsy series by Pimpl and colleagues mentioned in the previous paragraph, lethal pneumonia was identified twice as often in autopsies of splenectomized patients than in controls (57.9% vs 24.1%) and lethal sepsis with multiple organ failure occurred in 6.9% of splenectomized versus 1.5% of autopsies on controls. One consistent observation is that the risk for OPSI is greater after splenectomy for malignancy or hematologic disease than for trauma. The risk also appears to be greater in young children (younger than 4 years). The risk for fatal OPSI is estimated to be 1 per 300 to 350 patient-years follow-up for children, and 1 per 800 to 1000 patient-years follow-up for adults. The incidence of nonfatal infection and sepsis is likely to be significantly greater. A recent review of selected reported splenectomy series of 7872 total cases inclusive of both children and adults revealed 270 episodes of sepsis (3.5%), with 169 septic fatalities (2.1%). Infection may occur at any time after splenectomy; in one recent series, most infections occurred more than 2 years after splenectomy, and 42% occurred more than 5 years after splenectomy.

- OPSI typically begins with a prodromal phase characterized by fever and chills and nonspecific symptoms, including sore throat, malaise, myalgias, diarrhea, and vomiting. Patients may have had rigors for 1 to 2 days before seeking appropriate medical treatment. Pneumonia and meningitis may be present, but many cases have no identifiable focal site of infection and present with high-grade primary bacteremia. Progression of the illness is classically rapid, with the development of hypotension, disseminated intravascular coagulation, respiratory distress, coma, and death within hours of presentation. The mortality rate is between 50% and 70% for fully developed OPSI despite antibiotics and intensive care.

- *Streptococcus pneumoniae* is the most frequently involved organism in OPSI and is estimated to be responsible for between 50% and 90% of cases. Other organisms involved in OPSI include *Haemophilus influenzae, Neisseria meningitidis, Streptococcus* species and other than pneumococcal species, *Salmonella* species, and *Capnocytophaga canimorsus* (implicated in OPSI as a sequela of dog bites).

Prophylactic Treatment of Splenectomized Patients

- The spleen is important for generating responses to thymus-independent antigens. In elective procedures, immunization should be administered before splenectomy whenever possible; the Advisory Committee on Immunization Practices has recommended that the immunization precede splenectomy by at least 2 weeks. Presplenectomy immunization is not possible in cases of splenic trauma. The immunizations should be administered to these patients during the hospitalization in which their splenectomy occurred rather than waiting until they return for a follow-up visit. Many of these patients become lost to follow-up, and clinical studies have demonstrated adequate antibody response to immediate immunization. High-risk patients without spleens should be considered for revaccination if they received the earlier 14-valent vaccine rather than the more current 23-valent preparation or if more than 3 to 6 years have elapsed since primary immunization. Simultaneous immunization with *H. influenzae* type b, meningococcal serogroup C, and polyvalent pneumococcal vaccine is both immunogenic and well tolerated. Unfortunately, rare cases of OPSI have been reported in vaccinated patients.

CHAPTER 54

CHEST WALL AND PLEURA

CHEST WALL

Anatomy

- The bony thorax consists of 12 paired ribs, multiple cartilages, and the sternum and clavicles arranged about the thoracic vertebrae.
- The upper seven ribs (numbered 1 to 7) are true ribs because they articulate directly with the sternum by means of cartilages.
- The lower five ribs (numbered 8 to 12) are false ribs; they do not directly connect to the sternum anteriorly but, in most cases, connect with the costocartilage above them.
- Ribs 11 and 12 are floating ribs; they articulate only with the thoracic spine.
- The bony thorax is covered by three groups of muscles, the primary and secondary muscles of respiration and those attaching the upper extremity to the body.
- The 11 intercostal spaces are each associated numerically with the rib superior to it.

Chest Wall Deformities

Depression Deformities (Pectus Excavatum)

- Pectus excavatum (also called funnel chest) is the most common chest wall deformity, occurring in 1 out of 400 children.
- Males are affected more frequently than females (4:1).
- Pectus excavatum arises from imbalanced or excessive growth of the lower costal cartilages, causing posterior sternal depression.
- Most patients with pectus excavatum are asymptomatic at the time of presentation.
- In severe cases, decreased stroke volume and cardiac output have been documented, along with a restrictive pattern (decreased maximal breath capacity), on pulmonary function tests.

847

- The indications for operative intervention include cosmesis, psychosocial factors, and the presence of respiratory or cardiovascular insufficiency.
- Several surgical techniques for repair are practiced; the most common involves subperichondrial removal of the deformed anterior cartilaginous segments and transverse osteotomy with sternal straightening.

Protrusion Deformities (Pectus Carinatum)

- Pectus carinatum (also called pigeon breast) is a defect characterized by an anterior protrusion deformity of the sternum and costal cartilages.
- Three types of defects have been described in pectus carinatum.
  - The most common variant, an anterior displacement of the body of the sternum and symmetrical concavity of the costal cartilages, is termed chondrogladiolar protrusion.
  - The second variety involves a lateral depression of the ribs on one or both sides of the sternum; Poland s syndrome frequently is associated with this type.
  - The third and least common type, the pouter pigeon breast, consists of an upper or chondromanubrial prominence with protrusion of the manubrium and depression of the sternal body.
- In patients with chondrogladiolar or chondromanubrial deformity, the sternum can be straightened using an osteotomy (sometimes two) of the sternal table.

Poland's Syndrome

- Poland s syndrome is a rare, nonfamilial disease of unknown cause that occurs in 1 per 30,000 births.
- The components of the syndrome include the following:
  - Absence of the pectoralis major muscle.
  - Absence or hypoplasia of the pectoralis minor muscle.
  - Absence of costal cartilages.
  - Hypoplasia of breast and subcutaneous tissue (including the nipple complex).
  - A variety of hand anomalies.

Sternal Defects

- The upper sternal defects (cervical ectopia cordis) are associated with a broad defect that extends to the fourth costal cartilage in a U- or V-shaped appearance.

- Distal sternal clefts (thoracoabdominal ectopia cordis) are the most extensive defects and are associated with Cantrell s pentalogy.
- This group of anomalies is characterized by the following:
  - A distal cleft in the sternum.
  - Omphalocele.
  - Diaphragmatic cleft.
  - Pericardial defect.
  - Congenital heart defect (ventricular septal defect, tetralogy of Fallot).
- Bifid sternum is the least severe anomaly of the sternum and may be associated with facial hemangiomas.

Chest Wall Tumors

- Chest wall tumors are rare neoplasms that include tumors originating in the bone, cartilage, or soft tissue of the chest wall.
- Most bony chest wall tumors arise in the ribs (85%), with the remainder arising from the scapula, sternum, and clavicle.
- The correct treatment of chest wall tumors requires that pathologic confirmation be obtained.
- Excisional rather than incisional biopsy, with a minimum of a 1- to 2-cm margin, is preferred.
- Incisional biopsy occasionally may be necessary for a large tumor.
- Frequently, surgical resection is the treatment of choice and may require a multidisciplinary team approach (plastic surgery, neurosurgery, orthopedic surgery, and thoracic surgery).

Bone

Benign

- *Fibrous dysplasia* of bone accounts for more than 30% of benign chest wall tumors.
  - They are slow growing and most commonly present as an asymptomatic mass in the lateral or posterior aspect of the rib.
  - The diagnosis is assisted by the appearance of a lytic lesion in the posterior aspect of the rib with a characteristic soap bubble or ground glass appearance on chest x-ray examination.
  - Excision is indicated for symptom relief (pain) and to confirm the diagnosis.
- *Chondromas* account for 15% to 20% of benign chest wall lesions.

- The tumors can arise in the medulla (enchondroma) or the periosteum (periosteal chondroma).
- On chest x-ray examination, they appear as a lytic lesion with sclerotic margins that may be difficult to distinguish from chondrosarcomas.
- Wide excision of the lesion is necessary to rule out a malignant component.
- *Osteochondromas* present as a mass originating from the cortex of the rib.
- *Eosinophilic granuloma* is a benign component of malignant fibrous histiocytosis that primarily affects men.
  - Excisional biopsy is indicated for solitary lesions; radiotherapy is reserved for patients who present with multiple lesions.
- *Osteoid osteomas* are rare tumors that arise in the bony cortex of the rib or vertebral arches.
  - A small radiolucent nidus encircled by a sclerotic margin is frequently seen on chest x-ray film.
  - Indications for resection include cosmesis and relief of pain; resection of the entire rib is recommended.
- *Aneurysmal bone cysts* commonly occur in the ribs and may arise as the result of chest wall trauma.
  - The characteristic pattern of blow-out lytic lesion frequently is seen on chest x-ray film.
  - Complete excision is warranted for relief of pain.

Malignant

- *Chondrosarcoma* is the most common malignant tumor of the chest wall, accounting for 20% of all bone tumors.
  - On chest x-ray examination, a poorly defined tumor mass that is destroying cortical bone is observed.
  - The anterior costochondral junctions of the sternum most frequently are involved.
  - Resection with wide margins is the treatment of choice, with a 70% 5-year survival rate reported for complete excision.
  - Radiotherapy may be effective for control of local recurrences.
- *Osteosarcoma* (osteogenic sarcoma) is a tumor that arises in the long bones of adolescents and young adults.
  - In the chest, osteosarcomas account for 10% to 15% of malignant tumors.
  - Typically, the tumor presents as a rapidly enlarging mass with a characteristic sunburst pattern on chest x-ray examination.

- Because metastases are common at presentation, a complete radiographic evaluation of the lungs, liver, and bones is indicated.
- Five-year survival with complete excision and adjuvant chemotherapy approaches 60%.

- *Ewing s sarcoma* is a bone tumor that arises most commonly in the pelvis, humerus, or femur of young men.
  - It is the third most common malignant chest wall tumor (5% to 10%).
  - A mass that is intermittently painful is a common presentation in this disease.
  - A characteristic onion peel appearance caused by periosteal elevation and bony remodeling is seen on chest x-ray film.
  - Survival is approximately 50% at 5 years with multimodality therapy (chemotherapy, radiotherapy, and surgery).

- *Solitary plasmacytoma* is a rare tumor arising from plasma cells.
  - Multiple myeloma is the same tumor arising in more than one location.
  - The tumor commonly presents as pain without a mass in older men.
  - A diffuse, punched-out appearance of the bone caused by myelogenous deposits is seen in chest x-ray film.
  - Systemic disease can be confirmed using serum electrophoresis, urinalysis (Bence Jones protein), and bone marrow aspiration.
  - Incisional biopsy frequently is used to confirm the diagnosis, although a solitary plasmacytoma should be resected completely.
  - Radiotherapy is the primary mode of therapy, with a 5-year survival of 30% reported.

Metastatic

- Metastatic neoplasms may involve the chest wall by direct extension or by metastases from blood-borne deposits, with the latter being the most common.
- Tumors that involve the chest wall by direct extension include breast and lung cancer.
- In breast cancer, locoregional recurrence involving the chest wall can occur in more than 10% of stage II lesions after mastectomy.
- Chest wall invasion occurs in 5% of primary non-small cell lung cancer patients; nodal involvement is a strong prognostic determinant of survival.

- Pancoast or superior sulcus tumors are lung cancers characterized by arm pain, atrophy of hand muscles, bone destruction, and Horner s syndrome.
- Treatment of Pancoast tumors currently uses preoperative radiotherapy and chemotherapy, followed by surgery.
- Secondary chest wall metastases arise from sarcomas and breast, lung, kidney, and thyroid cancers; they are treated with palliative radiotherapy.

Reconstruction

- Defects in the anterior, superior, and lateral chest wall commonly are reconstructed if the defect is greater than 5 cm.
- Skeletal stabilization is obtained using a prosthetic mesh or patch or with methyl methacrylate.
- Posterior defects generally do not require reconstruction if they are adequately covered by the scapula.

Chest Wall Infections

- Soft tissue infections commonly include superficial abrasions, carbuncles, or furuncles.
- Herpes zoster (shingles) also may present with painful lesions distributed along cutaneous nerve dermatomes and usually is self-limited.
- Inflammatory breast carcinoma may mimic chest wall infection or breast abscess and requires a high index of suspicion to make the appropriate diagnosis.
- Cartilage and bony structures occasionally may be the source of a chest wall infection.
- Costochondritis usually is self-limited, as in Tietze s syndrome.
- Bone infections arise primarily from surgical interventions such as median sternotomy.
- Sternal wound infection or thoracotomy infection occurs in approximately 1% to 2% of operative cases.
- Treatment of sternal osteomyelitis includes radical d bridement, irrigation systems, systemic antibiotics, and muscle flap reconstruction.
- Occasionally, chest wall infections can arise from fungal infections, such as actinomycosis or nocardiosis, and frequently lead to chest wall fistulae.
- Radionecrosis is an injury that occurs secondary to radiotherapy and its severity is dose-dependent.

Thoracic Outlet Syndrome

- Thoracic outlet syndrome (TOS) refers to compression of the subclavian vessels and nerves of the brachial plexus in the region of the thoracic inlet.
- These neurovascular structures of the upper extremity may be compressed by a variety of anatomic structures, such as bone, muscles, trauma, fibrous bands, or neoplasm.
- Symptoms most commonly develop secondary to neural compromise; however, vascular or neurovascular symptoms are reported.
- The patient population most commonly affected by TOS is middle-aged women.
- The subclavian artery exits the chest behind the sternoclavicular joints and passes between the scalenus anticus and medius muscles.
- The trunks of the five spinal nerves (C5 to C8, T1) accompany the artery after they exit their intervertebral foramina.

Diagnosis

- The symptoms associated with TOS vary depending on the anatomic structures that is compressed.
- In more than 90% of cases, neurogenic manifestations are reported.
- Ulnar nerve (C8-T1) involvement is the most common neural involvement and is associated with motor weakness and atrophy of the hypothenar and interosseous muscles and pain and paresthesia along the medial aspects of the arm and hand, the fifth finger, and the medial aspect of the fourth finger.
- The Adson (scalene) test causes narrowing of the space between the scalenus anticus and medius, resulting in compression of the subclavian artery and the brachial plexus. The patient is instructed to inspire maximally and breath hold while the neck is fully extended and the head is turned toward the affected side; loss or decrease of radial pulse or the reproduction of neurologic symptoms suggests a positive test.
- Nerve condition velocities can be very useful in differentiating the causes of neurologic symptoms reported by patients and are an adjunct to diagnosing TOS.

Management

- Once the diagnosis of TOS has been confirmed, the initial method of management is nonsurgical.
- Improvements in postural sitting, standing, and sleeping positions are recommended first, along with behavior modification at work.
- Many patients also benefit from muscle stretching and strengthening exercises as instructed by physiotherapists.
- The initial operation for TOS should include complete removal of the first rib.

Chest Wall Trauma

- Approximately 30% of patients presenting with significant trauma have a chest wall injury.

Ribs

- A higher incidence of fractures is observed in the elderly because of the loss of chest wall compliance from ossification of costal cartilage and osteoporosis.
- Chest and rib x-ray films can help to confirm the diagnosis in an acute setting but cannot completely rule out this injury.
- The management of rib fractures depends on the number and location of the injuries.
- Fractures of the fist two thoracic ribs usually are seen in high-velocity injuries and can be associated with aortic disruption (6%).
- Fractures of the lower thoracic ribs (T11-T12) are uncommon because the ribs are short and less exposed.
- Injury to three or more ribs often requires hospitalization for analgesia and monitoring of respiratory status.
- Splinting from improperly controlled pain can lead to atelectasis, retained secretions, and pneumonia, especially in the elderly.
- Analgesia can be provided using oral, intravenous, or intramuscular opioid analgesics for mild to moderate injury or epidural analgesia or intercostal nerve blocks for more severe injuries.
- Flail chest is a unique injury in which rib fractures lead to an unstable chest wall that results in paradoxical motion during respiration.
- Pulmonary contusion is the most commonly associated injury in check wall trauma.
- Maintenance of adequate ventilation is the goal of therapy in flail chest injury.

Sternum

- A step deformity may be palpable if fracture dislocation of the sternum has occurred.
- The diagnosis is made by clinical evaluation with the assistance of a lateral chest x-ray film.
- Operative stabilization using internal fixation is indicated in isolated injuries to achieve analgesia or long-term cosmetic improvement.
- The main concern of sternal injuries is the potential for associated underlying injuries that can be life threatening, such as aortic disruption, cardiac contusion, and pericardial effusion.

PLEURA

Anatomy

- The pleural space is a potential cavity lining the chest wall and into which each lung protrudes.
- The parietal pleura lines the inner surface of the chest wall and covers the diaphragm and pericardium and other mediastinal structures.
- The visceral pleura covers both lungs and follows all fissures.
- The parietal pleura derives its arterial blood supply from systemic arteries.
- The dual blood supply of the visceral pleura is both systemic and pulmonary.
- Visceral pleural lymphatics form a subpleural plexus when they mesh with superficial lung lymphatics; this subpleural plexus subsequently drains into the mediastinal lymph nodes.
- Parietal pleura is richly innervated by the intercostal nerves, except the mediastinal and central diaphragmatic parietal pleurae, which are innervated by the phrenic nerves.
- The visceral pleural is insensitive and is innervated by vagal branches and the sympathetic system.

Pleural Effusions

- The movement of fluid across the pleural membranes is complicated but in general is governed by Starling s law of capillary exchange.
- This suggests that the flux of fluid is controlled by the balance of both oncotic and hydrostatic pressures within the pleural capillaries and pleural space.
- A small imbalance of accumulation and absorption of pleural fluid will lead to the development of a pleural effusion.

- The mechanisms of this imbalance include the following:
  - Increased hydrostatic pressure.
  - Increased negative intrapleural pressure.
  - Increased capillary permeability.
  - Decreased plasma oncotic pressure.
  - Decreased or interrupted lymphatic drainage.
- Approximately 300 mL of fluid is required for the development of costophrenic angle blunting seen on upright chest x-ray film.
- At least 500 mL of effusion is necessary for detection on clinical examination.
- Transudative effusions occur as the result of a change in fluid balance in the pleural space.
- Exudative effusions suggest the disruption or integrity loss of pleura or lymphatics.
- An effusion is considered exudative if it meets any one of the flowing criteria:
  - Pleural fluid protein-to-serum protein ratio greater than 0.5.
  - Pleural fluid lactate dehydrogenase (LDH)-to-serum LDH greater than 0.6.
  - Pleural fluid LDH 1.67 times normal serum.

Benign Effusion

- Treatment of benign pleural effusions is directed toward treatment of the underlying disease, such as congestive heart failure or ascites.
- Tube thoracostomy or thoracoscopic drainage with or without chemical pleurodesis is warranted for recurrent benign effusions.
- Pleurodesis can be carried out through the chest tube once chest tube outputs have decreased to less than 150 to 200 mL per day.
- Typically 300 mg of doxycycline or 2 to 5 g of talc in 100 to 200 mL of saline solution is instilled, and the chest tube is clamped at its exit site.
- The patient is turned at intervals for 1 hour to assist with distribution, and then the chest tube is replaced to suction drainage.
- Thoracoscopic drainage of effusions with intraoperative chemical pleurodesis is currently widely used with excellent results.

Malignant Effusion

- Most malignant pleural effusions are exudative.

- Metastatic breast and lung cancers are the most common malignancies that cause malignant effusions.
- A malignant pleural effusion is best approached with a combination of treatment of the underlying disease (if available) and specific intervention on the effusion itself.
- Surgical treatment options for malignant effusions are similar to those for benign effusions.

Empyema

- Empyema is a pyogenic or suppurative infection of the pleural space.
- They may be classified into three categories based on the chronicity of the disease process:
  - The acute phase is characterized by pleural effusion of low viscosity and cell count.
  - The transitional or fibrinopurulent phase, which can begin after 48 hours, is characterized by an increase in white blood cells in the pleural effusion and is associated with fibrin deposition on visceral and parietal pleurae and progressive lung entrapment.
  - The organizing or chronic phase occurs after as little as 1 to 2 weeks and is associated with an ingrowth of capillaries and fibroblasts into the pleural rind and inexpansible lung.
- Most often, empyemas are the result of a primary infectious process in the lung.
- Historically, these infections were commonly due to *Streptococcus* or *Pneumococcus pneumoniae;* today gram-negative and anaerobic organisms are common causes of empyema.
- Complications of empyema include empyema necessitatis (spontaneous decompression of pus through the chest wall), chronic empyema (with entrapped lung), osteomyelitis or chondritis of the ribs or vertebrae, pericarditis, mediastinitis, the development of a bronchopleural fistula, or disseminated infection of the central nervous system.
- In the acute and early fibropurulent phases, complete thoracentesis can be both diagnostic and therapeutic.
- Tube thoracostomy or VATS empyema drainage may be indicated for pleural drainage if thoracentesis fails or the empyema has progressed beyond its earliest stages.
- Occasionally, radiologically guided catheter drainage can be a useful adjunct to surgical procedures.
- Thoracotomy with d bridement or formal decortication in later stage empyema is reserved for treatment failures with persistent sepsis.

- Chronic empyema is the result of failure to recognize or properly treat acute pneumonia or acute empyema, or failure (or incompleteness) of earlier intervention, and usually is associated with lung entrapment by a thick pleural peel or fibrothorax.
- The open surgical approaches for chronic empyema include variations of an open thoracostomy with rib resection or full thoracotomy with empyema evacuation and lung decortication.
- The appropriate procedure depends on the patient s overall status and comorbidities.

Chylothorax

- Chylothorax is the accumulation of lymph within the pleural space.
- Chylothorax characteristically is milky white fluid that contains a high concentration of emulsified fats (triglycerides, chylomicrons) and a lymphocytic predominance on cell count.
- Chylothorax occurs when the contents of the thoracic duct empties into pleural space.
- Following diagnosis, management of chylothorax consists initially of tube, thoracostomy drainage (chest tube insertion) with complete lung re-expansion and supportive measures, such as a low-fat or fat-free diet supplemented by medium-chain triglycerides and aggressive fluid, electrolyte, and nutritional replacement or correction.
- The most common surgical procedures are ligation of the thoracic duct or mass ligation of tissue at the diaphragmatic hiatus (generally through a right thoracotomy) or direct closure of the duct injury.
- Instillation of olive oil or cream via nasogastric tube at the time of surgery can help to identify the duct and area of leakage.

Pneumothorax

- Pneumothorax is the accumulation of air within the pleural space.
- Pneumothoraces may be spontaneous or occur secondary to a traumatic, surgical, therapeutic, or disease-related event.
- If air enters the pleural space repeatedly (as with inspiration) and is unable to escape (i.e., tension pneumothorax), positive pressure develops in the pleural space, causing compression

of the entire lung, shifting of the mediastinum and heart away from the pneumothorax, and severe respiratory compromise with hemodynamic collapse.

- Tension pneumothorax is an emergency requiring immediate decompressive treatment.
- A primary spontaneous pneumothorax occurs without known cause or evidence of diffuse pulmonary disease or from subpleural blebs.
- A secondary spontaneous pneumothorax occurs as the result of an underlying pulmonary process that predisposes to pneumothorax.
- Iatrogenic pneumothoraces are common and may be caused by thoracentesis, central venous catheterization, surgery, mechanical ventilation, or diagnostic lung biopsy.
- Patients with pneumothorax most commonly present with chest pain.
- Dyspnea is the second most common symptom.
- Small pneumothoraces (<20%) that are stable may be monitored if the patient has few symptoms.
- Indications for intervention include progressive pneumothorax, delayed pulmonary expansion, or development of symptoms.
- Tube thoracostomy (chest tube insertion) and underwater seal drainage are the mainstays of treatment for moderate to large or symptomatic spontaneous pneumothorax.
- Complications of chest tube insertion for pneumothorax are infrequent, but include laceration of an intercostal vessel, laceration of the lung, intrapulmonary placement of the chest tube, and infection.
- Primary spontaneous pneumothorax tends to recur with increasing frequently after each episode.
- Surgery is recommended for a recurrence or the development of a contralateral pneumothorax.
- Surgery for primary spontaneous pneumothorax has evolved over recent years from open thoracotomy (axillary or posterolateral) to a minimally invasive video-assisted approach.
- Apical blebs are resected and the parietal pleura over the apex of the hemithorax can be removed (pleurectomy), abraded (mechanical pleurodesis), or treated with talc or tetracycline-like agents (chemical pleurodesis or poudrage).
- The recurrence rate for these procedures, performed open or closed, is less than 5%.
- Treatment options for primary and secondary spontaneous pneumothorax are similar, but treatment must be individualized.

Mesothelioma

- Mesothelioma is a rare neoplasm that arises from mesothelial cells lining the parietal and visceral pleurae and can present in a localized or diffuse manner.
- Typically, the lesions are diagnosed as an asymptomatic mass on chest x-ray film.
- The diffuse variant presents as a locally aggressive tumor that commonly is associated with asbestos exposure (75%).
- A long latency period between asbestos exposure and the development of disease has been reported.
- Dyspnea is the most commonly reported presenting symptom.
- A number of techniques are used to confirm the diagnosis of malignant pleural mesothelioma (MPM), including thoracocentesis of pleural effusion and pleural biopsy.
- With supportive care only, survival for mesothelioma ranges between 4 and 12 months.
- Treatment of this tumor using single-modality therapy such as radiotherapy, chemotherapy, or surgery has not demonstrated any improvement in survival.
- Two surgical cytoreductive procedures, extrapleural pneumonectomy (EPP) and pleural pneumonectomy and pleurectomy/decortication, have been used in the treatment of MPM.
- The published results of pleurectomy/decortication in a multimodality setting indicate a median survival between 9 and 21 months and a mortality rate ranging from 1.5% to 5%.
- Controversy surrounding the use of EPP is based on published trials that report high operative morbidity and mortality with no impact on patient survival when used as a single-modality therapy.
- Advances in perioperative management and the development of multimodality treatment approaches have led to long-term survival.
- Results from a recent series at Brigham and Women s Hospital treated with EPP followed by sequential chemotherapy and radiotherapy identified a favorable subgroup with a 46% 5-year survival.

CHAPTER 55

THE MEDIASTINUM

ANATOMY

- Many mediastinal tumors and cysts occur in characteristic locations; therefore, the mediastinum has been subdivided artificially for the convenience of localizing specific types of lesions. Some subdivide the mediastinum into four compartments superior, anterior, middle, and posterior; however, the frequency with which tumors occurring in the anterior or posterior compartments extend into the superior mediastinum has prompted a division of the mediastinum into three subdivisions: the anterosuperior, middle, and posterior.

MEDIASTINAL EMPHYSEMA

- Air may enter the mediastinum from the esophagus, trachea, bronchi, lung, neck, or abdomen, producing mediastinal emphysema or pneumomediastinum.

MEDIASTINITIS

- Infection of the mediastinal space is a serious and potentially fatal process.
- Mediastinitis occurs most often after median sternotomy for cardiac operations.

MEDIASTINAL HEMORRHAGE

- Mediastinal hemorrhage is most frequently caused by blunt or penetrating trauma, thoracic aortic dissection, rupture of aortic aneurysm, or surgical procedures within the thorax.

SUPERIOR VENA CAVA OBSTRUCTION

- A number of benign and malignant processes may cause obstruction of the superior vena cava, leading to superior vena caval syndrome.
- In adults the most frequent cause is a malignant neoplasm, usually a bronchogenic carcinoma.

PRIMARY NEOPLASMS AND CYSTS

- A large number of neoplasms and cysts may arise from multiple anatomic sites in the mediastinum and present as myriad clinical signs and symptoms.
- Although differences in the relative incidence of neoplasms and cysts exist in some series, the most common mediastinal masses are neurogenic tumors (20%), thymomas (19%), primary cysts (18%), lymphomas (13%), and germ cell tumors (10%).
- Malignant neoplasms represent 25% to 42% of mediastinal masses. Lymphomas, thymomas, germ cell tumors, primary carcinomas, and neurogenic tumors are the most common.
- The incidence of mediastinal masses varies in infants, children, and adults.

Clinical Features

- Of patients with a mediastinal mass, 56% to 65% have symptoms at presentation. Patients with a benign lesion are more often symptom free (54%) than are patients with a malignant neoplasm (15%).
- Infants and children are more likely to present with symptoms or findings (78%) because of the relatively small space within the mediastinum.

Diagnosis

- The initial diagnostic intervention should be a careful history and physical examination.
- Computed tomography (CT) scanning with contrast medium enhancement should be done routinely in patients with a mediastinal mass. In patients with a contraindication to the use of contrast dye and in those with surgical clips in the anatomic region of interest, magnetic resonance imaging (MRI) is useful.
- The 2-deoxy-2-(^{18}F)fluoro-D-glucose (FDG) positron-emission tomography (PET) scan has played an adjunctive role in evaluation of mediastinal neoplasms, especially in determining the malignant potential of a mediastinal mass.
- Male patients in their second through fifth decades who have an anterosuperior mediastinal mass should have alpha-fetoprotein and beta-human chorionic gonadotropin (beta-HCG) serologies obtained.
- Recent advances in immunohistochemical and core biopsy techniques have allowed it to become more accurate for

establishing the initial diagnosis of lymphoma, but it is probably better used for confirming recurrent disease.
- Mediastinoscopy is a useful technique to evaluate and biopsy lesions of the middle mediastinum.
- Thoracoscopic and thoracoscopically assisted procedures are increasingly attaining a leading role in diagnosing and treating a variety of mediastinal lesions in carefully selected patients.
- Although most patients undergo surgical procedures safely, patients with large anterosuperior or middle mediastinal masses, particularly children, have an increased risk for severe cardiorespiratory complications during general anesthesia.

Neurogenic Tumors

- Neurogenic tumors are the most common neoplasm, constituting 20% of all primary tumors and cysts.
- MRI is preferred to evaluate the presence and extent of the intraspinal component.

Neuroblastoma

- Biologically they can behave quite uniquely and have been known to spontaneously regress, mature, or proliferate aggressively. Unfortunately the majority presents at advanced stages and do not regress spontaneously or mature.
- Therapy is determined by the stage of the disease.
- Interestingly, mediastinal neuroblastomas appear to have a better prognosis than neuroblastomas occurring elsewhere.

Ganglioneuroblastoma

- Ganglioneuroblastomas exhibit an intermediate degree of differentiation between ganglioneuromas and neuroblastomas.
- Treatment of ganglioneuroblastomas ranges from surgical excision alone to various chemotherapeutic strategies depending on histologic characteristics, age at diagnosis, and stage of disease.

Ganglioneuroma

- Ganglioneuromas are benign tumors originating from the sympathetic chain that are composed of ganglion cells and nerve fibers.
- Surgical excision provides cure.

Neurilemoma, Neurofibroma, and Neurosarcoma

- The most common neurogenic tumor is the neurilemoma.
- With both neurilemoma and neurofibroma, surgical excision results in cure.

Paraganglioma (Pheochromocytoma)

- When appropriate, surgical resection is the optimal therapy.

Thymoma

- Thymoma is the most common neoplasm of the anterosuperior mediastinum and the second most common mediastinal mass.
- Differentiation between benign and malignant disease is determined by the presence of gross invasion of adjacent structures, metastasis, or microscopic evidence of capsular invasion.
- Whenever possible, the therapy for thymoma is surgical excision without removing or injuring vital structures.
- The perioperative management in patients with myasthenia gravis is extremely important to prevent complications.
- Because thymomas have been reported to have late recurrences, cure rates should be based on 10-year follow-up data.

Germ Cell Tumors

- Germ cell tumors are benign and malignant neoplasms thought to originate from primordial germ cells that fail to complete the migration from the urogenital ridge and come to rest in the mediastinum.
- Although these lesions are identical histologically to germ cell tumors originating in the gonads, they are not considered to be metastatic from primary gonadal tumors.

Teratomatous Lesions

- Teratomas are neoplasms composed of multiple tissue elements derived from the three primitive embryonic layers foreign to the area in which they occur.
- These tumors are located most commonly in the anterosuperior mediastinum, although 3% to 8% are found in the posterior mediastinum.
- The teratodermoid (dermoid) cyst is the simplest form.

- Malignant tumors are differentiated from benign tumors by the presence of primitive (embryonic) tissue or by the presence of malignant components. Immature teratomas contain combinations of mature epithelial and connective tissues with immature areas of mesenchymal and neuroectodermal tissues.
- Diagnosis and therapy rely on surgical excision.
- For malignant teratomas, chemotherapy and radiation therapy, combined with surgical excision, are individualized for the type of malignant components contained in the tumors. The overall prognosis is poor for malignant tumors.

Malignant Nonteratomatous Germ Cell Tumors

- Malignant germ cell tumors also occur predominantly in the anterosuperior mediastinum. Unlike benign teratomas, there is a marked male predominance.
- Serologic measurements of alpha-fetoprotein and beta-human chorionic gonadotropin (HCG) are useful for the following tasks: differentiating seminomas from nonseminomas, quantitatively assessing response to therapy in hormonally active tumors (the plasma half-life of alpha-fetoprotein and beta-HCG is 5 days and 12 to 24 hours, respectively), and diagnosing relapse or failure of therapy before changes that can be observed in gross disease.

Seminomas

- Seminomas constitute 50% of malignant germ cell tumors and 2% to 4% of all mediastinal masses.
- Treatment varies somewhat based on extent of disease and usually consists of chemotherapy with or without secondary surgery or combination chemotherapy and radiotherapy.
- As discussed in the subsequent section on nonseminomatous mediastinal germ cell tumors, residual disease should be surgically resected after chemotherapy.
- Excellent long-term survival rates have been seen with mediastinal seminoma, with a recent large multi-institutional series reporting an 88% 5-year survival.

Nonseminomatous Tumors

- Malignant nonseminoma tumors include choriocarcinomas, embryonal cell carcinomas, immature teratomas, teratomas with malignant components, and endodermal cell (yolk sac) tumors, of which 40% are a mixture of tissue types.

- The nonseminomas differ from seminomas in several aspects: they are more aggressive tumors that are frequently disseminated at the time of diagnosis, they are rarely radiosensitive, and more than 90% produce either beta-HCG or alpha-fetoprotein.

- The local invasiveness of these tumors and their frequent metastasis usually preclude surgical resection of all disease at the time of diagnosis.

- Treatment of these nonseminomatous tumors currently is with cisplatin and etoposide-based regimens. Evaluation of these regimens followed by high-dose chemotherapy (cyclo-phosphamide, carboplatin, etoposide) and peripheral blood stem cell support is ongoing.

- Serum markers, alpha-fetoprotein, and beta-HCG are followed to assess response to treatment. If a complete serologic and radiologic response is achieved, patients are closely observed. If the disease progresses during therapy, salvage chemother-apy is initiated. If there is a serologic response but a radio-graphic abnormality remains, the patient is taken to the operating room, and surgical removal of as much of the remaining tumor as possible is performed. The pathology of the resected postchemotherapy specimen appears to be the most significant predictor of survival.

- Overall 45% of patients with mediastinal nonseminomas are alive at 5 years.

Lymphomas

- Although the mediastinum is frequently involved in patients with lymphoma at some time during the course of their dis-ease (40% to 70%), it is infrequently the sole site of disease at the time of presentation.

- Characteristically, these tumors occur in the anterosuperior mediastinum or in the hilar region of the middle mediastinum.

Hodgkin's Lymphoma

- This updated classification, the Revised European-American Lymphoma (REAL) classification, incorporated new immuno-logic and molecular data and divides Hodgkin s disease into two main groups: nodular lymphocyte predominant and classic Hodgkin s disease. More recently the new World Health Organization (WHO) classification of hematologic malignancies has incorporated the REAL concepts.

- The nodular sclerosing type is the most common type of Hodgkin s lymphoma seen in the mediastinum, occurring 55% to 75% of the time, followed by the lymphocyte-predominant type (40%).
- The neoplastic cells in Hodgkin s disease are Reed-Sternberg cells.
- Treatment of Hodgkin s lymphoma is determined by the stage of disease and the prognostic factors related to the patient and the tumor.
- Treatment is based on radiation therapy and chemotherapy. Surgical excision of all disease is rarely possible, and the surgeon s primary role is to provide sufficient tissue for diagnosis and to assist in pathologic staging.
- Early and intermediate stage Hodgkin s disease is generally treated with combined chemotherapy and involved field radiation.
- Patients with more advanced disease at presentation or with adverse prognostic factors are treated with extensive chemotherapy alone or with multimodality therapy.
- If cure is not achieved with conventional dose chemotherapy, patients with Hodgkin s disease should be considered candidates for high-dose chemotherapy with hematopoietic support.
- Today most patients with Hodgkin s disease whether localized or advanced can be cured.
- Unfortunately, as the cure rate has improved over the past several decades the long-term complications of treatment (secondary malignancies, coronary artery disease, and late pulmonary toxicity) have become more apparent.

Non-Hodgkin's Lymphoma

- Non-Hodgkin s lymphoma, like Hodgkin s disease is classified now by the WHO classification of lymphoid malignancies adopting the REAL concepts to define clinically relevant entities. Mediastinal non-Hodgkin s lymphoma is usually of either lymphoblastic (60%) or large cell morphology (40%).
- Lymphoblastic lymphoma occurs predominantly in children, adolescents, and young adults and represents 60% of cases of mediastinal non-Hodgkin s lymphoma.
- Twenty percent of lymphoblastic lymphomas are from B-cell precursors; the remainder are from T-cell precursors and phenotypically express various stages of T-cell differentiation.
- Large cell non-Hodgkin s lymphomas of the mediastinum are a diverse group of lymphomas arising from both B-cell

and T-cell lineage. These tumors are subdivided into primary mediastinal (thymic) large B-cell lymphoma and anaplastic large cell lymphoma of T-cell and null cell types.

- Primary mediastinal B-cell lymphoma is by far the most common of the large cell lymphomas seen in the mediastinum.
- These lymphomas likely originate from a native population of B cells located in the thymus.
- Histologically, mediastinal large B-cell lymphoma tumors are often composed of large clear cells, which may appear compartmentalized by associated connective tissue (sclerosis).
- Treatment of non-Hodgkin s lymphoma consists of aggressive anthracycline-containing chemotherapeutic regimens. After intensive chemotherapy, consolidation involved field radiotherapy may be given.
- Patients in first response with poor prognostic factors, with refractory disease, or with recurrent lymphoma can be treated with high-dose chemotherapy and with either autologous bone marrow or peripheral stem cell transplantation.

Residual Masses After Lymphoma Treatment

- After treatment of lymphomas, residual abnormalities within the mediastinum are commonly noted radiographically (64% to 88%).
- Gallium-67 scintigraphy is a metabolic imaging technique and has proven valuable in the determination of neoplastic disease in residual mediastinal abnormalities post-therapy.
- Recently the use of metabolic imaging with FDG-PET has shown promise as a noninvasive way to detect active mediastinal disease and predict relapse in patients with lymphoma.

Primary Carcinoma

- Primary carcinomas of the mediastinum constitute between 3% and 11% of primary mediastinal masses in most series and represent 4% of the mediastinal masses in the collected series. The origin of these tumors is unknown.
- Extensive involvement within the thorax and often metastatic disease outside the thorax characterize this disease. Surgical excision is rarely possible. Unfortunately, the routine use of radiation therapy and chemotherapy has been unsuccessful in prolonging survival.

Endocrine Tumors

Thyroid Tumors

- Although substernal extension of a cervical goiter is common, totally intrathoracic thyroid tumors are rare and make up only 1% of all mediastinal masses in the collected series.
- Although there may be a demonstrable connection with the cervical gland (usually a fibrous connective tissue band), a true intrathoracic thyroid gland derives its blood supply from thoracic vessels.
- Substernal extensions of a cervical goiter can usually be excised using a cervical approach.

Parathyroid Tumors

- Although parathyroid glands may occur in the mediastinum in 10% of patients, they are usually accessible through the cervical incision.
- Most often, these adenomas are found in the anterosuperior mediastinum (80%) embedded in or near the superior pole of the thymus.
- The clinical manifestations of a mediastinal parathyroid tumor are similar to those that occur with tumors of the cervical region; symptoms are related to the excess secretion of parathyroid hormone causing the hyperparathyroid syndrome. Preoperative attempts at anatomic localization are indicated.
- In patients with persistent hyperparathyroidism following cervical exploration if localization studies show residual parathyroid in the mediastinum, mediastinal exploration using a median sternotomy is indicated. Alternatively successful removal has been performed thoracoscopically.

Neuroendocrine Tumors

- Mediastinal neuroendocrine tumors, previously known as carcinoid tumors, arise from cells of Kulchitsky located in the thymus. These tumors show a predilection for males in their 40s and 50s, are usually located in the anterosuperior mediastinum, and behave aggressively.
- The best chance for cure is surgical excision, but local invasion or metastatic spread often precludes complete excision.

Mesenchymal Tumors

- Mediastinal mesenchymal tumors originate from the connective tissue, striatal and smooth muscle, fat, lymphatic tissue, and blood vessels present within the mediastinum, giving rise to a diverse group of neoplasms.

Extramedullary Hematopoiesis

Giant Lymph Node Hyperplasia (Castleman's Disease)

- Giant lymph node hyperplasia was initially described by Castleman.
- Two distinct histologic entities exist.
- Castleman s disease may also be multicentric.

Chordoma

- Chordomas are rare malignant tumors that may occur in the posterior mediastinum and originate from the primitive notochord.

Primary Cysts

- Primary cysts of the mediastinum make up 18% of the mediastinal masses in the collected series. These cysts can be bronchogenic, pericardial, enteric, or thymic or may be of an unspecified nature. More than 75% of cases are asymptomatic, and these tumors rarely cause morbidity.
- In addition, these masses need to be differentiated from malignant tumors.
- Bronchogenic cysts are the most common primary cysts of the mediastinum.
- Surgical excision is recommended in all patients to provide definitive histologic diagnosis, alleviate symptoms, and prevent the development of associated complications.
- Pericardial cysts are the second most frequently encountered cysts within the mediastinum.
- Enteric cysts (duplication cysts) arise from the posterior division of the primitive foregut, which develops into the upper division of the gastrointestinal tract. These cysts are found less frequently than bronchogenic or pericardial cysts and are most frequently located in the posterior mediastinum, usually adjacent to the esophagus.

LUNG (INCLUDING PULMONARY EMBOLISM AND THORACIC OUTLET SYNDROME)

ANATOMY

- The development of the respiratory system begins at approximately 21 to 28 days' gestation as a ventral groove in the foregut; the bronchial tree is complete at approximately 16 weeks.
- Ciliated tall columnar epithelium lines the larger airways.
- The alveoli are composed of type I and type II cells in approximately equal number.
- Type I cells constitute approximately 40% of the number of cells lining the alveoli but cover more than 90% of the alveolar lining and are for gas exchange.
- Type II alveolar cells are the granular pneumocytes with lipid inclusion bodies and manufacture surfactant, a lipoprotein, which decreases surface tension.
- The right lung is composed of three lobes: the upper, middle, and lower; two fissures (major and minor) separate these lobes.
- The left lung has two lobes—the upper lobe and the lower lobe separated by a single fissure; the lingula is a portion of the left upper lobe and corresponds embryologically to the right middle lobe.
- The blood supply of the lung is twofold:
    - Unoxygenated blood is pumped to the lung from the right ventricle by the way of the pulmonary artery.
    - After oxygenation in the lung, the blood is returned to the left atrium by way of the pulmonary veins.
- Blood supply to the bronchi is from the systemic circulation by bronchial arteries arising from the aorta.
- Lymphatic vessels are present throughout the parenchyma and gradually coalesce toward the hilar areas of the lungs.

PULMONARY FUNCTION TESTS AND CARDIOPULMONARY EXERCISE TESTING

- Certain comorbidities are associated with increased pulmonary risk, including smoking, poor overall health, increasing age, poorer pulmonary function or chronic obstructive pulmonary disease, asthma, and obesity.
- Before pulmonary resection, patients are evaluated by a combination of spirometry and pulmonary function tests (Fig. 56–1).
- CO_2 retention is associated with increased risk; a $Paco_2$ greater than 45 mm Hg suggests severe disease with nearly a 50% functional loss of the lung.
- The predicted postoperative forced expiratory volume in 1 second (FEV_1) is the most common and important predictor of postoperative pulmonary reserve; typically, this should be greater than 0.8 L predicted postoperative value.
- For patients with marginal pulmonary function, a quantitative xenon ventilation-perfusion lung scan should be performed to evaluate the impact of the planned extent of resection on the specific lobe or lung to be resected and to estimate the remaining pulmonary reserve.

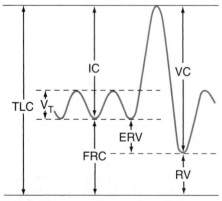

■ **FIGURE 56–1.** Spirometry. Subdivisions of lung volumes. ERV, expiratory reserve volume; FRC, functional residual capacity, that is, lung volume at end-expiration; IC, inspiratory capacity; RV, residual volume, that is, lung volume after forced expiration from FRC; TLC, total lung capacity; VC, vital capacity, that is, the maximal volume of gas inspired from RV; V_T, tidal volume.

- The surgeon can calculate or predict the postoperative FEV_1 with a ventilation/perfusion (V/Q) score by multiplying the preoperative FEV_1 of the noninvolved lung by the percentage of blood flow within the noninvolved lung.
- Other techniques of evaluating the patients for pulmonary reserve include obtaining maximal voluntary ventilation (MVV), stair climbing two flights or greater, carbon monoxide diffusing capacity (DLCO), and maximal oxygen consumption (VO_2 max).
- MVV describes the maximal movement of air into the lungs during a preset interval.
- If the patient can walk up one flight of stairs, a wedge resection is tolerated; if the patient can walk up two flights of stairs, a lobectomy is appropriate; if the patient can walk up three flights of stairs, a pneumonectomy is appropriate.
- The DLCO measures the rate at which test molecules such as carbon monoxide move from the alveolar space to combine with hemoglobin in the red blood cells; the DLCO is determined by calculating the difference between inspired and expired samples of gas.
- DLCO levels less than 50% are associated with increased perioperative risk.
- Low values of VO_2 max (<15 mL/minute/kg) are associated with increased risk of surgical morbidity and mortality.

LUNG CANCER

- Lung cancer is the most frequent cause of cancer death in both men and women and accounts for 14% of all cancer diagnoses and 28% of all cancer deaths.
- The decrease in lung cancer incidence and the mortality rate probably reflects decreasing cigarette smoking over the previous 30 years.
- One-year survival rates for lung cancer have improved from 32% in 1973 to 41% in 1994; however, the 5-year survival rate for all stages combined is only 14%.
- For localized disease, 5-year survival can approach 50% (stages I [60%] and II [40%]), for regional disease 20%, and for distant disease 2%; only a small percentage (15%) are discovered when localized.

Etiology

- Cigarette smoking is unequivocally the most important risk factor in the development of lung cancer.

- Other environmental factors include industrial substances such as asbestos, arsenic, chromium, or nickel; organic chemicals; radon or iatrogenic radiation exposure; air pollution; and other environmental (secondary) smoke in nonsmokers.

Pathology

Adenocarcinoma

- The most frequent histologic type and accounts for approximately 45% of all lung cancers.
- Derived from the mucus-producing cells of the bronchial epithelium; most of these tumors (75%) are peripherally located.
- Tends to metastasize earlier than squamous cell carcinoma of the lung.
- Bronchoalveolar carcinoma of the lung is a subcategory of adenocarcinoma but is a more indolent disease.

Squamous Cell Carcinoma

- Thirty percent of lung cancer.
- Approximately two thirds of these tumors are centrally located and tend to expand against the bronchus, causing extrinsic compression.
- Prone to undergo central necrosis and cavitation.
- Tends to metastasize later.

Large Cell Undifferentiated Carcinoma

- Ten percent of lung cancer.
- Tends to occur peripherally and may metastasize relatively early.
- Microscopically, these tumors show anaplastic, pleomorphic cells with vesicular or hyperchromatic nuclei and abundant cytoplasm.

Small Cell Lung Cancer

- Twenty percent of lung cancer; about 80% are centrally located; the disease is characterized by a very aggressive tendency to metastasize.
- Surgery is not the primary treatment for small cell carcinoma.

Lung Cancer Metastases

- Lung cancer with metastases is characterized as stage IV ($T_{any}N_{any}M_1$).
- Lung cancer may metastasize by direct (local) extension along the bronchus of origin, into the chest wall, across fissures, into the pulmonary vessels and the pericardium, and into the diaphragm.
- Hematogenous spread of lung cancer to the liver, adrenals, lung, bone, kidneys, and brain may occur; bone metastases are usually osteolytic.

Detection of Lung Cancer

- Patients with lung cancer typically are first seen with symptoms and in advanced stage (stages III and IV).
- No form of screening (sputum cytology, chest radiography, bronchoscopy, computed tomography [CT] scan) has proven cost effective.
- Most patients have bronchopulmonary symptoms such as cough, 75%; dyspnea, 60%; chest pain, 50%; and hemoptysis, 30%.
- Other symptoms may include hoarseness, superior vena cava syndrome, chest wall pain, Horner's syndrome, dysphagia, pleural effusion, or phrenic nerve paralysis.
- Paraneoplastic syndromes are distant manifestations of lung cancer (not metastases) as revealed in extrathoracic non-metastatic symptoms.

Staging of Lung Cancer

- Lung cancer can be roughly grouped into three major categories (Boxes 56–1 and 56–2):
  - Stages I and II tumors are contained within the lung and may be completely resected by surgery.
  - Stage IV disease includes metastatic disease and is not typically treated by surgery, except in those patients requiring surgical palliation.
  - "Resectable" stage IIIA and IIIB tumors are locally advanced tumors with metastasis to the ipsilateral mediastinal (N_2 lymph nodes; stage IIIA) or involving mediastinal structures ($T_4N_0M_0$).
- These tumors, by their advanced nature, may be mechanically removed with surgery; however, surgery does not control the micro-metastases that exist within the area of the operation, the lymphatics, or systemically (Boxes 56–3 and 56–4).

Box 56–1. TNM Definitions

T—Primary tumor

TX   Tumor proven by the presence of malignant cells in bronchopulmonary secretions but not visualized roentgenographically or bronchoscopically, or any tumor that cannot be assessed, as in a re-treatment staging

TO   No evidence of primary tumor

TIS   Carcinoma in situ

T1   A tumor that is 3 cm or less in greatest dimension, surrounded by lung or visceral pleura, and without evidence of invasion proximal to a lobar bronchus at bronchoscopy*

T2   A tumor more than 3.0 cm in greatest dimension, or a tumor of any size that either invades the visceral pleura or has associated atelectasis or obstructive pneumonitis extending to the hilar region. At bronchoscopy, the proximal extent of demonstrable tumor must be within a lobar bronchus or at least 2 cm distal to the carina. Any associated atelectasis or obstructive pneumonitis must involve less than an entire lung.

T3   A tumor of any size with direct extention into the chest wall (including superior sulcus tumors), diaphragm, or the mediastinal pleura or pericardium without involving the heart, great vessels, trachea, esophagus, or vertebral body, or a tumor in the main bronchus within 2 cm of the carina without involving the carina, or associated atelectasis or obstructive pneumonitis of entire lung

T4   A tumor of any size with invasion of the mediastinum or involving heart, great vessels, trachea, esophagus, vertebral body, or carina or presence of malignant pleural or pericardial effusion,[†] or with satellite tumor nodules within the ipsilateral, primary tumor lobe of the lung

N—Nodal involvement

NO   No demonstrable metastasis to regional lymph nodes

N1   Metastasis to lymph nodes in the peribronchial or the ipsilateral hilar region, or both, including direct extension

N2   Metastasis to ipsilateral mediastinal lymph nodes and subcarinal lymph nodes

---

Box 56–1. TNM Definitions—cont'd

N3   Metastasis to contralateral mediastinal lymph nodes, contralateral hilar lymph nodes, or ipsilateral or contralateral scalene or supraclavicular lymph nodes

M—Distant metastasis
M0   No (known) distant metastasis
M1   Distant metastasis present.[†] Specify site(s).

---

*The uncommon superficial tumor of any size with its invasive component limited to the bronchial wall, which may extend proximal to the main bronchus, is classified as T1.

[†]Most pleural effusions associated with lung cancer are due to tumor. There are, however, some few patients in whom cytopathologic examination of pleural fluid (on more than one specimen) is negative for tumor and the fluid is nonbloody and is not an exudate. In such cases in which these elements and clinical judgment dictate that the effusion is not related to the tumor, the patients should be staged T1, T2, or T3, excluding effusion as a staging element.

[†]Separate metastatic tumor nodules in ipsilateral nonprimary tumor lobes of the lung also are classified M1.

Data from Mountain CF: Revisions in the International System for Staging Lung Cancer. Chest 111:1710–1717, 1997; and Mountain CF, Dressler CM: Regional lymph node classification for lung cancer staging. Chest 111:1718–1723, 1997.

Radiographic Staging of Lung Cancer

● The chest x-ray film provides information on the size, shape, density, and location of the tumor in relation to the mediastinal structures.

● CT of the chest provides more detail than chest x-ray film on the surface characteristics of the tumor; relationships of the tumor to the mediastinum and mediastinal structures; and metastasis to lung, bone, liver, and adrenals.

● Enlargement of the mediastinal lymph nodes can be identified if present; when lymph nodes are greater than 1.5 cm in diameter, CT is approximately 85% specific in identifying metastasis to mediastinal lymph nodes.

Tissue-Based Staging

● Sputum cytology may yield a diagnosis of lung cancer but is not site-specific.

● Bronchoscopy, mediastinoscopy, or fine-needle aspiration (FNA) (bronchoscopic or CT-guided transthermic) is considered after obtaining a chest x-ray film or CT scan to obtain tissue for staging.

● Bronchoscopy is performed before resection to independently assess the endobronchial anatomy, exclude secondary

Box 56–2. Stage Grouping of the TNM Subsets

The TNM subsets are combined in seven stage groups, in addition to stage 0, reflecting fairly precise levels of disease progression and their implications for treatment selection and prognosis. Staging is not relevant for occult carcinoma TXN0M0.

Stage 0 is assigned to patients with carcinoma in situ, which is consistent with the staging of all other sites.

Stage IA includes only patients with tumors 3 cm or less in greatest dimension and no evidence of metastasis, the anatomic subset T1N0M0.

Stage IB includes only patients with a T2 primary tumor classification and no evidence of metastasis, the anatomic subset T2N0M0.

Stage IIA is reserved for patients with a T1 primary tumor classification and metastasis limited to the intrapulmonary including hilar, lymph nodes, the anatomic subset T1N1M0.

Stage IIB includes two anatomic subsets: patients with a T2 primary tumor classification and metastasis limited to the ipsilateral intrapulmonary, including hilar, lymph nodes the anatomic subset T2N1M0; and patients with primary tumor classification of T3 and no evidence of metastasis, the anatomic subset T3N0M0.

Stage IIIA includes four anatomic subsets that reflect the implications of ipsilateral, limited, extrapulmonary extension of the lung cancer. Patients included are those with a T3 primary tumor classification and metastasis limited to the ipsilateral intrapulmonary, including hilar, lymph nodes, T3N1M0 disease, and patients with T1, T2, T3 primary tumor classifications and metastasis limited to the ipsilateral mediastinal and subcarinal lymph nodes—the T1N2M0, T2N2M0, and T3N2M0 subsets.

Stage IIIB designates patients with extensive primary tumor invasion of the mediastinum and metastases to the contralateral mediastinal, contralateral hilar, and ipsilateral and contralateral scalene/supraclavicular lymph nodes. Patients with a T4 primary tumor classification or N3 regional lymph node metastasis, but no distant metastasis, are included.

> **Box 56–2. Stage Grouping of the TNM Subsets—cont'd**
>
> Stage IV is reserved for patients with evidence of distant metastatic disease, M1, such as metastases to brain, bone, liver, adrenal gland, contralateral lung, pancreas, and other distant organs, and metastases to distant lymph node groups such as axillary, abdominal, and inguinal. Patients with metastasis in ipsilateral nonprimary tumor lobes of the lung are also designated M1.

Data from Mountain CF: Revisions in the International System for Staging Lung Cancer. Chest 111:1710–1717, 1997; and Mountain CF, Dressler CM: Regional lymph node classification for lung cancer staging. Chest 111:1718–1723, 1997.

> **Box 56–3. Extrathoracic Nonmetastatic Symptoms (Paraneoplastic Syndromes)**
>
> **General**
> Weight loss/cachexia
> Fatigue
> General malaise
>
> **Endocrine**
> Cushing's syndrome from adrenocorticotropic hormone secretion
> Inappropriate antidiuretic hormone causing hyponatremia
> Carcinoid syndrome
> Hypercalcemia
> Rarely, hypoglycemia or ectopic gonadotropins
>
> **Skeletal**
> Clubbing, 10% to 20%
> Hypertrophic pulmonary osteoarthropathy—5% painful periosteal proliferation at the ends of long bones
>
> **Neuromuscular (approximately 15% and most common with small cell carcinoma)**
> Polymyositis
> Myasthenia-like syndrome (Eaton-Lambert)
> Peripheral neuropathy
> Subacute cerebellar degeneration
> Encephalopathy
>
> **Vascular thrombophlebitis**

Box 56–4. Criteria for Nonresectability

Recurrent laryngeal nerve paralysis
Superior vena cava syndrome
Involvement of main pulmonary artery
Contralateral or supraclavicular node involvement
Ipsilateral mediastinal nodes if high (2R)
Malignant (or bloody) pleural effusion, which may cause
  dyspnea or pleuritic chest pain or may be asymptomatic
Malignant pericardial effusion
Phrenic nerve paralysis (relative contraindication)
Extrathoracic metastatic disease typically involving the brain,
  bone, adrenals, or liver
Involvement of trachea, heart, great vessel
Insufficient pulmonary reserve
Other signs may suggest a more advanced tumor:
  Chest wall pain that may be described by the patient as
    dull, deep, and persistent
  Horner's syndrome causing compression of the splanchnic
    nerve with unilateral ptosis, meiosis, anhidrosis, and
    enophthalmos
  Phrenic nerve paralysis, with elevation of a hemidiaphragm
    from nerve paralysis
  Esophageal compression, yielding symptoms of dysphagia
    from extrinsic compression from enlarged subcarinal left
    nodes or direct invasion into the left mainstem/carina
    junction yielding a bronchoesophageal fistula

---

endobronchial primary tumors, and ensure that all known cancer will be encompassed by the planned pulmonary resection.

- Transbronchial biopsy may be performed with a special 21-gauge needle through the flexible bronchoscope; this technique may be used to biopsy mediastinal nodes or lung masses adjacent to the larger bronchi.
- An FNA via a transthoracic route may be approximately 95% accurate in patients with a poor operative risk.
- If the patient does have hard palpable lymph nodes in the cervical or supraclavicular area, FNA or biopsy may provide an accurate diagnosis of metastatic (N_3) involvement.
- A mediastinoscopy or anterior mediastinotomy (Chamberlain procedure) or video-assisted thoracic surgery (VATS) should be performed in all patients with enlarged (≥1 cm) mediastinal lymph nodes based on the location of the enlarged lymph nodes.

- Large mediastinal lymph nodes are more likely to be associated with metastasis (>70%); however, normal size lymph nodes (<1 cm) have a 7% to 15% chance of being involved.
- CT selects patients for mediastinoscopy with enlarged lymph nodes (≥1 cm) because 90% of patients with a normal mediastinum have negative N_2 lymph nodes after mediastinoscopy and pathologic examination (10% harbor cancer in normal-sized lymph nodes).
- Mediastinoscopy is recommended before the planned resection if the cancer is proximal, if pneumonectomy may be required, if the patient is at increased risk for the planned surgery or resection, if enlarged lymph nodes are noted on CT scan, or if neoadjuvant therapy is planned.
- Positron-emission tomography evaluation is being investigated as an alternative to mediastinoscopy for defining metastatic involvement of mediastinal nodes with lung cancer and other occult sites of metastases.
- Transesophageal ultrasound may assist the clinician in evaluating lung cancer that may abut the esophagus, heart, or aorta; directed transesophageal biopsies of subcarinal or posterior mediastinal lymph nodes may also be obtained.
- In patients with resectable lung cancer (stages I and II), a bone scan or a CT scan of the brain is not recommended in the absence of related symptoms such as bone pain or neurologic findings.
- In superior sulcus tumors with or without the first and second or third rib involvement, magnetic resonance imaging scanning may provide additional information as to the extent of the tumor's involvement with the brachial plexus, thoracic inlet, great vessels, or other mediastinal structures.

Solitary Pulmonary Nodule (SPN)

- An SPN may be defined as an asymptomatic mass within the lung parenchyma that is less than 3 cm in size.
- Overall, 33% of these masses are malignant; 50% are malignant if the patient's age is greater than 50 years.
- In general, a patient with an SPN should undergo resection for definitive diagnosis and treatment.
- The exceptions to this general statement are:
  - Those patients who have a mass unchanged for greater than 2 years (documented upon serial radiographic examinations).
  - Patients with benign patterns of calcification such as in hamartoma.

- Patients with masses clearly caused by an inflammatory process such as tuberculosis (TB).
- Those patients with prohibitive operative risk.
- Those patients in whom small cell carcinoma is suspected.
- If the FNA is positive for cancer, lobectomy is recommended; if the result is nondiagnostic, the results should not be trusted; consider repeat FNA then wedge resection for diagnosis; if positive, complete a lobectomy.
- A pneumonectomy should never be performed without a cancer diagnosis.

Molecular Markers

- K-*ras* mutation is the most frequent mutation with an associated poor survival outlook.
- DNA aneuploidy overexpression of *HER2* oncogenes and mutations in the retinoblastoma *(RB)* gene are also associated with poor survival.

Treatment of Lung Cancer

- Treatment options include surgery for localized disease, chemotherapy for metastatic disease, and radiation therapy for local control in patients whose condition is not amenable to surgery.
- Radiation therapy and chemotherapy together are better than chemotherapy or radiation therapy alone for primary treatment of advanced stage lung cancer.
- Protocols evaluating chemotherapy, radiation, and surgery for advanced stage lung cancer are ongoing.
- Surgery is not the primary treatment for small cell carcinoma; used for stage I only.
- Chemotherapy can provide patients with a survival advantage (12 months) over no treatment (6 months).

Treatment of Early-Stage Lung Cancer:
Stages IA, IB, IIA, IIB, and Early IIIA

- Early-stage lung cancer (stages I and II) may successfully be treated with surgery alone and, in most patients, yields long-term survival rates.
- Lobectomy with lymph node dissection or sampling is the procedure of choice for lung cancer confined to one lobe.
- En bloc resection of the lung and involved chest wall with mediastinal lymphadenectomy results in approximately a 40% 5-year survival rate.

- Based on favorable results with advanced stage disease, application of chemotherapy in earlier stages of lung cancer may improve survival expectations.

Treatment of Advanced Stage Lung Cancer (Stages IIIA [N2], IIIB, IV)

- Most patients with histologically confirmed N_2 disease (ipsilateral mediastinal nodes) have a biologically aggressive tumor with probable occult metastatic disease.
- Surgery alone for stage IIIA (N_2), IIIB, or IV lung cancer is infrequently performed because the risks of surgery usually exceed the benefits of surgery.

Chemotherapy

- Induction chemotherapy followed by radiation appears to improve survival in patients with locally advanced lung cancer in prospective randomized studies but morbidity increases.
- Cis platinum-based combination chemotherapy has been shown to improve survival expectation over and above that achieved with radiation alone.

Radiation Therapy

- Radiation therapy is a local control treatment modality.
- Postoperative radiation therapy may provide a local control advantage but no survival advantage in patients with complete resection of lung cancer.
- Radiation therapy can be effective palliative therapy in patients with symptomatic disease such as metastases to the bones or brain.
- Complications of radiation therapy include esophagitis and fatigue.

PULMONARY METASTASES

- The primary must be completely resected (controlled) before consideration of pulmonary metastasectomy.
- Patients who have complete resection of all metastases have associated longer survival expectations than those patients whose metastases are unresectable.
- Long-term survival (greater than 5 years) may be expected in approximately 20% to 30% of all patients with completely resectable pulmonary metastases (Box 56–5).

Box 56–5.   Criteria for Resection of Pulmonary Metastases

Pulmonary parenchymal nodules or changes consistent with metastases
Absence of uncontrolled extrathoracic metastases
Control of the patient's primary tumor
Potential for complete resection
Sufficient pulmonary parenchymal reserve following resection

Additional criteria for partial or complete resection
Provide a diagnosis
Evaluate the effects of chemotherapy on residual disease
Obtain tumor for markers, immunohistochemical studies, vaccine, and so on
Palliate symptoms
Decrease tumor burden

MISCELLANEOUS LUNG TUMORS

- Benign tumors of the lung account for less than 1% of all lung neoplasms and arise from mesodermal origins.
- Carcinoid tumors (1% of lung neoplasms) arise from Kulchitsky (amine precursor uptake and decarboxylation [APUD]) cells in bronchial epithelium.
- These "typical carcinoid" tumors (least malignant) are the most indolent of the spectrum of pulmonary neuroendocrine tumors that include atypical carcinoid, large cell undifferentiated carcinoma, and small cell carcinoma (most malignant).
- Carcinoid syndrome is uncommon with lung carcinoids, although it might occur with very large or metastatic tumors.
- Surgical resection of typical carcinoid and atypical carcinoid is standard, with complete removal of the tumor and as much preservation of lung as possible; lobectomy is the most common procedure.
- Adenoid cystic carcinoma is a slow-growing malignancy involving the trachea and mainstem bronchi that is similar to salivary gland tumors; treatment is wide en bloc resection with conservation of as much lung tissue as possible.

TRACHEA

- The location of the carina is at the level of the angle of Louis anteriorly and the T4 vertebra posteriorly.

- The blood supply to the trachea is lateral and segmental from the inferior thyroid, the internal thoracic, the supreme intercostal, and the bronchial arteries.
- Primary neoplasms of trachea include squamous cell carcinoma (two thirds) and adenoid cystic carcinoma (one third).

Tracheal Trauma

- Penetrating injuries to the trachea are usually cervical; penetrating injuries that involve the mediastinal trachea are usually lethal.
- Penetrating cervical injuries often involve the esophagus, and concurrent esophageal injury should be excluded by barium esophagram or esophagoscopy.
- Clinical features of a cervical injury are suggested by subcutaneous air in the neck, respiratory distress, and hemoptysis; diagnosis is made by bronchoscopy.
- Management of tracheal injuries includes control of airway by endotracheal intubation (using flexible bronchoscopy as a guide) or emergency tracheostomy.
- For injuries to the mediastinal trachea, the surgical approach is thoracotomy through the right fourth intercostal space or median sternotomy; associated esophageal injuries should be repaired primarily.
- Various techniques may be considered for diagnosis of tracheal abnormalities; plain x-ray films of the trachea and routine chest roentgenograms (posteroanterior), lateral, and obliques are critical first steps.
- CT of the trachea is good for examining luminal compromise; however, it is less suitable than linear tomograms for longitudinal abnormalities.
- If the patient has symptoms of dysphagia or if an esophageal cancer is suspected, a barium swallow is helpful to evaluate the extent of esophageal involvement.
- A tracheoinnominate fistula may result from prolonged cuff erosion inferiorly and anteriorly to the trachea.

EMPHYSEMA

- Emphysema is defined as dilation and destruction of the terminal air spaces.
- These air cavities may be defined as blebs (subpleural air space separated the lung by a thin pleural covering with only minor alveolar communications) or bulla (larger than a bleb with some destruction of the underlying lung parenchyma).

- Pneumothorax may occur with emphysema; conservative therapy often requires days to weeks of suction with chest tubes to obtain pleural symphysis.
- Indications for surgical intervention include a significantly large bulla (one third to one half of a hemithorax) with symptoms and only mild diffuse lung disease.
- Lung volume reduction surgery attempts to remove areas of lung with severe emphysema, allowing the remaining lung to expand better by decreasing hyperinflation and allowing the functional bronchioles to "expand" their diameter, giving improved elastic recoil with improved aeration and perfusion of the remaining lung.
- Lung transplantation is performed for chronic obstructive pulmonary disease (COPD) (especially alpha$_1$-antitrypsin deficiency), pulmonary fibrosis, primary pulmonary hypertension, and cystic fibrosis.
- Survival rate after lung transplantation is approximately 75% at 1 year, 60% at 2 years, and 50% at 5 years.
- Unilateral lung transplantation is more readily tolerated than double lung transplant.

ACUTE RESPIRATORY DISTRESS SYNDROME

- Approximately 50,000 cases occur each year in the United States, with a mortality rate of 30% to 70%.
- The initial clinical presentation of dyspnea, tachypnea, hypoxemia, and hypercapnia is nonspecific.
- A chest x-ray film may show diffuse bilateral infiltrates secondary to increased interstitial fluid.
- The underlying mechanism is increased pulmonary capillary permeability with extravasation of intravascular fluid and protein into the interstitium and alveoli.
- This process causes hypoxemia; pulmonary hypertension; CO_2 retention; secondary infections; and eventually right heart failure, hypoxia, and death.
- Criteria include impaired oxygenation with the PaO_2/FIO_2 ratio of less than 200 mm Hg and an estimated shunt fraction of more than 30%.
- Noncardiogenic pulmonary edema is present, and the pulmonary capillary wedge pressure is less than 18 mm Hg.
- Treatment is directed to improve oxygenation with optimal pulmonary hygiene, intubation, and pressure-controlled ventilation (peak pressure <35 mm Hg).
- Maintaining an inspired oxygen concentration as low as possible and positive end-expiratory pressure (<50%) 10 to 15 mm Hg to maintain the alveolar opening pressure and

functional residual capacity to maintain adequate oxygenation and carbon dioxide exchange.

BACTERIAL INFECTIONS

- Bronchiectasis is an infection of the bronchial wall and surrounding lung with sufficient severity to cause destruction and dilation of the air passages.
- With use of antibiotics, it has become rare to see an emaciated febrile patient coughing up large amounts of foul sputum accompanied by clubbing, cyanosis, and hemoptysis; currently, frequent respiratory infections are typical.
- Chest x-ray film and CT scan reveal extent.
- Bronchoscopy can be performed to clear secretions and, when the diagnosis is suspected, to rule out cancer, foreign body, or stricture.
- Cultures may be obtained to facilitate antibiotic treatment.
- Surgery is indicated if there is failure of medical therapy, recurrent pneumonia, or hemoptysis affecting a normal lifestyle.

Lung Abscess

- The infection is usually anaerobic and associated with aspiration from alcohol abuse, a debilitated or elderly individual, or esophageal disease.
- With aspiration progressing to lung abscess, the location is more commonly found on the right than the left.
- Lung abscess may also be superimposed on structural abnormalities (bronchogenic cyst, sequestration, bleb, or TB or fungal cavities).
- Clinical features are similar to those of chronic pneumonia, including fever, cough, leukocytosis, pleuritic pain, and sputum production.
- The chest x-ray film and the CT scan of the chest may demonstrate a rounded area of consolidation early and an air-fluid level on upright or decubitus chest x-ray later.
- The differential diagnosis includes loculated emphysema, which may be treated with drainage, epiphrenic diverticulum (in which the patient is not septic), or TB or fungus cavity.
- Medical management is with antibiotics and pulmonary toilet (e.g., re-expansion).
- Bronchoscopy to assist in drainage also rules out foreign body, stenosis, or cancer.
- Patients (85% to 95%) respond to medical management with rapid decrease in fluid, collapse of the walls, and complete healing in 3 to 4 months.

- Surgical therapy is indicated for persistent cavity (>2 cm and thick walled) after 8 weeks of medical therapy, failure to clear sepsis, and hemoptysis (often small sentinel bleed before a massive bleed).

Mycobacterial Infections

- TB tends to occur in apical and posterior segments of the upper lobes and superior segments of the lower lobes.
- Bronchoscopy may be required for patients not responding to medical management.
- Cancer should be excluded with a newly identified mass on chest x-ray film even with a positive TB skin test and an acid fast bacillus (AFB)-negative sputum.
- Medical management (five drugs) is with isonicotinic acid hydrazide (INH), rifampin, ethambutol, streptomycin, or pyrazinamide (Box 56–6).
- Surgical options include resection; preservation of lung tissue should be a goal of the treatment.
- A chest tube or open drainage may be used to control a large cavity with positive sputum.

Box 56–6. Potential Indications for Surgery for Pulmonary Tuberculosis

Open positive cavity after 3 to 6 months of chemotherapy, especially if resistant mycobacteria

Persistent positive sputum with pathology (destroyed lung, atelectasis, bronchiectasis, bronchostenosis) amenable to resection

Negative sputum but destroyed lung, blocked cavity, tuberculoma—consider for resection

Localized infection with atypical mycobacteria

Tuberculous bronchiectasis of lower and middle lobes (usually occurs in upper lobes—good drainage: lower and middle lobes do not drain well)

Open negative cavities if thick walled, slow response, or unreliable patient

To exclude cancer

Recurrent or persistent hemoptysis: resection if greater than 600 mL of blood is lost in 24 hours or less

Pleural disease where indicated

Fungal and Parasitic Infections

- Histoplasmosis is the most common of all fungal infections in the United States and is most frequently systemic; the localized form is usually an acute pneumonia, self-limited, and rarely severe.

- The lymphogenous reaction to *Histoplasma* causes mediastinal lymph node enlargement and may cause middle lobe syndrome, bronchiectasis, esophageal traction diverticulum, tracheoesophageal fistula, constrictive pericarditis, or fibrosing mediastinitis.

- Coccidiomycosis is endemic to the Southwest; inhaling the organism results in a primary lung disease that is usually self-limited.

- Treatment for symptomatic fungal infections is with amphotericin.

- Indications for surgery are cavitary disease (thick-walled or greater than 2-cm cavities, enlarging cavities, ruptured cavities), secondary bacterial infections, and severe recurrent hemoptysis.

- Cryptococcosis is the second most frequent lethal fungus after histoplasmosis; lungs are frequently involved; surgery may be required for open biopsy for diagnosis.

- Aspergillosis is an opportunistic infection; cavities may form because of destruction of the underlying pulmonary parenchyma; debris and hyphae may coalesce and form a fungus ball, which lies free in the cavity and can roll around; resection is indicated if isolated disease is present in good-risk patients.

- Mucormycosis is rare, opportunistic, and rapidly progressive; medical management with cessation of steroids and anti-neoplastic drugs and initiation of amphotericin and control of diabetes is undertaken.

- Actinomycosis is a chronic anaerobic endogenous infection deep within a wound; "sulfur granules" draining from infected sinuses are microcolonies; the cervicofacial form is the most common, and treatment is most commonly penicillin.

- Nocardiosis is an aerobic bacterium widely disseminated in soil; it resembles actinomycosis in invading the chest wall and produces subcutaneous abscesses and sinuses draining sulfur granules; surgery is performed to exclude cancer, to obtain a diagnosis, or to treat complications of the disease.

- Infections with *Entamoeba histolytica* are usually confined to the right lower thorax and are related to extension from a liver abscess below the diaphragm; metronidazole is usually effective.

- Infection with *Echinococcus* may occur; the hydatid cyst may rupture, flooding the lung or producing a severe hypersensitivity reaction.
- *Pneumocystis carinii* is an opportunistic infection that is positive on silver methenamine stain; bronchoalveolar lavage obtains the diagnosis in more than 90% of patients; seen especially in acquired immunodeficiency syndrome (AIDS) patients.

MASSIVE HEMOPTYSIS

- Massive hemoptysis is defined as greater than 500 to 600 mL of blood loss from the lungs in 24 hours; the most common etiologies are shown in Box 56–7.
- Diagnosis and treatment of massive hemoptysis typically include a chest x-ray examination and CT scan; emergency bronchoscopy is usually frustrating; bronchial artery embolization by transfemoral aortic catheter is most effective.
- Management may consist simply of bronchoscopy, clearing the airway of blood, cough suppression (with codeine), and rest if bleeding resolves.
- CT scan to identify etiology and elective bronchoscopy on resolution will allow planned surgical resection.

PULMONARY EMBOLISM

- Thrombi most commonly develop in the veins of the lower leg from stasis and a hypercoagulable state and propagate proximally to the deep veins of the leg and pelvis.

Box 56–7. Causes of Hemoptysis

Lung cancer
Lung abscess
Cavitary aspergillosis
Tuberculosis
Bronchiectasis
Swan-Ganz catheterization
Cystic fibrosis
Broncholithiasis
Foreign body
Transbronchial lung biopsy
Tuberculosis

- As these clots enlarge, the propensity for these clots to dislodge and embolize to the lungs increases.
- Vasoactive agents are released with further elevation of pulmonary vascular resistance, a shunt develops as the pulmonary blood flow is redistributed, and pulmonary edema may occur.
- Risk factors for pulmonary embolus may include high body-mass index, cigarette smoking, hypertension, and surgery.
- Resistance to activated protein C may be transmitted as an autosomal dominant trait in some patients with a propensity for venous thrombosis.
- The clinical presentation of pulmonary embolus ranges from dyspnea, tachypnea, and chest pain to instant death.
- Physical examination may include signs of right ventricular dysfunction.
- The electrocardiogram may demonstrate right ventricular hypertrophy with strain, right bundle branch block, tachycardia, and T-wave inversion in the anterior chest leads (V_1 to V_4).
- The D-dimer is elevated in a number of conditions other than pulmonary embolism; however, a negative D-dimer assay suggests the likelihood of pulmonary embolism is low.
- Other studies include ultrasound examination or impedance plethysmography of the lower extremities, ventilation perfusion lung scan, echocardiography, high-resolution spiral CT of the chest, and pulmonary angiogram.
- Pulmonary arteriogram images the obstructed pulmonary arteries and remains the "gold standard" for diagnosis.

Treatment of Pulmonary Embolus

- Untreated pulmonary embolism has a 30% hospital mortality rate, whereas treated patients have a mortality rate estimated at approximately 2%.
- Treatment includes systemic anticoagulation with heparin, oxygen, and analgesia; intravenous fluids may be required.
- Oral anticoagulation may be started with warfarin; the duration of warfarin therapy should be 3 months or longer.
- Use of an inferior vena cava filter should be considered in patients with pulmonary embolism, when anticoagulation would carry increased risk (e.g., recent surgery), or in patients with recurrent pulmonary emboli.
- In patients with a serious hemodynamic and hypoxic response, thrombolytics (streptokinase or urokinase) may be given; the value of such treatment must be weighed against the risk of major hemorrhage.

- Venous (suction) or open (surgical) embolectomy may be performed to extract or obliterate the clot in patients with life-threatening hypoxia or hemodynamic instability.

Prevention

- Subcutaneous heparin is most commonly used for perioperative prophylaxis and effectively reduces the rate of fatal pulmonary embolism.
- Mechanical compression devices to stimulate fibrinolysis (from stimulation of the venous endothelium) are effective in patients who are bed-bound.

THORACIC OUTLET SYNDROME

- Thoracic outlet syndrome includes compression of the subclavian artery, the subclavian vein, or the brachial plexus where it passes between the scalene muscles and over the first rib.
- Diagnosis is primarily clinical; clinical features include intermittent symptoms of nerve compression, which include pain, paresthesias, and weakness.
- Electromyelogram or nerve conduction studies are helpful to rule out carpal tunnel syndrome.
- Noninvasive arterial studies may be helpful.
- Angiography may be performed if aneurysm, thrombus, or emboli are suspected.
- Initial treatment is physical therapy for 2 to 12 months.
- Surgery is used as a last resort for severe pain, impaired motor function or atrophy, or treatment failure.
- Transaxillary first rib resection allows complete decompression with a good cosmetic result; cervical ribs are also removed; the supraclavicular approach is preferred by some.

CHAPTER 57

CONGENITAL HEART DISEASE

LESIONS RESULTING IN INCREASED PULMONARY BLOOD FLOW

- The amount of increased pulmonary blood flow will depend on the absolute size of the defect, the resistances of the pulmonary and systemic vascular beds, and the total pumping capacity of the ventricular mass.

Patent Ductus Arteriosus (PDA)

- Common isolated defect affecting 1 in 2000 births, with an increased incidence in premature neonates.

Anatomy and Pathophysiology

- Fetal structure that allows blood to divert away from the lungs and into the descending aorta.
- Functional closure is reversible and occurs first, mediated by the removal of the placental source of prostaglandin and its metabolism in the lungs.
- Physiology of a PDA that fails to close is left-to-right shunting and increased pulmonary blood flow with left atrial and ventricular volume overload.
- Complications of a PDA in older patients include aneurysm formation, infective endocarditis, calcification, and the risk of pulmonary vascular obstructive disease.

Diagnosis and Intervention

- Typical machinery murmur older children.
- Pulmonary congestion and failure to thrive neonates and infants.
- Difficulty in weaning from ventilatory support premature infants.
- Echocardiography is diagnostic.
- Cardiac catheterization if irreversible pulmonary hypertension is suspected in older patients.

Closure of the Patent Ductus Arteriosus

- Premature infants by indomethacin (inhibition of prostaglandin synthesis).
- Older children using coils and occluder devices.
- Surgery when other interventions fail or are inappropriate:
  - Left posterolateral thoracotomy.
- Duct is ligated or clipped (premature) or divided.
- Complications:
  - Bleeding.
  - Recurrent laryngeal nerve injury.
  - Pneumothoraces and chylothorax.

Aorticopulmonary Window

- Conotruncal anomaly, window, or communication between the aorta and the pulmonary artery.

Anatomy and Pathophysiology

- Associated lesions:
  - Ventricular septal defect (VSD).
  - Coarctation of the aorta.
  - Aortic arch interruption.
- Physiology is similar to large PDA with pulmonary overcirculation, pulmonary hypertension, left ventricular volume overload, and possible diastolic steal from the coronary circulation.

Diagnosis and Indications for Intervention

- Heart failure when the pulmonary vascular resistance (PVR) falls after birth.
- Echocardiography diagnostic.
- Intervention at the time of diagnosis, unless irreversible pulmonary vascular obstruction disease is already established.

Intervention

- Median sternotomy and cardiopulmonary bypass (CPB).
- Direct suture closure or patch closure with branch pulmonary artery reconstruction.

Atrial Septal Defects (ASD)

- Most common isolated cardiac defect.

Anatomy and Pathophysiology

- Atrial septum consists of the septum primum and the septum secundum.
- Defects failure of the septum primum to develop or regression of the interatrial folds.
- Four types:

  1. Ostium secundum.
  2. Ostium primum.

  - Form of atrioventricular (AV) canal defect.

  3. Sinus venous type.

  - Defect at the level of the superior vena cava or inferior vena cava.

  4. Coronary sinus type.

  - Unroofed coronary sinus as it traverses left atrium.

Direction and Amount of Shunting

- Depends on the size of the defect and the relative diastolic compliance of the ventricles.
- Congestive heart failure usually after the second or third decade.
- Older patients risks:
  - Paradoxical embolism and stroke.
  - Atrial fibrillation and flutter.
  - Sinus node dysfunction.
  - Pulmonary vascular obstructive disease.

Diagnosis Indications for Intervention

- Transthoracic echocardiography usually diagnostic.
- Cardiac catheterization to assess pulmonary pressure and PVR if pulmonary hypertension suspected and to exclude coronary artery disease in older patients.

Surgery

- Closure indicated all symptomatic patients, all children with a significant ASD.
- Adults with a left-to-right shunt greater than 1.5:1.
- Severe pulmonary vascular obstructive disease (resistance greater than 8.0 Wood units.m^2) is contraindication to closure.
- May be closed surgically or by percutaneous transcatheter device closure.

Postoperative Complications

- Pericardial effusions.
- Postpericardiotomy syndrome.
- Postoperative dysrhythmias.
- Residual ASDs.

Ventricular Septal Defects

- May be single, multiple, or part of more complex cardiac anomalies.

Anatomy and Pathophysiology

- Classified by the position they occupy in the ventricular septum.

Perimembranous or Paramembranous Defects

- Around the membranous septum and fibrous trigone of the heart near the aortic valve and annulus of the tricuspid valve.
- Conduction tissue passes along the posteroinferior rim of the defect.

Muscular Defects

- Single but commonly multiple.

Subarterial, Outlet, or Conal Defects

- Located in the outlet portions of the left and right ventricles.
- Superior edge is the conjoined annulus of the aortic and pulmonary valves.
- Also called juxta-arterial or supracristal defects.
- Associated with prolapse of the unsupported aortic valve cusps and progressive aortic regurgitation.

Malalignment Defects

- Malalignment between the infundibular and the trabecular muscular septum.
- Malalignment can be anterior, as in tetralogy of Fallot (TOF) or posterior.
- Associated defects:
  - PDA.

- Pulmonary stenosis.
- ASD.
- Persistent left superior vena cava.
- Coarctation of the aorta.

Hemodynamic Effect

- Left-to-right shunting leading to increased pulmonary blood flow, left atrial dilatation, and left ventricular volume overload.
- Size of the shunt determined by the size of the defect and the PVR.
- Quantify shunt by the ratio of systemic to pulmonary blood flow (Qp:Qs).
- In time, as the PVR increases, histologic changes occur within the pulmonary vascular bed, which may be irreversible.
- As the PVR increases, left-to-right side shunt decreases then a reversal of the flow occurs, leading to a right-to-left shunt with the development of increasing cyanosis (Eisenmenger s syndrome).

Diagnosis and Indications for Intervention

- Clinical picture varies:
  - Asymptomatic patient with a murmur, patient in fulminant heart failure, and cyanosed patient with irreversible pulmonary vascular obstructive disease.
- Echocardiogram is diagnostic.
- Cardiac catheterization when reversibility of the pulmonary artery pressure (PAP) is questionable.
- PVR of more than 8.0 Woods units.m^2 after interventions to produce pulmonary vasodilatation is inoperable.

Management

- Intervene when the likelihood of spontaneous VSD closure is lowest and the risk of irreversible pulmonary vascular disease and ventricular dysfunction are minimized.
- Eighty percent of VSDs seen at 1 month of age will close spontaneously.
- When the defect is large and congestive heart failure and failure to thrive is present, early closure is warranted.
- Subarterial VSDs (risk of irreversible aortic valve cusp prolapse) leads to earlier intervention.
- Large VSD without signs of spontaneous closure should be closed by age 1 year.

- Multiple VSDs: if large shunt presents beyond 6 to 8 weeks, pulmonary artery banding and removal after 2 years of age with an attempt at septation is a reasonable option.

Surgery

- Most VSDs can be repaired through a right atrial approach.
- Mortality and morbidity increase with multiple VSDs, pulmonary hypertension, and complex associated anomalies.

Atrioventricular Canal Defects

- Also known as endocardial cushion defects or AV septal defects.
- High incidence of Down s syndrome.
- Spectrum of anomalies depending on the presence of atrial and ventricular defects.
- Partial atrioventricular canal (PAVC) or complete atrioventricular canal (CAVC) defects.

Anatomy and Pathophysiology

- Three principal components in a CAVC defect:
  - Defect of the AV septum.
  - Defect of the interventricular septum.
  - An abnormal AV valve.
- Ostium primum defect or PAVC defect consists of ASD associated with abnormal AV valve anatomy, a cleft leaflet of the left-sided and right-sided AV valves.
- Classification of CAVC Rastelli types A, B, and C relates to the superior AV valve leaflet chordal attachments to the ventricular septum.
- In PAVC defect, the pathophysiology is that of an ASD, with or without left-sided AV valve regurgitation.
- CAVC defect, the pathophysiology is that of a VSD with an associated ASD.

Diagnosis

- Heart failure uncommon in PAVC before 6 months of age but is quite common in CAVC by the age of 2 months.
- Irreversible pulmonary vascular obstructive disease may occur before 1 year of age.
- Echocardiography is diagnostic.
- Cardiac catheterization is indicated when elevated PVR is suspected.

Surgery

- PAVC surgery at preschool age or earlier.
- CAVC age for surgery relates to the risk for the development of pulmonary vascular obstructive disease: repair by 3 months of age is a reasonable compromise.
- Careful suture placement for the ASD and VSD patch is essential to avoid heart block.

Truncus Arteriosus

- Single arterial trunk arises from both ventricles, from which the coronary and pulmonary arteries originate.
- Usually associated with conotruncal VSD.

Anatomy and Pathophysiology

- Associated lesions include aortic arch obstruction, right aortic arch, interrupted aortic arch, and ASDs.
- Pathophysiology relates to a pressure and volume overload to both right and left ventricles, with pulmonary overflow dependent on the PVR.
- PVR fall after birth causes significant pulmonary overflow and congestive heart failure.
- Heart failure is more severe with truncal valve regurgitation.

Diagnosis and Presentation

- Echocardiography is diagnostic.
- Cardiac catheterization in older infants when pulmonary vascular disease is suspected.

Surgery

- Complete repair is recommended in the neonatal period but can be safely delayed up to 3 months in patients with easily controlled heart failure.
- VSD is closed and a conduit is placed from the right ventricle to the transected pulmonary arteries.

ABNORMALITIES OF VENOUS RETURN: SYSTEMIC AND PULMONARY

Abnormal Systemic Venous Return

- Persistent left superior vena cava to the coronary sinus.

Anomalous Pulmonary Venous Return

Partial

- Right upper pulmonary veins draining to the superior vena cava.
- Right-sided pulmonary veins to the inferior vena cava.
- Left upper pulmonary veins draining to the left innominate vein via a vertical vein.

Diagnosis and Presentation

- Depends on the magnitude of the associated shunt.
- Degree of systemic desaturation.
- Presence or absence of pulmonary vein obstruction.

Surgery

- Redirection of the pulmonary venous return with closure of the ASD.

Cor Triatriatum

- Diaphragm or membrane separating the left atrium into two chambers.
- Presentation is that of obstructed mitral inflow.
- Operative correction:
  - Excision obstructing membrane.
  - Closure of the ASD.

Total Anomalous Pulmonary Venous Connection (TAPVC)

- Abnormal drainage of all the pulmonary veins directly or indirectly to the systemic venous atrium.
- Supracardiac, cardiac, infracardiac, or mixed.

Pathophysiology

- Depends on whether or not the veins or ASD is obstructed.

Diagnosis and Presentation

- Obstructed TAPVC present with cyanosis, various levels of pulmonary venous congestion, respiratory compromise, and acidosis requires immediate surgical intervention.
- Unobstructed TAPVC similar to that of a large ASD with some degree of cyanosis.

Surgery

- Supracardiac TAPVC.
  - Anastomosis between the retropericardial pulmonary venous confluence and the left atrium.
- Intracardiac type.
  - Huge coronary sinus unroofed into the left atrium.
- Infracardiac type.
  - Pulmonary venous confluence and left atrium are anastomosed in a side-to-side fashion.
  - Descending vertical vein is divided.

LESIONS RESULTING IN DECREASED PULMONARY BLOOD FLOW

- Reduce pulmonary blood flow by obstruction at, below, or above the pulmonary valve.

Tetralogy of Fallot

- Conotruncal defect resulting from anterior malalignment of the infundibular septum.
- Four components of TOF:
  - The VSD.
  - Aortic valve override.
  - Narrowing of the right ventricular outflow tract.
  - Secondary right ventricular hypertrophy, resulting from narrowing of the right ventricular outflow tract.

Anatomy and Pathophysiology

- Right ventricular outflow tract obstruction (RVOTO) subpulmonary level, pulmonary valve level, main pulmonary artery level, pulmonary artery bifurcation level.
- Physiology depends on the degree of RVOTO.
  - Minimal obstruction left-to-right shunt (acyanotic TOF).
  - Severe obstruction pulmonary blood flow causes profound cyanosis.

Indications for Intervention

- Nature of the RVOTO dictates management.
- Hypercyanotic episodes (Tet spells) may occur with agitation or irritability.
- Chest x-ray examination may be classic boot-shaped heart.
- Echocardiography diagnostic.

- Cardiac catheterization.
  - TOF with previous palliation.
  - Presence of aortic pulmonary collaterals and pulmonary artery branching abnormalities are suspected.
- Asymptomatic patients elective repair from the neonatal period up until 1 year of age.
- Symptomatic or cyanotic patients complete repair as a single-stage procedure or two-stage approach, initial systemic-to-pulmonary artery shunting.

Surgical Intervention

Palliation

- A systemic-to-pulmonary artery shunt if risk of complete repair is considered to be higher than two-stage approach.

Complete Repair

- Closure of the VSD and relief of the RVOTO.

Pulmonary Atresia and Intact Ventricular Septum

- Spectrum ranges from patients with small right ventricles, small tricuspid valves, and associated coronary artery abnormalities, at high risk.
- Other end of the spectrum, nearly normal-sized right ventricles, well-developed infundibulum, and a favorable prognosis.

Anatomy and Pathophysiology

- Atresia of the pulmonary valve.
  - Intact ventricular septum.
  - Variable hypoplasia of the right ventricle and tricuspid valve.
- Pulmonary blood flow is supplied by a PDA.
- Physiology is similar to that of other forms of functional single ventricle with a duct-dependent pulmonary circuit.
- Cardiac catheterization for an assessment of coronary artery anatomy when sinusoids and fistula formation are suspected.

Management

- Staged approach toward either a univentricular or a biventricular repair, based initially on the size of the infundibulum.

- Fontan-type track is chosen if right ventricle will be inadequate.

Pulmonary Valve Stenosis

- Unicuspid, bicuspid, or tricuspid valve with commissural fusion.
- Balloon valvuloplasty is the initial procedure of choice.

Transposition of the Great Arteries (TGA)

- Aorta arising from an anatomic right ventricle and the pulmonary artery rising from an anatomic left ventricle.

Simple Transposition

- Interventricular septum is intact or almost intact.
- Dominant physiologic abnormality is reduced oxygenation with increased right and left ventricular volume load.

Complex Transposition of the Great Arteries

- VSD or VSDs allow mixing at an additional level, adding congestive heart failure.

Diagnosis

- Diagnosis with echocardiography.
- If balloon atrial septostomy is required, it is usually done under echocardiographic guidance.

Surgical Intervention

- Arterial switch operation.
- Surgery usually by 2 weeks but should be achieved by 3 months of age.
- Postoperatively, re-evaluation for supravalvar, aortic, and pulmonary stenosis should be followed with echocardiography.

Double-Outlet Right Ventricle (DORV)

- Conotruncal malformation in which both great arteries arise or mostly arise from the right ventricle.

Anatomy and Pathophysiology

- All of one and more than 50% of the other great artery arises from the right ventricle.
- Four types of DORV based on the relationship of the VSD to the great vessels.
- Physiology will depend on the nature of the VSD, state of the AV valves, and the degree of pulmonary stenosis.

Surgery

- Type of operation depends on VSD location and presence of pulmonary outflow obstruction.

LEFT VENTRICULAR OUTFLOW TRACT OBSTRUCTION (LVOTO)

- LVOTO can occur at any level from the subaortic area to the descending aorta.
- Significant hypoplasia of the left ventricle, mitral valve, and aortic valve may preclude a biventricular repair.

Aortic Stenosis

Valvar Aortic Stenosis

- Symptoms are usually seen only when the stenosis is severe.
- Multiple additional levels of LVOTO may accompany valvar stenosis.

Diagnosis and Presentation

- Echocardiogram is usually diagnostic.
- Neonates and infants present with congestive heart failure or circulatory collapse.
- Older infants present with signs of congestive heart failure or a murmur.

Surgery

- Balloon dilatation is a valid alternative to surgical valvotomy.
- Aortic valve replacement is the less preferable option.

Subaortic Stenosis

- Three groups:
  - Discrete membranous.
  - Fibromuscular tunnel type.

- Hypertrophic type.
- Associated lesions include malalignment VSD defects, coarctation of the aorta, and CAVC.

Physiology

- Pressure overload on the left ventricle associated with progressive left ventricular hypertrophy and eventual dysfunction.
- Echocardiography can identify the anatomic site of obstruction and the degree of obstruction.

Surgery

- Indications:
  - A gradient of more than 25 mm Hg.
  - The presence of underlying aortic insufficiency.
  - Coexisting lesions.
- Surgery removes the LVOTO and preserves the aortic valve.

Supravalvar Aortic Stenosis

- Localized or diffuse narrowing from the level of the sino-tubular junction.
- Coronary orifices may be obstructed by the thickened right of tissue at the sino-tubular junction.
- Pathophysiology is that of pressure overload and progressive left ventricular hypertrophy and eventual dysfunction.

Diagnosis

- Cardiac catheterization to identify coronary artery origin narrowing, other systemic artery origin stenosis, and peripheral pulmonary artery stenosis.

Surgery

- Indications:
  - Gradient of more than 50 mm Hg in an asymptomatic patient.
  - Positive exercise testing.
- Under CPB, patch angioplasty of the ascending aorta.

Aortic Arch Interruption

- Loss of continuity between the ascending and the descending aorta.

- Descending aorta flow is maintained through a large ductus arteriosus.
- Associated large, malalignment VSD.

Anatomy and Pathophysiology

- Aortic arch interruption is classified into three types:
  - Type A (25%): interruption beyond the left subclavian artery.
  - Type B (70%): interruption between the left carotid and the subclavian arteries.
  - Type C (5%): interruption between the innominate and the left carotid arteries.
- Present within the first few days of life.
- Reduced systemic blood flow to the lower extremities causes acidosis, renal failure, hepatic ischemia, and necrotizing enterocolitis.
- Pulmonary circulation is flooded as the PVR drops.
- Treatment with prostaglandin E_1 (PGE_1) allows reopening of the duct, providing a period for recovery before undertaking complete repair.
- DiGeorge syndrome in 15% to 30% of infants.
  - Hypocalcemia can be problematic, and blood products should be irradiated.

Surgery

- Single-stage complete repair is preferable to a staged approach.
- Resection of all ductal tissue followed by anastomosis between the separated aortic segments is performed.

Coarctation of the Aorta

- Congenital narrowing of the thoracic aorta, usually occurring distal to the left subclavian artery, at the point of insertion of the ductus arteriosus.

Anatomy and Pathophysiology

- Site of coarctation is always juxtaductal, with or without associated arch or isthmic hypoplasia.
- Severe coarctation and duct-dependent descending aortic flow present with cardiovascular collapse at the time of spontaneous ductal closure.
- Treatment with PGE_1 opens and maintains the patency of the ductus arteriosus, preserving distal organ perfusion.

- Older patients often asymptomatic or have claudication on exercise or upper body hypertension.

Diagnosis and Indications for Intervention

- Absent femoral pulses and poor distal perfusion are highly suspicious for the diagnosis in an infant.
- Older child upper extremity hypertension and a differential between upper and lower body pressures.
- Echocardiogram in most instances will confirm the diagnosis.

Surgery

- Surgical options include resection and end-to-end anastomosis, prosthetic patch aortoplasty (rarely done associated with late aneurysms), and subclavian flap aortoplasty.

UNSEPTATABLE HEARTS AND THE FONTAN PRINCIPLE

- One of the ventricles is inadequate for supporting total cardiac output.
- Fontan principle requires:
  - Total resistance to blood flow through the lungs and into the ventricular cavity is nearly normal.
  - Systemic venous return can be connected directly to the pulmonary arteries without an intervening pump.
- Often used preliminary procedure before completing the Fontan connection is the bidirectional cavopulmonary shunt (superior vena cava connected to pulmonary artery) or bidirectional Glenn shunt.
- Complications of the Fontan procedure are frequent and can include atrial arrhythmias and pleural effusions.
- With bad Fontan physiology, ascites with protein-losing enteropathy and progressive ventricular dysfunction.

Tricuspid Atresia

Anatomy and Physiology

- Three types:
  - Type 1 (70%): great arteries are in concordance with the ventricles.
  - Type 2 (20%): hearts with TGA.
  - Type 3 (<10%): hearts with AV discordance and TGA.

Diagnosis and Management

- Echocardiography diagnostic in infant.
- Cardiac catheterization required for assessment of PVR and to assess the anatomy of the pulmonary arteries if previous pulmonary artery banding or previous shunt placement before second stage.

Surgery

- Ultimate goal for these patients is to achieve anatomy and physiology favorable for an eventual Fontan circuit.
- Infants with inadequate pulmonary blood flow will require shunting.
- In infants with unobstructed pulmonary blood flow, a pulmonary artery band is applied.

Hypoplastic Left Heart Syndrome

- Severe aortic valve hypoplasia or atresia, hypoplasia of the ascending aorta, stenosis or atresia of the mitral valve, and hypoplasia or atresia of the left ventricle.
- Diagnosis made by echocardiography.
- Staged operative strategy for long-term palliation involves the following:
  - Creation of an unobstructed outlet to the systemic circuit and adequate pulmonary blood flow.
  - Followed a few months later by a bidirectional cavopulmonary shunt.
  - Finally, completion of the Fontan.

Physiology

- In neonates, the duct must be kept open with PGE_1 infusion.
- Key to managing these patients is to balance the pulmonary and systemic blood flows.

CORONARY ARTERY ANOMALIES

- Anomalous left coronary artery rising from the pulmonary artery (ALCAPA).

Pathophysiology

- After birth, the PAP falls and left coronary artery perfusion decreases.

- Ischemia causes impaired ventricular function and myocardial infarcts and leads to left ventricular dilatation.
- ALCAPA should be suspected in any infant with mitral regurgitation, ventricular dysfunction, or dilated cardiomyopathy.

Surgery

- Direct reimplantation of the ALCAPA into the ascending aorta is currently the procedure of choice.

Vascular Rings and Pulmonary Artery Sling

- Abnormalities of the aortic arch and its branches, compressing the trachea and/or esophagus.
- Pulmonary artery sling occurs when the left pulmonary artery arises from the right pulmonary artery, passing leftward between the trachea and the esophagus.

Complete Vascular Rings

- Double arch: equal arches or left or right arch dominant.
- Right arch: left ligamentum arteriosus from anomalous left subclavian artery.
- Right arch: mirror image branching, with left ligamentum from descending aorta.

Partial Vascular Rings

- Left arch: aberrant right subclavian artery.
- Left arch: innominate artery compression.

Diagnosis

- Symptoms reflect the degree of tracheal and esophageal compression and the presence of coexistent tracheomalacia or stenosis from complete rings.
- Echocardiography can document an abnormal head and neck vessel branching pattern.
- Magnetic resonance imaging study provides complete anatomic detail.

Surgery

- Division of the ring and, in the case of double arch, preservation of the dominant arch is performed.

- Pulmonary artery slings are approached through the midline.
  - Use of CPB facilitates tracheal reconstruction and relocation of the right pulmonary artery.

Ebstein's Anomaly of the Tricuspid Valve

- Rare defect in which the tricuspid valve attachments are displaced into the right ventricle.
- Associated abnormalities are an ASD, pulmonary atresia, and congenitally corrected transposition.
- Major hemodynamic issue is tricuspid incompetence with decreased pulmonary blood flow and, if an ASD is present, right-to-left shunting causing cyanosis.

Diagnosis and Intervention

- Critically ill neonates have poor survival rates, and surgery is indicated only after stabilization with PGE_1 and controlled ventilation.
- In older patients, cyanosis and heart failure are indications to intervene.

Surgery

- Critically ill neonates, after stabilization, palliation with a systemic-to-pulmonary artery shunt may be required.
- In older patients, options include tricuspid valve repair and tricuspid valve replacement.

Mitral Stenosis

- Mitral stenosis is caused by obstruction at a supravalvar, valvar or subvalvar level, singly or in combinations.
- Supravalvular stenosis is due to a ring of fibrous tissue above the annulus of the mitral valve or attached to the proximal leaflets.
- Three types of subvalvular stenosis have been recognized:
  - Parachute mitral valve.
  - Hammock valve.
  - Absence of one or both papillary muscles.
- Surgical intervention in children is aimed at preserving the mitral valve.
- Prosthetic valves are the least desirable option.

Heart Transplantation

- Pediatric heart transplant candidates fall into two categories:
  - Primary or secondary cardiomyopathy.
  - Congenital heart disease not amenable to standard surgery.

Lung and Heart-Lung Transplantation

- Potential candidates for lung transplantation are those with end-stage pulmonary vascular disease or bronchopulmonary pathology.
- Bronchopulmonary pathology includes those patients with cystic fibrosis and severe bronchopulmonary dysplasia.
- Patients with repairable congenital heart lesions who have Eisenmenger s syndrome with long-standing, irreversible cardiomyopathy are candidates for heart-lung transplantation.

Results

- Heart transplantation for children has a 30-day perioperative mortality of 15% to 20% and 1- and 5-year actuarial survival rates of 75% to 80% and 60% to 75%, respectively.

CHAPTER 58

Surgical Treatment of Coronary Artery Disease

CORONARY ARTERY ANATOMY

- The left anterior descending (LAD) supplies the anterior and left lateral portions of the left ventricle.
- The right coronary artery (RCA) supplies most of the right ventricle and the posterior part of the left ventricle.

CORONARY CIRCULATION AND REGULATION OF BLOOD FLOW

Coronary Blood Flow

- In response to strenuous exercise, the healthy heart can increase myocardial blood flow four- to sevenfold.

Factors Influencing Coronary Vascular Resistance

- Metabolic. Local myocardial metabolism is the primary regulator of coronary blood flow.
- Physical. The coronary vasculature can compensate and maintain normal coronary perfusion pressures between systolic pressures of 60 and 180 mm Hg via the process of autoregulation.
- Neural and neurohumoral.

MECHANICS OF PUMP FUNCTION

- Pressure-volume loops are useful in understanding various physiologic and pathophysiologic conditions. The shape of the pressure-volume loop during systole is determined by the contractility of the heart and the afterload against which the ventricle is ejecting.

CORONARY ARTERY DISEASE (CAD)

Pathogenesis

- In the final stages of the disease, patients become symptomatic or die from a myocardial infarct because of marked narrowing or closure of the vessel lumen, plaque rupture, or coronary artery thrombosis.

Role of Inflammation

- The primary causes of atherosclerotic CAD are endothelial injury induced by an inflammatory wall response and lipid deposition.

Plaque Rupture

- Seventy percent to 80% of coronary thrombi occur where the fibrous cap of an atherosclerotic plaque has fissured or ruptured.

Lipid Metabolism

Fixed Coronary Obstructions

- Once the cross-sectional area of the vessel decreases by 75% or more, however, coronary blood flow is significantly compromised.

ISCHEMIA AND MYOCARDIAL CELL INJURY

- Ischemia of 15 to 20 minutes duration is associated with postischemic myocardial dysfunction that lasts from hours to days despite the restoration of normal coronary blood flow. This reversible injury is referred to as myocardial stunning.
- Reversible contractile dysfunction that matches a reduction in resting coronary artery blood flow is termed hibernating myocardium.
- Myocardial infarction represents cell death and necrosis. It is an irreversible injury that is associated with ischemia lasting more than 20 minutes.
- Another cause of cardiomyocyte cell loss associated with ischemia is apoptosis or programmed cell death.
- There is preclinical and circumstantial evidence in humans that an ischemic adaptive phenomenon exists in the human heart. This phenomenon is known as ischemic preconditioning (IPC).

CLINICAL MANIFESTATIONS AND DIAGNOSIS OF CORONARY ARTERY DISEASE

Clinical Presentation

- Angina is not, however, always present with myocardial ischemia. As many as 15% of patients with significant CAD do not present with angina.

Physical Examination

Laboratory Studies

- Elevated serum cholesterol is associated with an elevated risk of coronary heart disease.
- High sensitivity C reactive protein (hs-CRP) adds to the predictive value of total and high-density lipoprotein (HDL) cholesterol in determining risk of future myocardial infarction.

Diagnostic Studies

Chest X-Ray Examination

Electrocardiogram (ECG)

- For detection of CAD, the sensitivity and specificity of an exercise ECG approaches 70% and 80%.

Echocardiography

- The sensitivity and specificity of echocardiography can be enhanced with the administration of intravenous dobutamine in incremental doses and is helpful in differentiating stunned, hibernating, and infarcted myocardium.

Single-Photon Emission Computed Tomographic (SPECT) Imaging

- ^{201}TI or ^{99m}Tc-sestamibi SPECT imaging has a sensitivity for detecting CAD of 85% to 96%, and when gated with ECG has a specificity of 90%.

Positron-Emission Tomography (PET)

- 18F-2-fluoro-2-deoxyglucose (FDG) PET is a highly accurate predictor of improvement in regional wall motion and global left ventricular ejection fraction (EF) after myocardial revascularization.

Magnetic Resonance Imaging (MRI)—Gadolinium MRI

- These findings suggest that cardiac MRI is an excellent alternative diagnostic method that can be used to determine the presence and extent of CAD and myocardial viability.

ECG-Gated Multi-Detector Spiral Computed Tomography (MDCT)/Electron Beam Computed Tomography (EBCT)

Cardiac Catheterization

- High-quality coronary angiography is essential for the identification of CAD and the assessment of its extent and severity.

CORONARY ARTERY BYPASS SURGERY: TECHNICAL ASPECTS

Cardiopulmonary Bypass (CPB)

- Use of CPB requires suppression of the clotting cascade with heparin because the components of the bypass pump and the surgical wound are powerful stimuli for thrombus formation.
- The mean oxygen consumption of the body decreases by 50% for every 10¡C decrease in body temperature.

Myocardial Protection Techniques

- The cornerstone, however, is the use of systemic hypothermia and the infusion of cold hyperkalemic crystalloid or blood solutions directly into the proximal ascending aorta after placement of the aortic cross-clamp.

Conduits for Coronary Artery Bypass Grafting

- The internal thoracic arteries (ITA) (left and/or right) are the preferred conduits because their patency rates exceed 90% at 10 years.
- Because there is some evidence that there may be a survival benefit associated with using only arterial grafts, the radial artery is often used in conjunction with ITA grafts to revascularize the heart.
- The most commonly used conduit is the greater saphenous vein.
- Vein graft patency rates have been reported to be 88% early after grafting, 81% at 1 year, 75% at 5 years, and 50% at 15 years. Venous graft occlusion rate is approximately 2% per year.

Anesthesia for Myocardial Revascularization

- Also, real-time cerebral bispectral index monitoring, although somewhat controversial, can be used to predict anesthetic depth and avoid excess narcotic anesthesia.
- The use of intraoperative transesophageal echocardiography (TEE) represents another major advance in cardiac anesthesia.
- With off-pump coronary artery bypass graft surgery (OPCAB), there is, in general, a greater requirement for increased monitoring and circulatory support.

The Operation

- Distal anastomoses.
- Proximal anastomoses.
- Termination of cardiopulmonary artery bypass.
  - Once the patient has been adequately rewarmed (approximately 36.5°C), normal sinus rhythm has been restored, and ventilation has been re-established, then the patient is weaned from CPB by gradually reducing the pump flow rates to zero while maintaining adequate intravascular volume via transfusion.
- Postoperative care.
  - The primary considerations during the first 12 hours after the operation should be the maintenance of adequate blood pressure, cardiac output, correction of coagulation defects, correction of ionized hypocalcemia, stabilization of intravascular volume, and normalization of the peripheral vascular resistance.
  - Significant hypertension results in increased myocardial oxygen consumption and tension on arterial suture lines.
  - The most common causes of low cardiac output are myocardial ischemia, hypovolemia, abnormal heart rate and rhythm, myocardial dysfunction, and cardiac tamponade.
  - In the immediate postoperative period, most patients are tachycardic.
  - Arrhythmias are common and may result from abnormal electrolytes, acidosis, high circulating catecholamine levels, and myocardial ischemia.
- Intra-aortic balloon pump (IABP).
- Tamponade.
  - Pericardial tamponade is due to formation of pericardial clot and compression of the heart.
- Postoperative bleeding.

- Bleeding, greater than 500 mL in the first hour or persistent bleeding greater than 200 mL/hour for 4 hours are indications for mediastinal exploration. Exploration is also indicated if a large hemothorax is identified on chest x-ray film or if pericardial tamponade occurs.
- Extubation.

INDICATIONS FOR CORONARY ARTERY BYPASS GRAFT (CABG) SURGERY AND OUTCOMES AFTER REVASCULARIZATION

Chronic Stable Angina

- CABG surgery versus medical management.
  - They also helped to identify specific categories of patients with angina who were most likely to benefit from CABG surgery, namely patients with left main coronary artery disease; one, two, or three-vessel disease with proximal LAD involvement; and three-vessel disease with impaired left ventricular function.
  - Nevertheless, as a direct result of these clinical studies, CABG surgery is now accepted as an appropriate therapeutic modality for the treatment of specific subsets of patients with chronic stable angina.
- Percutaneous transluminal coronary angioplasty (PTCA) versus medical management.
  - Patients with angina may be treated relatively safely with either medical management or PTCA intervention.
- CABG surgery versus PTCA.
  - Despite these limitations, it appears that CABG surgery clearly confers a survival benefit to diabetic patients that is superior to angioplasty.
  - Patients with stable angina can safely undergo PTCA as a first intervention for CAD. CABG surgery confers a superior long-term survival benefit in patients with specific anatomic lesions and is associated with an increased freedom from angina, a significant reduction in antianginal medications, and fewer subsequent percutaneous coronary interventions (PCIs). CABG surgery is the treatment of choice in diabetic patients.

Acute Coronary Artery Syndromes

Unstable Angina (UA)/Non-ST-Elevation Myocardial Infarction (NSTEMI)

- PCI versus medical management.
  - It appears that although PTCA may be an acceptable therapeutic option in patients with unstable angina, it is

associated with the need for repeat revascularization procedures.
- Adjunctive therapy to PCI.
  - It does appear, however, that coronary stenting and anti-platelet therapy improves the efficacy and durability of PCI in managing patients with UA/NSTEMI.
- CABG surgery versus medical management.
  - These and other studies demonstrate that CABG surgery is an effective treatment for the management of unstable angina and is associated with sustained symptom relief and excellent long-term survival.
- CABG surgery versus PCI.
  - Whether long-term survival and symptom relief in unstable angina patients with multivessel disease treated with stented angioplasty will be comparable to CABG surgery is unknown.

ST-Elevation Myocardial Infarction (STEMI)/Acute Myocardial Infarction (AMI)

- PCI versus medical management for AMI.
  - These findings suggest that PTCA has a survival advantage over thrombolytics as an initial treatment for STEMI/AMI and that use of delayed PTCA as an adjunct to therapy, including thrombolytics, does not effect survival.
  - Although PTCA may confer a short-term benefit over medical management and thrombolytics, the benefit does not persist over time.
  - There appears to be no major advantage to PTCA for patients with STEMI/AMI.
- Role of CABG surgery.
  - The controversial aspect is the timing, because early operative mortality may be as low as 5% in patients with a subendocardial infarction or as high as 25% in patients with poor ventricular function.
  - CABG surgery after uncomplicated MI can be accomplished with acceptable mortality rates provided appropriate supportive interventions, including IABP, are used early to stabilize the patient before surgery.

Coronary Artery Bypass Graft Surgery and Special Patient Populations

- Diabetes.
  - CABG surgery that includes ITA grafts appears to be the treatment of choice for diabetic patients.

- Women.
  - Although still controversial, the preponderance of evidence indicates that female gender is an independent risk factor for increased morbidity and mortality after CABG surgery.
- Renal disease.
  - Although CABG surgery in patients with renal insufficiency and failure is associated with increased morbidity and mortality, CABG surgery is associated with better survival when compared with PCI.
- Obesity.
  - Although obesity may affect morbidity, its impact on mortality is unclear. This may be due to the marked variability of the definition of obesity, a reliance on anecdotal experience, and the observational nature of the studies to date.

Reoperation for Coronary Artery Disease

- Although reoperative CABG surgery can be performed safely, overall patient survival and freedom from angina over time are diminished.

Complications of Coronary Artery Disease Amenable to Surgery

- In general, surgical repair and resection in conjunction with CABG surgery results in angina relief and resolution of heart failure symptoms for most patients.
- Patients who are considered candidates for surgery should be managed early with closure of the defect and concomitant CABG surgery. In the absence of refractory heart failure and hemodynamic instability, the survival rate may be as high as 75%.
- The hospital mortality may be as high as 50% although in selected patients the mortality may be as low as 10% to 15%.

ALTERNATIVE METHODS FOR MYOCARDIAL REVASCULARIZATION
Off-Pump Coronary Artery Bypass Graft Surgery

- It appears that the operation may be a safe alternative to conventional CABG surgery with CPB.
- Whether OPCAB surgery results in greater cerebral protection will have to await the results of the VA Prospective Randomized Cooperative Study when it concludes in 2007.

- It is unclear whether OPCAB surgery actually reduces the risk of significant clinical renal failure compared with CABG surgery with CPB.

Robotics

- Although only a few preliminary studies have been initiated, the results to date suggest that CABG surgery can be safely performed with satisfactory graft patency rates.

Transmyocardial Laser Revascularization (TMLR)

- TMLR therapy is associated with a reproducible improvement in symptoms; patients undergoing TMLR have shown a persistent improvement in angina class using the Canadian Cardiovascular System.

CHAPTER 59

ACQUIRED HEART DISEASE: VALVULAR

DIAGNOSTIC CONSIDERATIONS

- Valvular heart disease may be suggested by a patient's history or by a heart murmur detected on physical examination. Regardless of the valve lesion in question, echocardiography should be used to assess the severity of the stenosis, regurgitation, or both.
- Although most valve lesions may be accurately diagnosed by echocardiography, cardiac catheterization may be necessary to confirm the diagnosis or to provide additional information pertaining to ventricular function.

MITRAL VALVE

Surgical Anatomy of the Mitral Valve

- There are three important surgical landmarks (Fig. 59–1). First, the circumflex coronary artery runs along the epicardial surface of the heart overlying the posterior mitral annulus. Just millimeters of left atrial muscle separate the artery from the annulus, making it susceptible to injury during mitral valve surgery. Second, the aortic valve is in close approximation to the anterior leaflet of the mitral valve (aortomitral continuity). The noncoronary leaflet of the aortic valve is, therefore, susceptible to injury during mitral surgery. Third, the atrioventricular node is located deep to the posteromedial commissure of the mitral valve.

Mitral Stenosis

Etiology

- Rheumatic fever is the principal cause of mitral stenosis, and about two thirds of patients with rheumatic mitral stenosis are female.

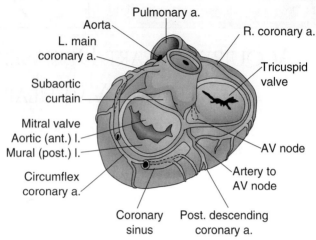

■ FIGURE 59–1. Anatomy of the mitral valve as it relates to other cardiac structures. Important surgical landmarks include the relationship of the mitral valve to the aortic valve, the circumflex coronary artery, and the atrioventricular (AV) node. *(From Buchanan SA, Tribble CG: Reoperative mitral replacement. In Kaiser LR, Kron IL, Spray TL [eds]: Mastery of Cardiothoracic Surgery. Philadelphia, Lippincott-Raven, 1998, p 351.)*

Pathophysiology

- The cross-sectional area of the normal mitral valve is 4 to 6 cm². A mitral valve area of 2 cm² is considered moderate mitral stenosis, and an area of 1 cm² is considered severe mitral stenosis.

Diagnosis

- Dyspnea is the principal symptom of mitral stenosis.
- The echocardiogram is the principal tool used to confirm the diagnosis.

Balloon Mitral Valvuloplasty

- First performed in 1984, balloon mitral valvuloplasty has become the treatment of choice for selected patients with mitral stenosis.

Mitral Valve Replacement

● If mitral valve replacement is required, efforts should be made to preserve the posterior and, in some cases, the anterior leaflets of the native mitral valve.

Mitral Regurgitation

Etiology

● Papillary muscles. Worldwide, rheumatic fever remains the most common cause of mitral regurgitation; it results in deformity and retraction of the leaflets and shortening of the chordae.

Pathophysiology

● In fact, *normal* parameters of systolic function indicate significant contractile dysfunction of the left ventricle. An ejection fraction (EF) of less than 40% in the setting of mitral regurgitation indicates significant left ventricular contractile dysfunction.

Diagnosis

● The symptoms of mitral regurgitation are those of heart failure: shortness of breath, dyspnea on exertion, orthopnea, pulmonary edema, and diminished exercise tolerance. Symptoms are determined by the degree of mitral regurgitation, the rate of its progression, the degree of pulmonary hypertension, and the magnitude of left ventricular contractile dysfunction.

Natural History of Mitral Regurgitation

● The natural history of the disease is variable, determined by the cause of mitral regurgitation, the regurgitant volume, and the magnitude of left ventricular systolic dysfunction.

Treatment

● The cornerstone of medical management is diuresis and afterload reduction with angiotensin-converting enzyme inhibitors.
● Even in the absence of symptoms, therefore, patients should be referred for surgery when the left ventricular EF is less

than 60% or when the left ventricular end systolic diameter (ESD) is more than 45 mm Hg.

● When possible, the valve should be repaired.
● The operative mortality rate associated with mitral valve repair (0% to 2%) is significantly less than that for replacement (4% to 8%).

Aortic Stenosis

Etiology

● Acquired aortic stenosis usually results from calcification of the aortic valve associated with advanced age. Although the process is most often idiopathic, rheumatic fever may affect the aortic valve in a process similar to that of the mitral valve.

Pathophysiology

● For quick calculations, this simplifies to the following:

$$\text{Aortic valve area (AVA)} = \text{Cardiac output} \div \sqrt{\text{Mean pressure gradient}}$$

● As the valve area decreases to 1 cm^2, there is little change in the transvalvular gradient needed to generate the same flow, and patients frequently experience no symptoms. With a valve area of 0.8 cm^2, patients invariably develop symptoms.

Diagnosis

● The classic symptoms of aortic stenosis are angina, syncope, and heart failure.
  ● Gradient = $4V^2$.

Natural History

● Angina is usually the earliest symptom, and the mean survival of a patient with aortic stenosis and angina is 4.7 years. When a patient experiences syncope, survival is typically less than 3 years. Patients with dyspnea and congestive heart failure, in keeping with their associated left ventricular dysfunction, have a mean survival of 1 to 2 years. Congestive heart failure is the presenting symptom in nearly one third of patients.
● Therefore, aortic valve surgery should be recommended to patients with symptomatic and asymptomatic disease

who have evidence of left ventricular decompensation or a transvalvular gradient of more than 4 m/second.

Pathophysiology

● Unlike aortic stenosis, in which the pathologic process is left ventricular pressure overload, the pathophysiology of aortic insufficiency derives from left ventricular volume overload.

Diagnosis

● The compensatory mechanisms of aortic regurgitation may permit patients to remain symptom free for long periods. When these compensatory mechanisms begin to fail, however, left ventricular dysfunction becomes manifest, and patients experience symptoms of heart failure.

Natural History

● Because of the compensatory mechanisms discussed previously, patients with chronic aortic regurgitation may be symptom free for long periods. In fact, patients with mild to moderate aortic regurgitation have an excellent long-term prognosis; 10-year survival rate after diagnosis is about 85% to 95%.

Treatment

● Medical therapy for aortic regurgitation is based on a combination of afterload reduction and diuretics.

SURGICAL OUTCOMES

● The operative mortality rate for valve replacement surgery is influenced by several variables, including which valve is replaced, whether coronary bypass surgery is performed at the same operation, and other patient-specific variables.
● The choice of prosthetic valve must be patient specific. Mechanical valves have excellent durability and will perform indefinitely without structural deterioration. However, because they are thrombogenic, mechanical valves obligate the patient to lifelong anticoagulation (warfarin sodium). Hence, the patient with a mechanical valve incurs the risks of chronic anticoagulation. Bioprosthetic valves do not require anticoagulation but will undergo structural deterioration.

CHAPTER 60

THORACIC VASCULATURE (WITH EMPHASIS ON THE THORACIC AORTA)

EMBRYONIC DEVELOPMENT

- The systemic arterial system originates from the heart and aortic sac as six pairs of ventrally situated arteries, or aortic arches.
- The six paired embryonic aortic arches develop and regress during maturation to eventually become distinct structures of the thoracic aorta.
- Embryonic veins.

FUNCTIONAL ANATOMY

- Aortic root.
- Ascending aorta.
- Aortic arch.
- Descending thoracic aorta.
- Artery of Adamkiewicz.
- Thoracoabdominal aorta.

Congenital Anomalies

- The most common right-to-left branching pattern of the aortic arch is brachiocephalic artery, left common carotid artery, and left subclavian artery (75%).
- Vascular ring.
- Left retroesophageal subclavian artery.
- Aberrant right subclavian artery.
- Patent ductus arteriosus.
- Coarctation.
- Persistent left superior vena cava.

AORTIC DISEASES AND ETIOLOGY

- The most common diseases of the aorta are aneurysm and dissection.
- An aortic aneurysm is defined as a localized or diffuse aortic dilatation that exceeds 50% of the normal aortic diameter.
- A tear in the intima allows blood to escape from the true lumen of the aorta, dissects the aortic layers, and reroutes some of the blood through a newly formed false channel.
- Marfan's syndrome.
- Aortic dilatation observed in Marfan's patients is the result of defects in a specific component of elastic fibers known as fibrillin-1 *(FBN1)*.
- Primary tumors of the aorta are extremely rare with less than 100 cases reported in the English literature.
- Sarcomas.
- Because tumors may mimic aneurysm or aortic occlusive disease, diagnoses are often made postmortem or intra-operatively.

DIAGNOSTIC IMAGING

- Aortography.
- Computed tomography (CT) evaluates systemic vasculature, defining aortic anomalies, dissection aneurysm, clots, and calcification, and pulmonary vasculature, depicting lung disease and thoracic venous anomalies such as pulmonary arteriovenous malformation.
- Helical, (spiral), CT.
- CT angiography (CTA).
- Magnetic resonance (MR).
- An image is detected by radio frequency signals when the body's hydrogen atoms react to the MR's strong magnetic field.
- Other imaging modalities for thoracic vasculature include transesophageal echocardiography (TEE), intravascular ultra-sound (IVUS), and intraoperative epiaortic ultrasound (IEUS).

THORACIC AORTIC ANEURYSMS

- This study reported a population incidence of detected tho-racic aortic aneurysms estimated to be 5.9 new aneurysms per 100,000 person-years in 1982.
- These authors estimated the incidence to be 10.4 per 100,000 person-years, or three times higher than the 1951 to 1980 rate after age adjustment.

- Untreated, 75% to 80% of thoracic aortic aneurysms will eventually rupture.
- Aneurysm size significantly influences the rate of rupture.
- Chronic back pain.
- Hoarseness.
- Dyspnea.
- Pulmonary hypertension.
- Dysphagia.
- Hemoptysis or hematemesis.
- Intestinal angina.
- Arterial hypertension.
- Widened pulse pressure.
- Patients who are diagnosed with aneurysms greater than or equal to 5 cm, or with rapid aneurysm enlargement, are considered for surgical repair.

THORACIC AORTIC DISSECTION

- Abrupt excruciating pain epitomizes the onset of acute aortic dissection.
- Acute type A dissection most often requires emergency surgical repair because of the associated high risk of death because of rupture, tamponade, and/or aortic valve insufficiency.
- For acute type B aortic dissection, the treatment of choice is generally medical therapy aimed at pain control and the correction of hypertension.
- Serial imaging of the dissected aorta should be obtained before discharge from the acute-care hospital and then at 1 month, 3 months, 6 months, 12 months, and yearly thereafter.

SURGICAL TREATMENT AND RESULTS: PROXIMAL THORACIC AORTA

- Wheat technique.
- Composite valve graft.
- Bentall technique.
- Christian Cabrol.
- Modification of the Cabrol technique.
- Button technique.
- Repair of a diseased aortic root can be accomplished safely, depending on risk factors, with an overall operative mortality rate in the range of 2% to 15%.
- Closed technique.
- Open distal anastomosis technique—with profound hypothermic circulatory arrest.

- Another technique that has been used for cerebral protection during the circulatory arrest period is antegrade cerebral perfusion. This technique uses cannulae inserted directly into the ostia of the innominate and left common carotid arteries during the period of arrest.
- Before profound hypothermic circulatory arrest became a regular part of aortic surgery, arch replacement carried an extremely high mortality rate of up to 75%. The introduction of profound hypothermia and circulatory arrest reduced operative mortality to between 10% and 15%. The development of additional circulatory adjuncts has reduced operative mortality to around 5%.

SURGICAL TREATMENT AND RESULTS: DISTAL THORACIC AORTA

- Distal aortic perfusion.
- Cerebrospinal fluid (CSF) drainage to provide spinal cord protection.
- Modified thoracoabdominal incision.
- Full thoracoabdominal exploration.
- Mortality rates for repair of descending thoracic and thoracoabdominal aortic aneurysms currently range between 5% and 21%, depending on the series and the patient's condition at the time of surgery.
- Immediate neurologic deficit.
- Delayed-onset neurologic deficit.
- Renal failure increases morbidity, length of stay, and mortality.
- Acute aortic dissection substantially raises the risk of paraplegia following graft replacement of the descending thoracic or thoracoabdominal aorta.
- Chronic dissection undoubtedly makes surgical repair of descending thoracic and thoracoabdominal aortic aneurysms more difficult, but survival and neurologic outcome do not differ from that of aneurysm surgery without dissection.

EXTENSIVE AORTIC ANEURYSM AND THE ELEPHANT TRUNK TECHNIQUE

- Extensive aortic aneurysm (also known as mega aorta) refers to aneurysmal involvement of the entire ascending, transverse aortic arch and thoracoabdominal aorta.
- Elephant trunk technique.
- Mortality rates range from 5% to 9% after stage 1 and 6% to 7% for stage 2.

CHAPTER 61

ENDOVASCULAR SURGERY

VASCULAR ACCESS

- Percutaneous access can be achieved by a single- or double-wall puncture technique.
- Patients with scarred access sites from prior interventions or with decreased pulses because of occlusive disease may benefit from ultrasound guidance with Doppler insonation or B-mode visualization of the target vessel.
- The femoral artery is the most commonly used site of arterial entry and allows access to almost any arterial bed with an associated low complication rate.
- In the absence of femoral pulses or for those patients in need of visceral or arch vessel intervention, the brachial artery may provide a preferable point of entry.
- Care is required when accessing the brachial artery to minimize the risk of median nerve injury resulting from brachial sheath hematoma or, rarely, needle-induced nerve trauma.

GUIDEWIRES AND CATHETERS

- Multipurpose angled (MPA) or Berenstein catheters are often used to assist passage of a wire across a stenosis or occlusion or into a branch vessel.
- If unable to cross a stenosis with a standard wire, use of guidewires or catheters with hydrophilic coatings is indicated, although use of these systems carry a greater risk of arterial dissection.
- Guidewires range from 0.014 to 0.035 inches in diameter with a recent trend toward increased use of systems that use 0.014-inch or 0.018-inch wires.
- Hydrophilic wires are not suitable for performing interventions because they are easily dislodged during placement or withdrawal of angioplasty balloons or vascular stents.
- Stiff wires may exist for specific interventions. For example, the Rosen wire has a stiff body and floppy J-tip, which is used for renal artery angioplasty and stenting. The J-tip design prevents the wire from perforating the renal parenchyma as the wire is advanced into the terminal arterial branches.

- When using a coaxial balloon catheter or stent delivery system in which the wire passes through a central lumen, guidewire lengths should be twice that of the intended catheter.
- Use of a monorail system in which the wire passes through a distal side lumen of the balloon catheter or stent deployment device allows use of wires of shorter length.
- Catheters have been designed for specific arterial beds and designated by configuration, length, and French size.

BALLOON CATHETERS

- For patients with an elevated serum creatinine (≥ 1.4 mg/dL), preintervention hydration, minimization of contrast load have been advocated to limit the nephrotoxic effects of the contrast agent.
- Options for lesion localization when the baseline serum creatinine exceeds 2 mg/dL, includes use of gadolinium, CO_2 contrast, or intravascular ultrasound (IVUS).
- The total administered volume of gadolinium should not exceed 0.2 to 0.4 mmol/kg, which is equivalent to 30 to 60 mL in a 75-kg individual.
- A mean pressure gradient of greater than 10 mm Hg is sufficiently significant to require treatment. If a pressure gradient is not detected in the resting state, then 100 µg of nitroglycerin can be infused intra-arterially to mimic the increased demand that occurs with walking.
- Appropriate preinterventional therapy is a prerequisite for optimizing the likelihood of a successful treatment outcome.
- Patients are routinely hydrated overnight and no oral intake is permitted 8 hours before the procedure.
- Aspirin (81 mg) is initiated 24 hours before intervention.
- Before angioplasty or stenting, we administer 5000 units of heparin intravenously, and a single dose of cefazolin or vancomycin is administered, if a vascular stent or prosthesis is to be inserted.
- After angioplasty and/or stenting, all patients are placed on aspirin and clopidogrel (Plavix) with an initial 300-mg loading dose followed by 75 mg/day for 3 to 6 months.
- A balloon catheter is selected based on balloon diameter (millimeters) and length (centimeters), as well as the length of the catheter shaft, which is dictated by lesion location and chosen access site.
- Pressure required for inflation may vary widely from 4 to 16 atmospheres and is dependent on the compliance of the vascular lesion to be dilated. Higher pressures are typically required for relatively stiff venous stenoses.

- Balloons that are composed of a compliant plastic, such as silastic, have a much greater range of potential final diameters, with continued balloon expansion dictated as a function of the inflated volume.
- Cutting balloon technology is under investigation for applications in peripheral arterial disease.
- IVUS provides a very accurate means for defining vessel size, and marker catheters that contain radiopaque marks at known intervals can also be used for an assessment of vessel diameter.

INTRAVASCULAR STENTS AND ENDOPROSTHESES

- Vascular stents are commonly used following an inadequate angioplasty with dissection or elastic recoil of an arterial stenosis.
- Vascular stents are classified into two basic categories: balloon-expandable and self-expanding.
- Balloon-expandable stents are usually composed of stainless steel, mounted on an angioplasty balloon, and deployed by balloon inflation.
- Self-expanding stents are deployed by retracting a restraining sheath and usually consist of Elgiloy (a cobalt, chromium, nickel alloy) or Nitinol, a shape memory alloy composed of nickel and titanium, which will contract and assume a heat-treated shape above a transition temperature that depends on the composition of the alloy.
- Self-expanding stents will expand to a final diameter that is determined by stent geometry, hoop strength, and vessel size. If the vessel diameter is significantly less than that of the stent, final stent length may be longer than the anticipated unconstrained length.
- Covered stents have been designed with either a surrounding polytetrafluorethylene (PTFE) or polyester fabric and have been used for treatment of traumatic vascular lesions, including arterial disruption and arteriovenous fistulas and iliac or femoral arterial occlusive disease and popliteal aneurysms.
- Drug-eluting stents transiently release antiproliferative agents into the vessel wall to reduce intimal hyperplasia and restenosis. Efficacy has been demonstrated for local delivery of selected agents, such as rapamycin and paclitaxel, in the coronary circulation.
- Intravascular brachytherapy may play an important adjunctive role in reducing postangioplasty restenosis.

- Endovascular infrarenal aneurysm repair require that patients have an infrarenal aneurysm with at least a 1.5 cm neck and not greater than 60 degrees of angulation.
- Clinical trials are underway with devices that will expand indications to aneurysms involving the visceral segment of the abdominal aorta.
- Thoracic aortic devices have been used to treat descending thoracic aneurysms, traumatic aortic transections, and aortic dissections.

IMAGE-GUIDED THERAPY

- Fluoroscopy functions via an image intensifier that receives, concentrates, and brightens an x-ray image to produce an electronic image that can be displayed on a screen, and it is the modality used for digital subtraction angiography.
- The road map technique allows for a representation of the arterial tree by contrast angiography on one digital screen with real-time fluoroscopy on another screen.
- It is important that everyone exposed to the radiation field be protected by appropriate lead gowns, glasses, and gloves to minimize their exposures and risks from the radiation.

CHAPTER 62

CEREBROVASCULAR DISEASE

STROKE EPIDEMIOLOGY

- Stroke mortality is the third leading cause of death in the United States, accounting for 1 in every 15 deaths in 1992.
- There has been a 60% decline in U.S. stroke mortality between 1960 and 1990; despite this, nearly 150,000 Americans died of stroke during 1995.
- Twenty-five percent of those patients who have strokes die in the year after the stroke; morbidity in the 3 million surviving stroke victims is substantial; it is the leading cause of serious disability in the United States.
- Internal carotid artery atherosclerosis is the most common and treatable cause of atherosclerotic stroke.

PATHOLOGY AND PATHOPYSIOLOGY

- Atherosclerosis of arteries supplying the brain is the leading cause of ischemic stroke in North America and Europe.
- Large artery atherosclerosis, most often involving the carotid bifurcations, causes stroke by three principal mechanisms: embolization of atherosclerotic and thrombotic material (artery-to-artery emboli); thrombotic occlusion; and hypoperfusion from advanced, hemodynamically significant stenoses.
- Aortic arch atherosclerosis may also be a source of cerebral emboli.
- Small vessel atherosclerosis in the brain is the leading cause of subcortical or lacunar infarcts.
- Plaque destabilization with rupture of the plaque results in embolization of debris from the central core, producing symptoms of transient ischemic attack (TIA), amaurosis fugax, and stroke.
- Cardiac sources of emboli can produce TIAs anywhere in the brain; in contrast, emboli of the carotid artery cause predominantly middle cerebral or ophthalmic artery territory TIAs unless the contralateral carotid artery is severely stenosed or occluded.

CLINICAL PRESENTATION AND WORKUP: TRANSIENT ISCHEMIC ATTACK

- Symptomatic patients present with TIAs, amaurosis fugax, or stroke.
- TIAs are defined as brief episodes of focal loss of brain function resulting from ischemia that can usually be localized to that portion of the brain supplied by one vascular system.
- Episodes lasting less than 24 hours are classified as TIAs; they commonly last 2 to 15 minutes, are rapid in onset, leave no persistent defect, and multiple attacks occur often.
- Left carotid system TIAs manifest as the following:
  - Motor dysfunction (dysarthria, weakness, paralysis, or clumsiness of the right extremities and/or face).
  - Loss of vision in the left eye (amaurosis fugax) or, rarely, the right field of vision (homonymous hemianopsia).
  - Sensory symptoms (numbness, including loss of sensation or paresthesias involving the right upper and/or lower extremity or face).
  - Aphasia (language disturbance).
- Right carotid system TIAs produce similar symptoms on the opposite side, except that aphasia occurs only when the right hemisphere is dominant for speech (left-handed individual).
- Vertebrobasilar system TIAs are characterized by the rapid onset of the following:
  - Motor dysfunction (weakness, paralysis, or clumsiness) of any combination of upper and lower extremities and face, left and/or right.
  - Sensory symptoms (loss of sensation, numbness, or paresthesia involving the left, right, or both sides).
  - Loss of vision in one or both homonymous visual fields.
  - Loss of balance, vertigo, unsteadiness or disequilibrium, diplopia, or dysarthria.
  - In general, these symptoms are not associated with carotid artery TIAs.
- The following symptoms are generally considered TIAs:
  - March of a sensory deficit.
  - Unconsciousness without other symptoms.
  - Vertigo alone.
  - Dizziness alone.
  - Dysarthria alone.
  - Diplopia alone.
  - Incontinence of bowel or bladder.
  - Loss of vision associated with alteration of level of consciousness.
  - Focal symptoms associated with migraines.

- Confusion alone.
- Amnesia alone.
- Drop attacks (loss of consciousness associated with collapse) alone.
- A reversible ischemic neurologic deficit (RIND) or small stroke has similar symptoms to TIA but lasts longer than 24 hours; full neurologic function returns within 48 to 72 hours.
- *Amaurosis fugax* is defined as a transient monocular visual disturbance.
  - Symptoms of amaurosis fugax are sudden in onset and last for minutes; they are usually shorter than cortical TIAs.
  - Patients often describe the visual disturbance as being like a curtain shade descending to the horizontal mid-visual field and then ascending; the opposite can occur with the curtain shade ascending to the mid-horizontal visual field and then descending.
  - Almost complete loss of vision in the eye can occur, as well as telescoped vision or looking out of a tunnel.
  - The visual impairment itself may be complete absence of vision in the involved portion or blurriness or "graying" of vision.
  - The pathophysiology of amaurosis fugax is an embolus that originates in the internal carotid artery, travels through the ophthalmic artery, and lodges in the central retinal artery or one of its branches.
- The diagnosis of TIA and amaurosis fugax is based on history.
- Once the diagnosis of TIA, amaurosis fugax, or small stroke is established, urgent workup is required because these are warning symptoms of major stroke.
- The first priority is to rule out carotid artery occlusive disease using duplex ultrasonography.
- If advanced carotid stenosis is present ipsilateral to the symptoms, carotid endarterectomy is generally indicated and no further testing is required except for a brain imaging study to rule out intracranial pathology.
- Contrast arteriography is helpful for lesser degrees of stenosis; contrast arteriography is also indicated when more proximal atherosclerotic disease is suspected involving the branches coming off the aortic arch.
- In patients with negative findings on duplex ultrasonography, arteriography is useful to eliminate intracranial vascular disease and unusual arteriopathies such as fibromuscular dysplasia.
- If the source for TIA has not been identified after duplex ultrasonography, brain imaging tests, and complete arteriography, cardiac sources must be ruled out with echocardiography and

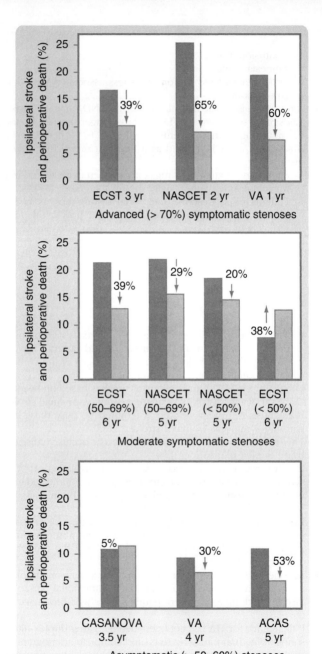

Continued

■ FIGURE 62–1. Randomized trials comparing carotid endarterectomy *(cross-hatched bars)* to medical therapy *(open bars)* in symptomatic *(top and middle graphs)* and asymptomatic *(bottom graph)* patients. Principal endpoints include ipsilateral stroke and death with operation or initiation of medical treatment. The percentage relative risk reduction from carotid endarterectomy is indicated by the *downward-pointing arrows.* The length of follow-up for each trial is indicated below the bars. ACAS, Asymptomatic Carotid Atherosclerosis Study; CASANOVA, Carotid Artery Stenosis with Asymptomatic Narrowing: Operation Versus Aspirin; ECST, European Carotid Surgery Trial; NASCET, North American Symptomatic Carotid Endarterectomy Trial; VA, Veterans Administration Trial.

arrhythmia monitoring; workup for hypercoagulable disorder may also be indicated.

CAROTID ENDARTERECTOMY IN MODERN TIMES

- Important randomized trials are presented in Figure 62–1; in all trials, carotid endarterectomy was compared with best medical therapy (antiplatelet or anticoagulant mediation and risk factor reduction).
- The risk of stroke and death with medical therapy was greater in symptomatic patients than in asymptomatic patients, thereby yielding a more striking relative risk reduction with endarterectomy.
- Because of the more benign prognosis with medical therapy in asymptomatic patients, it was more difficult to demonstrate a clear-cut, positive benefit of operation.
- The Asymptomatic Carotid Atherosclerosis Study (ACAS) showed conclusive benefit of carotid endarterectomy in asymptomatic patients.
- In contrast, almost all trials in symptomatic patients demonstrated an important benefit of carotid endarterectomy that was most apparent in patients with advanced, high-grade stenoses.
- The most influential trial was the North American Symptomatic Carotid Endarterectomy Trial (NASCET) in which patients were randomized to either medical or surgical therapy for TIA or mild, disabling stroke ipsilateral to a 70% to 99% narrowing of the internal carotid artery.
- Carotid endarterectomy reduced the overall risk of fatal and nonfatal stroke from 26% in the medical group to 9% in the surgical patients; this represented an absolute risk reduction of 17% in favor of surgery and a relative risk reduction of 65%.

- The absolute risk reduction for all ipsilateral stroke at 2 years was 26% among patients with a stenosis of 90% to 99% at entry, 18% among those patients with a stenosis of 80% to 89%, and 12% among patients with stenosis of 70% to 79%.
- More recent results of the NASCET trial showed that carotid endarterectomy reduced the risk of ipsilateral stroke from 23% to 16% in patients with 50% to 69% stenoses.
- For patients with less than 50% stenoses, carotid endarterectomy offered no advantage over medical therapy in preventing stroke; it is not recommended for these patients.
- Commonly recognized risk factors associated with stroke included age (>70 years); gender (male); systolic hypertension (>160 mg Hg); diastolic hypertension (>90 mm Hg); degree of stenosis (>70%); presence of ulceration as determined by arteriography; and history of smoking, hypertension, myocardial infarction, congestive heart failure, diabetes, intermittent claudication, or elevated blood lipid levels.
- The long-term benefit of surgery is greater and the risk of stroke with medical treatment is higher for men than for women and for patients who have had stroke rather than for those with TIAs.
- The major risk of carotid endarterectomy is stroke; this risk should be 2% or less, and individual surgeons whose stroke rate is higher should not perform carotid endarterectomy.

CURRENT INDICATIONS FOR CAROTID ENDARTERECTOMY

- Operation is recommended in patients with carotid stenosis 50% or greater with ipsilateral TIAs, amaurosis fugax, a reversible neurologic deficit, or small stroke and in selected cases of recurrent, symptomatic carotid stenosis.
- Patients with less degrees of symptomatic stenosis may be considered for operation if they have failed medical therapy, particularly if there is evidence of ulceration of the lesion or if contralateral occlusion is present.
- Individualized patients may require surgery for progressive stroke, progressive retinal ischemia, acute carotid occlusion, symptomatic carotid stump syndrome, and global cerebral ischemia and in certain cases of symptomatic carotid dissection and true or false aneurysm.
- The procedure is generally not indicated in patients with vertebrobasilar distribution TIAs or multi-infarct dementia, those with severe neurologic deficits, and those with evidence of intracranial hemorrhage or large infarcts.

- Indications for endarterectomy in asymptomatic patients remain less clear-cut; it is likely that those with advanced stenoses (≥70%) benefit most.
- It is appropriate to reserve carotid endarterectomy only for *good-risk,* asymptomatic patients with advanced stenoses; the presence of ulceration may lower the threshold for recommending operation.

OPERATIVE MANAGEMENT

Preoperative Evaluation

- The overall incidence of myocardial infarction after carotid endarterectomy is low (0.3% from NASCET data), and extensive preoperative cardiac testing is unnecessary and cost ineffective.
- Aspirin therapy should be started at the time of diagnosis of TIA, amaurosis fugax, or stroke; low-dose aspirin (80 to 325 mg per day) is optimal in preventing thromboembolic events during and after carotid endarterectomy.

Surgical Procedure

- The common carotid, internal carotid, and external carotid arteries are all exposed in sequence, and dissected with minimal manipulation of the disease-bearing carotid bifurction area.
- To ensure adequate cerebral perfusion during carotid artery clamping, brain function can be monitored using electroencephalography or somatosensory-evoked potentials, or the operation can be performed under regional anesthesia with direct assessment of the patient's neurologic status; in the event that adequate perfusion is not present during clamping, a shunt can be inserted to direct blood to the brain.

POSTOPERATIVE COMPLICATIONS

Stroke or Transient Neurologic Deficit

- Neurologic deficits within the first 12 hours of operation are almost always the result of thromboembolic phenomena stemming from the endarterectomy site.
- Immediate heparinization and exploration are indicated without the need for confirmatory arteriography or noninvasive tests.

- Deficits occurring 12 to 24 hours should be promptly investigated with a computed tomography (CT) scan and duplex ultrasound or arteriography.

Hyperperfusion Syndrome and Intracerebral Hematoma

- The incidence of hyperperfusion syndrome after carotid endarterectomy is 0.3% to 1.0%.
- The pathophysiology is secondary to paralysis of autoregulation from chronic ischemia.
- Restoration of internal carotid flow leads to hyperperfusion in the ipsilateral cerebrovascular bed.
- Pathologic changes include mild cerebral edema, petechial hemorrhages, frank intracerebral hemorrhage, and seizures.
- This syndrome is often heralded by ipsilateral frontal headache within the first week after endarterectomy; headache may be followed by focal motor seizures that are often difficult to control.
- Seizures are usually successfully treated with phenytoin (Dilantin); aspirin and anticoagulants should be avoided and hypertension carefully controlled.

Hypertension and Hypotension

- Fluctuations in blood pressure with postoperative hypertension or hypotension are common after endarterectomy performed under general anesthesia, occurring in one third to one half of patients; this usually disappears within 12 to 24 hours.

Wound Complications

- Bleeding complications, particularly wound hematomas, occur in 1.4% to 3.0% of patients undergoing endarterectomy.
- An important symptom suggesting the presence of a significant hematoma that may lead to airway embarrassment is the inability to swallow.

Operative Damage to Nerves

- The sensory branches of the cervical plexus, the transverse cervical nerve and the greater auricular nerve, are frequently severed or injured during the course of carotid endarterectomy, resulting in ipsilateral numbness of the upper face, lower neck, and lower ear.
- Permanent hyperesthesia in this area is common after carotid endarterectomy.

- Other nerves can be damaged, such as the vagus, hypoglossal, facial, glossopharyngeal, and spinal accessory; damage can occur as a result of high exposure, by traction, or by the cautery.

ONGOING ISSUES

Outcome

- Carotid endarterectomy should be performed with low morbidity and mortality in selected patients with appropriate symptoms, and the limits of perioperative morbidity and mortality should be categorized by clinical presentation.
- The combined morbidity and mortality of the procedure should not exceed 3% for asymptomatic patients, 5% for TIAs, and 7% for ischemic stroke; in addition, the 30-day mortality rate from all causes related to endarterectomy should not exceed 2%.

Increasing the Benefit-to-Cost Ratio of Carotid Endarterectomy

- Duplex ultrasonography alone or in combination with magnetic resonance imaging (MRI) is often sufficient for preoperative evaluation of carotid stenosis and eliminates the need for contrast angiography.
- Contrast angiography is expensive and carries with it a 1% to 1.5% risk of stroke; it also results in complications at the arterial puncture site in 5% of patients and contrast agent-induced renal dysfunction in 1% to 5%.
- Indications for adjunctive arteriography include the following:
  - A discrepancy among the history, physical examination, duplex scan, and CT scan.
  - Patients presenting with vertebrobasilar symptoms.
  - Symptomatic patients suspected of proximal disease involving branches of the aortic arch or intracranial disease (normal duplex scan of the carotid bifurcation).
  - Patients with duplex evidence of carotid occlusion in the presence of ongoing ipsilateral hemispheric symptoms.
  - Patients with nonatherosclerotic disease, such as fibromuscular dysplasia, and patients with recurrent carotid stenosis because plaque morphology and extent of disease are sometimes unusual in these patients.
  - Patients with duplex scans that are equivocal or of poor quality.

Recurrent Carotid Stenosis

- Recurrent stenosis is infrequent, but not rare.
- The overall risk appears to be about 10% in the first year after primary endarterectomy, 3% in the second year, and 2% in the third year; long-term risk has been estimated to be approximately 1% per year.
- Symptomatic recurrent carotid disease occurs in about 0.6% to 3.0% of patients after endarterectomy.
- In general, the mean risk of stroke with reoperation is approximately 4%, with a death rate of approximately 1.2% and cranial nerve injury of approximately 12%.

Carotid Shunt and Monitoring

- The benefit of using an internal shunt during carotid endarterectomy is the re-establishment of cerebral blood flow in the minority of patients who need it.
- The major risks are the introduction of emboli into the internal carotid artery resulting in cerebral embolization and intimal injury.
- Patients who undergo surgery under regional and local anesthesia can have shunts placed selectively if neurologic status deteriorates when the carotid arteries are clamped; this occurs in 10% to 15% of cases.
- Patients who undergo surgery under general anesthesia can have cerebral perfusion monitored by measurement of internal carotid artery back-pressure ("stump pressure" of less than 50 mm Hg is the generally accepted criterion for need for shunt placement), isotopic regional blood flow measurements, transcranial Doppler monitoring, somatosensory-evoked potential monitoring, or electroencephalographic monitoring; alternatively, some surgeons shunt all patients undergoing surgery under general anesthesia.

Timing of Operation After Stroke

- The early experience with carotid endarterectomy resulted in a policy to delay the operation for 4 to 6 weeks in patients diagnosed with acute stroke for fear of clinical deterioration associated with conversion of an ischemic infarct into a hemorrhagic one.
- It is now believed that an early operation without waiting 4 to 6 weeks is safe in patients with minor, nondisabling stroke;

a compelling reason for not delaying the operation is that patients may be placed at risk for recurrent stroke during the waiting period.

- Patients with severe neurologic deficits, including altered consciousness, are not candidates for early carotid endarterectomy, unless they have considerable clinical recovery and, therefore, have brain tissue that can be preserved.

- Patients with a small stroke on CT without significant midline shift, a stable neurologic deficit, and a normal level of consciousness have low risk with early surgery; if these individuals have an advanced (>70%) stenosis, they should undergo early operation; if the stenosis is moderate (50% to 69%), delaying operation for 4 to 6 weeks may be prudent.

- Patients with large strokes on CT with a midline shift may be at higher risk, particularly if they have a depressed level of consciousness; operation should be delayed until these patients improve and plateau in their clinical recovery.

Simultaneous Carotid Endarterectomy and Coronary Artery Bypass

- One fourth to one third of patients undergoing carotid endarterectomy have severe underlying coronary artery disease.

- The incidence of hemodynamically significant carotid stenosis in screening studies of patients undergoing coronary artery bypass is 5% to 11%.

- The overall stroke and death rate with combined carotid endarterectomy and coronary artery bypass procedures is higher than with either procedure alone.

- Staged approaches are appropriate in most patients.

- Initial carotid endarterectomy followed by coronary artery bypass is frequently applied to patients who present with symptomatic, high-grade carotid lesions who have stable coronary artery disease.

- In patients undergoing urgent or emergent coronary artery bypass grafting who have advanced carotid disease, a reversed staged approach may be used, whereby carotid endarterectomy is carried out later; alternatively, carotid endarterectomy can be performed first under regional and local anesthesia, which is safer for the heart.

Carotid Angioplasty and Stent Placement

- Major trials are currently proposed and underway; until data from such trials are available, the procedure of carotid angioplasty and stenting should be considered experimental.
- Studies to date suggest that stroke rates of up to 20% occur with stenting and angioplasty; early restenosis from intimal hyperplasia also occurs frequently in the setting of small arteries such as the internal carotid artery.

CHAPTER 63

ANEURYSMAL VASCULAR DISEASE

- Aneurysm—most commonly found in the human aorta, iliac, popliteal, and femoral arteries.
- Arterial ectasia—enlargement less than 50% of normal diameter.
- Arteriomegaly.
- Rupture.
- Thrombosis or embolism.
- Morphology is a fusiform.
- Saccular.
- Etiology.
- Atherosclerotic.
- Multifactorial.
- Genetic predisposition, aging, atherosclerosis, inflammation, and localized proteolytic enzyme activation.
- Mycotic aneurysms.
- Aortic dissection.
- Intimal tear and separation of the layers of the aortic wall.
- Dissecting aneurysm.
- Poststenotic arterial dilatation or arteriovenous fistulas.
- Pseudoaneurysms.
- Trauma, vascular intervention, or anastomotic disruption.

HISTORICAL PERSPECTIVE

- Modern repair of an abdominal aortic aneurysm—1951.
- Aneurysmectomy.
- Dacron polyester graft.
- Thoracoabdominal—1954.
- Endovascular approach—1991.

PATHOGENESIS

- Interaction of multiple factors rather than a single process.
- Decrease in the amount of medial and adventitial elastin.
- Atherosclerotic aneurysms.

Genetic

- Ten percent to 20% of first-degree relatives.
- With Marfan's syndrome.
- Ehlers-Danlos type 4.

Proteolytic

- Marked decrease in the quantity of elastin in the aneurysm wall while the quantity of collagen remains unchanged.
- Matrix metalloproteinase (MMP) 9 or other proteases.

EPIDEMIOLOGY

Distribution of Aortic Aneurysms

- The infrarenal aorta.
- Juxtarenal aneurysms.
- Thoracoabdominal.
- The iliac arteries.

Prevalence of Abdominal Aortic Aneurysms

- More than threefold increase in overall and age-specific prevalence of abdominal aneurysms.
- A male-to-female ratio of approximately 8:1.
- Prevalence of aneurysms is approximately 10% in men with hypertension or with clinical evidence of peripheral, carotid, or coronary arterial disease.
- Thirteenth most common cause of death.
- Thoracic aortic aneurysms.
- Aortic dissection.

NATURAL HISTORY

Abdominal Aortic Aneurysms

- Rupture of an abdominal aortic aneurysm.
- Overall mortality rate of 78% to 94%.

RISK OF RUPTURE

- The single most important factor associated with rupture is maximal cross-sectional aneurysm diameter.
- The risk of rupture is estimated at 1% to 3% per year for aneurysms 4 to 5 cm, 6% to 11% per year for 5- to 7-cm aneurysms, and 20% per year for aneurysms greater than 7 cm.

- Chronic obstructive pulmonary disease (COPD) and pain.
- Advanced age, female gender, and renal failure.

ABDOMINAL AORTIC ANEURYSMS

Clinical Presentation

- Asymptomatic before rupture.
- Palpation of a pulsatile abdominal mass.
- Abdominal ultrasound, computed tomography (CT), magnetic resonance imaging (MRI), or plain abdominal radiograph.
- Inflammatory aneurysms.

Diagnosis

- "Eggshell."
- Ultrasound is accurate in demonstrating the presence of an aortic aneurysm and in measuring transverse aneurysmal diameter.
- Screening and for surveillance.
- CT is the most precise test for imaging aortic aneurysms.
- Three-dimensional image.
- MRI.
- Arteriography provides reliable information on artery lumen caliber and branch vessel disease.
- Assessment of the size of the aneurysm by arteriography is unreliable.

Preoperative Evaluation

- Coexisting cardiac, pulmonary, or renal disease.
- The most important step in preparing for invasive treatment of aortic disease is the cardiac evaluation.
- Exercise electrocardiogram (ECG) testing.
- Detsky modified Goldman risk index, Eagle's criteria, and the recommendations of the American Heart Association.
- COPD and impaired renal function.
- Selection of patients for aneurysm repair.
- When the maximal diameter reaches 5.5 cm, risk of rupture increases rapidly; an aneurysm repair is indicated.
- Open surgical repair or endovascular repair.

Operative Technique of Open Surgical Repair

- Open surgical repair of abdominal aortic aneurysms is performed through a transperitoneal or retroperitoneal exposure.
- The transabdominal approach.

- The retroperitoneal exposure.
- The inferior mesenteric artery.
- Reimplantation.
- Juxtarenal aneurysms.
- "Tube graft" reconstruction.

Endovascular Aortic Aneurysm Repair

- Endovascular aneurysm repair.
- Self-expanding or balloon-expandable stents.
- Morbidity related to the procedure is much reduced.
- Early tubular grafts have been replaced by modular bifurcated grafts.
- The appropriately sized primary module is inserted under fluoroscopic guidance and deployed just below the renal arteries.
- Proximal infrarenal neck at least 1.5 to 2 cm in length and common iliac arteries for proximal and distal fixation of an endograft, without excessive tortuosity and with appropriate iliofemoral access.
- Long-term survival after endovascular aneurysm repair has been comparable to that with open repair.

RUPTURED ABDOMINAL AORTIC ANEURYSM

- Into the peritoneal cavity or into the retroperitoneum.
- Acute excruciating back and abdominal pain, accompanied by pallor, diaphoresis, syncope, and other symptoms and signs related to blood loss and hypovolemic shock.
- Patients with ruptured aortic aneurysms require immediate surgical repair.
- Acutely expanding aneurysms may present with abdominal pain and tenderness on palpation. These are prone to rupture and should be repaired on an emergent basis.
- Progressive multiorgan dysfunction.
- Endovascular repair.
- Restricted fluid resuscitation.

RESULTS AND COMPLICATIONS OF AORTIC ANEURYSM REPAIR

- The overall population-wide mortality rate for open aneurysm repair is 5% to 10%.
- Perioperative mortality rate for thoracoabdominal aortic aneurysm repair is 8.5% to 15%.
- Overall, morbidity rate after elective aneurysm repair is 10% to 30%.

- Myocardial infarction is also the most common cause of postoperative death.
- Evidence of ongoing postoperative bleeding should lead to early re-exploration.
- Emboli or thrombosis.
- Microemboli.
- Postoperative paralytic ileus.
- Colon ischemia occurs after 1% of aneurysm repairs.
- Paraplegia is rare after infrarenal aortic aneurysm repair, with an incidence of 0.2%.
- Sexual dysfunction.
- Late complications.
- Pseudoaneurysms.
- Graft or graft limb thrombosis, and graft infection.
- Late deaths are generally due to cardiac causes.
- The mean duration of survival has been reported to be 7.4 years after aortic aneurysm repair.
- Endoleak.
- Endoleaks can often be fixed by endovascular methods.
- Graft migration and stent graft occlusion.
- Endograft limb occlusion.
- Persistent renal impairment.
- Conversion to open repair.
- Kaplan-Meier estimates for the freedom from all-cause rupture has been 99.5% at 1 year, 98.5% at 2 years, 98.4% at 3 and 4 years.

Iliac Aneurysms

- Occur in conjunction with aortic aneurysms.

COMPLICATING FEATURES OF ANEURYSM REPAIR

- Complicated by a concurrent disease process.
- Emergencies such as a ruptured or symptomatic aneurysm when preoperative images (CT scan) are unavailable, the aneurysm always takes priority.

Horseshoe Kidney

- Creatinine.
- Furosemide and mannitol.
- Endovascular repair.
- The left retroperitoneal approach.

Accessory Renal Arteries

- Accessory renal arteries should be preserved when possible during aortic reconstruction.
- By reimplanting.

Venous Anomalies

- Left-sided vena cava and retroaortic left renal vein are the most common anomalies.
- Bilateral inferior vena cava.

Inflammatory Aneurysms

- Dense fibroinflammatory rind that is usually adherent to the fourth portion of the duodenum and often involves the inferior vena cava and left renal vein. One or more ureters may also be involved.

Associated Abdominal Malignancy

- Liver tumors.
- Incidental discovery of a liver mass.
- Colonic neoplasm.
- Concurrent renal or bladder neoplasm.
- Incidental ovarian cysts and tumors.
- Solid ovarian abnormality.
- Uterine tumors.
- Tubo-ovarian abscess and pelvic inflammatory disease.

THORACIC AORTIC ANEURYSMS

- Thoracic aortic aneurysms may involve the ascending, arch, or descending thoracic aorta or a combination of these segments.
- Atherosclerotic or degenerative.
- Marfan's syndrome.
- Ehlers-Danlos syndrome.
- CT angiography.
- Magnetic resonance (MR) angiography.
- Three-dimensional reconstruction.
- Endovascular repair.
- Woven polyester tube grafts.
- Paraplegia.
- Thoracic aortic stent grafts.

- Endovascular repair appears to have a promising role in the treatment of descending thoracic aortic aneurysms.

THORACOABDOMINAL ANEURYSMS

- First thoracoabdominal aneurysm repair—1955.
- Type I.
- Type II.
- Type III.
- Type IV.
- CT scanning and MR angiography.
- The risk of rupture must be weighed against the risk of serious operative morbidity and death, and patients who undergo repair must have optimization of their cardiac and pulmonary function preoperatively.
- The technique of open surgical repair.
- To minimize the risk of paraplegia.
- The risk of paraplegia was highest in patients with Type I and II.

FEMORAL AND POPLITEAL ARTERY ANEURYSMS

- Together they constitute 90% of the peripheral aneurysms not involving the aortoiliac arteries.
- Asymptomatic.
- In 10% of femoral aneurysms, evidence of distal embolization is found.
- Limb-threatening in 44% of cases.
- Rupture of these aneurysms is rare and occurs at a rate of 1% to 14% in femoral aneurysms and at a rate less than 5% in popliteal aneurysms.
- Venous thrombosis or edema.
- A Baker cyst or tumor.
- Duplex ultrasonography.
- Angiography.
- Forty percent of patients have abdominal aortic aneurysm, and 70% have contralateral femoral popliteal aneurysms.
- Transverse diameter greater than 2 cm for popliteal aneurysms and greater than 2.5 cm for common femoral aneurysms.

UPPER EXTREMITY ANEURYSMS

- Subclavian artery aneurysms.
- Atherosclerosis, compression at the thoracic outlet, and trauma.

- Fifty percent of patients have aortoiliac or other peripheral aneurysms.
- Horner's syndrome.
- Duplex ultrasound or CT.
- Surgical repair.
- Decompression of the thoracic outlet.
- An aberrant right subclavian artery.
- Kommerell diverticulum.
- Axillary arteries.
- History of previous blunt or penetrating trauma.
- The ulnar artery.

VISCERAL ARTERY ANEURYSMS

- Involved arteries and their relative frequencies include the:
  - Splenic (60%).
  - Hepatic (20%).
  - Superior mesenteric (5.5%), and other arterial (each less than 5%).
- Splenic artery aneurysms occur most frequently in females with a female-to-male ratio of 4:1.
- Women of childbearing age who have splenic artery aneurysms are at particularly high risk of death as a result of aneurysm rupture and should have elective repair.
- Symptomatic or ruptured aneurysms also warrant immediate repair.
- Surgical techniques for treating splenic artery aneurysms include simple proximal and distal ligation without arterial reconstruction; for proximal aneurysms and splenectomy versus aneurysm exclusion and vascular reconstruction for salvage of the spleen.

MYCOTIC ANEURYSMS

- Localized infection.
- *Salmonella* and *Staphylococcus*.
- Pulsatile mass accompanied by fever and chills.
- Septic emboli.
- CT and MR study.
- In the groin, duplex ultrasonography.
- Eradication of the infection and preservation of adequate blood supply.
- *In situ* reconstruction following aggressive débridement and wound care.
- Autologous veins including superficial femoral veins.

PSEUDOANEURYSMS

- Pseudoaneurysms are contained arterial disruptions that can be categorized to two main types: those that result from a perforation of an artery by traumatic or iatrogenic injury and those that result from dehiscence of a surgical vascular anastomosis.
- Management includes direct surgical repair or exclusion of the pseudoaneurysm with a stent graft.
- Pseudoaneurysms arising in small, nonvital arteries may be treated with ligation, compression, or coil embolization.
- *Iatrogenic* pseudoaneurysms occur most commonly after arterial puncture for vascular intervention, and the most frequently affected site is the common femoral artery.
- Pseudoaneurysms manifest with pain, a pulsatile mass, and compression of adjacent structures.
- The imaging modality of choice is duplex ultrasonography.
- Pseudoaneurysms less than 2 cm in diameter have a 70% likelihood of spontaneous thrombosis with compression therapy; whereas larger ones and those in anticoagulated patients are likely to persist.
- *Anastomotic* pseudoaneurysms occur as a result of partial or complete disruption of a vascular anastomotic suture line.
- Surgical repair of anastomotic pseudoaneurysms is indicated and consists of patching or, preferentially, graft replacement of the disrupted region.
- Bacterial cultures should be obtained at the time of reconstruction, and, if gross evidence of infection exists, proper débridement and appropriately planned reconstruction must be performed.

HUMAN IMMUNODEFICIENCY VIRUS-RELATED ARTERIAL ANEURYSMS

- Multiple and occur at unusual sites.

CHAPTER 64

PERIPHERAL ARTERIAL OCCLUSIVE DISEASE

BASIC CONSIDERATIONS

- Arterial occlusive diseases are highly prevalent in Western societies, where they constitute the leading overall cause of death.

Atherosclerosis

General Observations and Risk Factors

- Atherosclerosis is a complex, chronic inflammatory process that affects the elastic and muscular arteries. The disease is both systemic and segmental.
- The most important independent risk factors for atherosclerosis are hypercholesterolemia, hypertension, cigarette smoking, and diabetes mellitus.
- Studies have demonstrated a strong positive correlation between atherosclerotic cardiovascular disease and elevated total and low-density lipoprotein (LDL) cholesterol and an equally strong negative correlation with high-density lipoprotein (HDL) levels.
- Cigarette smoking is strongly associated with the incidence of atherosclerosis.
- Mechanism for the effects of smoking is likely to involve direct toxicity of tobacco metabolites on the vascular endothelium, probably by creating oxidant stress. Diabetic patients are also at markedly increased risk for atherosclerosis, often manifesting a particularly virulent form of the disease, leading to higher rates of myocardial events, stroke, and amputation.
- Age and gender also demonstrate an important influence.
- Prevalence will continue to increase with the advancing age of people in the United States.

Pathology and Theories of Atherogenesis

- The pathologic hallmark of atherosclerosis is the atherosclerotic plaque. There are several major components of plaque—smooth muscle cells (SMCs), connective tissue (matrix), lipid, and inflammatory cells (predominantly macrophages).

- An important concept linking plaque morphology with clinical events is the relationship between the fibrous cap—a layer of SMCs and connective tissue of variable thickness—and the underlying necrotic lipid core, composed of amorphous extracellular lipid, plasma proteins, and hemostatic factors.

- Anatomic distribution of atherosclerosis is remarkably constant and is thought to reflect an important role for hemodynamic stresses.

- Plaques tend to be concentrated at bifurcations or bends, where local alterations in shear stress, flow separation, turbulence, and stasis are known to occur. The infrarenal abdominal aorta, proximal coronary arteries, iliofemoral arteries (especially the superficial femoral artery), carotid bifurcation, and popliteal arteries are commonly involved.

- Atherosclerotic plaques are dynamic lesions that may undergo progression or regression over time. Similarly, the underlying arterial wall also undergoes adaptive remodeling.

- The "response to injury" hypothesis and its more recent modifications, which include the concept of endothelial cell dysfunction, is the leading theory of pathogenesis. This hypothesis incorporates important roles for lipid, inflammation, and thrombosis in addition to proliferation and dysfunction of the residing cells in the arterial wall. In the earlier versions of this theory, the triggering event was thought to be a focal denuding injury to the endothelium.

- The final common pathway is a loss of the numerous atheroprotective effects of normal endothelium, which include its barrier function, potent antiadhesive properties, and antiproliferative influence on the underlying SMCs.

- The SMC plays a central role in the developing lesion. Migration and proliferation of medial SMCs result in a cellular neointima.

- An important role for platelets and their growth-promoting and vasoactive products has long been espoused. The prototypic growth factor platelet-derived growth factor (PDGF).

- An alternative explanation is offered by the "monoclonal hypothesis," which hinges on the intriguing observation that many atherosclerotic plaques appear to contain a clonally expanded population of SMCs.

Other Arteriopathies

- Buerger's disease is exclusively associated with cigarette smoking.
  - Occlusive lesions are predominantly seen in the muscular arteries, with a predilection for the tibial vessels. Rest pain, gangrene, and ulceration are the typical presentations. Recurrent superficial thrombophlebitis ("phlebitis migrans") is a characteristic feature.
  - Reveals diffuse occlusion of the distal extremity vessels.
- Takayasu's arteritis ("pulseless disease") commonly afflicts younger female patients.
  - Prodrome marked by systemic inflammatory signs and symptoms. The arterial pathology is focused on the aorta and its major branches.
  - Brachiocephalic vessels.
- Temporal arteritis (sometimes referred to as giant cell arteritis) predominantly afflicts patients older than 50 years, with a slight (2:1) female preponderance.
  - Headache is a common symptom. Blindness, usually irreversible, is a dreaded complication.
  - High-dose corticosteroid therapy.
- Raynaud's phenomenon is characterized by recurrent, episodic vasospasm of the digits brought on by cold exposure or emotional stress.
  - Produces pallor of the digits, followed by cyanosis, and accompanied by pain and paresthesias. Rewarming leads to marked rubor caused by a hyperemic response.
  - Secondary Raynaud's phenomenon has been associated with a variety of rheumatologic, hematologic, and traumatic disorders, as well as a number of drugs and toxins.

Diagnostic Modalities in Peripheral Arterial Occlusive Disease

Noninvasive Hemodynamic Assessment

- Atherosclerotic plaques produce local and downstream alterations in pressure and flow that may be quantitated by a variety of noninvasive methods.
- In the lower extremities, measurement of pressure plays a central role in the assessment of disease severity. Segmental pressure measurements.
- The ankle pressure.
- Because the ankle pressure varies with central aortic pressure, it is commonly indexed to the brachial artery pressure as a ratio (ankle-brachial index [ABI]). The ABI is quite reproducible

in a given patient and is, therefore, extremely useful for longitudinal surveillance of obstructive disease. In normal resting subjects, the ABI is slightly greater than unity (1.0 to 1.2).

- Claudicants usually fall in the 0.5 to 0.7 range, whereas critical ischemia (rest pain or tissue necrosis) most commonly is associated with an ABI less than 0.4.
- False elevation resulting from extensive vascular.
- A more complete assessment of infrainguinal arterial disease may be obtained by the segmental pressure technique.
- A toe pressure of greater than 30 mm Hg is predictive of successful healing in approximately 90% of cases, whereas values less than 10 mm Hg are highly predictive of poor outcome.
- Exercise (treadmill) testing may be used in patients with claudication.
- Patients with calf claudication resulting from superficial femoral arterial disease uniformly demonstrate a marked decrease in ankle pressure at the time of symptom occurrence as a result of the increased gradient produced by a fixed resistance in the setting of increased blood flow.
- Limb plethysmography, which measures the fluctuation in limb volume during the cardiac cycle, is a useful adjunct to segmental pressure measurements.
- Transmetatarsal peripheral vascular resistances (PVRs), obtained with a cuff across the forefoot, are particularly useful in diabetic patients with falsely elevated segmental limb pressures.

Doppler and Duplex Ultrasonography

- Ultrasound technology has revolutionized vascular imaging.
- Duplex ultrasound combines the traditional B-mode two-dimensional image with Doppler measurement of blood flow parameters. Doppler relies on a measured frequency shift, which correlates with the velocity of flow. The B-mode image is used to guide placement of the Doppler sampling volume at different locations, and the resulting frequency or velocity profile can be used to grade the severity of obstructive lesions.
- The most common application is for carotid bifurcation disease.
- Color-flow imaging facilitates the examination by allowing the technician to rapidly identify deeper vessels and by demonstrating areas of turbulence where high-grade lesions are likely to reside.

Transcutaneous Oximetry

- Transcutaneous measurement of oxygen tension ($tcPO_2$) is another technique for assessing tissue perfusion.
- The electrodes measure oxygen diffused to the skin, which is a reflection of underlying tissue perfusion.
- Normal $tcPO_2$ levels in the foot are in the 50 to 60 mm Hg range. Values greater than 40 mm Hg are predictive for healing of foot lesions or primary forefoot amputations; values less than 10 mm Hg are almost universally associated with failure to heal.

Arteriography

- The modern era of arterial reconstruction was made possible by the development of contrast arteriography (Moniz 1927, dos Santos 1929), which allowed for anatomic localization of aneurysmal and occlusive lesions and their relationship to symptoms.
- Aortic and lower extremity arteriograms are generally performed by needle puncture of the femoral or brachial arteries, followed by guide wire placement and catheter insertion using the Seldinger technique. Most diagnostic studies are performed using catheters passed through 5-French (1.7 mm outer diameter) sheaths.
- A large variety of highly specialized guide wires and catheters have been developed to assist radiologists in selective cannulation of remote vessels (e.g., renal, mesenteric, cerebral, and pulmonary vasculature).
- Complications of arteriography.
- Atheroembolization and puncture site problems.
- "Blue toe syndrome."
- Pseudoaneurysm formation.
- Arteriovenous (AV) fistula.
- Contrast agents may produce both minor and major adverse reactions.
- Idiosyncratic reactions to contrast occur in approximately 4% of patients.
- Anaphylaxis
- Nausea, urticaria, pruritus.
- Renal toxicity is an important adverse consequence of contrast arteriography.
    - Ischemia resulting from the osmotic diuresis produced or direct toxic effects on tubular epithelium.
    - Factors associated with elevated risk include chronic renal insufficiency (baseline creatinine >1.5 mg/dL), diabetes,

dehydration, age older than 60 years, recent surgery, and larger doses of contrast medium.
- Computed tomography (CT) with intravenous contrast administration can also delineate vascular anatomy.
- Magnetic resonance angiography (MRA) is an important technique that is gaining application by virtue of rapidly improving technology. It offers the distinct advantages of being noninvasive and avoiding contrast exposure.
- Obtaining vascular enhancement is time-of-flight (TOF), in which brightness is directly related to the velocity of blood entering the slice. As a result, lesion severity is often over-estimated, which is an important limitation.

Therapeutic Interventions in Arterial Occlusive Disease

Medical Management

- The medical management of atherosclerosis is targeted to reduce progression, induce regression, and prevent morbid endpoints of lesion formation.
- Lipid-lowering therapy.
  - Dietary treatment.
  - Drugs include niacin, bile acid–binding resins, 3-hydroxl-3-methylglutaryl (HMG)-CoA reductase inhibitors (the statins), clofibrate, and gemfibrozil.
- Smoking cessation is clearly of paramount importance.
- Antiplatelet therapy.
  - Aspirin remains the cornerstone of antiplatelet therapy, with a well-established record of accomplishment of compliance, low risk, and minimal cost.
  - Ticlopidine and clopidogrel.

Basic Techniques of Arterial Surgery

- Technical success in arterial reconstructive surgery hinges on the meticulous application of basic techniques of handling and suturing blood vessels.
- Vessel wall spared of disease.
- The choice of orientation (i.e., longitudinal or transverse) of the arteriotomy depends on the vessel size, the local extent of disease, and the reconstructive technique being used.
- Suture materials for vascular surgery are nonabsorbable (e.g., polypropylene).
- Right angle, then be gently rotated along its curvature to draw the suture through. Shallow angled bites, levering of

the needle, or rough handling of the suture can produce a localized linear tear in an atherosclerotic vessel.

- Slight, gentle eversion of the edges is important.
- Flushing and backbleeding by release of clamps is an important maneuver to be done before completing the anastomosis, to remove any small amounts of thrombus, air, or debris.

Surgical Bypass Grafting

- Surgical bypass grafting has evolved as the most widely applicable technique for the treatment of arterial occlusive lesions. It has found broad application in the coronary, abdominal, and peripheral vascular beds. In comparison to other techniques such as angioplasty, stenting, or endarterectomy, bypass is far less restrictive in terms of the anatomic nature of lesions amenable to treatment.
- The specific choice of percutaneous or surgical approach must be tailored to the individual patient, lesion, and the skill and experience of the operator.
- Anatomic exposure of the selected inflow and outflow arteries is obtained through standard incisions in the abdomen or extremities.
- Despite arteriographic appearances, the presence of significant plaque or calcification may require modifying the original operative strategy. Whenever possible, segments bearing minimal disease are selected for anastomotic sites because this greatly facilitates both vascular occlusion and suturing.
- Shorter grafts are preferable.
- Application of atraumatic vascular clamps, elastic vessel loops, intraluminal occluders, or an extremity tourniquet.
- Systemic anticoagulation, by intravenous administration of heparin sodium, is achieved before vascular occlusion. Standard heparin doses are in the range of 70 to 100 units/kg as a bolus.
- The half-life of heparin ranges from 60 to 90 minutes in most patients.
- The arteriotomy is preferably made in a disease-free area.
- Anastomoses are most commonly performed either in an end-to-side or end-to-end configuration.
- End-to-end anastomoses are facilitated by slightly beveling the two ends (45 degrees) to enlarge the opening.
- End-to-side configurations are usually made at an entry angle of less than 45 degrees to minimize turbulence.
- The optimal choice of graft material depends on the anatomic location, size, and hemodynamic environment of the bypass. The ideal vascular graft would be characterized by

both its mechanical attributes and postimplantation healing responses.

- Mechanical strength.
- Availability, suturability, and simplicity of handling.
- The graft should be resistant to both thrombosis and infection and, optimally, would be completely incorporated by the body to yield a neovessel resembling a native artery in structure and function.
- Large-caliber arterial reconstructions, currently available synthetic grafts.
- Whereas graft infection, occlusion, and dilatation are important clinical problems, most patients can expect durable patency and a low frequency of repeat procedures.
- Prosthetic grafts have generally proven unfavorable as small-caliber (<6 mm) arterial substitutes. In these demanding, low-flow environments, the primary factor influencing long-term patency is the conduit itself, and the thromboresistance of endothelialized autogenous materials becomes paramount.
- Autogenous vein, particularly the greater saphenous, has proven to be a durable and versatile arterial substitute. In the lower extremity, long-term results with saphenous vein bypass (used in either the *in situ* or reversed configurations) to below-knee popliteal, tibial, and even pedal arteries have been excellent and serve as the standard of reference for other conduits. Ectopic (i.e., lesser saphenous, arm veins) or composite vein grafts for infrapopliteal bypass are generally inferior to a single segment saphenous vein, although they are still superior to the performance of synthetic grafts in the hands of most surgeons.
- The most important complications of surgical bypass are graft occlusion and infection.
- Infection of vascular grafts may be catastrophic and poses immediate threat to both life and limb. Death may occur by sudden and massive hemorrhage internally or externally. Limb loss may result from secondary thrombosis or failure of attempted re-do procedures following graft removal.

Surgical Endarterectomy

- Endarterectomy is a direct disobliterative technique that takes advantage of the pathologic localization of atherosclerosis to the intima and inner media.
- The most common and technically simplest technique is the open method, performed by way of a longitudinal arteriotomy with direct vision of both endpoints and the entire endarterectomized surface. Extraction, eversion, and

semiclosed methods are applicable in specific situations as well.

● Is most feasible and durable when applied to focal stenotic lesions in large-caliber, high-flow vessels. The carotid bifurcation, visceral artery origins, and common femoral artery are particularly well suited to this approach.

● Early failures are due to technical problems with the imperfect endpoints or to *in situ* thrombosis on the exposed nonendothelialized surface. Platelet aggregation to the collagenous matrix is a particular problem, and antiplatelet therapy is usually used. Late failures are due to exuberant intimal hyperplasia.

Percutaneous Angioplasty, Stenting, and Other Endovascular Techniques

● Percutaneous techniques for treating arterial occlusions, including balloon dilatation, stenting, and atherectomy, have undergone tremendous development in the past quarter century and are assuming an increasingly important role.

● The mechanism of dilation in balloon angioplasty is thought to involve fracture and displacement of plaque and overstretch of the media and perhaps the adventitia as well.

● Crossing of the lesion with a guide wire.

● Percutaneous transluminal angioplasty (PTA) has found its greatest success in the treatment of focal stenoses in large-caliber, high-flow arteries. The 5-year patency rate for PTA (without stenting) of common iliac lesions, for example, is in the 70% to 80% range. Excellent results have also been reported for suitable aortic, arch vessel, renal, and mesenteric lesions. Results in the femoropopliteal system are inferior to bypass overall, but carefully selected lesions, primarily in claudicants, may be durably treated.

● Restenosis following angioplasty.

● Intravascular stents.

● Maintain luminal patency by exerting persistent radial force on the vessel. Metallic stents come in a variety of design configurations and sizes.

● Stents are most commonly used as an adjunct to PTA, although their application as a primary modality is increasing. Localized dissections, elastic recoil, or residual stenoses following PTA are situations in which stent placement can often improve the technical result.

● The anatomic sites most suitable for stenting are similar to those mentioned for endarterectomy.

● Catheter-directed atherectomy.

- For debulking of restenotic lesions, particularly in the coronary circulation, but repeated treatments are not infrequently required as a result of recurrence of the hyperplastic response.

Thrombolytic Therapy

- Fibrinolytic drugs enhance conversion of plasminogen to plasmin, which is then capable of degrading fibrin clot.
- Except for acute embolic events, thrombolytic therapy for arterial occlusive disease is not a sole modality. Instead, it is used as an important adjunct to PTA or surgical interventions.
- Urokinase and tissue plasminogen activator (tPA).
- For arterial occlusions, regional therapy by means of an angiographically guided catheter is most effective.
- An initial high-dose infusion (lacing dose) is followed by a lower dose regimen, with frequent follow-up angiograms to document progressive lysis to a satisfactory endpoint.
- Because of the significant risks of bleeding and the need for careful monitoring of the infusion catheters, patients requiring extended therapy (in some cases up to 48 hours) are best managed in an intensive care setting.
- Appropriate selection of patients is critical for reducing the incidence of serious complications and improving the likelihood of successful lysis.
- Relative contraindications include remote gastrointestinal bleeding, hemostatic disorders, severe hypertension, or intracardiac thrombus. The risk of serious bleeding (5% to 15%) is increased with longer durations of therapy and a decrease in fibrinogen levels to less than 100 mg% or to less than 50% of baseline; all are associated with the development of a systemic lytic state. Fresh thrombi are the most easily lysed.
- In addition, patients with acute, rapid deterioration to advanced ischemia are often poorly collateralized and may not tolerate the time required to achieve reperfusion with this approach.

ACUTE THROMBOEMBOLIC DISEASE

- The management of acute extremity ischemia remains a major surgical challenge.
- Limb loss rates of 8% to 22% and perioperative mortality rates of 10% to 17% continue to be reported. Maximization of limb salvage, while minimizing associated morbidity and mortality, requires expeditious diagnosis and restoration of perfusion.

Pathophysiology

- Unlike the brain, which suffers infarction after only 4 to 8 minutes of ischemia, or the myocardium, which infarcts after 17 to 20 minutes, the lower extremity may be salvaged after up to 5 to 6 hours of profound ischemia.
- Nervous tissue is generally the most sensitive component of the extremity to the effects of ischemia.
- Skeletal muscle is the major structural component of the extremity and, for a variety of reasons, plays a key role in the pathophysiology of extremity ischemia.

Reperfusion Syndrome

- The resulting myonephropathic syndrome, with its associated hemodynamic instability, lactic acidosis, and hyperkalemia, is well recognized by surgeons. Myoglobin released from injured muscle cells into the circulation is cleared through the kidneys, resulting in dark urine (without red blood cells).
- Acute renal failure may be produced.
- Myocardial contractility may become depressed.
- Life-threatening dysrhythmias.
- Intracellular edema results.
- Interstitial edema results.
- Acute compartment syndrome results as pressure increases beyond capillary perfusion pressure (30 mm Hg), and tissue perfusion is impaired. Unless recognized and decompressed by fasciotomy, compartment syndromes will lead to prolonged tissue ischemia despite apparent successful revascularization.
- "Reperfusion injury" (i.e., cellular injury that occurs or is manifested at the time perfusion is restored to ischemic tissue).
- Oxygen-derived free radicals.

Etiology

Embolism

- Embolic occlusion of a previously unobstructed vessel generally results in the most severe forms of acute ischemia.
- More recently, atherosclerotic cardiovascular disease has become the major contributor. Approximately 70% of patients with cardiogenic emboli have atrial fibrillation with the emboli arising in atrial mural thrombus. Atrial fibrillation is currently the most common source of cardiogenic emboli. Acute myocardial infarction is the second most common

cause of cardiogenic emboli, preceding approximately one third of peripheral embolic events.

- Peripheral embolization may often be the first sign of a previously "silent" myocardial infarction.
- *Paradoxical embolization.*
- Circulation through the patent foramen ovale.
- In most situations, such atheroembolization results in diffuse microembolization, resulting in the picture of painful, bluish discoloration of the toes with cutaneous gangrene, livido reticularis, and often transient muscular pain. This so-called blue toe syndrome generally appears in the setting of palpable peripheral pulses right down to the pedal level.
- In approximately 10% to 15% of cases, the source of embolization ultimately cannot be determined. Such emboli should not be designated as idiopathic until a detailed history and physical, as well as complete cardiac and peripheral imaging, fail to identify an embolic source.
- The emboli tend to lodge at branch points where vessel diameter decreases. Approximately 10% to 15% of large cardiogenic emboli lodge at the aortic bifurcation. Such "saddle emboli" may result in profound bilateral lower extremity ischemia and neurologic ischemic injury. Another 15% embolizes to the iliac bifurcation. The most common site of lower extremity embolization is the femoral bifurcation constituting more than 40% of cases. Smaller emboli lodge at the distal popliteal artery level at the level of the tibioperoneal artery trunk in approximately 10% to 15% of cases.
- Embolization to the cerebral circulation occurs in approximately 13% of cases with potentially devastating results. Mesenteric and renal embolization to the vessels occurs in approximately 5% of peripheral emboli.

Thrombosis

- Acute thrombosis generally occurs in vessels affected by preexistent atherosclerosis.
- The most common extremity vessel affected is the superficial femoral artery, which is often affected by long segments of atherosclerosis. Popliteal artery aneurysms are also prone to thrombosis and may result in severe ischemia, particularly when associated with embolization to the tibial vessels.
- With hypercoagulable states.
- Antithrombin III deficiency, lupus anticoagulant (antiphospholipid antibody), and protein C deficiency. Although usually associated with venous thrombosis, activated protein

C resistance caused by the spontaneous mutations of factor V Leiden may also cause arterial thrombosis.
- Heparin-induced antibodies.

Presentation and Evaluation

- The classic presentation of patients with acute ischemia of the extremities may be recalled by the "five Ps": *pain, pallor, pulselessness, paresthesias,* and *paralysis.*
- Pain is the most common complaint in alert patients.
- Pallor is a common but relative finding that depends on the degree of ischemia and the underlying skin color.
- The absence of arterial pulses on examination will alert the surgeon to both the location of the arterial occlusion and the degree of ischemia.
- The presence of normal arterial pulses in the contralateral extremity is most suggestive of an acute embolus because patients with acute thrombosis generally have some degree of symmetrical pulse deficit owing to long-standing atherosclerosis. A handheld continuous-wave Doppler examination plays an important role in the initial evaluation of patients with acute vessel occlusion.
- Neurologic dysfunction is a sensitive barometer of the degree of ischemia. With mild ischemia, the findings may be subjective and subtle. Early paresthesias may be characterized as a numbness of the toes or a slight decrease of sensation of the foot compared with the contralateral extremity to light touch or pinprick. With severe ischemia, however, profound sensory loss may lead to complete anesthesia of the foot, indicative of impending tissue loss without early revascularization.
- Weakness of the extremity is another important sign of neurologic ischemia.
- The acute embolic occlusion of an extremity artery can be accurately diagnosed by a careful history and physical examination in most cases; emboli to the cerebral and visceral bed may be more difficult to identify and treat.
- Patients with emboli tend to have risk factors (e.g., atrial fibrillation, recent myocardial infarction, prosthetic heart valve), a more sudden onset of symptoms (no prior claudication), and unilateral findings (normal contralateral extremity).
- When the history and physical examination implicates an embolus as the source of occlusion, the subsequent evaluation should be simple and direct. Routine preoperative blood work and chest x-ray film are obtained, and a 12-lead electrocardiogram is performed to document atrial fibrillation,

cardiac ischemia, or a previous (and perhaps unsuspected) myocardial infarction. Because arterial emboli are removed by direct arterial cutdown and removal of the embolus (as described later), there is generally no need for preoperative arteriography.

- The surgical management of patients with acute arterial thrombosis is generally more complex than the simple arteriotomy and clot extraction used for embolic occlusion.
- These patients are best evaluated with complete arteriography to define the optimal approach to revascularization. Rarely, arterial thrombosis results in such profound ischemia that the patient is taken immediately to the operating room and intraoperative arteriography is performed after arterial exposure.

Management

Embolic Occlusion

- Patients with acute arterial occlusion should be anticoagulated with an intravenous heparin bolus (5000 to 10,000 units) and begun on a continuous infusion at 1000 units/hour.
- Recurrent embolization occurs in approximately 7% of patients who are chronically anticoagulated versus 21% of those who are not.
- The most important initial decision focuses on the viability and potential salvage in the ischemic limb. Rarely, patients have such longstanding and severe ischemia that irreversible ischemic injury to the extremity (manifesting as rigor of the muscles or frank gangrenous changes to the foot) has occurred. Such cases are best treated with primary extremity amputation.
- In most cases, however, early revascularization for restoration of limb function is indicated.
- A standard longitudinal or oblique skin incision is made with the common femoral artery as well as profunda femoris and superficial femoral arteries all independently controlled. Normal arteries, free of significant atherosclerosis, are best incised transversely just above the femoral bifurcation. In patients with significant atherosclerosis, however, longitudinal arteriotomies afford the best exposure and most reliable closure (often with an arterial patch). Patients with iliac level emboli often have an absence of a femoral pulse. Inflow is restored by retrograde passage of a number 4 or 5 balloon thrombectomy catheter. The catheter is passed in 10-cm increments. Gentle inflation of the catheter as it is withdrawn

engages and extracts the thrombus without causing arterial wall injury. Each passage should extend an additional 10 cm until pulsatile arterial inflow is restored. Passages are continued until no additional thrombus is recovered. Attention is then turned to the outflow vessels. Antegrade passage of a number 3 Fogarty catheter, 3 to 5 cm down the profunda, generally extracts any impacted thrombus and restores good backflow. The catheter is then passed down the superficial femoral artery in increments until no further thrombus is extracted. This may necessitate passage to the popliteal level or beyond. Blind passage of the Fogarty catheter from the groin to below the popliteal artery almost always results in cannulation of the peroneal artery. Specific cannulation of the anterior tibial and posterior tibial arteries requires more distal, below the knee popliteal artery exposure. Alternatively, selective passage of balloon catheters over guidewires using fluoroscopic control has facilitated selective cannulation of distal vessels. When good inflow and backbleeding has been restored, the transverse arteriotomy is closed with 5-0 polypropylene sutures and flow is restored.

- For patients with a palpable popliteal pulse and a distal emboli, exposure is best obtained at the level of the below-knee popliteal artery through a standard medial incision.

- Patients with a saddle embolus to the aortic bifurcation with bilateral lower extremity ischemia are approached through simultaneous bilateral femoral artery cutdowns.

- Patients with upper extremity emboli are approached in a similar fashion. The entire extremity is prepped and draped into the field. Usually the entire embolectomy can be performed under local anesthesia through a longitudinal incision performed just above the elbow. The brachial artery is carefully dissected from its companion structures, and a transverse arteriotomy is performed. Most emboli impact just above the elbow and are easily extracted by passage of a number 3 Fogarty catheter both proximally and distally. Emboli that have lodged at the subclavian level are generally easy to remove by retrograde passage of the number 3 Fogarty catheter from the elbow proximally to the subclavian level. Arterial closure and assessment are similar to that performed for the lower extremity.

Thrombotic Occlusion

- In patients with a satisfactory inflow and outflow vessel with a long segment of occluded vessel, the best option is generally to proceed to surgery and perform a surgical bypass procedure.

- When short segment thrombotic occlusions are identified, a catheter-directed infusion of thrombolytic therapy may recanalize the vessel, revealing an appropriate underlying lesion for balloon angioplasty.
- When the arteriogram reveals no distal arterial reconstitution appropriate for bypass, catheter-based thrombolysis may restore sufficient perfusion to establish or reveal a distal vessel suitable for bypass.

Compartment Syndrome

- As described previously, extremities subjected to prolonged periods of ischemia followed by reperfusion suffer reperfusion injury manifesting as both intracellular and interstitial edema. This reperfusion injury occurs regardless of the cause of arterial occlusion (embolus or thrombosis) or mode of revascularization (balloon embolectomy, surgical bypass, or catheter-based thrombolytic recanalization). When muscular swelling occurs within the confines of an unyielding osseofascial bound space, increased compartmental pressures occur.
- In the lower extremity, the calf is the most frequently affected area. The anterior compartment of the calf, followed by the lateral, deep posterior, and superficial posterior compartments are involved with decreasing frequency. Within the thigh, the anterior quadriceps compartment is the most frequently involved area. In the upper extremity, the anterior or volar forearm compartment is most frequently involved, but the dorsal forearm and hand and upper arm may also be involved by reperfusion edema.
- Capillary perfusion may become impaired.
- The diagnosis of compartment syndrome is based on a high degree of suspicion and careful evaluation for signs and symptoms. Extremities that are revascularized after 4 to 6 hours of severe ischemia are most at risk for development of compartment syndrome. The early signs and symptoms must be carefully watched for, particularly in patients with decreased sensorium. The typical clinical findings of early compartment syndrome are severe pain that is disproportionate to the relative paucity of physical findings. Patients usually have marked tenderness on compression of the edematous calf and severe discomfort on passive extension of the calf with dorsiflexion or plantarflexion of the foot. Because the anterior compartment is the most commonly affected space within the calf, the first neurologic findings are often numbness in the area of the great toe web space, attributable to pressure on the deep peroneal nerve. Palpable pulses and strong Doppler signals

may be well preserved despite progressive compartment syndrome and should not lead to a false sense of security. When the diagnosis of compartment syndrome is in question, direct measures of the pressure within the compartment may be performed. A needle cannula placed directly into the compartment and attached to a pressure transducer gives an accurate measure of the intracompartmental pressure. There are also portable, handheld devices designed for measurement of intracompartmental pressures. Although somewhat controversial, it is generally agreed that, as compartmental pressure reaches 30 mm Hg, capillary perfusion is impaired and neurologic and muscular injury occurs.

- Changes necessitates early and effective decompression to prevent a permanent and disabling injury. Most vascular surgeons prefer a two-incision, four-compartment fasciotomy. The medial-based longitudinal incision is made just posterior to the tibia and is carried down through the fascia into the superficial posterior space. The soleus muscle is then incised longitudinally, near its tibial insertion, and the deep fascia incised longitudinally to decompress the deep posterior compartment. A second anterolateral calf incision is made longitudinally and carried down through the fascia into the anterior compartment. A second longitudinal fascial incision is made over the lateral compartment, decompressing the peroneus muscles. Severe compartment syndrome is manifest by an immediate pouting of the muscles as they swell beyond the fascial incision.
- Prophylactic fasciotomies.

CHRONIC OCCLUSIVE DISEASE OF THE LOWER EXTREMITIES

Presentation and Natural History

- Patients with arterial claudication suffer from reproducible ischemic muscle pain resulting from inadequate oxygen delivery during exercise. Studies suggest that patients with claudication, although having an increased risk of cardiovascular mortality, have a low risk of limb loss (Table 64–1).
- The annual risk of mortality and limb loss in patients with claudication is approximately 5% and 1%, respectively. More than half of these patients either remain stable or have improvement in their symptoms with conservative management, consisting of increased exercise, weight loss, and risk factor modification. Approximately 20% to 30% of patients with claudication come to operation within 5 years because of disease progression.

TABLE 64–1. Natural History of Intermittent Claudication

Study	Patients (n)	Follow-up (yr)	Stable/Improved (%)	Amputation (%)	Survival (%)
Boyd	1476	5	80	7.2	73
		10	60	12	38
Imparato	104	2.5	79	5.8	—
McAllister	100	6	78	7.0	89

Adapted from Braunwald E: Atlas of heart diseases. In Craeger MA (ed): Vascular Disease, vol VII. Philadelphia, Current Medicine, 1996, p 3.5.

- Rest pain occurs when blood flow is inadequate to meet metabolic requirements. In the lower extremity, ischemic rest pain is localized to the forefoot and should be easily distinguished from benign nocturnal muscle cramps in the calf, which are also common in older patients. The patient with rest pain is often awakened by severe discomfort in the forefoot and hangs the affected extremity off the bed for temporary relief of symptoms. Patients often have trophic changes, such as muscle wasting, thinning of skin, thickening of nails, and hair loss in the distal affected limb.
- The patient with critical ischemia is at risk for tissue infection or gangrene resulting from arterial insufficiency. Patients with diabetes or renal failure are more susceptible to the development of ischemic pedal ulcers. Minor trauma to the forefoot leads to ulcer formation and skin breakdown that, with diminished tissue perfusion, are unable to heal. The simple friction between adjacent ischemic toes may result in breakdown termed "kissing ulcers." Bacterial superinfection of pedal and leg ulcers, as well as osteomyelitis of the underlying bone, frequently complicate the management of these patients. The depth and pattern of ulcer penetration, the degree of bone involvement, the location of the ulcer, the presence of infection, the presence of neuropathy, and the degree of arterial insufficiency all may affect the management of the complex patient with lower extremity arterial insufficiency.

Evaluation

Vascular Laboratory

- Noninvasive testing may aid in predicting the location and severity of atherosclerotic occlusive disease.

Angiography

- The standard angiographic approach for patients with lower extremity occlusive disease should be by transfemoral catheterization. The aorta, iliacs, femorals, and distal runoff arteries from both lower extremities should be evaluated.
- Both MRA and duplex ultrasonography are assuming an increased role in the delineation of central and peripheral vascular anatomy.

Cardiac Risk Assessment

- Because myocardial ischemia remains the leading cause of death following vascular surgery, patients should undergo preoperative risk factor assessment and selective stress testing before undergoing major vascular surgery. The initiation and optimization of medical therapy (particularly beta-adrenergic blockade) before elective vascular surgery has been of paramount importance in minimizing perioperative morbidity and death in this group of patients.

Management

Aortoiliac Occlusive Disease (AOD)

Percutaneous Transluminal Angioplasty

- During the 1990s, the indications for PTA have become more liberal as the effectiveness of PTA of the iliac arteries has been increasingly well documented. PTA is performed under local anesthesia with minimal sedation, as a day surgery admission, with significantly less morbidity and productivity reduction. Although initially performed only in the common iliac artery for stenosis, PTA is routinely used to treat short segment occlusions and external iliac lesions. Iliac artery PTA may be particularly useful to help improve inflow before a more distal surgical reconstruction.
- Iliac artery stents have also begun to play an increasing role in the management of patients with AOD.
- Five-year patency rates for common iliac PTA alone are typically in the range of 80% and are notably inferior (50% to 60%) for external iliac disease. Importantly, complication rates are low and failure rarely changes the available surgical options.

Aortofemoral Bypass

- Aortofemoral bypass is performed under general endotracheal anesthesia. An epidural catheter is placed preoperatively to improve pain control and facilitate early postoperative extubation. The patient is prepped and draped from the chest to the mid-thighs with the groins exposed. The femoral vessels are exposed first through bilateral longitudinal, oblique incisions. Preliminary exposure of the femoral vessels minimizes the time that the abdomen is open and improves the efficiency of the operation. In patients with significant occlusive disease of the femoral arteries, a broad exposure of the profunda femoris for potential profundaplasty should be performed before entry into the abdomen.
- The proximal anastomosis may be completed with either an end-to-end or end-to-side configuration.

- The end-to-side technique for the proximal anastomosis of the aortofemoral bypass graft is generally reserved for patients with occlusion of the external iliac arteries who would lack retrograde perfusion of important collaterals in the pelvis.
- Many patients with AOD have associated occlusive disease of the femoral arteries, and it is essential that blood flow to the profunda femoris artery be optimized. In this instance, the toe of anastomosis is placed onto the profunda femoris artery.
- Aortobifemoral bypass grafting has generally resulted in patency rates among the highest reported for any major arterial reconstruction. Primary patency rates of ABF grafts at 5 years are reported to be 70% to 88% with 10-year rates of 66% to 78%.

Extra-Anatomic Bypass

- Extra-anatomic bypass is most useful when femoral inflow is required and a direct transabdominal reconstructive approach is contraindicated because of patient comorbidities or intra-abdominal pathology or because the aorta is thought to be an unsatisfactory inflow source. Extra-anatomic bypass grafting may also be preferable in patients with uncontrolled malignancy or in patients in whom other diseases might limit their life expectancy.
- Axillofemoral (or bifemoral) bypass.
- The axillary artery on the side with the least evidence of upper extremity atherosclerosis (higher blood pressure, strongest pulse) is selected as the donor site. If the disease burden is equal in both upper extremities, the right axillary artery should be used as the preferred donor vessel because it has a lower risk of developing subclavian occlusive disease than the left.
- The tunnel should course laterally from the axillary artery deep to the pectoralis major, inferiorly along the midaxillary line (superficial to the external oblique fascia), and then medial to the anterior superior iliac spine.
- A 6- or 8-mm externally supported polytetrafluoroethylene (PTFE) graft is the preferred conduit.
- If an axillobifemoral graft is to be performed, the inflow for the femorofemoral bypass originates off the hood of the femoral anastomosis of the axillofemoral graft. Flow is re-established, hemostasis is attained, and the wounds are irrigated with antibiotic solution and closed with an absorbable suture. Because patients undergoing axillofemoral grafting often have increased comorbidities, the mortality rate following

axillofemoral bypass grafting ranges up to 13%. Five-year primary patency rates vary widely in the literature and range from 19% to 79%, with secondary patency rates as high as 85%.

Femorofemoral Bypass

● In the patient with unilateral iliac occlusive disease, the contralateral femoral artery may serve as a source of inflow. Although a femorofemoral bypass is best performed under general or regional anesthesia, it may be completed under local anesthesia in selected circumstances. Bilateral groin incisions are employed.
● Cumulative patency rates range from 60% to 80% at 5 years after femorofemoral bypass.

Iliofemoral Bypass

● In addition to femorofemoral bypass, iliofemoral bypass may be used to treat unilateral iliac artery disease. An iliofemoral bypass is best suited for patients with occluded or stenosed external iliac arteries and a relatively disease-free proximal common iliac artery.
● Three-year patency rates for iliofemoral bypass are 90% or greater in several reports.

Infrainguinal Occlusive Disease

● Infrainguinal arterial occlusive disease represents the most common manifestation of chronic arterial occlusive disease confronted by the vascular surgeon.
● Patients with multilevel occlusions of the superficial femoral, popliteal, and tibial arteries generally have rest pain or ischemic tissue loss. These ischemic ulcerations initially present as small, dry ulcers of the toes or heel area but may progress to frank gangrenous changes of the forefoot or heel. Most smokers initially have isolated superficial femoral artery occlusive disease and claudication. On the other hand, diabetics more often harbor distal occlusions of the popliteal and tibial arteries; these patients may initially have frank tissue necrosis with no prior history of claudication if the superficial femoral artery is spared.
● Patients with truly disabling claudication, such as those who are unable to perform their occupation because of claudication symptoms, should be considered for arteriography and interventional therapy. Once the ischemic symptoms have progressed to the point of rest pain or tissue ulceration,

surgical therapy is generally indicated for the purposes of pain relief and limb salvage. In the patient considered a candidate for interventional therapy, an arteriogram is performed to delineate the anatomy.

- In general, infrainguinal bypass surgery is best performed with autogenous vein conduit, preferably the ipsilateral greater saphenous. The superiority of autogenous vein reconstructions is most evident for bypass grafts performed to the below-knee popliteal, tibial, or pedal vessels.

Reversed Vein Graft

- The original technique for infrainguinal bypass surgery, an approach still preferred by many surgeons, uses the greater saphenous vein in a reversed configuration.

In Situ Greater Saphenous Vein Bypass

- The *in situ* greater saphenous vein bypass technique differs in that the saphenous vein is left in its own bed (i.e., *in situ*) rather than removing it and reversing its orientation. This approach requires disruption of the competent saphenous vein valves to allow flow down the vein.
- There are several practical advantages to the *in situ* technique, however, which offer technical benefits to the surgeon. Maintaining the vein graft in the *in situ* configuration allows the surgeon to sew the large end of the greater saphenous vein to the larger femoral vessels and to sew the smaller distal saphenous vein to the smaller tibial vessels. This size match at the proximal and distal ends facilitates the completion of precise technical anastomoses. Preservation of the saphenous vein hood offers particular advantages when sewing to a thick-walled, diseased femoral artery. Given these technical advantages, it is possible to successfully use smaller greater saphenous veins, which may not be serviceable for the reversed.
- A valvulotome is then used to lyse the valves and therefore allow antegrade flow through the graft.
- On completion of the bypass with either a reversed or *in situ* saphenous vein, flow through the graft and outflow arteries is assessed with a continuous-wave Doppler. A completion arteriogram is performed by direct cannulation of the proximal graft to demonstrate the bypass conduit, distal anastomosis, and outflow bed. Unsuspected technical defects, such as intraluminal thrombus, kinking or twisting of the graft, or unlysed valves, should be immediately repaired.

Prosthetic Bypass

- As mentioned previously, both polyester (Dacron) and PTFE graft material may be selectively used for infrainguinal arterial reconstructive surgery, particularly when the distal anastomosis is to the above-knee popliteal artery.
- To large-caliber vessels with good outflow.
- A variety of surgical adjuncts, including the creation of a distal AV fistula, the patching of the distal prosthetic graft to native artery bypass with a vein patch, and the creation of a cuff of autogenous vein interposed between the native artery and prosthetic graft at the distal anastomotic site, have all been proposed as useful techniques for improving the results of prosthetic bypass grafts performed to the below-knee level.

Reoperative Bypass Surgery

- Increasingly, patients are having failure of previous arterial reconstructions and recurrence of their limb-threatening ischemia symptoms. Reoperative infrainguinal arterial reconstruction offers a number of challenges. In most cases, the ipsilateral greater saphenous vein has previously been used and is no longer available for the secondary bypass procedure. Extensive scarring around the inflow and outflow vessels resulting from the previous surgical dissection complicates the surgical exposure. A number of strategies are useful in dealing with these complex cases. Whenever possible, alternative arterial inflow sites above or below the previous scarred arteries should be used to avoid dissection in areas of previous scarring.
- The contralateral greater saphenous vein, if available, constitutes the optimal conduit for secondary bypass surgery.
- Cephalic and basilic veins are often of excellent caliber and quality.
- Venovenostomy to create composite vein grafts.
- Despite improvements in operative techniques, the results of re-do infrainguinal bypass surgery remain inferior to those obtained with primary operation. When autogenous vein is available for secondary bypass, 5-year patency rates of 60% and limb salvage rates of 72% have been achieved.
- Early failure vein grafts (within 30 days) generally represents a judgmental or technical error within the conduct of surgery.
- Intermediate failures (30 days to 2 years) are generally due to intimal hyperplastic lesions that form at anastomotic sites or valve sites within the graft. Late graft failures (beyond 2 years)

are most often due to progression of atherosclerotic occlusive disease within the inflow or outflow vessels.

- Serial postoperative examinations with a duplex scan have proven extremely accurate in identifying significant vein graft lesions that threaten the graft patency.
- The role of PTA in the management of infrainguinal occlusive disease is considerably more limited than in the management of AOD.
- Unlike the management of iliac lesions in which stents have proven to be useful after technically complicated angioplasties, stents have not significantly improved the patency of femoral or popliteal angioplasties.

CHRONIC VISCERAL ISCHEMIA

Renovascular Occlusive Disease

- Chronic occlusive disease of the main renal artery results in reduced blood flow to the kidney. When the level of occlusion exceeds 60% of the diameter of the main renal artery, changes in pressure and flow distally result in increased secretion of renin and subsequent shifts in peripheral vasoconstriction and extracellular fluid volume, which result in hypertension.
- Among patients with diastolic blood pressure greater than 115 mm Hg, the prevalence of renovascular hypertension is 15% to 20%, and, among children younger than 5 years, the prevalence approximates 75%.
- When there is significant bilateral renal artery involvement, total glomerular filtration rate is reduced sufficiently to decrease creatinine clearance. Renal insufficiency from reduced renal perfusion is a late manifestation of advanced arterial occlusive disease involving both kidneys.
- Recognition and correction of large artery renal occlusive disease can result in impressive improvement in blood pressure control and preservation of renal function.

Pathology

- Atherosclerosis accounts for nearly 90% of cases of renovascular hypertension.
- Atherosclerotic process begins in the adjacent aorta with "spillover" plaque that encroaches into the proximal renal artery, resulting in "orificial" renal artery stenosis.
- Studies using serial angiography and renal ultrasound have elucidated the natural history of atherosclerotic renal

occlusive disease. Arteries detected to have more than 60% stenosis progress over the next several years to increased stenosis and ultimate occlusion.

- Fibromuscular dysplasia is the second most common type of renal artery disease.
- Multiple stenoses with intervening dilatations that may appear like a "string-of-beads."
- True aneurysms may occur in approximately 10% of patients with this condition, most often at branch points of the peripheral arterial arcade. Lesions are bilateral in 70% and medial fibroplasia can also affect other arteries, most commonly the internal carotid and external iliac arteries.

Pathophysiology

- Hypertension occurs after reduction in mean renal artery perfusion pressure by greater than 60% diameter or 75% cross-sectional area of the proximal renal artery. Renal baroreceptors in the afferent arterioles sense the reduction in mean arterial pressure, leading to release of renin by the juxtaglomerular apparatus. Renin appears in the renal vein and hydrolyzes angiotensinogen, produced in the liver, to form angiotensin I. This decapeptide is inactive but is converted to the octapeptide angiotensin II in the lungs by angiotensin-converting enzyme (ACE). Angiotensin II is a strong vasoconstrictor with a half-life of 4 minutes and acts directly on vascular smooth muscle. ACE inhibitors such as captopril are particularly effective in treating hypertension related to high renin and subsequent high angiotensin II levels (Fig. 64–1).
- Angiotensin II also facilitates formation of aldosterone by the adrenal cortex. Aldosterone causes conservation of salt and water by the kidney, resulting in increased extracellular fluid volume contributing to hypertension. Diuretics are beneficial in controlling hypertension because they help correct hypervolemia.
- When one renal artery is involved with occlusive disease, increased renin secretion from the affected kidney results in hypertension, which suppresses renin secretion from the contralateral kidney.
- When both kidneys are involved, or in circumstances of a solitary affected kidney, overall renal hypoperfusion results in hypervolemic hypertension. With increasing severity, decreased creatinine clearance occurs and azotemia supervenes.
- Renovascular hypertension has a significant impact on the heart and vascular tree.

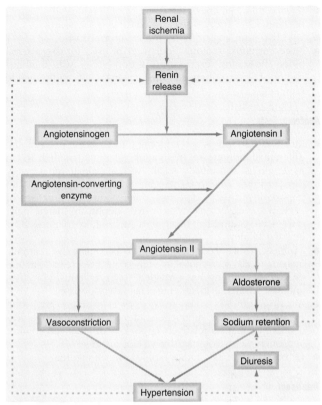

■ FIGURE 64–1. Consequences of renin hypersecretion as result of renal ischemia. Dotted arrows represent inhibitory influence.
(Adapted from Pickering TG: Renal vascular disease. In Braunwald S, Creager MA [eds]: Atlas of Heart Diseases, vol. 7. St. Louis, CV Mosby, 1996, p. 4.3.)

- In the presence of bilateral renal artery occlusive disease and resulting hypervolemia superimposed on hypertension, a sudden hypertensive crisis may occur with acute left ventricular failure precipitating so-called flash pulmonary edema.

Diagnosis

- Hypertensive patients in the pediatric age group.
- Women between the ages of 25 and 50 years should similarly be considered.

- If azotemia becomes worse on antihypertensive therapy, bilateral renal artery disease should be suspected.
- Selective sampling of blood from each renal vein.
- More currently, radionuclide tracer is used to assess renal blood flow and excretory function. The ACE inhibitor captopril has enhanced the accuracy of radionuclide scanning.

Anatomic Tests

- Renal ultrasound is an important method of determining differential kidney size. In an adult, a kidney less than 10 cm in length is abnormally small, with proximal renal artery disease being one possible cause. Renal ultrasound is an important means of detecting other contributing causes of azotemia, such as renal cysts or hydronephrosis. Increasingly, duplex ultrasound has been used successfully to assess flow into the kidney.
- Magnetic resonance imaging (MRI) is becoming the anatomic imaging modality of choice in many centers where gadolinium-enhanced scanning has provided an expeditious, objective, and safe means of identifying renal artery disease.
- Arteriography is the most precise diagnostic tool. Intravenous digital subtraction arteriography, although less invasive, requires a relatively large dose of iodinated contrast and often yields comparatively poor images.
- Carbon dioxide as a radiographic contrast medium.

Treatment

- Initial therapy of renovascular hypertension is medical. Beta-adrenergic blockers, diuretics, vasodilators, and ACE inhibitors are commonly used with success. A more aggressive therapeutic approach is justifiable if blood pressure control requires increasing doses of two or three medications or if renal function deteriorates while on antihypertensive medications, particularly ACE inhibitors (Fig. 64–2). Under these circumstances, noninvasive imaging with ultrasound or MRI should be performed, followed by arteriography as appropriate with plans to proceed at the same sitting with percutaneous endovascular renal artery therapy if favorable lesions are confirmed.
- Balloon dilatation is the procedure of choice for patients with fibromuscular dysplasia involving the main renal artery, reserving surgical revascularization for more complicated lesions involving branches of the renal artery.

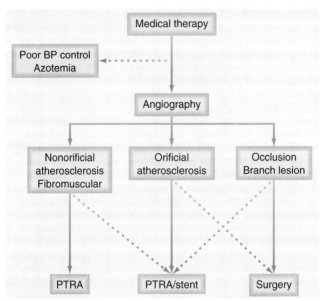

■ FIGURE 64–2. Therapeutic scheme for patients with proven renal artery occlusive disease. Dotted arrows represent secondary therapeutic options.

- Technical success for orificial atherosclerosis is no greater than 50%, and the long-term success rate is 40% among those initially successfully treated by angioplasty. The immediate and long-term success of balloon angioplasty can be improved by using arterial stenting. Although not necessary for most nonorificial lesions, stents have extended the usefulness of percutaneous therapy to orificial atherosclerosis.
- Transaortic endarterectomy.
- Occlusive lesions may be bypassed with proximal anastomosis in the aorta, the iliac artery, or an aortic prosthesis. Prosthetic material or autogenous vein are equally satisfactory for anastomosis to the proximal renal artery. Autogenous vein is preferred for more distal anastomoses or when small kidneys are involved.
- The presence of an occluded artery is not necessarily a contraindication to revascularization. Percutaneous therapy may be attempted and, if a wire can be passed through the occlusion, balloon angioplasty and stent may succeed.

More typically, surgery is necessary, at which time a short segmental occlusion is usually found with reconstitution of a virtually normal artery within 1 to 2 cm. If the kidney is more than 7 to 8 cm in length, there is a significant chance of recovery of function and reduction in renin secretion following revascularization.

Results of Revascularization

- Recurrent stenosis occurs in approximately 10% of patients.
- Among patients with atherosclerosis, hypertension is cured in roughly one third and improved in 50%, with failure in 10% to 20%. Endarterectomy of the renal artery orifice is a very durable procedure. Serial study of bypass patency indicates as many as 88% of grafts remain patent for as long as 20 years following surgery.
- Renal function has been reported to improve in 40% of patients who had revascularization for azotemia. Such patients almost always underwent revascularization bilaterally or had a solitary kidney, with the therapeutic goal of increasing blood flow to as much renal parenchyma as possible.

Mesenteric Ischemia

- Vascular occlusive disease of the mesenteric vessels is a relatively rare but often catastrophic problem.
- Chronic intestinal ischemia often presents a diagnostic challenge, but results are gratifying with timely therapy.

Pathophysiology

- Mesenteric arterial anatomy is notable for rich collateral flow (Fig. 64–3). As a result, gradual occlusion of one or even two of the main mesenteric trunks is usually tolerated, as long as there is time for collateral from uninvolved branches to enlarge. On the other hand, sudden occlusion of a main branch or more peripherally beyond the largest collaterals may be poorly tolerated, with profound consequences.
- Compromised bowel mucosa allows unrestricted influx of toxic materials from the bowel lumen with systemic consequences. If serosal surfaces are affected by full-thickness necrosis, bowel perforation and peritonitis ensue.
- Acute mesenteric artery occlusion most frequently results from a cardiogenic embolus and usually involves the superior mesenteric artery. Embolic occlusion most often occurs distal to the origin of the superior mesenteric artery because

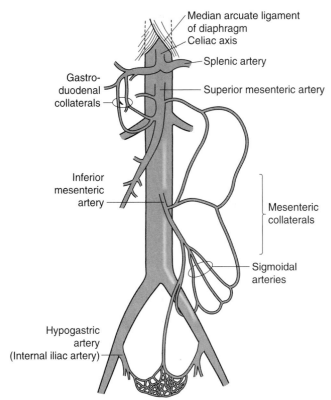

■ FIGURE 64–3. Mesenteric arterial anatomy demonstrating extensive collateral channels between major branches. *(Adapted from Stoney RJ, Wiley EJ: Surgery of celiac and mesenteric arteries. In Haimovici HH [ed]: Vascular Surgery: Principles and Techniques. New York, McGraw-Hill, 1976, pp 668–679.)*

the embolus is pushed into the artery to a point where arborization reduces the lumen to a diameter less than that of the embolus (Fig. 64–4). Less commonly, thrombotic occlusion at the site of chronic atherosclerotic plaque occurs at the origin of the vessel adjacent to ostial disease. In both instances, secondary stasis thrombosis may occur in adjacent proximal and distal vessels to the point where flow from collaterals is maintained. Acute embolic occlusion is generally a more profound and damaging insult than thrombosis at the site of chronic disease because of (1) lack of

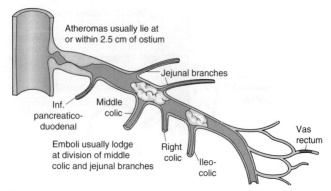

■ **FIGURE 64–4.**   Typical location of superior mesenteric artery obstruction in patients with embolic and thrombotic occlusion. *(From Donaldson M: Mesenteric vascular disease. In Creager MA, Braunwald E [eds]: Atlas of Heart Diseases, vol VII. St. Louis, Mosby, 1996, pp 5.1–5.16.)*

protection by chronically enlarged collateral from the other mesenteric arteries, (2) occlusion at levels beyond the point of inflow of larger collaterals, and (3) occlusion of multiple branches to adjacent segments at the point of arterial arborization.

- Chronic mesenteric insufficiency is almost exclusively a problem in the older age group with diffuse atherosclerosis that involves the aorta and the proximal mesenteric arteries.
- Relative ischemia occurs after meals when there is increased demand for flow into the mesenteric bed. Vasodilation after eating reduces peripheral resistance, but flow cannot increase in the presence of proximal fixed occlusive lesions creating transient ischemic pain, which has been appropriately termed "intestinal angina."

Presentation and Management

Acute Mesenteric Arterial Occlusion

- The most common cause of acute mesenteric arterial occlusion is embolus to the superior mesenteric artery and rarely the celiac artery. Severe pain is always present and prominent, centered in the periumbilical region (Box 64–1). Abdominal examination typically reveals relatively little tenderness during the early stages, only to become more impressive as

---

Box 64–1. Presentation of Acute Mesenteric Ischemia

Concurrent cardiac or debilitating disease
Pain out of proportion to tenderness
Abdominal distention, gastrointestinal dysfunction
Evidence of "third" spacing—oliguria, hemoconcentration
Blood in stool
Elevated white cell count—often >20,000
Metabolic acidosis
Elevated serum enzymes
Bowel distention, wall thickening on kidney-ureter-bladder
  imaging and computed tomography
Endoscopic findings in colon
Specific findings on arteriogram

---

ischemic bowel produces visceral peritonitis and finally parietal peritonitis.

- Underlying cardiac disease is responsible for the embolus in 90% of cases, and manifestations of arrhythmia, recent myocardial infarction, or valvular disease may be present.
- Surgery offers the best chance of successful treatment. Exploratory laparotomy allows rapid confirmation of the diagnosis and exclusion of other conditions.
- Most often, the proximal superior mesenteric artery should be opened longitudinally and thromboembolectomy performed using a patch angioplasty to close the artery.
- In patients with significant associated chronic arterial disease in whom thrombosis has occurred, a simple thromboembolectomy may fail to restore normal inflow. In such cases, the superior mesenteric artery arteriotomy is used as the site for distal anastomosis of a bypass.
- A "second look" operation.

Nonocclusive Mesenteric Insufficiency

- Patients suffering from nonocclusive mesenteric insufficiency are frequently seriously ill and often have been in an intensive support setting before development of mesenteric insufficiency.
- Classic arteriographic findings include absence of large vessel occlusion and a pattern of sequential focal vasospasm with "beading" of the major mesenteric branches and a "pruned tree" appearance to the distal vasculature.

Mesenteric Venous Occlusion

- Mesenteric venous occlusion occurs in patients with a number of concurrent illnesses, including liver disease and portal hypertension, pancreatitis, intraperitoneal inflammatory conditions, hypercoagulable states, and systemic low-flow states (Box 64–2). Venous thrombosis is less dramatic than arterial occlusion, and early diagnosis is typically difficult because the presentation is subtle (Table 64–2). Abdominal pain is usually vague and tenderness mild or equivocal. CT scan may demonstrate thickened bowel wall with delayed passage of intravenous contrast into the portal system and lack of opacification of the portal vein. Arteriography may demonstrate venous congestion and lack of prompt filling of the portal system.

Box 64–2. Conditions Associated With Mesenteric Venous Thrombosis

PORTAL HYPERTENSION
Cirrhosis
Congestive splenomegaly

INFLAMMATION
Peritonitis
Inflammatory bowel disease
Pelvic or intra-abdominal abscess
Diverticular disease

POSTOPERATIVE STATE AND TRAUMA
Splenectomy and other postoperative states
Blunt abdominal trauma

HYPERCOAGULABLE STATES
Neoplasms (colon, pancreas)
Oral contraceptives
Pregnancy
Migratory thrombophlebitis
Antithrombin III, protein C/S deficiency
Peripheral deep vein thrombosis
Polycythemia vera
Thrombocytosis

OTHER CONDITIONS
Renal disease (nephrotic syndrome)
Cardiac disease (congestive failure)

TABLE 64–2. Presentation of Mesenteric Venous Thrombosis Pancreatic Cancer

Pain (insidious)	81%
Gastrointestinal bleed	19%
Guaiac + stool	63%
Anorexia	44%
Previous deep vein thrombosis	44%
Pancreatic cancer	13%
Hepatitis	25%
Thrombocytosis	25%
Increased fibrinogen	13%
Decreased proteins C, S	50%

Chronic Mesenteric Insufficiency

- Patients with advanced chronic mesenteric artery disease most commonly have a stereotypical pattern of postprandial pain in a periumbilical location that occurs within 30 minutes of a meal (Table 64–3). It gradually resolves thereafter, only to recur with subsequent meals. Because eating causes pain, patients reduce the size of meals and develop a pattern of "food fear" abstinence that results in weight loss. Malabsorption is rarely, if ever, a component of this disease.
- The definitive diagnostic study is arteriography, which invariably reveals occlusion of at least two of the three major mesenteric arteries. Patterns of collateral are often prominent, including a large meandering artery in the mesentery of the colon.
- In selected circumstances, revascularization by balloon angioplasty or stent placement may be successful, a strategy particularly applicable among elderly patients who may be poor candidates for surgery. More commonly, definitive

TABLE 64–3. Signs and Symptoms of Chronic Mesenteric Arterial Insufficiency

Pain	100%
Weight loss	80%–98%
Abdominal bruit	68%–75%
Nausea, vomiting	54%–84%
Diarrhea	35%
Constipation	13%–26%
Hemoccult + stool	8%

therapy requires surgery using either a direct approach to proximal arterial occlusions via transaortic endarterectomy or bypass grafting. Bypass may be performed using a prosthetic graft originating in the supraceliac aorta and connecting to both the celiac and superior mesenteric arteries. Alternatively, retrograde bypass from the infrarenal aorta or iliac artery may be used. Surgical exploration and therapy is usually facilitated because the patient has lost a significant amount of weight preoperatively.

- A small subset of patients without atherosclerosis and generally of younger age experience postprandial pain on the basis of celiac artery compression from the median arcuate ligament of the diaphragm.

- Evaluation using MRI or arteriography reveals extrinsic compression of the proximal celiac artery with poststenotic dilatation. Images during inspiration and expiration demonstrate a dynamic constriction of the artery. Therapy should be directed at highly selected patients.

CHAPTER 65

VASCULAR TRAUMA

KEY CONCEPTS

- The fundamental difference between elective vascular surgery and vascular trauma is the physiology of the wounded patient.
- The surgeon must keep in mind that, although major hemorrhage (typical of truncal vascular injuries) is an immediate threat to the patient's life, ischemia (commonly from peripheral arterial injury) is a threat to limb viability, a much lower priority.

Patterns of Injury

- Vascular trauma occurs in a limited number of patterns, which are determined primarily by the mechanism of injury.
- Dramatic increase in iatrogenic vascular trauma.

Minimal Injury and Nonoperative Management

- Nonocclusive intimal flaps, segmental narrowing, small false aneurysms, and small arteriovenous fistulae generally have a benign natural history and are very likely to either heal or improve without intervention.

Endovascular Therapy

- In the hemodynamically stable patient with a nonbleeding traumatic arterial lesion, percutaneous placement of an endovascular stent-graft across a defect in the arterial wall is a low-morbidity solution to a problem that may otherwise require a technically challenging surgical procedure.
- For some arterial injuries, the endovascular option is proving to be the preferred approach.
- The endovascular approach to blunt injuries to the descending thoracic aorta is currently the focus of much interest.

OPERATIVE PRINCIPLES

Access, Exposure, and Control

- Direct pressure over the bleeding site typically using digital or manual compression.
- The surgeon can then choose which definitive hemostatic technique to deploy from the wide array of hemostatic options.
- Balloon catheter tamponade using a Foley catheter inserted into the missile tract is a very useful adjunct to obtaining rapid temporary control.
- A cardinal operative principle in managing major vascular trauma is to first obtain proximal (and if possible also distal) control of the injured vessel.
- In the chest, control of a vascular injury hinges on correct selection of a thoracotomy incision.
- In the abdomen, the major vessels are located in the retroperitoneum and, therefore, exposure is based on operative maneuvers that mobilize the intraperitoneal viscera off the underlying retroperitoneal structures.

Assessing the Injury and the Patient

- External inspection often does not reflect the full extent of intimal damage.
- Selection of the vascular repair technique is heavily influenced not only by the anatomic situation but also by the patient's physiologic condition.
- Self-propagating triad of hypothermia, coagulopathy, and acidosis.
- The hypothermia-coagulopathy-acidosis syndrome effectively marks the boundaries of the patient's physiologic envelope.
- The operative management of a vascular injury must focus not only on restoration of anatomy but also on the patient's physiologic envelope.

Simple and Complex Repairs

- Simple repairs are very rapid and include ligation, lateral repair, and shunt insertion. Complex repairs are patch angioplasty, end-to-end anastomosis, and graft interposition.
- Ligation of an injured vessel in a critically injured patient is a marker of good surgical judgment rather than an admission of defeat.

Temporary Intraluminal Shunts

TRUNCAL VASCULAR TRAUMA

The Neck

- Injuries to major cervical vessels are frequently associated with trauma to adjacent structures.

Clinical Presentation and Immediate Concerns

- Two immediate concerns are the focus of clinical attention.

Diagnostic Studies

- Asymptomatic patients with penetrating injuries to the base of the neck (zone I) require a four-vessel arch angiography.
- The same applies to penetrating injuries above the angle of the mandible (zone III), where both exploration and distal control are technically difficult.
- Patients with asymptomatic midcervical injuries (zone II) may undergo either formal neck exploration (a straightforward procedure associated with very low morbidity) or a combination of four-vessel angiography, esophagoscopy, and barium swallow to rule out significant arterial and esophageal injury.

Operative Management

- The standard cervical incision is along the anterior border of the sternocleidomastoid muscle.
- Carotid arteries.
  - There are no good data to support preference for vein or synthetic interposition grafts in the neck nor is there evidence to support routine shunting.
- Vertebral artery injuries.
  - The artery is best controlled by simple means, such as tightly filling the bleeding hole in the transverse process with bone wax.

Blunt Carotid and Vertebral Artery Injury

- It is possible to identify these injuries in up to 1% of blunt trauma admissions.
- The key pathophysiologic event is an intimal tear that can remain asymptomatic or progress to local thrombosis, embolization, or distal dissection.

- A salient clinical feature of this injury is that in approximately one half of the patients there are latent period of hours or days before neurologic deficit appears.
- The standard diagnostic modality is angiography.
- Most patients are treated with systemic anticoagulation (if not prohibited by associated injuries), although the benefits of intravenous heparin are less clear in low-grade nonobstructing luminal irregularities.

Penetrating Thoracic Vascular Trauma

Choice of Incision

- In stable patients, the choice of thoracotomy incision is dictated by angiographic findings. In the actively bleeding, hemodynamically unstable patient, the incision is based on the presumed location of the vascular injury. Generally, an anterolateral thoracotomy on the injured side is the incision of choice for patients with ongoing bleeding into the pleural cavity.
- Right-sided injuries to the base of the neck are approached through a median sternotomy.
- A supraclavicular incision is used to gain access to the more distal parts of both subclavian arteries.

Management of Specific Injuries

- Penetrating injuries to the innominate vessels and proximal carotid arteries present intraoperatively as a mediastinal hematoma.

Blunt Thoracic Vascular Trauma

The Aorta

- It is a lethal injury that provides the surgeon with a window of opportunity for effective surgical intervention. This window may be missed because the injury remains asymptomatic until catastrophic bleeding suddenly occurs.
- The dominant pathophysiologic event in blunt aortic injury is sudden deceleration with creation of a shear force between a relatively mobile part of the thoracic aorta and an adjacent fixed segment.
- Eighty-five percent of patients with a full-thickness blunt thoracic aortic injury die before arrival to a hospital. Most of the

remaining 15% have a contained rupture and are candidates for operative repair. However, 15% of patients with blunt aortic injury who arrive at a trauma center die before operative intervention.

- Generally, a contained blunt aortic injury is not an explanation for hemodynamic instability. If the patient with a suspected or proven blunt aortic injury is hemodynamically unstable, the explanation usually lies in other associated injuries, typically in the abdomen.
- The most important aspect of the physical examination is not to miss associated injuries.
- Several radiographic findings on a supine chest x-ray film should suggest the diagnosis of blunt aortic injury. The most significant ones are a widened mediastinum (>8 cm) and an obscured or indistinct aortic knob.
- Helical computed tomography (CT) angiography is rapidly becoming an imaging modality that rivals aortography as being more expedient and noninvasive.
- Aortography remains the "gold standard" imaging modality to which all other modalities are compared.
- The management of blunt aortic injury is prompt operative repair of the injured aortic segment. However, in some patients, a purposeful delay or even nonoperative management may be indicated.
- The standard operative repair of aortic injuries uses clamp and direct reconstruction and can be achieved by using one of three adjuncts: pharmacologic control of central hypertension, a temporary passive shunt, or pump-assisted atriofemoral bypass.
- The most dreaded complication is paraplegia or paraparesis, occurring in approximately 8% of patients. The incidence of spinal cord damage is affected neither by choice of operative technique nor by the method chosen to deal with central hypertension and distal ischemia.

The Innominate Artery

- Blunt innominate artery injury is akin to a side hole in the thoracic aorta.
- The operative repair of blunt innominate artery injury is based on the bypass and exclusion principle, thus eliminating the need for cardiopulmonary bypass, shunts, or the use of heparin.

ABDOMINAL VASCULAR INJURIES

- Vascular injuries are much more common following abdominal gunshot wounds (25% of patients) as compared with stab wounds (10%).
- The patient with free hemorrhage usually presents in shock, whereas the patient with a contained retroperitoneal hematoma may be hemodynamically stable or unstable but responsive to fluids.

Immediate Concerns

- Temporary control of hemorrhage is the obvious first priority.
- The natural urge to immediately proceed with definitive repair is the worst possible mistake at this point. Instead, the time interval should be used to transfuse and resuscitate the patient, to obtain additional instruments and an autotransfusion device, to optimize exposure, and to organize the operating room team.
- Once the total injury burden of the patient is determined, the surgeon must choose between the traditional operative profile of definitive repair and a "damage control" profile.
- The damage control approach temporarily sacrifices anatomic integrity to avoid the irreversible physiologic insult that presents as the hypothermia-coagulopathy-acidosis syndrome.

Aortic Clamping

- The supraceliac aorta is most expediently clamped at the diaphragmatic hiatus.

Maneuvers for Retroperitoneal Exposure

- Left-sided medial visceral rotation (Mattox maneuver) exposes the entire length of the abdominal aorta and its branches (except the right renal artery).
- Right-sided medial visceral rotation ("extended Kocher" maneuver) consists of medial reflection of the right colon and duodenum by incising their lateral peritoneal attachments.

Approach to Retroperitoneal Hematoma

- The location of a retroperitoneal hematoma and mechanism of injury guide the decision to explore the hematoma.
- Any hematoma in zone 1 mandates exploration for both penetrating and blunt injury.

- A supramesocolic hematoma is the result of injury to the suprarenal aorta, celiac axis, proximal superior mesenteric artery, or the proximal part of a renal artery.
- A hematoma in zone 2 is the result of injury to the renal vessels and/or parenchyma and mandates exploration for penetrating trauma.

Specific Abdominal Vascular Injuries

- *Abdominal aorta.*
- The mortality rates for abdominal aortic injuries range between 50% to 90%, with injuries to the perirenal aortic segment being the most lethal (>80% mortality).
- Despite theoretical concerns that spillage of intestinal content may cause synthetic graft infection, a synthetic graft is the only practical option.
- Penetrating injuries to the *iliac vessels* carry high mortality rates (25% to 40%), because exposure and control can be difficult and associated injuries to adjacent abdominal organs are the rule rather than the exception.
- The use of a polytetrafluoroethylene (PTFE) graft for iliac artery reconstruction in the presence of peritoneal contamination is a cause for concern.
- A low threshold for fasciotomy should be maintained following iliac vessel injuries.
- *Superior mesenteric vessels.*
- The origin of the superior mesenteric artery is exposed by left-sided medial visceral rotation, whereas the infrapancreatic part of the vessel is accessed by pulling the small bowel down and to the left and incising the peritoneum of the root of the mesentery. Another option for exposure of the infrapancreatic part is the Cattel-Braasch maneuver.
- If graft interposition is required to reconstruct the superior mesenteric artery, a takeoff from the distal aorta above the bifurcation keeps the suture line away from an injured pancreas.
- Penetrating injuries to the *renal arteries* usually result in nephrectomy, because associated injuries make complex vascular reconstruction of the renal artery an unattractive option.
- Because blunt renovascular trauma is characteristically associated with more life-threatening injuries, a significant diagnostic delay is common, and attempted renal salvage by major vascular reconstruction is usually not an option.

Inferior Vena Cava (IVC)

- Retrohepatic IVC injuries.
- There is no optimal solution for the technical challenge of retrohepatic IVC trauma. Several authors have reported successful packing of these injuries, and this simple solution, if performed early and effectively, may prove the most practical approach to injuries in this low-pressure system.

PERIPHERAL VASCULAR TRAUMA

Initial Assessment

- In an ischemic extremity, the severity of ischemia and the arterial segment involved are the key considerations.
- Although it is stated that restoration of arterial perfusion in less than 6 hours improves limb salvage rates, the window of opportunity for salvage is not a rigid interval.
- Of all the symptoms and signs of acute limb ischemia, a sensory-motor deficit conveys the greatest urgency.

Noninvasive Vascular Diagnosis

- The handheld Doppler is a reliable screening tool for significant arterial obstruction following both blunt and penetrating trauma.
- The routine use of Duplex ultrasonography in the acute admission area of many trauma centers is limited by logistical constraints.

Role of Arteriography

- It is indicated when the information gained can alter or facilitate the operative approach.
- The use of arteriography to rule out arterial trauma in asymptomatic patients with penetrating wounds in proximity to the neurovascular bundle has changed in the last decade.

The Mangled Extremity

- The mangled extremity is defined as injury to an extremity that involves at least three of the four major tissue systems of a limb, consisting bone, soft tissue, vessels, and nerves.
- In practice the decision to proceed with amputation hinges on surgical judgment and the patient's individual circumstances.

Operative Technique

- It is preferable to achieve bone alignment before vascular reconstruction.
- If the limb is not grossly ischemic, reduction and fixation of fractures are performed first. If the limb is ischemic, a temporary intraluminal shunt can be inserted.
- First priority with peripheral vascular injuries is to obtain proximal and distal control.
- Most injuries require end-to-end anastomosis or an interposition graft.
- There is some controversy surrounding graft interposition of the femoral artery.
- Considerable evidence has accumulated to support the use of PTFE grafts in a contaminated operative field because the material is resistant to dissolution by bacterial collagenase and fares better than a vein graft if soft tissue cover is lost.
- Graft protection by adequate soft tissue cover is a fundamental principle in vascular surgery that is especially relevant in trauma.

Vein Injuries

- The available evidence supports the repair of venous injuries encountered during exploration for an associated arterial trauma but only if the patient is hemodynamically stable and the repair will not jeopardize or delay management of other significant injuries.

Fasciotomy

- Compartment syndrome is common in these patients but is also notoriously difficult to diagnose early.
- Arbitrary definitions of ischemic times are poor guidelines to the need for fasciotomy.
- The safest course of action is to maintain a low threshold for fasciotomy and decide based on individual clinical circumstances and operative findings.
- In lower extremity fasciotomy, the four compartments of the leg should all be decompressed and is most commonly achieved through two longitudinal incisions.

Iatrogenic Trauma

- Ongoing hemorrhage into the subcutaneous tissue presents as an expanding hematoma, in which the major concern is not so much massive blood loss as pressure necrosis of the skin overlying the expanding hematoma and compression of the branches of the cutaneous branches of the femoral nerve with a resulting painful neuralgia.

- Initial treatment is by ultrasound-guided manual compression.
- The underlying mechanism is an intimal flap or fracture of a small segment of the arterial wall that leads to thrombosis. Understanding this pathophysiologic mechanism is the key to an effective repair because simple thrombectomy will not suffice.

Management of Specific Injuries

- Common or superficial femoral arteries.
  - Popliteal artery injuries result in limb loss more often than any other peripheral vascular injury.
  - A full fasciotomy is performed before the vascular exploration in a grossly ischemic leg.
- Lower leg arteries.
  - Patients with severe blunt trauma to the lower leg usually present with a combination of extensive bone and soft tissue damage and diminished or absent pedal pulses.
  - The traditional teaching that it is advisable to maintain patency of at least two shank arteries following blunt trauma is unproved.
  - Exposure of the lower leg arteries is best begun proximally, away from the area of injury.
- The anterior tibial artery is approached through a separate anterolateral incision between the tibialis anterior and the extensor hallucis longus muscles.
- Axillary artery injuries.
- Injuries to the brachial artery account for 20% to 30% of peripheral arterial injuries, making this vessel the most frequently injured artery in the body.
- Ulnar or radial artery injuries.

CHAPTER 66

VENOUS DISEASE

INTRODUCTION

- Disorders of the vascular system can broadly be classified, in anatomic terms, into arterial, venous, or lymphatic diseases.
- Disorders of the venous system can be divided into thrombotic or thromboembolic disease and venous insufficiency.
- Another factor in truly assessing the prevalence of venous disease, in particular venous insufficiency, is that the range of venous insufficiency can span a vast array of manifestations, from mildly symptomatic varicose veins to severe chronic venous insufficiency with ulceration.

ANATOMY

- The nomenclature of the venous system of the lower limb has undergone a revision and the most relevant changes are addressed here. The revised nomenclature is shown in Boxes 66–1 and 66–2 and is used in this chapter.
- Superficial venous system.
- Deep venous system.
- Specific disorders of the veins.
  - Varicose veins.
  - Risk factors.

Anatomy and Physiology of Venous Function

- The majority of the capacitance of the vascular tree is in the venous system. Because of the thin walls relatively devoid of elastin, the venous system is able to accommodate large changes in volume with virtually no increase in pressure up to a point.
- The calf muscles augment venous return by functioning as a pump.
- The return of the blood to the heart from the lower extremity is facilitated by the muscle pump function of the calf—a mechanism whereby the calf muscle, functioning as a bellows during exercise, compresses the gastrocnemius and soleal sinuses and propels the blood toward the heart. The

Box 66–1. Superficial Veins

Terminologica Anatomica	Proposed Terminology
Greater or long saphenous vein	Great saphenous vein
	Superficial inguinal veins
External pudendal vein	External pudendal vein
Superficial circumflex vein	Superficial circumflex iliac vein
Superficial epigastric vein	Superficial epigastric vein
Superficial dorsal vein of clitoris or penis	Superficial dorsal vein of clitoris or penis
Anterior labial veins	Anterior labial veins
Anterior scrotal veins	Anterior scrotal veins
Accessory saphenous vein	Anterior accessory great saphenous vein
	Posterior accessory great saphenous vein
	Superficial accessory great saphenous vein
Smaller or short saphenous vein	Small saphenous vein
	Cranial extension of small saphenous vein
	Superficial accessory small saphenous vein
	Anterior thigh circumflex vein
	Posterior thigh circumflex vein
	Intersaphenous veins
	Lateral venous system
Dorsal venous network of the foot	Dorsal venous network of the foot
Dorsal venous arch of the foot	Dorsal venous arch of the foot
Dorsal metatarsal veins	Superficial metatarsal veins (dorsal and plantar)
Plantar venous network	Plantar venous subcutaneous network
Plantar venous arch	
Plantar metatarsal veins	Superficial digital veins (dorsal and plantar)
Lateral marginal vein	Lateral marginal vein
Medial marginal vein	Medial marginal vein

Box 66-2. Deep Veins

Terminologica Anatomica	Proposed Terminology
Femoral vein	Common femoral vein
	Femoral vein
Profunda femoris vein or deep vein of thigh	Profunda femoris vein or deep femoral vein
Medial circumflex femoral vein	Medial circumflex femoral vein
Lateral circumflex femoral vein	Lateral circumflex femoral vein
Perforating veins	Deep femoral communicating veins (accompanying veins of perforating arteries)
	Sciatic vein
Popliteal vein	Popliteal vein
	Sural veins
	Soleal veins
	Gastrocnemius veins
	Medial gastrocnemius veins
	Lateral gastrocnemius veins
	Intergemellar vein
Genicular veins	Genicular venous plexus
Anterior tibial veins	Anterior tibial veins
Posterior tibial veins	Posterior tibial veins
Fibular or peroneal veins	Fibular or peroneal veins
	Medial plantar veins
	Lateral plantar veins
	Deep plantar venous arch
	Deep metatarsal veins (plantar and dorsal)
	Deep digital veins (plantar and dorsal)
	Pedal vein

normally functioning valves in the venous system prevent retrograde flow; it is when one or more of these valves become incompetent that symptoms of venous insufficiency can develop.

VENOUS INSUFFICIENCY

● The anatomy of venous drainage of the lower extremity is such that the superficial and the deep venous system independently or in concert may exhibit valvular dysfunction and insufficiency of a degree severe enough to cause symptoms.

- Symptoms.
  - The patient with symptomatic varicose veins will relate, most often, symptoms of aching, heaviness, discomfort, and sometimes outright pain in the calf of the affected limb. This is particularly worse at the end of the day, most likely resulting from prolonged sitting or standing that results in venous distension and associated pain. The symptoms are typically reduced or absent in the morning because the limb has not been in a dependent position through the night.
- Pathogenesis.
  - Pressure studies show that two sources of venous hypertension exist. The first is gravitational and is a result of venous blood coursing in a distal direction down linear axial venous segments.
  - The second source of venous hypertension is dynamic. It is the force of muscular contraction, usually contained within the compartments of the leg.

DIAGNOSTIC EVALUATION OF VENOUS DYSFUNCTION

- The most important of all noninvasive tests available to study the venous system are the physical examination and a careful history that elucidates the symptoms mentioned earlier.
- Duplex technology more precisely defines which veins are refluxing by imaging the superficial and deep veins.
- Phlebography.

Nonoperative Management

- The cornerstone of therapy for patients with chronic venous insufficiency (CVI) is external compression and most patients are treated nonoperatively.
- Compression that relieves the leg edema generally controls the CVI.

Venous Ablation

- Sclerotherapy.
- Surgery.
  - Modern treatment of varicose veins is fundamentally centered on the principle of ablation of the reflux source, sometimes termed the "escape point."

- Surgery for severe CVI.
  - Surprisingly, superficial reflux may be the only abnormality present in advanced chronic venous stasis.
  - Maintaining that all venous ulcers are surgically incurable is not reasonable when these data suggest that superficial vein surgery holds the potential for ameliorating the venous hypertension.
- Direct venous reconstruction.

DEEP VENOUS THROMBOSIS (DVT)

- The triad of venous stasis, endothelial injury, and hypercoagulable state first posited by Virchow in 1856 has held true a century and a half later.
- The thrombotic process initiating in a venous segment can, in the absence of anticoagulation or in the presence of inadequate anticoagulation, propagate to involve more proximal segments of the deep venous system, thus resulting in edema, pain, and immobility. The most dreaded sequel to an acute DVT is that of pulmonary embolism, a condition of potentially lethal consequence.
- Etiology.
  - The triad of stasis, vessel injury, and hypercoagulable state exists in most surgical patients.
- Stasis.
- The hypercoagulable state.
  - The standard array of conditions screened for when searching for a hypercoagulable state is listed in Box 66–3. Should any of these conditions be identified, a treatment regimen of anticoagulation is instituted for life, unless specific contraindications exist.
  - Increases in platelet count, adhesiveness, changes in coagulation cascade, and endogenous fibrinolytic activity

---

Box 66–3. Hypercoagulable States

- Factor V Leiden mutation
- Prothrombin gene mutation
- Protein C deficiency
- Protein S deficiency
- Antithrombin III deficiency
- Homocysteine
- Antiphospholipid syndrome

all result from physiologic stress such as major operation or trauma and have been associated with an increased risk of thrombosis.
- Vein injury.

Diagnosis

- Incidence.
  - Venous thromboembolism occurs for the first time in approximately 100 persons per 100,000 each year in the United States. This incidence increases with increasing age with an incidence of 0.5% per 100,000 at age 80. More than two thirds of these patients have DVT alone and the rest have evidence of pulmonary embolism.
- Clinical diagnosis.
  - Major venous thrombosis involving the iliofemoral venous system results in a massively swollen leg with pitting edema, pain, and blanching, a condition known as phlegmasia alba dolens.
- Venography.
- Impedance plethysmography.
- Fibrin fibrinogen assays.
  - The D-dimer test measures cross-linked degradation products, which is a surrogate of plasmin's activity on fibrin. It is shown that in combination with clinical evaluation and assessment, the sensitivity exceeds 90% to 95%.
  - It is important to know that after an operation (i.e., in the postoperative patient) that D-dimer is causally elevated because of surgery, and as such, a positive D-dimer assay for evaluating for DVT is of no utility.
- Duplex ultrasound.
  - The modern diagnostic test of choice for the diagnosis of DVT is the duplex ultrasound, a modality that combines Doppler ultrasound and color flow imaging.
- Magnetic resonance venography (MRV).

Prophylaxis

- The methods of prophylaxis can be mechanical or pharmacologic.
- The most likely mechanism for the efficacy of this device is from prevention of venous stasis.
- Low-molecular-weight heparin (LMWH) inhibits factor Xa and factor IIA activity, with the ratio of anti-factor Xa to anti-factor IIA activity ranging from 1:1 to 4:1. LMWHs have a

longer plasma half-life and have significantly higher bioavailability.

- Comparison of LMWH with mechanical prophylaxis demonstrates superiority of LMWH in reduction of the development of venous thromboembolic disease.
- In short, LMWH should be considered the optimal method of prophylaxis in moderate and high-risk patients.

TREATMENT

- Any venous thrombosis involving the femoropopliteal system should be treated with full anticoagulation.
- The incidence of recurrent venous thromboembolism increases if the time to therapeutic anticoagulation is prolonged.
- If, however, the patient has a known hypercoagulable state or has experienced episodes of venous thrombosis, then lifetime anticoagulation is required, in the absence of contraindications.
- Oral anticoagulants are teratogenic and thus cannot be used during pregnancy.
- Thrombolysis.
  - One exception is the patient with phlegmasia in whom thrombolysis is advocated for relief of significant venous obstruction. In this condition, thrombolytic therapy probably results in better relief of symptoms and less long-term sequelae than heparin anticoagulation alone.
- Vena cava filter.
- The most worrisome and potentially lethal complication of DVT is pulmonary embolism.
- The gold standard for diagnosis of pulmonary embolism remains the pulmonary angiogram, but increasingly this is being displaced by the computed tomography (CT) angiogram.
- Adequate anticoagulation is usually effective in stabilizing venous thrombosis, but if a patient should develop a pulmonary embolism in the presence of adequate anticoagulation, a vena cava filter is indicated.
- The distinction between the hypovolemia of caval occlusion versus the right heart failure from pulmonary embolism can be arrived at by measuring filling pressures of the right side of the heart.

CHAPTER 67

THE LYMPHATICS

EMBRYOLOGY AND ANATOMY

● Figure 67–1.

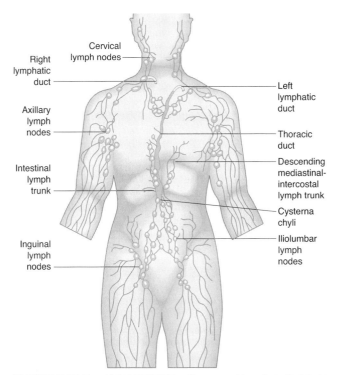

■ FIGURE 67–1. Major anatomic pathways and lymph node groups of the lymphatic system.

FUNCTION AND STRUCTURE

- The lymphatic system is composed of three elements: (1) the initial or terminal lymphatic capillaries, which absorb lymph; (2) the collecting vessels, which serve primarily as conduits for lymph transport; and (3) the lymph nodes, which are interposed in the pathway of the conducting vessels, filtering the lymph and serving a primary immunologic role.
- The lymphatic system has three main functions. First, tissue fluid and macromolecules ultrafiltrated at the level of the arterial capillaries are reabsorbed and returned to the circulation through the lymphatic system. Every day, 50% to 100% of the intravascular proteins are filtered this way in the interstitial space. Normally, they then enter the terminal lymphatics and are transported through the collecting lymphatics back into the venous circulation. Second, microbes arriving in the interstitial space enter the lymphatic system and are presented to the lymph nodes, which represent the first line of the immune system. Finally, at the level of the gastrointestinal tract, lymph vessels are responsible for the uptake and transport of most of the fat absorbed from the bowel.

PATHOPHYSIOLOGY AND STAGING

- Lymphedema is the result of an inability of the existing lymphatic system to accommodate the protein and fluid entering the interstitial compartment at the tissue level. In the first stage of lymphedema, impaired lymphatic drainage results in protein-rich fluid accumulation in the interstitial compartment. Clinically, this manifests as soft pitting edema.
- In the second stage of lymphedema, tissue edema is more pronounced and nonpitting and has a spongy consistency.
- In the third and most advanced stage of lymphedema, there is excessive subcutaneous fibrosis and scarring with associated severe skin changes characteristic of lymphostatic elephantiasis.

DIFFERENTIAL DIAGNOSIS

- In most patients with second- or third-stage lymphedema, the characteristic findings on physical examination can usually establish the diagnosis. The edematous limb has a firm and hardened consistency. There is loss of the normal perimalleolar shape resulting in a "tree trunk" pattern. The dorsum of the foot is characteristically swollen, resulting in the appearance of the "buffalo hump," and the toes become thick and squared. In advanced lymphedema, the skin undergoes characteristic changes such as lichenification, development of peau d'orange, and hyperkeratosis. In addition, the patients give a history of recurrent episodes of cellulitis and lymphangitis after trivial trauma and frequently present with fungal infections affecting the forefoot and toes.

- The evaluation of a swollen extremity should start with a detailed history and physical examination. The most common causes of bilateral extremity edema are of systemic origin. The most common etiology is cardiac failure, followed by renal failure. Hypoproteinemia secondary to cirrhosis, nephrotic syndrome, and malnutrition can also produce bilateral lower extremity edema. Another important cause to consider with bilateral leg enlargement is lipedema. Lipedema is not true edema but rather excessive subcutaneous fat found in obese women. It is bilateral, nonpitting, and greatest at the ankle and legs, with characteristic sparing of the feet. There are no skin changes, and the enlargement is not affected by elevation. The history usually indicates that this has been a lifelong problem that "runs in the family."

- Once the systemic etiologies of edema are excluded, in the patient with unilateral extremity involvement, edema secondary to venous and lymphatic pathology should be entertained. Venous pathology is overwhelmingly the most common cause of unilateral leg edema. Leg edema secondary to venous disease is usually pitting and is greatest at the legs and ankles with a sparing of the feet. The edema responds promptly to overnight leg elevation. In the later stages, the skin is atrophic with brawny pigmentation. Ulceration is associated with venous insufficiency occurs above or posterior and beneath the malleoli.

CLASSIFICATION

DIAGNOSTIC TESTS

- The diagnosis of lymphedema is relatively easy in the patient that presents in the second and third stages of the disease. It can, however, be a difficult diagnosis to make in the first stage, particularly when the edema is mild, pitting, and relieved with simple maneuvers such as elevation. For patients with suspected secondary forms of lymphedema, computed tomography (CT) and magnetic resonance imaging (MRI) are valuable and indeed essential for exclusion of underlying oncologic disease states. In patients with known lymph node excision and radiation treatment as the underlying problem of their lymphedema, additional diagnostic studies are rarely needed except as these studies relate to follow-up of an underlying malignancy. For patients with edema of unknown etiology and a suspicion for lymphedema, lymphoscintigraphy is the diagnostic test of choice. When lymphoscintigraphy confirms that lymphatic drainage is delayed, the diagnosis of primary lymphedema should never be made until neoplasia involving the regional and central lymphatic drainage of the limb has been excluded through CT or MRI. If a more detailed diagnostic interpretation of lymphatic channels is needed for operative planning, then contrast lymphangiography may be considered.

- Lymphoscintigraphy.
- Direct contrast lymphangiography.

THERAPY

- Most lymphedema patients can be treated with a combination of limb elevation, a high-quality compression garment, complex decongestive physical therapy, and compression pump therapy. A new class of medications known as benzopyrones is still under investigation in the United States, but it may find a place in the care of lymphedema in the near future. Operative treatment may be considered for patients with advanced complicated lymphedema that fail management with nonoperative means.

General Therapeutic Measures

- All patients with lymphedema should be educated in meticulous skin care and avoidance of injuries. The patients should always be instructed to see their physicians early for signs of infections because these may progress rapidly to serious systemic infections. Infections should be aggressively and promptly treated with appropriate antibiotics directed at gram-positive cocci.
- Finally, the patients should make every effort to maintain ideal body weight.

Elevation and Compression Garments

- For lymphedema patients in all stages of disease, management with high-quality elastic garments is necessary at all times except when the legs are elevated above the heart. The ideal compression garment is custom fitted and delivers pressures in the range of 30 to 60 mm Hg. Such garments may have the additional benefit of protecting the extremity from injuries such as burns, lacerations, and insect bites. The patients should avoid standing for prolonged periods and should elevate their legs at night by supporting the foot of the bed on 15-cm blocks.

Complex Decongestive Physical Therapy (CDP)

- This specialized massage technique for patients with lymphedema is designed to stimulate the still functioning lymph vessels, evacuate stagnant protein rich fluid by breaking up subcutaneous deposits of fibrous tissue, and redirect lymph fluid to areas of the body where lymph flow is normal·

- This kind of therapy is appropriate for patients with all stages of lymphedema.

- When the patient is first referred for CDP treatment, the patient undergoes daily to weekly massage sessions for up to 8 to 12 weeks. Limb elevation and elastic stockings are a necessary adjunct in this phase. After maximal volume reduction is achieved, then the patient returns for maintenance massage treatments every 2 to 3 months.

Drug Therapy

- Benzopyrones have attracted interest as potentially effective agents in the treatment of lymphedema. This class of medications including 1,2-benzopyrone (Coumarin) is thought to reduce lymphedema through stimulation of proteolysis by tissue macrophages and stimulation of the peristalsis and pumping action of the collecting lymphatics. Benzopyrones have no anticoagulant activity.

- The enthusiasm for use of benzopyrones in the United States has been tempered. Additional trials should be undertaken to clarify the potential effects of the medications on primary and secondary lymphedemas in different extremities and stages.

Operative Treatment

- Ninety-five percent of patients with lymphedema can be managed nonoperatively. Surgical intervention may be considered for patients with stage II and III lymphedema who have severe functional impairment, recurrent episodes of lymphangitis, and severe pain despite optimal medical therapy. Two main categories of operations are available for the care of patients with lymphedema: reconstructive and excisional.

- **Reconstructive operations** should be considered for those patients with proximal (either primary or secondary) obstruction of the extremity lymphatic circulation with preserved, dilated lymphatics distal to the obstruction. In these patients, the residual dilated lymphatics can be either anastomosed to nearby veins or to transposed healthy lymphatic channels (usually mobilized or harvested from the contralateral extremity) in an attempt to restore effective drainage of the lymphedematous extremity.
- For those patients with primary lymphedema who have hypoplastic and fibrotic distal lymphatic vessels such reconstructions is not an option. For such patients, surgical strategy involving transfer of lymphatic bearing tissue (portion of the greater omentum) into the effected limb has been attempted.
- Alternatively a segment of the ileum can be disconnected from the rest of the bowel, stripped of its mucosa and mobilized to be sewn onto the cut surface of residual ilioinguinal nodes in an attempt to bridge lower extremity with mesenteric lymphatics.
- **Excisional operations** are essentially the only viable option for patients without residual lymphatics of adequate size for reconstructive procedures. For patients with recalcitrant stage II and early stage III lymphedema where the edema is moderate the skin is relatively healthy, an excisional procedure that removes a large segment of the lymphedematous subcutaneous tissues and overlying skin is the procedure of choice. This palliative procedure was introduced by Kontoleon in 1918 and was later popularized by Homan as "staged subcutaneous excision underneath flaps".
- When the lymphedema is extremely pronounced and the skin is unhealthy and infected, the simple reducing operation of Kontoleon is not adequate. In this case, the classic excisional operation originally described by Charles in 1912 is performed. The procedure involves complete and circumferential excision of the skin, subcutaneous tissue, and deep fascia of the involved leg and dorsum of the foot. The excision is usually performed in one stage and coverage is provided preferably by full-thickness grafting from the excised skin.

CHYLOTHORAX

- Chylous pleural effusion is usually secondary to thoracic duct trauma (usually iatrogenic after chest surgery) and rarely a manifestation of advanced malignant disease with lymphatic metastasis. Presence of chylomicrons on lipoprotein analysis and a triglyceride level of more than 110 mg/dL in the pleural fluid are diagnostic. Initially, patients can be treated nonoperatively with tube thoracostomy and medium-chain triglyceride diet or total parenteral nutrition. For patients with thoracic duct injury and an effusion that persists after 1 week of drainage, video-assisted thoracoscopy or thoracotomy should be used to identify and ligate the thoracic duct above and below the leak.

CHYLOPERITONEUM

- In contrast to chylothorax, the most common cause of chylous ascites is congenital lymphatic abnormalities in children and malignancy involving the abdominal lymph nodes in adults. Postoperative injury to abdominal lymphatics resulting in chylous ascites is rare.

TUMORS OF THE LYMPHATICS

- **Lymphangiomas** are the lymphatic analog of the hemangiomas of blood vessels. They are generally divided into two types including (1) simple or capillary lymphangioma and (2) cavernous lymphangioma or cystic hygroma.
- The treatment of lymphangiomas should be surgical excision, taking care to preserve all normal surrounding infiltrated structures.
- **Lymphangiosarcoma** is a rare tumor that develops as a complication of long-standing (usually more than 10 years) lymphedema. Clinically the patients present with acute worsening of the edema and appearance of subcutaneous nodules that have a propensity toward hemorrhage and ulceration. The tumor can be treated, as other sarcomas, with preoperative chemotherapy and radiation followed by surgical excision, which usually may take the form of radical amputation. Overall, the tumor has a very poor prognosis.

CHAPTER 68

ACCESS AND PORTS

VASCULAR ACCESS

Overview

- Frequent access to the bloodstream is required for patients undergoing the following:
  - Parenteral nutrition.
  - Chemotherapy for malignant disease.
  - Plasmapheresis.
  - Short-term and long-term dialysis.
- Hemoaccess:
  - Fistula, jump graft, or external angioaccess.
  - Frequent access to the vascular system.
  - High-flow system.
  - Multiple needle punctures.
  - Sclerotic solutions.
- Cost:
  - End-stage renal disease budget, maintaining and placing vascular access devices and fistulas cost approximately $1 billion per year in the United States (17% of the budget).

External Angioaccess

Dialysis Through Major Vessels

- Short-term: subclavian, external jugular, internal jugular, or femoral vein percutaneously placed catheters.
- Dual-lumen, silicone rubber catheters low incidence of recirculation (2% to 5%).
  - Single catheter more recirculation (20% to 40%).
- Two separate catheters placed through two separate needle sticks (Tesio); blood flows of up to 400 mL/minute.
- Locations of tip: right atrium, junction of superior vena cava, and right atrium.
- Problems:
  - Subclavian catheter for approximately 2 weeks up to 50% significant stenosis; fistulas clot or arms swell up; only less than 10% when using internal jugular; if central

catheter in place, get a Doppler study before placing permanent access. Gold standard is the venogram.
- Catheters clot and get infected causing line sepsis and endocarditis.
● Femoral catheters at the patient s bedside; removed after dialysis, to prevent infection or venous thrombosis. Problems with repeated use are iliofemoral thrombosis, local bleeding, or arterial puncture and injury.

Nutrition, Blood Access, and Chemotherapy

● Sites: subclavian, internal jugular, external jugular, basilic veins, or inferior vena cava.
● Catheter type: totally implantable or external, such as Broviac, Hickman, and Groshung.

Complications

● Early complications (subclavian or internal jugular; most commonly on right).
  - Pneumothorax (4% incidence).
  - Arterial injury.
  - Thoracic duct injury.
  - Air embolus.
  - Inability to pass the catheter.
  - Bleeding.
  - Nerve injury.
  - Great vessel injury (less than 1%).
● Late complications:
  - Thrombosis (4% to 10%).
  - Treatment: urokinase transluminal (4000 U), contrast angiography, or urokinase (40,000 U/hour for 12 hours).
  - Infection (7% to 39%).
  - Avoidance: insert sterilely; keep exit site covered with gauze and iodophor ointment; change every 3 days.
  - Treatment: intravenous (IV) antibiotics for exit-site infections; removal in tunnel infections and sepsis.

Internal Angioaccess

Natural Fistulas

● Brescia-Cimino fistula (radial artery to cephalic vein at wrist) patency 65% at 1 year and 55% to 89% at 2 years.
  - Allen s test to minimize hand ischemia.
  - Methods: side-to-side, end artery to side vein, side artery to end vein, and end artery to end vein.

Types of Natural Fistulas

- Snuff-box fistula (new name: autogenous radial-cephalic direct wrist access).
- Ulnar artery to basilic vein.
- Antecubital vein to brachial artery.
- Brachiobasilic fistula.
- Brachiocephalic fistula (patency: 80% 1 year) (new name: autogenous brachial-cephalic upper arm direct access).
- Basilic vein transposition (upper arm) patency 73% 2 year (new name: autogenous brachial-basilic upper arm transposition).
- Basilic (or ulnar) vein transposition (forearm) to radial artery.
- Saphenous vein loop to superficial femoral artery.
- Saphenous vein transposition to forearm.
- National Kidney Foundation s Dialysis Outcome Quality Initiative Guidelines:
  - Fifty percent new access should be natural fistulas.
  - Vein mapping by Doppler ultrasound: artery greater than 2 mm; vein greater than 2.5 mm and continuous.

Complications

- Failure to mature: poor vessels, poor venous outflow.
- Thrombosis (9%): excessive dehydration; hypotension.
- Stenosis at the proximal venous limb (48%).
- Aneurysms (7%) from repeated needle punctures.
- Heart failure: a marginal cardiac reserve and a fistula flow rate of more than 500 mL/minute.
- Arterial steal syndrome with ischemia (1.6%) treat by banding or ligation.
- Venous hypertension distal to the fistula: distal tissue swelling, hyperpigmentation, skin induration, and eventual skin ulceration; treat ligation of the distal venous limb.
- Infection (<3%).

Prosthetic Grafts

- Ideal material:
  - Easy to handle and to suture.
  - Allow graft-host biocompatibility.
  - Minimally thrombogenic.
  - Inexpensive.
  - Seal after repeated needle punctures.
  - Allow tissue ingrowth.

- Currently: polytetrafluorethylene (PTFE) (patency: 80% at 1 year and 69% at 2 years).
  - Usual sizes used are a 6-mm graft or a rapid-taper 4- to 7-mm graft.
  - Mature for 1 to 2 weeks avoids problem of hematoma formation if graft stuck immediately.

Placement

- Nondominant arm.
- Start as distal in the arm as possible.
- Forearm loop (patency: 78% at 1 year) or upper arm loop (patency 60% at 1 year) (higher incidence of ischemia).
- Interposition grafts in the lower extremity: only if no viable upper extremity sites.
- Last resort: axillary artery to axillary vein across the chest (necklace graft), loop on the anterior chest, and axillary artery to iliac vein.

Complications

- Early hemorrhage: at the anastomotic site.
- Late hemorrhage: needle puncture.
- Early thrombosis: technical reasons.
- Later thrombosis:
  - Venous intimal hyperplasia at or distal to the anastomosis.
  - Treatment: patch graft, balloon dilatation of the strictured area, or graft bypass of the obstruction.
- Low blood pressure.
- Excessive external pressure.
- Hypercoagulability: protein S, protein C, antithrombin III, plasminogen, factor V, and antiphospholipid antibodies.
- Infection.
  - Treatment.
  - Local drainage and wound care, if suture line not involved.
  - Bypassed with a short graft.
  - Removal of the entire graft.
  - Involvement of the suture line.
  - Tunnel infection.
  - Clotting of the graft.
  - Lack of success with local wound therapy (50% to 75%).
- False aneurysms:
  - Multiple needle sticks lacerates the graft.

Patency

- Appears to be related to the magnitude of arterial inflow and the size and distensibility of the venous outflow.

Radiographic Intervention and Screening for Stenosis

- Schwab: early intervention for graft stenosis with percutaneous luminal angioplasty reduced the incidence of graft thrombosis.
- Test: pressure greater than 150 mm Hg on three separate occasions equals venous stenosis greater than 50%.
- Monitoring:
  - Doppler examination.
  - Checking venous pressure.
  - Checking of recirculation.
  - Feeling for a thrill: if felt over entire length, then blood flow is greater than 450 mL/minute.
- Clotted graft: dissolved with urokinase or broken up mechanically.
  - Occasionally, pulmonary emboli.
  - Surgical thrombectomy equals radiologic.
- Stenosis management:
  - Venous stenosis only: surgical intervention not greater or less than percutaneous angioplasty (patency 40% 1 year).
  - With both venous stenosis and long-segment venous outflow stenosis; surgery greater than radiology.
  - Central stenosis: angioplasty with or without stents.

Physiology

- Possible consequences of a large, functioning arteriovenous fistula:
  - Fall in both systolic and diastolic blood pressure.
  - An increase in cardiac output.
  - An increase in venous blood pressure both proximal and distal to the fistula.
  - An increase in pulse rate.
  - Slight increase in the size of the heart.
  - Increases blood volume.
  - Progressive lengthening and dilatation of both the proximal artery and the vein with smooth muscle hypertrophy then eventually smooth muscle atrophy leads to aneurysmal dilatation and a tortuous vessel.

PERITONEAL DIALYSIS

Physiology

- The exact surface and mechanism responsible for hemofiltration in peritoneal dialysis remain unknown.
  - Theory: diffusion across the capillary membrane being the primary transport barrier.
  - Effective surface area depends on the number of transcellular pores available for transport corresponding to the number of perfused capillaries (peritoneal surface approximates the total body surface area).
- Clearance:
  - Urea: 100 L/week in hemodialysis versus 70 L/week continuous ambulatory peritoneal dialysis (CAPD) versus 604 L/week for normal kidneys.
  - CAPD better at clearing large solutes (>500 daltons) than small solutes compared with hemodialysis.
  - Ultrafiltration in CAPD depends on Starling forces and lymphatic drainage.

Indications

- Inability to undergo hemodialysis.
  - Poor vascular access.
  - An unstable cardiovascular system.
  - Bleeding diatheses.
- Relative advantages:
  - Increased patient mobility and independence.
  - Fewer dietary restrictions, lower incidence of anemia.
  - Increased patient satisfaction.
  - No requirement for systemic anticoagulation.
- Absolute contraindications:
  - Obliteration of the peritoneal space from previous surgery.
  - Inadequate peritoneal clearance.
  - Lack of diaphragmatic integrity.
- Relative contraindications:
  - Respiratory insufficiency secondary to dialysate infusion.
  - Large abdominal hernias.
  - Malignant peritoneal disease.

Technical Procedures

- Catheters.
  - Straight versus coiled intra-abdominal configurations.
  - Single and double cuffs.
  - Preformed intercuff bends (Swan neck).

- Placement:
  - Open surgical technique, percutaneously, or laparoscopically.
  - Incision.
  - Tip: directed toward the pelvis.
  - First cuff placed in muscle on posterior fascia.
  - Second Dacron cuff at least 1 inch from the skin surface.
  - Omentectomy may also be necessary in some instances (especially children).
- Complications:
  - Malfunction ranges from 12% to 73%.
    Obstruction.
  - Evaluation and salvage of malfunctioning catheters:
    Peritoneoscopy.
    Laparoscopic manipulation (salvage rates between 50% and 80%).

Dialysis Fluids

- Osmotic forces secondary to glucose concentrations.
  - Low osmolarity (1.5%) causes little fluid removal (200 mL per 2-L exchange).
  - Greatest concentration (4.5%) treats or prevents fluid overload (800 mL per 2-L exchange). High-concentration dialysis fluid is more irritating.
- Glycosylation of the peritoneal vascular walls leads to reduces the intrinsic filtering ability.
- A typical exchange is 2 L four times per day.

Complications

Surgical Placement

- Leakage of dialysate.
- Intraperitoneal bleeding.
- Bowel or bladder perforation.
- Subcutaneous bleeding with hematoma formation from tunnel construction.
- Ileus.

After Placement

- Exit-site infection.
  - Rate of 0.80 per patient-year.
  - Gram-positive organisms (80%); *Staphylococcus aureus* 90%.
  - Exit site infection precedes peritonitis in about 20% of cases.

- Peritonitis (incidence of 1.3 to 1.4 episodes per patient-year).
  - Routes:
    Through the dialysis tubing and peritoneal catheter.
    From tissue around the catheter.
    From fecal contamination, such as in diverticulitis.
    Blood-borne infections.
    Ascending infection from the fallopian tubes in women.
  - Pathogen:
    Usually single.
    Sixty percent to 70% gram-positive cocci with coagulase-negative *Staphylococcus* the most common.
    Gram-negative bacilli 20% to 30%.
    Pseudomonas aeruginosa 5% to 10%.
    Uncommon causes are tuberculosis and fungal infection.
    Risk factors for fungal peritonitis include recent hospitalization, immunologic compromise, and bacterial peritonitis.
  - Treatment:
    By peritoneal and parenteral antibiotics.
    Synergistic double coverage is indicated for *P. aeruginosa*.
    Catheter removal is usually required for fungal infections.
- Mechanical failure:
  - Poor inflow:
    Displacement.
    Omental wrapping.
    Partial blockage of the catheter holes.
  - Total obstruction:
    Kinking of the catheter.
    Blockage of all catheter holes.
    Omental wrapping of the entire intra-abdominal portion of the catheter.

Catheter Longevity

- One year in 85%.
- Significantly shorter in patients with diabetes.
- Infection is the leading reason for discontinuation of CAPD.
- Abdominal surgical events and social reasons have surpassed infection as a cause of treatment failure in some centers.

SUMMARY

- Renal transplantation is still the therapy of choice for suitable patients with end-stage renal failure. Superb patient compliance is a basic requirement of paramount importance.

CHAPTER 69

PEDIATRIC SURGERY

NEWBORN PHYSIOLOGY

- Before the ductus arterious is closed, there may be a higher partial pressure and saturation of oxygen in the blood when sampled from the right arm (preductal) when compared with the other extremities (postductal) because of the flow of unoxygenated blood from the pulmonary artery through the ductus into the aorta.
- Cardiac perfusion is best monitored clinically by capillary refill, which should be less than 1 second.
- Neonates that are cold-stressed respond by nonshivering thermogenesis. Metabolic rate and oxygen consumption are augmented by brown fat mobilization.

FLUIDS, ELECTROLYTES, AND NUTRITION

- The margin for error is narrower when compared with adults.
- On a body weight basis, protein and energy requirements are much greater in younger children, and the requirements decrease with age.
- Infants who are losing weight, or even failing to gain weight, require a careful reassessment of metabolic needs and amount of nutrition provided.
- In the first 3–5 days of life, there is a physiologic water loss of up to 10% of the body weight of the infant.
- This is the singular exception to the general principle that infants are expected to gain weight each day.
- The best two indicators of sufficient fluid intake are urine output and osmolarity.
- The daily requirements for sodium are 2 to 4 mEq/kg and for potassium are 1 to 2 mEq/kg.
- The parameter that is most indicative of sufficient provision of calories in neonates is daily weight gain.
- The absolute minimum intravenous glucose infusion rate for neonates is 4 to 6 mg/kg/minute.
- In infants with unconjugated hyperbilirubinemia, fat administration should be done with caution, because fatty acids may displace bilirubin from albumin (Table 69–1).

TABLE 69–1. Daily Fluid Requirements for Neonates and Infants

Weight	Volume
Premature <2.0 kg	140-150 mL/kg/day
Neonates and infants 2-10 kg	100 mL/kg/day for first 10 kg
Children between 10-20 kg	1000 mL + 50 mL/kg/day for weight 10 – 20 kg
Children >20 kg	1500 mL + 20 mL/kg/day for weight >20 kg

Adapted from Coran AG: The Pediatric Surgical Patient, *Scientific American Surgery*, Wilmore DW, Cheung LY, Harken AH, Holcroft JW, Meakins JL (eds), Sect. VII, Subsect. 12, Healtheon/WebMD New York, 2000.

EXTRACORPOREAL LIFE SUPPORT (ECLS)

- The major indications for initiation of neonatal ECLS include meconium aspiration, respiratory distress syndrome, persistent pulmonary hypertension, sepsis, and congenital diaphragmatic hernia.
- An infant must have at least 80% predicted mortality with continued conventional medical management to justify this high-risk therapy.
- Exclusion criteria include prematurity (less than 24 weeks' gestation), the presence of cyanotic congenital heart disease or other major congenital anomalies that preclude survival, intractable coagulopathy or hemorrhage, sonographic evidence of a significant intracranial hemorrhage (greater than a grade I intraventricular hemorrhage), and more than 10 to 14 days of high-pressure mechanical ventilation.

TRAUMA

- In children between 1 and 15 years of age, trauma is the leading cause of death.
- If endotracheal intubation is required, an uncuffed endotracheal tube should be used in children younger than 8 to 10 years.
- The appropriate endotracheal tube size can be estimated visually as being equivalent to the diameter of the child's little finger. Alternatively the appropriate endotracheal tube inner diameter can be calculated by the following formula: 4 + (patient's age in years) ÷ 4.
- Crystalloid is given as a rapid intravenous bolus in increments of 20 mL/kg.

- In children younger than 6 years in whom an intravenous line cannot be secured within a reasonable period, intraosseous access should be considered.
- An estimate of a child's entire blood volume is roughly 80 mL/kg.
- The indications for computed tomography (CT) include the presence of a distracting injury such as an associated arm or leg fracture or significant closed head injury or if the examination is unclear or cannot be obtained because of an uncooperative or very young child or if the serum glutamine-oxaloacetic transaminase (SGOT) or serum glutamic-pyruvic transaminase (SGPT) are greater than 200 or 100 IU/L, respectively.
- The major indications for laparotomy in these circumstances include obvious hemodynamic instability, the need for blood transfusion in amounts greater than half the child's calculated blood volume (40 mL/kg) within the first 24 hours following injury, or obvious extravascular blush of intravenously administered contrast material.

LESIONS OF THE NECK

Cystic Hygroma

- Because hygromas are not neoplastic tumors, radical resection with removal of major blood vessels and nerves is not indicated.

Branchial Cleft Remnants

- All branchial remnants are present at the time of birth, although they may not become clinically evident until later in life.
- Remnants from the second branchial cleft are the most common.

Thyroglossal Duct Cyst

- Thyroglossal remnants are involved with the embryogenesis of the thyroid gland, tongue, and hyoid bone and produce midline masses extending from the base of the tongue (foramen cecum) to the pyramidal lobe of the thyroid gland.
- The classic treatment has remained unchanged since it was described by Sistrunk in 1928 and involves complete excision of the cyst in continuity with its tract, the central portion of

the hyoid bone, and the tissue above the hyoid bone extending to the base of the tongue.

Torticollis

● Congenital torticollis should be distinguished from acquired torticollis.

Cervical Lymphadenopathy

● Nontender, fixed nodes in the supraclavicular region are worrisome for malignancy.
● If a diagnostic lymph node biopsy is indicated, a preoperative chest radiograph should be performed to exclude associated mediastinal adenopathy.
● If significant airway compression is seen, every attempt should be made to perform the biopsy under local anesthesia.

ALIMENTARY TRACT

Esophageal Atresia and Tracheoesophageal Fistula (EA/TEF)

● There is a nonrandom, nonhereditary association of anomalies in patients with EA/TEF that must be considered under the acronym VATER (*V*ertebral, *A*norectal, *T*racheal, *E*sophageal, *R*enal or *R*adial limb). Another acronym that is commonly used is VACTERL (*V*ertebral, *A*norectal, *C*ardiac, *T*racheal, *E*sophageal, *R*enal, and *L*imb).
● The inability to pass a nasogastric tube into the stomach of the neonate is a cardinal feature for the diagnosis of EA.
● A preoperative echocardiogram is essential to evaluate the presence or absence of congenital heart disease and to define the side of the aortic arch.
● The blood supply to the upper esophageal pouch is generally robust and based on arteries derived from the thyrocervical trunk. On the other hand, the blood supply to the lower esophagus is more tenuous and segmental, originating from intercostal vessels.
● In patients with pure EA, the gap between the two esophageal ends is frequently wide, thus preventing a primary anastomosis in the newborn period.
● In patients with pure TEF without EA, the site of the TEF is usually in the region of the thoracic inlet. As such, the surgical approach is via a cervical incision.
● The mortality of EA/TEF is directly related to the associated anomalies.

Gastroesophageal Reflux (GER)

- In a child with documented GER, an episode of near-miss sudden infant death syndrome (SIDS) is an absolute indication for antireflux surgery.
- The limitation of this study is that it nicely delineates risk for acid injury to the esophagus but may fail to detect pathologic GER in patients who have symptoms related to pulmonary aspiration.
- Indications for surgical intervention include severe GER that is unresponsive to aggressive medical management. In addition, surgery is generally warranted in patients with life-threatening near-miss SIDS episodes, failure to thrive (FTT), or esophageal stricture.
- The risk for recurrent GER and other morbidity are highest in the neurologically impaired population.

Hypertrophic Pyloric Stenosis

- This condition is most common between the ages of 2 and 8 weeks.
- Gastric outlet obstruction leads to nonbilious, projectile emesis; loss of hydrochloric acid with the development of hypochloremic; metabolic alkalosis; and ultimate dehydration.
- The clinical presentation of infants with HPS present is projectile and/or frequent episodes of *nonbilious* emesis.
- Because the infant with underlying metabolic alkalosis will compensate with respiratory acidosis, postoperative apnea may occur. Thus, the serum HCO_3^- should be normalized before surgery.

Intestinal Atresia

- Duodenal atresia (DA) is felt to occur as a result of failure of vacuolization of the duodenum from its solid cord stage.
- The classic plain abdominal radiograph of DA is termed the "double bubble" sign.

Anomalies of Intestinal Rotation and Fixation

- Rotates around the axis of the superior mesenteric artery (SMA) for 270 degrees in a counterclockwise direction.
- Complete nonrotation of the midgut is the most frequently encountered anomaly and occurs when neither the duodenojejunal limb nor the cecocolic limb undergoes rotation.
- Most patients develop symptoms during the first month of life.

- The sudden appearance of bilious emesis in a newborn is the classic presentation.
- Occasionally, plain abdominal radiographs may reveal evidence for intestinal obstruction; however, the most common findings are nonspecific. The upper gastrointestinal (GI) contrast series remains the gold standard for the diagnosis.
- The operative management for most rotational anomalies of the intestine is the Ladd's procedure.
- If a volvulus is encountered, it should be remembered that in most cases, the volvulus twists in a clockwise direction; thus, it should be untwisted in a counterclockwise manner.

Necrotizing Enterocolitis (NEC)

- The radiographic hallmark of NEC is pneumatosis intestinalis (Fig. 69–1).

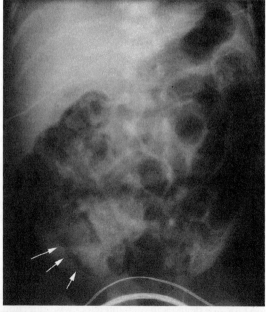

■ **FIGURE 69–1.** Plain abdominal radiograph of an infant with necrotizing enterocolitis demonstrating diffuse pneumatosis intestinalis. In addition to the typical ground glass appearance, linear gas corresponding with the submucosal plane of the bowel wall is easily visualized (arrows).

- The absolute indication for operative management of NEC is the presence of intestinal perforation as revealed by the identification of free air on plain abdominal radiographs.
- Intestinal strictures may develop after either medical or surgical management of NEC in roughly 10% of infants.

Meconium Syndromes

- In patients with simple meconium ileus, important plain abdominal radiographic findings include dilated, gas-filled loops of small bowel; absence of air-fluid levels; and a mass of meconium within the right side of the abdomen mixed with gas to give a "ground glass" or "soap bubble" appearance.

Intussusception

- In most pediatric intussusceptions, the cause is unknown, the location is at the ileocecal junction, and there is no identifiable pathologic lead point.
- Although frequent bowel movements may occur with the onset of pain, the progression of the obstruction results in bowel ischemia with passage of dark blood clots mixed with mucus commonly referred to as "currant jelly" stool.
- When the clinical index of suspicion for intussusception is high, hydrostatic reduction by contrast or air enema is the diagnostic and therapeutic procedure of choice.
- Recurrence rates after hydrostatic reduction are roughly 11% and usually occur within the first 24 hours.

Hirschsprung's Disease

- The abnormal bowel is the contracted, distal segment, and the normal bowel is the proximal, dilated portion.
- The aganglionosis always involves the distal rectum and extends proximally for variable distances.
- Failure to pass meconium in the first 24 hours is highly significant and a cardinal feature of this condition.
- The initial diagnostic step in a newborn with radiographic evidence for a distal bowel obstruction is a barium enema.
- A rectal biopsy is the gold standard for the diagnosis of Hirschsprung's disease.
- Absent ganglia, hypertrophied nerve trunks, and robust immunostaining for acetylcholinesterase are the pathologic criteria to make the diagnosis.

Imperforate Anus

- The most common defect is an imperforate anus with a fistula between the distal colon and the urethra in boys or to the vestibule of the vagina in girls.
- Clinically, if an anocutaneous fistula is seen anywhere on the perineal skin of a boy or external to the hymen of a girl, a low lesion can be assumed, which allows a primary perineal repair procedure to be performed, without the need for a stoma.
- In general, the higher the anorectal malformation, the greater the frequency of associated urologic abnormalities.
- Infants with intermediate or high lesions traditionally require a colostomy as the first part of a three-stage reconstruction.
- Globally, 75% of all patients have voluntary bowel movements. Half of this group still soils their underwear occasionally and the other half are considered totally continent.

ABDOMINAL WALL

Abdominal Wall Defects

- In contrast with omphalocele, the defect seen with gastroschisis is always on the right side of the umbilical ring with an intact umbilical cord, and there is never a sac covering the abdominal contents.
- In contrast with gastroschisis, karyotype abnormalities are present in roughly 30% of infants, including trisomies 13, 18, and 21.
- Because the viscera are covered by a sac, operative repair of the defect may be delayed to allow thorough evaluation of the infant.
- In contrast to patients with an omphalocele, the risk for associated anomalies with gastroschisis is infrequent.

Inguinal Hernia (IH)

- Virtually all IH in children are indirect and congenital in origin.
- This is distinguished from a *noncommunicating* hydrocele by the history of variation in size throughout the day and palpation of a thickened cord above the testicle on the affected side.
- Considering these factors, most pediatric surgeons perform herniorrhaphy before the neonate is discharged to home from the nursery.

- In girls, the most common structure present in an IH that cannot be reduced is an ovary.
- The IH repair should be done after the period of observation to allow tissue edema to subside.

Undescended Testes (UDT)

- In the former, the testicle cannot be manipulated into a scrotal position, whereas in the latter the testicle can be pulled down into the scrotum.
- The effect of higher temperatures and other factors on the developing UDT result in several abnormalities, including attenuated spermatogenesis, infertility, and increased risk for malignancy.
- The customary surgical procedure for treatment of UDT that are palpated within the inguinal canal is by orchidopexy along with repair of the associated inguinal hernia.

Umbilical Hernia (UH)

- Exceptions to this general rule are a large UH defect (>2 cm) because the likelihood for spontaneous resolution is lower. Furthermore, a history of incarceration, a large skin proboscis, or a patient with a ventriculoperitoneal shunt are other relative indications for repair.

Epigastric Hernia

CONGENITAL DIAPHRAGMATIC HERNIA (CDH)

- Most CDH defects are on the left side (80%); however, up to 20% may occur on the right side.
- The exact survival rate for CDH is difficult to determine but in the range of 60% to 70%.
- The posterolateral location of this hernia is known as a Bochdalek hernia and distinguished from the congenital hernia of the anteromedial, retrosternal diaphragm, which is known as a Morgagni hernia.
- The most frequent clinical presentation of CDH is respiratory distress because of severe hypoxemia.
- It is important to remember that the pneumothorax in patients with CDH always occurs on the side *contralateral* to the side of the CDH.
- Most pediatric surgeons wait for a variable period of time (24 to 72 hours) to allow for stabilization of the infant before embarking on surgical repair.

CONGENITAL CHEST WALL DEFORMITIES

- The most common indication for surgery in patients with pectus deformities is cosmetic.
- Notwithstanding many decades of experience with this condition, no appreciable consensus has been reached regarding the degree of cardiopulmonary impairment, if any, that this common chest wall deformity produces.
- The surgical correction of a pectus excavatum should not be done before the age of 5 years.

BRONCHOPULMONARY MALFORMATIONS

- Cysts within the pulmonary parenchyma typically communicate with a bronchus, whereas those in the mediastinum usually do not.
- Usually no bronchial communication and there is frequently an aberrant systemic blood supply.
- In approximately 85% of cases, the intralobar sequestration is supplied by an anomalous systemic vessel arising from the infradiaphragmatic aorta and located within the inferior pulmonary ligament.
- Within a histologically normal lung resulting from abnormal cartilaginous support of the feeding bronchus.
- Single lobe and represents a multicystic mass of pulmonary tissue in which there is proliferation of bronchial structures at the expense of alveoli.
- Type III congenital cystic adenomatoid malformations (CCAM) are often associated with mediastinal shift, the development of nonimmune hydrops, and a generally poor prognosis.

HEPATOBILIARY

Biliary Atresia (BA)

- Bile duct proliferation, severe cholestasis with plugging, and inflammatory cell infiltrate are the pathologic hallmarks of this disease.
- A serum direct bilirubin level greater than 2.0 mg/dL or greater than 15% of the total bilirubin level defines cholestasis and is distinctly abnormal; further evaluation is mandatory.
- Thus, the initial opportunity for success in the management of this disease relies on the *early* recognition of abnormal direct hyperbilirubinemia.
- The classic technique for correction of BA is the Kasai hepatoportoenterostomy.

Choledochal Cyst

- The triad of a right upper quadrant mass, abdominal pain, and jaundice is highly suggestive of the diagnosis.
- Total cyst excision with Roux-en-Y hepaticojejunostomy is the definitive procedure for management of type I and II choledochal cysts.

CHILDHOOD SOLID TUMORS

Neuroblastoma (NBL)

- NBL is the most common abdominal malignancy in children.
- Approximately 25% of patients present with a solitary mass that may be cured by surgical therapy, whereas most present with extensive locoregional or metastatic disease.
- The most common presentation is a fixed, lobular mass extending from the flank toward the midline of the abdomen.
- A spot urine should be tested for the catecholamine metabolites homovanillic and vanillylmandelic acid.
- Amplification of the N-*myc* oncogene is one of the classic factors associated with rapid tumor progression and poor prognosis.
- Surgical resection of the primary tumor and adjacent lymph nodes should be the goal and may be curative for localized stage 1 and 2 disease.

Wilms' Tumor (WT)

- WT is an embryonal tumor of renal origin and is the most common primary malignant kidney tumor of childhood.
- The goals for operative therapy for WT are to confirm the diagnosis; assess the opposite kidney and other abdominal organs for metastatic spread; and completely resect the primary tumor, ureter, and adjacent lymph nodes.

Rhabdomyosarcoma (RMS)

- The prognosis for a child or adolescent with RMS is related to patient age, site of origin, extent of tumor at time of diagnosis or after surgical resection, and tumor histology.
- From a histologic standpoint, the botryoid and spindle cell subtypes are associated with a more favorable outcome.
- The basic surgical principles for the treatment of RMS are complete resection of the primary tumor with a surrounding margin of normal tissue, coupled with sampling of the adjacent lymph nodes.

Liver Tumors

- Hepatoblastomas (HBL) usually occur before 3 years of age, whereas hepatocellular carcinoma (HCC) may be found in children and adults of all ages.
- HBL is associated with hemihypertrophy, very low birth-weight, and the Beckwith-Wiedemann syndrome.

Teratoma

- Teratomas are tumors that contain elements derived from more than one of the three embryonic germ layers.

CHAPTER 70

NEUROSURGERY

CEREBROVASCULAR

Spontaneous Subarachnoid Hemorrhage

- Can range from a small focal amount of blood to a large diffuse subarachnoid hemorrhage.
- Most frequent cause is rupture of an intracranial aneurysm.
- Subarachnoid hemorrhage accounts for approximately 10% of all strokes.

Symptoms and Signs

- A sudden explosive onset of very severe headaches.
- Depending on the severity of the bleed, the patient's neurologic condition may vary from completely awake and oriented to moribund with severe neurologic deficits.
- Subarachnoid blood can cause sterile meningitis, leading to a stiff neck, a minor fever, and photophobia.
- Most patients are hypertensive after a subarachnoid hemorrhage, and electrocardiographic changes are frequent, including prolonged QT intervals, elevated or depressed ST segments, and ventricular arrhythmias.

Cerebral Aneurysms

- Cerebral aneurysms (berry aneurysms) account for slightly more than half of all cases of spontaneous subarachnoid hemorrhage.
- Can occur almost anywhere along the circle of Willis, especially common at the junction of the posterior communicating artery and one of the anterior cerebral arteries, or at the first major branches of the middle cerebral artery.
- In the posterior fossa, the most common location is at the terminal bifurcation of the basilar artery.
- Multiple aneurysms are found in approximately 20% of all patients.
- Rebleeding is the single most important cause of death.
- Vasospasm is a major cause of complications and death.

- Risk of vasospasm is related to the amount of blood in the subarachnoid space.

Diagnosis and Management of Subarachnoid Hemorrhage

- Unenhanced computed tomography (CT) scans have become the procedure of choice for the detection of subarachnoid hemorrhage and are positive in more than 90% of patients.
- In cases in which there is a high clinical suspicion of a subarachnoid hemorrhage and a diagnosis cannot be confirmed by CT scanning, a lumbar puncture should be performed.
- The presence of xanthochromia in the supernatant fluid demonstrates that bleeding has occurred and that bloody cerebrospinal fluid (CSF) is not the result of a traumatic lumbar puncture.

Surgical Treatment of Aneurysms

- Most authorities advocate early surgical intervention, within the first 48 hours after hemorrhage.
- Treatment involves the placement of a surgical aneurysm clip around the neck of the aneurysm.
- Patients at high risk for conventional surgery may undergo endovascular coiling of their aneurysm.

Spontaneous Hypertensive Intracerebral Hemorrhage

- Blood clot in the parenchyma of the brain without preceding trauma.
- Ten percent of all strokes.
- Deterioration may occur secondary to progressive brainstem compression and obstructive hydrocephalus.
- Most frequently occurs in the putamen, thalamus, cerebellum, or pons from the small perforating arteries of the brain.
- Hemorrhages in the putamen typically produce a rapidly progressive hemiparesis, hemisensory loss, and hemianopsia contralateral to the hemorrhage.
- A thalamic hemorrhage usually manifests a hemisensory loss greater than the patient's motor deficit.
- Pontine hypertensive hemorrhages demonstrate small pupils, bilateral pyramidal signs, and a rapid loss of consciousness.
- Cerebellar hemorrhage characteristically presents with headache, dizziness, nausea, and vomiting.
- Diagnosis of hypertensive intracerebral hematoma is made by a CT scan of the brain.

Treatment

- Hypertension should be controlled, but care should be taken to preserve cerebral perfusion pressure to at least 70 to 80 mm Hg.
- Patients with an initial good neurologic examination who are deteriorating are candidates for surgery.
- The goal of surgery is to remove the hematoma, therefore, removing the pressure on the surrounding brain and restoring the intracranial pressure (ICP) to normal.
- Two basic surgical methods for removing intracerebral hematomas: stereotactic needle aspiration and craniotomy with open removal of the hematoma.
- Surgical therapy should be used for the evacuation of cerebellar hematomas causing brainstem compression.

Vascular Malformations

- Capillary telangiectasias and venous angiomas rarely bleed.
- Cavernous angiomas that have caused a clinically significant bleed should be removed.
- Arteriovenous malformations (AVMs) are treated by microsurgery, embolization, or radiosurgery.

CENTRAL NERVOUS SYSTEM TUMORS

Intracranial Tumors

- The incidence of primary brain tumors in the United States is 11.5 per 100,000, or approximately 35,000 per year.
- Metastatic brain tumors present in 150,000 to 250,000 patients per year.

Clinical Presentation

- Two major presentations: generalized increase in ICP, and focal compression or irritation of the brain.
- The most common symptoms of increased ICP are headache, nausea, vomiting, and reduction in the level of consciousness.
- Focal compression may cause a focal neurologic deficit.
- Irritation of the cerebral cortex by a tumor can cause a seizure.

Radiology

- The recommendation for initial screening is a gadolinium-enhanced magnetic resonance imaging (MRI).

- CT scans are more sensitive for detecting bony abnormalities and are less costly and time consuming to perform, and they are useful in the postoperative period.
- Cerebral angiography is indicated when highly vascular tumors are suspected.

Surgery

- First goals are diagnosis and reduction of tumor mass effect; complete removal is ideal but not always possible.
- Image-guided (CT or MRI) stereotactic techniques allow highly accurate biopsies.

Primary Brain Tumors

- Arise from either within the brain parenchyma (intra-axial) or outside the parenchyma (extra-axial).

Intra-Axial Brain Tumors

- Gliomas arise from astrocytes, oligodendrocytes, and ependymal cells.

Astrocytomas

- Most common type of glioma and accounts for 50% of all primary brain tumors.
- Recent investigations into the genetic abnormalities of astrocytomas have shown frequent mutations in the *p53* gene, abnormalities on chromosome 10, and overexpression of the epidermal growth factor receptor.
- The most common grade 1 astrocytoma is the *pilocytic astrocytoma*; pilocytic astrocytomas in the cerebrum and cerebellum are well circumscribed, surgically accessible, and therefore curable by complete resection; chemotherapy and radiation do not normally play a role in treatment.
- Low-grade astrocytomas (grade 2) are infiltrative; complete surgical resection is impossible.
- There is some evidence supporting radiation therapy but no evidence that chemotherapy plays a role in treatment; underscoring the fact that these are not benign tumors, the median survival time is 5 to 7 years.
- High-grade astrocytomas appear as irregularly enhancing areas on MRI.
- There is a mass effect and extensive areas of edema and infiltrating tumor cells; the best treatment involves surgical

resection followed by fractionated external beam radiation to a dose of 60 Gy (6000 rads).

- Chemotherapy may slightly improve survival in selected patients.
- Bischloroethylnitrosurea (BCNU) impregnated absorbable wafers also offer a small survival advantage and may replace intravenous chemotherapy in some patents.

Oligodendrogliomas

- Treatment is similar to astrocytomas with the exception that chemotherapy may be more effective.

Ependymomas

- Typically found in the fourth ventricle in children.
- Treatment is maximum surgical resection followed by radiation therapy.

Medulloblastomas

- The most common primary brain tumor in children.
- Derived from an undifferentiated precursor to both astrocytes and neurons, medulloblastomas are most often found in the cerebellar vermis.
- Present with symptoms of hydrocephalus.
- Treatment consists of surgical resection followed by radiation therapy.
- Because these tumors are at risk for spread through the CSF system, craniospinal radiation is advocated.

Extra-Axial Brain Tumors

Meningiomas

- After astrocytomas, most common primary brain tumor.
- Meningiomas do not invade the brain unless they are malignant, but they can invade and erode the skull or cause a hyperostotic reaction.
- Usually found in adults and are more common in women.
- Appear isointense to brain on T1 and T2 MRI sequences but enhance strongly and homogeneously with gadolinium.
- Primary treatment should be surgery because cure is possible if a complete resection is accomplished.
- Stereotactic radiosurgery offers a new tool for the control of residual tumor growth.

- Large (>4 cm) residual or recurrent meningiomas may require treatment with conventional fractionated radiation therapy.
- Chemotherapy does not now play a significant role in the treatment of this tumor.

Schwannomas

- Most commonly arise from cranial nerve VIII (vestibuloacoustic nerve).
- Bilateral acoustic tumors in young adults suggest neurofibromatosis 2 (NF2).
- Treatment is surgical resection or radiosurgery.

Pituitary Adenomas

- Cells in the anterior pituitary may give rise to benign pituitary adenomas.
- Described as functional or nonfunctional, depending on whether the tumor secretes an anterior pituitary hormone.
- The most common functional tumor is the *prolactinoma,* which causes amenorrhea and galactorrhea in women; dopamine agonists such as bromocriptine can shrink prolactinomas in 80% of cases.
- Overproduction of adrenocorticotrophic hormone by a pituitary adenoma causes Cushing's disease.
- A growth hormone–secreting adenoma causes acromegaly, which results in growth of the hands, feet, lower jaw, and supraorbital ridge; most serious effects of acromegaly are hypertension, cardiomegaly, and hyperglycemia.
- Nonfunctional pituitary adenomas typically present with mass effect on adjacent structures, notably the optic chiasm, and manifests a bitemporal field cut.
- Tumors can be approached through the nose via a trans-septal, trans-sphenoidal opening in the sella; no scalp incisions or brain retraction is required for complete removal of pituitary tumors.

Secondary Brain Tumors

Metastatic Brain Tumors

- By virtue of disproportionately high blood flow, the brain is a common site for metastases.
- Most common primary origins are lungs (35%), breast (20%), skin (melanoma) (10%), kidney (10%), and gastrointestinal tract (5%).

- MRI is the preferred screening study.
- Management is dependent on the number of lesions, their size, and the condition of the patient.
- A large (>4 cm) metastasis causing neurologic compromise should be resected, if surgically accessible, and then followed with whole-brain radiation therapy (WBRT).
- A smaller, single metastasis causing neurologic deficit may be removed or treated with radiosurgery and WBRT or with WBRT alone.
- Prognosis is improved when the primary tumor is controlled and the extent of metastatic disease is limited.
- Chemotherapy is not useful in most brain metastases, with the exception of small cell lung cancer and seminomas.

TRAUMATIC HEAD INJURY

- Trauma causes approximately 150,000 deaths in the United States annually.
- In addition, there are 10,000 new spinal cord injuries annually.

Initial Evaluation of the Patient with Severe Head Injury

- Using the well-established Glasgow Coma Scale (GCS), patients who will not open their eyes even to a painful stimulus, will not utter words, or will not follow even the simplest commands are considered to be in a coma.
- A dilated pupil, particularly in cases in which traumatic injury of the globe can be excluded, often indicates the side of a mass lesion, such as a hematoma where the clot has displaced the mesial-temporal lobe structures compressing the ocular motor nerve.
- The CT scan can be used to assess the presence and location of hematomas, contusions, and brain swelling and the presence of herniation either across the midline or across the tentorium where there is actual or incipient compression of the upper brainstem (Table 70–1).

Primary and Secondary Injuries

- Primary injury includes diffuse axonal injury, contusion, hematoma, and traumatic subarachnoid hemorrhage.
- Although contusions and hematomas usually are evident immediately after an impact, they can increase in size particularly over the first 12 to 24 hours, and very early CT scan may not be sufficient to evaluate their full effect; in most centers a second, delayed CT scan is then the routine.

TABLE 70–1. Scoring with the Glasgow Coma Scale

Eye-Opening Response		Verbal Response		Motor Response	
Score	Response	Score	Response	Score	Response
4	Spontaneous	5	Oriented	6	Obeys commands
3	To speech	4	Confused	5	Localizes to painful stimulus
2	To pain	3	Inappropriate responses	4	Withdraws to painful stimulus
1	No response	2	Incomprehensible responses	2	Extension to painful stimulus
		1	No response	1	No response

- Extra-axial clots include acute subdural hematoma and epidural hematoma.
- Secondary injuries are potentially preventable and treatable and include the effects of hypotension and hypoxia and herniation with elevated ICP resulting from mass effect.
- The correction of shock and hypoxia is the first level of management of head-injured patients, and any head-injured patient who is suspected of having poor ventilation should be intubated urgently.
- Secondary brainstem injury frequently occurs from mass effect, which is usually supratentorial; herniation then occurs across the tentorium with secondary brainstem compression.

Intracranial Pressure

- Evaluation of the patient with severe head injury during the acute period relies on rigorous and frequent monitoring of the patient's neurologic examination; GCS score; the pupils; arterial blood gases; and, in many cases, ICP.
- ICP monitoring is usually started after the initial CT scan in patients not taken to the operating room for evacuation of a mass lesion; even patients taken to the operating room frequently have ICP monitors placed at the end of the operation.

Nonoperative Management

- Initial management is assessment and treatment of shock and hypoxia, a search for other injury, or coagulopathy.
- A lateral cervical spine x-ray film that visualizes the cervical spine from the cranial cervical junction to the C7-T1 interspace is extremely important.
- A patient with a significant clot or contusion should be taken to the operating room for evacuation provided there is no severe coagulopathy.
- When no operative lesion is found by CT, which occurs in approximately 70% of cases, the patient is treated by medical management primarily directed at normalization of ICP.
- A repeat CT scan should be made routinely during the first 12 to 24 hours and again if ICP becomes elevated.
- In patients without significant mass effect and in patients after evacuation of the mass, the following steps should be taken:
  - The head of the bed is elevated to 30 degrees, and the head is placed in a neutral position.
  - A firm collar should be used until stability of the cervical spine can be shown later by flexion and extension views of the neck.

- ICP should be maintained below 20 mm Hg, and cerebral profusion pressure (CPP) should be maintained above 70 mm Hg.
- Hypotension, particularly a mean arterial blood pressure of less than 90 mm Hg, should be prevented or treated.
- ICP elevations of more than 20 mm Hg should be actively treated.
- The first line of management is the drainage of ventricular fluid when possible, that is, there has been placement of a ventricular catheter and the use of short-acting sedatives and muscle relaxants even though neurologic examination is lost and greater reliance is placed on ICP monitoring and CT scanning; these drugs can be intermittently discontinued and the patient evaluated periodically.
- If ICP elevations still occur, mannitol or other diuretics are used.
- The role of hyperventilation has become controversial; the mechanism of action is reduction in brain blood volume and thereby mass effect via a change in cerebrovascular tone (vasoconstriction); although brain blood volume is reduced, so is cerebral blood flow, and ischemia has been shown to be a common event in patients with severe head injury.
- When ICP becomes refractory to these strategies, a CT scan is mandatory.
- In cases without new mass lesions, barbiturate therapy to lower ICP has been advocated.
- Another option is decompressive craniotomy.

Operative Management

- Clots or contusions larger than 25 to 30 cm^3 are generally considered to cause significant mass effect capable of causing neurologic deterioration and progressive brain injury.

DEGENERATIVE DISORDERS OF THE SPINE

Lumbar Radiculopathy

- As individuals age, the annulus normally desiccates, and because of this process, it becomes more susceptible to tearing or rupture.
- Disc herniations can occur in any direction, but the most clinically significant are those that occur posterolaterally.
- Disc material extruded in this location may compress a nerve root or the cauda equina, causing radicular symptoms and signs in the anatomic distribution of the affected nerve root.

- Large, central herniations may compress the cauda equina or result in bilateral radicular symptoms.
- Desiccation of the herniated disc material can lead to shrinkage of the herniated fragment with resolution of the patients' signs and symptoms.
- In the lumbar spine, at least 90% of disc herniations occur at the L5-S1 or L4-L5 levels (Table 70–2).
- Radicular pain on flexion of the straight leg at the hip (Laségue sign) is one of the most important tests in the diagnosis of a herniated disc.
- Unless the patient's signs are associated with sphincter disturbance or significant weakness in a radicular distribution, most patients are treated medically for 2 weeks.
- A large number of nonoperative therapies are available and include rest, analgesics, muscle relaxants, and the application of heat.
- After the acute period of pain has resolved, physical therapy with attention to lumbosacral exercises may prevent recurrences.
- If conservative measures fail to relieve the patient's symptoms or if sphincter disturbances or weakness occurs, imaging of the spine is indicated.
- MRI is the preferred method for imaging the spine, but in selected patients postmyelography CT may be helpful.
- Indications for surgery include radicular pain that does not improve with conservative measures, recurrent episodes of incapacitating pain, disc herniations associated with significant weakness in the appropriate muscle groups, and massive midline herniations with signs of cauda equina compression.

Degenerative Cervical Lesions

Clinical Presentation

Cervical Radiculopathy

- The usual history is that of a proximal radiating arm pain with numbness and paresthesias distally in the nerve root distribution.
- The pain and paresthesias may be intensified by neck movement.
- The most common root compression syndromes are those involving the sixth and seventh cervical roots.
- With C6 root compression, the pain is in a radicular distribution down the arm, distal to the elbow, and paresthesias

TABLE 70–2. Clinical Findings of Common Lumber Disc Herniations

Disc	Nerve Root	Pain	Sensory Change	Motor Deficits	Reflex Loss
L3–4	L4	Anterior thigh, anterior leg, medial ankle	Anterior leg	Quadriceps	Knee jerk
L4–5	L5	Posterior hip and posterolateral thigh and leg	Medial dorsum of foot and occasionally medial ankle	Foot and toe extension	None
L5–S1	S1	Hip, buttock, and posterior thigh and leg	Lateral foot and ankle	Plantar flexion	Ankle jerk

or sensory loss over the thumb and index finger; biceps weakness (flexion of the elbow) and weakness in extension of the wrist, is present, and diminution of the biceps and brachioradialis reflex may be present.

- With C7 root compression, the pain radiates down the back of the arm distal to the elbow; triceps muscle weakness (extension of the elbow) and weakness in flexion of the wrist are hallmarks of this nerve root compression.
- Eighth nerve root compression causes pain down the arm and sensory changes that involve the ulnar side of the hand, but they usually present with intrinsic hand muscle weakness.

Myelopathy

- Compression of the spinal cord can lead to cervical myelopathy, which is manifested by motoneuron dysfunction at the level of compression and upper motoneuron dysfunction (spasticity, clonus, increased deep tendon reflexes, Babinski's sign, and Hoffmann's sign) below the level.
- These patients usually complain of poor muscle coordination, especially in their hands and when walking.

Diagnostic Studies

- MRI is the procedure of choice as an initial diagnostic tool to evaluate cervical radiculopathy and myelopathy.
- In some cases in which the diagnosis is not immediately apparent, a cervical myelogram followed by CT scanning could yield definitive information.
- In cases in which the clinical diagnosis is in doubt and other causes, such as plexopathies or peripheral nerve compression, must be excluded, electromyography and nerve conduction studies are helpful.

Treatment

- The initial treatment of a patient with acute radiculopathy is conservative and consists of restriction of activity, soft cervical collar, and medication for pain and muscle spasm.
- Anti-inflammatory and antispasmodic medication may be of value over a prolonged period to reduce the discomfort of cervical spondylosis.
- The majority of the patient's symptoms will improve with conservative treatment.

- There are two indications to perform surgery in patients with cervical radiculopathy.
  - Failed medical management with intolerable arm pain.
  - Progressive and significant motor loss.
- The aim of surgery is to provide nerve root decompression, and this can be accomplished by either a posterior approach through a foraminotomy or by an anterior approach through the intervertebral disc.
- Cervical myelopathy poses a far greater surgical challenge.
- Conservative therapy plays only a minor role in these patients, and surgery is indicated far more urgently than radiculopathy because compression of the spinal cord poses a significant risk to the patient's spinal cord function.

FUNCTIONAL NEUROSURGERY

Stereotactic Neurosurgery

- *Stereotactic neurosurgery* is defined as the use of a coordinate system to provide accurate navigation to a point or region in space.
- The coordinate system may be a fixed stereotactic frame that is rigidly attached to the skull, or it may be based on a frameless system that uses fiducial markers placed on the scalp that are then correlated with MRI or CT results.
- Medically intractable patients with Parkinson's disease may be treated by deep brain stimulation in the subthalamic nucleus.
- Radiosurgery uses multiple beams of radiation focused to a single point to treat brain tumors, vascular malformations, and trigeminal neuralgia.

Epilepsy Surgery

- Epilepsy is a complex condition with recurrent seizures not resulting from an active provoked cause.
- In the United States, there are more than 100,000 new cases a year.
- Of these, 60,000 are temporal lobe epilepsy, characterized most frequently by partial complex seizures, and of these, 25% are medically intractable.
- Of the intractable group, one third are probably candidates for seizure surgery—in this particular case, a partial anterior temporal lobectomy.
- Other types of operations include excision of seizure foci at sites other than the temporal lobe, hemispherectomy, and section of the corpus callosum (callosal callosotomy).

The Workup

- The initial workup is the search for remediable or treatable causes for the chronic recurrent seizures.
  - Structural lesions.
  - Brain tumors.
  - Cerebrovascular abnormalities such as AVMs or cavernous malformations.
- When seizures are associated with structural lesions, removal of the lesion itself, or lobectomy (early in the course of the seizures), is frequently sufficient to result in a seizure-free life.
- CT or, in most cases, MRI is an important part of the initial workup.

Surgery

Resection of a Seizure Focus

- The most frequent operation of this kind is *temporal lobectomy*.
- The second most common site after a temporal lobectomy is the frontal cortex.
- The results here, however, are in general less predictable than with temporal lobe resections.

Other Cranial Operations for Generalized Seizures

- Section of the corpus callosum callosotomy is used to interrupt the spread of severe seizures and mitigate generalization; indications are otherwise not specific, but the operation is usually reserved for severe cases, frequently where there are drop attacks (atonic seizures) and thereby a significant risk of injury.
- Hemispherectomy is an operation usually restricted to children with extensive unilateral epileptiform activity.

Vagal Nerve Stimulator

- Reduction in seizure frequency is usually 50%, which is similar to the result of many drugs but without drug side effects.
- Only 1% of patients with vagal nerve stimulators become seizure free.

Neurosurgical Treatments for Pain

- There are two broad categories of pain: nociceptive and neuropathic.

- *Nociceptive pain* is caused by the activation of peripheral sensory receptors by an unusually strong stimulus.
- *Neuropathic pain* is poorly understood and is characterized by a lack of peripheral stimulation, such as central pain that occurs after a stroke; it frequently contains elements of burning, tingling, or electric shocks and is poorly responsive to narcotic medications.
- Neurosurgical treatments may be either neuroablative or neuroaugmentive.

Trigeminal Neuralgia

- Characterized by brief episodes of severe, lancinating pain in the distribution of the trigeminal nerve.
- The cause is unknown, but patients usually have arterial compression of the trigeminal nerve near the root entry zone.
- Surgical treatments include microvascular decompression, glycerol rhizotomy, and gamma knife radiosurgery.

Neuroablation Procedures

Neurectomy

- Transection of a peripheral nerve results in numbness and may temporarily relieve pain, but it is not a viable long-term therapy.
- The pain may recur and become neuropathic in nature.
- Because most peripheral nerves are mixed sensorimotor, neurectomy will result in motor loss as well.

Rhizotomy

- Open ablation of the sensory root can be performed via an intradural or extradural approach or percutaneously using radiofrequency coagulation or phenol injection.
- Rhizotomy may be useful for pain with distribution in a limited number of dermatomes.

Dorsal Root Entry Zone Lesion

- This treatment is most successful for nerve root or brachial plexus avulsion and spinal cord injury.
- It has also been used for postherpetic neuralgia and post-thoracotomy pain.

- Extension of this concept to the trigeminal nucleus caudalis has been used to treat anesthesia dolorosa, atypical facial pain, and postherpetic neuralgia.

Cordotomy

- Performed percutaneously with radiofrequency lesioning of the spinothalamic tract in the anterior portion of the cervical spinal cord.

Myelotomy

- This procedure is most often used for bilateral nociceptive pain resulting from cancer.

Midbrain Tractotomy

- This procedure ablates the spinothalamic tract in the brainstem with the use of stereotactic guidance.
- The most common indication is for face and shoulder pain from head and neck cancer.

Cingulotomy

- This procedure is most useful when depression is the dominant feature of the pain syndrome.

Sympathectomy

- Indicated for the treatment of causalgia, reflex sympathetic dystrophy, or Raynaud's phenomenon.
- The endoscopic approach is preferred.

Neuroaugmentation Procedures

Spinal Cord Stimulation

- Spinal cord stimulation is indicated for neuropathic pain syndromes, including peripheral nerve injury, reflex sympathetic dystrophy, deafferentation pain, and postherpetic neuralgia.
- Short-term success is seen in 80% of patients, with 50% having long-term pain relief.

Deep Brain Stimulation

- Two primary deep brain sites have been used for the relief of pain.
  - Periaqueductal gray.
  - Sensory thalamus.
- Periaqueductal gray has been used primarily for nociceptive pain and likely activates endogenous opioids.
- Thalamic stimulation is based on the gate control theory and is used for neuropathic pain.

Intrathecal Narcotic Infusion

- Continuous delivery of intrathecal morphine is made possible by an implantable, programmable pump.
- This treatment modality is usually used for nociceptive cancer pain.

SURGERY FOR CONGENITAL ABNORMALITIES

Myelomeningoceles

- Myelomeningoceles represent the most important clinical example of disordered neurulation because most affected infants survive.
- The essential defect is a failure of closure of the caudal neuropore.
- The resulting lesion by definition involves the spinal cord, a deficient axial skeleton, and an incomplete meningeal and dermal covering.
- The thoracolumbar junction is the most common level affected (45%), followed by lumbar (20%), lumbosacral (20%), and sacral (10%).
- Improvements in prenatal screening for neural tube defects and folic acid supplementation have contributed to a world-wide decline in the birth prevalence of myelomeningocele.
- Virtually all children born with a myelomeningocele will also have a constellation of associated anomalies of the skull, brain, spine, and spinal cord that have been collectively described as the *Chiari II malformation.*
- Between 80% and 90% of children born with myelomeningocele will develop hydrocephalus and require shunting.
- Myelomeningocele is repaired shortly after birth, usually within the first 48 hours.
- Surgical goals include elimination of CSF leakage, preservation of neurologic function, and prevention of infection.

Encephaloceles

- Disordered closure of the cranial neuropore can also result in various defects that are known to cause substantial neurologic dysfunction; the worldwide incidence is nearly 1 in 5000 live births.
- One of the extreme forms, anencephaly, results from failure of cranial neuropore closure; this affects both the forebrain and brainstem and is not compatible with survival.

Hydrocephalus

- Results from an imbalance between the production and absorption of CSF.
- Communicating hydrocephalus is present when an obstruction to the flow of the CSF occurs outside of the ventricular system, usually at the level of the basal subarachnoid cisterns or at the arachnoid granulations.
- Noncommunicating hydrocephalus results from lesions that create an obstruction to CSF flow within the ventricular system.
- In nearly all cases, hydrocephalus results from the decreased absorption of CSF. Only in the rare case of a choroid plexus papilloma has increased CSF production been implicated.
- Aqueductal stenosis is a major cause of hydrocephalus in the newborn and is responsible for nearly one third of congenital cases.
- Nearly 80% to 90% of children born with myelomeningocele will develop hydrocephalus because of fourth ventricular outlet obstruction and compromise of the posterior fossa subarachnoid cisterns.
- The Dandy-Walker malformation is another cause of congenital hydrocephalus and is characterized by the absence of the cerebellar vermis, cystic expansion of the fourth ventricle, and hydrocephalus.
- Viral and parasitic exposure *in utero* is a well-known cause of congenital hydrocephalus, with cytomegalovirus and toxoplasmosis having been implicated in many cases.
- *Acquired* forms of hydrocephalus usually occur after intraventricular hemorrhage or after an episode of meningitis.
- The clinical features of hydrocephalus are related to the development of elevated ICP.
- In the newborn, excessive head enlargement with an enlarged, tense anterior fontanelle and open cranial sutures are common presentations.

- The presentation in an older child is more acute because the moderating effects of open cranial sutures are not present; severe headache, vomiting, and lethargy are the usual presenting signs in these children.
- CT scanning remains the most commonly used imaging technique for screening or emergent indications and is preferred when a more detailed assessment of intracranial morphology is required.
- MRI is becoming the imaging modality of choice in many clinical situations.
- Most cases are treated by diversion of CSF from the cerebral ventricles to the peritoneal cavity via a ventriculoperitoneal shunt; other less favored sites for diversion include the pleural cavity and the superior vena cava.

CENTRAL NERVOUS SYSTEM INFECTIONS

- Acute bacterial meningitis is an infection of the subarachnoid spaces and meninges.
- Bacteria responsible may spread to the subarachnoid space from an infection of contiguous structure such as the paranasal sinuses or through the bloodstream.
- The causative organism will vary depending on the patient's age.
    - Newborns tend to be infected by gram-negative enteric organisms such as *Escherichia coli* and *Klebsiella*.
    - In children, *Haemophilus influenzae* pneumococci and meningococci are the predominant organisms.
    - Meningitis in adults is usually caused by either pneumococcal or meningococcal infection.
- Symptoms are due to leptomeningeal irritation and elevated ICP and usually include fever, neck stiffness, and headache.
- Once meningitis is suspected, treatment should begin immediately, sometimes even before obtaining a CSF specimen if the clinical suspicion is high.
- Surgery is usually reserved for cases complicated by hydrocephalus.

CHAPTER 71

PLASTIC SURGERY

INTRODUCTION

- "The specialty of plastic surgery deals with the repair, replacement, and reconstruction of physical defects of form or function involving the skin, musculoskeletal system, craniomaxillofacial structures, hand, extremities, breast and trunk, and external genitalia. It uses aesthetic surgical principles not only to improve undesirable qualities of normal structures, but in all reconstructive procedures as well."

GENERAL PLASTIC SURGICAL PRINCIPLES AND TECHNIQUES

Skin Incisions and Excisions

- Skin creases and hair bearing areas are useful places to camouflage incisions.
- Tension should be avoided across skin incisions, because it will result in wide and unsightly scars.
- When possible, incisions should be placed perpendicular to the long axis of the underlying muscle.
- The most favorable excision design is the double lenticular or elliptical design with a 4:1 length-to-width ratio.

Open Wounds

- Wound closure by primary healing or first intention involves closure of the wound by direct skin approximation, flap, or skin graft.
- Spontaneous healing, or secondary intention, involves wound healing without surgical manipulation. Tertiary healing, healing by third intention, or delayed primary closure combines tenants of both primary healing and spontaneous healing.
- Wound healing is negatively affected by systemic, regional, or local factors (Fig. 71–1).
- Two common problems encountered in chronic open wounds are malnutrition and bacterial inoculation.

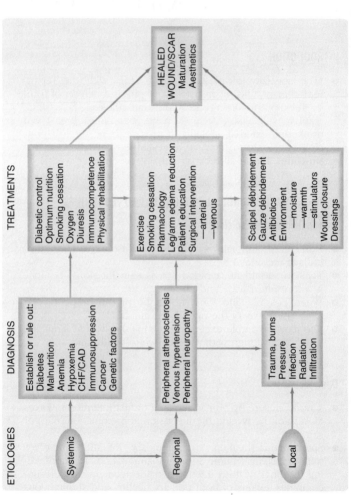

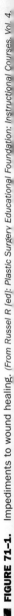

FIGURE 71–1. Impediments to wound healing. *(From Russel R [ed]: Plastic Surgery Educational Foundation: Instructional Courses, Vol. 4.*

Wound Closure

- In general, expeditious closure of wounds is one of the goals of plastic surgery and should follow a reconstructive ladder beginning with the simple and advancing to the complex as the wound dictates (Box 71–1). An optimal linear closure is seen when the skin edges are coapted under minimal tension without redundant skin mounds (dog-ears) at the incisional poles.
- Dermal approximation is of paramount importance, because it should bear most of the tension dispersed across the skin interface.
- Epidermal skin sutures function for fine alignment of skin edges.

Débridement and Irrigation

- Although technically easy, proper wound débridement requires astute surgical judgment and careful inspection. Débridement implies the removal of devitalized and contaminated tissues while preserving critical structures such as nerves, blood vessels, tendons, and bone. Extent of débridement is modified according to wound type.
- In addition to débridement, wound irrigation, with or without antibiotics, should be a mainstay of infection control.

Grafts and Flaps

- Skin grafts can be divided based on thickness: full-thickness and split-thickness grafts (Fig. 71–2).
- Split-thickness grafts are especially valuable to close larger wounds.
- Thin split-thickness grafts contract to a greater extent than thick split-thickness or full-thickness grafts.
- There are three steps in the "take" of a skin graft: imbibition, inosculation, and revascularization.
- The most common causes of skin graft failure are hematoma (or seroma), infection, and movement (shear).

Box 71–1. Reconstructive Ladder	
Linear closure	Myocutaneous flaps
Skin grafts	Free flaps
Skin flaps	

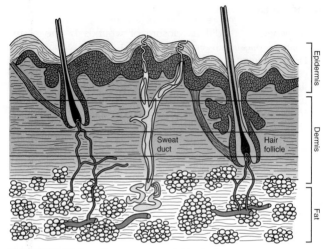

■ FIGURE 71–2.   Cross section of skin depicting levels contained in split-thickness and full-thickness skin grafts. *(Modified from Townsend CM [ed]: Sabiston Textbook of Surgery: The Biological Basis of Modern Surgical Practice, 16th ed. Philadelphia, WB Saunders, 2000, p 1553.)*

- Special considerations in choosing a skin graft donor site include skin quality and color from the donor region that will best match the recipient site.

Flaps

- A flap is defined as a partially or completely isolated segment of tissue perfused with its own blood supply.
- Flaps vary greatly in terms of complexity from simple skin flaps with a random blood supply to microvascular free flaps containing composite tissue.
- Random flaps rely on the low perfusion pressures found in the subdermal plexus to sustain the flap and not a named blood vessel.
- Advancement and rotation flaps represent commonly used random patten skin flaps (Figs. 71–3 and 71–4).
- An axial flap is based on a named blood vessel and can provide a reproducible and stable skin or skin and muscle (myocutaneous) flap. Flaps can also be raised with the underlying fascia (fasciocutaneous), which recruits the fascial

Advancement   Rotation

■ **FIGURE 71–3.** Graphic representation of commonly used local flaps: advancement and rotation flaps.

blood supply thereby increasing the predictable vascularity to the flap.

- An axial flap that remains attached to its proximal blood supply and is transposed to a defect is known as a pedicled flap.
- Microsurgery.
  - The relatively recent advent of microsurgery has dramatically altered the practice of plastic surgery and allows the surgeon a plethora of reconstructive options that were not previously available.
- Clinical assessment remains the gold standard for free flap monitoring.
- The most common cause of flap failure is venous congestion.

HEAD AND NECK: CONGENITAL AND CRANIOMAXILLOFACIAL

Cleft Lip and Palate

- Epidemiologic analysis is important when advising expectant parents. Cleft lip and palate occurs in approximately 1 in 1000 live births.
- An isolated cleft palate occurs in approximately 1 in 2000 live births.
- The etiology of clefting of the lip and palate remains unknown, but a multifactorial combination of heredity with environmental factors seems most plausible.
- Cleft patients require a wide variety of specialists.
- Principles of cleft lip repair include layered repair of the skin, muscle, and mucous membrane to restore symmetric length and function.
- The goal of cleft palate repair is to establish a competent valve that can isolate the oral and nasal cavities, thus re-creating the muscular sling necessary for palatal elevation.

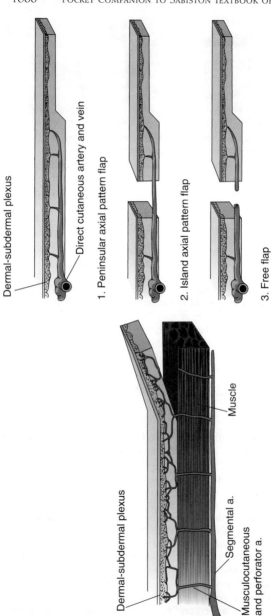

A Random pattern skin flap

Dermal-subdermal plexus

Muscle

Segmental a.

Musculocutaneous
and perforator a.

Dermal-subdermal plexus

Direct cutaneous artery and vein

1. Peninsular axial pattern flap

2. Island axial pattern flap

3. Free flap

B Axial pattern skin flaps

FIGURE 71–4.   Vascular patterns of random pattern and axial skin flaps. *(From Place MJ, Herber SC, Hardesty RA: Basic techniques and principles in plastic surgery. In Aston SJ, Beasley RW, Thorne CHM [eds]: Grabb and Smith's Plastic Surgery, 5th ed. Philadelphia, Lippincott-Raven, 1997, p 21.)*

Other Congenital Anomalies

- Embryologic development of the head and neck begins at the fourth week with the formation of the branchial apparatus.
- Ear deformities are commonly encountered in newborn infants and vary widely in severity.
- Minor abnormalities in ear shape can sometimes be overcome with early splinting or taping of the newborn's ear.
- For anotia or microtia, surgical repair is recommended at age 7.
- When ears protrude excessively from the temporal scalp, otoplasty provides the surgical correction.

Less Common Anomalies

- Craniofacial surgery is a reconstructive discipline that addresses the skull, the facial skeleton, and soft tissues of the face.
- Access to the craniofacial skeleton is accomplished through inconspicuous incisions.
- Premature fusion of the cranial sutures is known as craniosynostosis, and occurs 1 in 2000 live births. Craniosynostosis can limit the skull's volume and increase intracranial pressure.
- When premature skull fusion is documented, surgical correction is performed in conjunction with a neurosurgeon.
- Maxillofacial surgery addresses dental occlusion with selective osteotomies of facial bones.

Trauma

- For more severe injuries, a trauma evaluation is mandatory with establishment of a secure airway and cervical spine clearance before management of the facial injury.
- Physical examination should include careful attention to facial nerve (cranial nerve VII) function and parotid duct integrity.
- Meticulous reapproximation of the anatomy should be undertaken as soon as the patient's general medical condition allows.
- Tetanus prophylaxis should be administered.
- Common fractures of the facial skeleton include nasal fractures, mandible fractures, zygomatic complex (ZMC), maxilla (Le Fort I, II, and III), naso-orbital-ethmoid complex (NOE), and frontal sinus fractures. Nasal fractures are the most common facial fractures.
- It is mandatory to assess the nasal septum for a possible septal hematoma.

- Naso-orbital-ethmoid fractures.
  - Present with a complex nasal fracture including a saddle nose deformity, a wide nasal root with loss of anterior projection, and telecanthus.
- Fractures of the frontal sinus.
  - Damage to the nasofrontal duct and posterior wall of the frontal sinus must be identified.
  - Cerebrospinal fluid rhinorrhea indicates fracture involvement of the posterior wall of the frontal sinus.
- Facial height and projection depend on a complex bony buttressing system.
- Fractures of the zygoma, or malar bone, are known as zygomatic complex or ZMC fractures.
- These patients present with eye findings.
- For fractures involving the orbital floor, indications for surgical exploration include diplopia, extraocular muscle entrapment, and enophthalmos. Orbital injury that affects the superior orbital fissure is a surgical emergency.
- Superior orbital fissure syndrome.
- Orbital apex syndrome.
- Midface fractures involving the maxilla can be classified by fracture patterns known as Le Fort I, II, and III.
- This procedure known as interdental or intermaxillary (IMF) fixation is necessary to re-establish the proper dento-skeletal relationships, immobilize the fractured bones, and ensure normal postoperative occlusion.
- Mandible fractures are second only to nasal fractures in frequency.
- Cervical spine clearance is recommended because up to a 10% coincident of cervical spine trauma is reported in association with mandible fractures.
- The airway can be compromised in patients with bilateral subcondylar mandible fractures.
- As in midface fractures, restoration of dental occlusion forms the foundation for fracture management.
- Many patients with mandibular fractures experience trauma to the inferior alveolar nerve (a branch of the trigeminal nerve).
- Condylar and subcondylar mandible fractures are most often treated by IMF alone.

HEAD AND NECK

Facial Nerve Palsy

- The facial nerve, cranial nerve VII, is responsible for innervating muscles of facial expression (mimetic muscles).

- There are five distinct branches of the facial nerve: frontal (temporal), zygomatic, buccal, marginal mandibular, and cervical.
- A three-dimensional understanding of facial nerve anatomy is essential to identify or protect a nerve branch.
- The most common cause of facial paralysis is Bell's palsy.
- Most patients with Bell's palsy have a complete remission.
- Trauma in the form of temporal bone fractures or deep facial lacerations is the second most frequent cause of facial palsy.
- Immediate exploration and primary repair of the facial nerve affords the best chance to regain nerve function.

TRUNK AND EXTERNAL GENITALIA

Chest Wall Reconstruction

- More complex defects usually require flap reconstruction.
- Larger defects, greater than 10 cm with loss of more than three adjacent ribs, can risk flail chest with attendant compromised respiratory function.
- Wound infection and dehiscence occurs in approximately 2% of median sternotomies.
- A muscle flap will also recruit much needed blood supply to the area to assist in healing and controlling infection.

Breast Reconstruction

- Breast cancer is the most common malignant neoplasm in women affecting approximately 1 in 8 females in the United States.
- The reconstructive surgeon must account for this deficient skin envelope in an attempt to recreate the breast mound.
- The simplest form of breast reconstruction is tissue expansion followed by placement of permanent breast implants.
- This is the most popular mode of breast reconstruction.
- The breast mound can be created using myocutaneous flaps such as the transverse rectus abdominis myocutaneous (TRAM) flap or the latissimus dorsi myocutaneous flap. The TRAM flap uses the infraumbilical and suprapubic fat, which derives its blood supply from the underlying rectus abdominis muscle.
- Latissimus dorsi muscle.
- Based on the thoracodorsal vessels.
- The contralateral breast should always be considered as part of the total reconstructive procedure.

Abdominal Wall Reconstruction

- Prosthetic fabrics such as polytetrafluoroethylene (PTFE) and polypropylene are widely used to span preperitoneal defects.
- In the case of infection, the mesh must be removed and the infection cleared before closure is attempted.
- Large abdominal hernias, which have failed mesh repair, may be amenable to closure by component separation.

Pressure Sores

- One of the most costly problems in modern medicine is pressure sores, which are derived from prolonged immobility.
- Pressure sores commonly occur over pressure-bearing surfaces such as the occipital scalp, elbows, heels, iliac crests, greater trochanters, ischial tuberosities, and the sacrum. Pressure sores result from tissue ischemia occurring from prolonged pressure exceeding capillary arterial pressure of 32 mm Hg.
- Treatment of these wounds requires a multidisciplinary approach with focus on prevention of reoccurrence.
- The simplest involves four grades: grade I (skin erythema), grade II (skin ulceration with necrosis into subcutaneous tissue), grade III (necrosis involving the underlying muscle), and grade IV (exposed bone/joint).

External Genitalia

- For those infants with ambiguous external genitalia, gender reassignment (usually female) should be done by 18 months of age.
- Fournier's gangrene is a mixed aerobic and anaerobic infection that spreads rapidly along fascial planes.

LOWER EXTREMITY

Trauma

- Re-establishment of normal or near normal ambulation in a sensate extremity is the goal in lower extremity trauma.
- Fasciotomy is often required to prevent ischemic changes in muscle and nerve tissues following high-energy or crush injuries.
- Thigh injuries can generally be managed with delayed primary closure or skin grafting alone.

TABLE 71-1. Gustilo Classification of Open Fractures of the Tibia

Type	Description
I	Open fracture with a wound <1 cm
II	Open fracture with a wound >1 cm without extensive soft tissue damage
III	Open fracture with extensive soft tissue damage
IIIA	III with adequate soft tissue coverage
IIIB	III with soft tissue loss with periosteal stripping and bone exposure
IIIC	III with arterial injury requiring repair

- Fractures of the lower leg are most often classified according to the Gustilo system (Table 71–1).

Venous Stasis, Ischemic, and Diabetic Ulcers

- Lower extremity ulcers may have a similar appearance but often have differing etiologies and treatment needs.
- Venous stasis ulcers result from venous hypertension, which is usually caused by valvular incompetence.
- Treatment regimens focus on increasing venous return and decreasing edema.
- Arterial inflow should be checked using noninvasive Doppler studies that record the ankle/brachial index.
- Ischemic lower extremity ulcers are due to arterial insufficiency from proximal arterial occlusion.
- Associated with very low ankle/brachial index readings between 0.1 to 0.3.
- These ulcers will not heal without surgical revascularization of the extremity.
- Diabetic ulcers commonly result from decreased protective sensation.
- Treatment is focused on preventing further damage to the area.

Lymphedema

- Lymphedema is an accumulation of protein and fluid in the subcutaneous tissue.
- Lymphedema praecox.
- Lymphedema tarda.
- Surgical techniques offer only symptomatic relief, and there is no procedure that reliably produces a cure.

BREAST AND AESTHETIC SURGERY

- Macromastia (abnormally large breasts) is a functionally difficult and psychology devastating problem for some women (Fig. 71–5).
- For males, the problem of large breasts (gynecomastia) can be psychologically devastating.
- Gynecomastia can be due to abnormal hormone levels.
- Breast augmentation is usually accomplished through discrete incisions placed around the areola, at the inframammary fold, or in the axilla.
- With age and childbearing, breasts will sag below the level of the inframammary crease resulting in breast ptosis.
- Breast ptosis is classified as grade I (nipple areolar complex [NAC] position at the level of the inframammary fold), grade II ptosis (NAC position below the inframammary fold), and grade III ptosis (NAC position well below the inframammary fold and pointing down).
- Lipodystrophy, excess fatty deposits in distinct anatomic areas, and redundant skin can be addressed through suction-assisted lipectomy (SAL) or excisional techniques, respectively.
- Although large-volume liposuction has been reported in the literature, the surgeon must be cautious because large

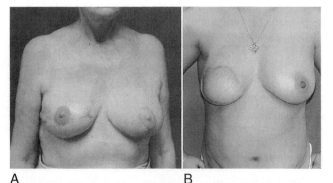

A   B

■ **FIGURE 71–5.**   *A,* A 63-year-old woman after right mastectomy with tissue expander followed by implant reconstruction, right nipple reconstruction with tattooing of the nipple areolar complex, and contralateral full-scar mastopexy. *B,* A 43-year-old woman after right mastectomy with autologous tissue reconstruction with transverse rectus abdominis myocutaneous (TRAM) flap.

intravascular fluid shifts may occur when volumes in excess of 5000 mL are aspirated.

- Excision techniques are necessary in cases in which redundant skin, abundant striae, or ptotic changes are present.
- Brachioplasty.
- Thigh lift.
- Abdominoplasty.
- Facial aging, although unavoidable, can be drastically hastened with sun exposure, smoking, and poor skin care.

CHAPTER 72

HAND SURGERY

CLINICAL ANATOMY

- The hand has five digits: the thumb and four fingers (note that the thumb is not called a finger).
- The four fingers are called the index, long, ring, and small fingers.
- The anatomic structures of the hand can be broadly classified into six groups depending on the principal function that they perform: covering, supporting, restraining, feeding, controlling, and moving.

Covering Structures

- The skin of the hand is highly specialized.
- The palmar skin, especially at the fingertips, is endowed with a profusion of sensory end organs, such as pacinian bodies, Merkel discs, and Meissner corpuscles.
- The palmar skin is fixed to the underlying aponeurosis by retinacula cutis at the skin creases.
- The nail is a hardened keratinous outgrowth from skin and protects the dorsal aspect of the sensitive fingertip.

Supporting Structures

- The skeletal elements of the hand comprise the distal radius and ulna, 8 carpal bones, 5 metacarpals, and 14 phalanges.
- The thumb has only two phalanges, whereas the other four digits have three each.
- The wrist joint is a complex articulation of the distal radius and ulna with the carpal bones.
- The proximal carpal row comprising the scaphoid, lunate, and triquetrum (with the exception of the outlying pisiform) is devoid of any muscular insertion.
- The distal carpal row is formed by the trapezium, trapezoid, capitate, and hamate.
- Flexion and extension of the wrist principally occur at the midcarpal joint, whereas radial and ulnar deviations occur mainly at the radiocarpal articulation.

- The carpometacarpal joint (CMCJ) of the thumb is the most mobile of all joints in the hand.
- The metacarpophalangeal joints (MCPJs) are condyloid joints and can move in three planes.
- Flexion-extension occur on a transverse axis in the sagittal plane, abduction-adduction take place on an anteroposterior axis in the coronal plane, and a small amount of rotation occurs on the longitudinal axis of each metacarpal in the transverse plane.
- The interphalangeal joints (IPJs) are essentially hinge joints and principally permit flexion and extension.
- The capsules of the MCPJs and IPJs are reinforced on either side by collateral ligaments.
- The volar capsules of these joints display a specialized fibro-cartilaginous thickening termed the *volar plate*.

Restraining Structures

- The palmar aponeurosis consists mainly of three components: a central triangular portion with thenar and hypothenar slips on either side.
- The fibrous flexor sheath is a specialized osteofibrous tunnel through which the long flexor tendons of the digits pass.
- The flexor sheath of each finger displays localized thickenings known as pulleys that are particularly important in preventing bowstringing of the tendons.
- These pulleys may be annular or cruciate.
- The flexor retinaculum spans the transverse arch of the carpus and forms the roof of the carpal tunnel; it prevents bowstringing of the long flexor tendons during flexion of the wrist.
- On the dorsal side, this function is taken over by the extensor retinaculum, which restrains the long extensors of the wrist and digits.

Feeding Structures

- The blood supply to the hand is principally from the radial and ulnar arteries.
- The radial and ulnar arteries each divide in the proximal part of the wrist into superficial and deep branches.
- The superficial palmar arch is usually dominated by the ulnar artery.
- In contrast, the deep palmar arch is usually dominated by the radial artery.

- The digital arteries of the thumb are located entirely on the volar aspect of the thumb.
- On the other hand, the digital arteries of the fingers are located on either side of the flexor sheath.

Controlling Structures

- The *radial nerve* provides extrinsic extensors of the hand, the wrist extensors, and the supinator.
- The *median nerve* innervates the flexor digitorum superficialis (FDS), the flexor pollicis longus, the two radial flexor digitorum profundus (FDP), the two radial lumbricals, and most of the thenar musculature.
- The *ulnar nerve* provides motor innervation to the flexor carpi ulnaris, the two ulnar FDP and lumbricals, the hypothenar musculature and interossei, the adductor pollicis, and the deep portion of the flexor pollicis brevis.

Moving Structures

Extrinsic Muscles

- The extensor muscles are located dorsally and divided into three subgroups:
  - The first subgroup consists of the brachioradialis, extensor carpi radialis longus, and extensor carpi radialis brevis (ECRB).
  - The second subgroup forms a superficial layer and consists of three muscles: the extensor carpi ulnaris extends and ulnarly deviates the wrist; the extensor digit quinti and extensor digitorum communis act primarily to extend the MCPJs of the small and remaining fingers, respectively.
  - The third subgroup is deep and consists of four muscles: the abductor pollicis longus, extensor pollicis brevis, and extensor pollicis longus act on the thumb, and the extensor indicis proprius acts on the index finger.
- The flexor muscles are arranged in three layers:
  - The first superficial group consists of the pronator teres, flexor carpi radialis, flexor carpi ulnaris, and palmaris longus muscles.
  - The intermediate group consists of the FDS, which independently flexes the proximal interphalangeal (PIP) joints.
  - The deep group contains three muscles: flexor pollicis longus, which flexes the IPJ of the thumb; FDP, which flexes the distal interphalangeal (DIP) joints of the fingers;

and pronator quadratus, which lies between the radius and ulna.

Intrinsic Muscles

- The intrinsic muscles originate at or distal to the wrist.
- Four *dorsal interossei* muscles and three *palmar interossei* muscles provide abduction and adduction, respectively.
- Four *lumbricals* originate on the FDP tendons and insert on the radial side of the extensor mechanism.

CLINICAL EVALUATION OF THE INJURED HAND

- Evaluation of the hand should be carried out in a systematic manner.
- Active and passive range of motion are ascertained; the vascularity of the hand is determined.
- Active bleeding suggests arterial injury and should be controlled with pressure and elevation.
- The ligation and clamping of vessels should be avoided.
- The Allen test should be performed in which the radial and ulnar arteries are occluded by the examiner and the patient is asked to open and close the hand a few times; pressure is then released from one artery, and perfusion is assessed; capillary refill should occur throughout the entire hand within 5 seconds; the test is then repeated for the other artery.
- Nerves are assessed for both sensory and motor function using the two-point discrimination test in which a paper clip is folded so that its ends are 4 mm apart; a patient is able to distinguish one and two ends of the paper clip in a noninjured digit; a two-point sensibility greater than 8 mm suggests nerve injury.
- The FDP is examined by holding the MCPJ and PIP joint in extension while asking the patient to flex to DIP joint; the FDS is assessed by holding the adjacent fingers in extension and the MCPJ of the involved finger in extension; the patient is then asked to flex the PIP joint.

Diagnostic Aids

Radiographs

- In general, anteroposterior, lateral, and oblique views are obtained.

Arteriography

- Operative intervention should not be delayed for arteriography when urgent surgery is indicated.

Computed Tomography (CT) and Magnetic Resonance Imaging (MRI)

- Injuries of carpal bones can be missed in conventional radiographs.
- CT helps pick up most of these fractures.
- Intraosseous lesions are best delineated by CT.
- Soft tissue lesions, subtle ligamentous disruptions, early avascular necrosis of bones, and tumors can often be detected only by MRI.

Ultrasound and Doppler Scans

- Ultrasound scans can help detect soft tissue lesions, picking up occult ganglia and intramuscular masses.

ANESTHESIA

- Most upper extremity anesthesia is performed with local or regional anesthetics.
- Lidocaine or bupivacaine without vasoconstrictive agents is used to perform digital nerve blocks.
- The hand can be anesthestized with a wrist block or an axillary block.

Tourniquet

- A tourniquet promotes visualization and minimizes blood loss.
- Upper extremity tourniquets should remain inflated no more than 2 hours, and the interval between deflation and reinflation should be at least 5 minutes for every 30 minutes of tourniquet ischemia.

SOFT TISSUE INJURIES

Fingertip Injuries

- Fingertip injuries are the most common hand injuries.
- A nail bed injury should be explored if a hematoma occupies more than 25% of the nail plate surface area; they are repaired with 7-0 chromic sutures with the aid of loupe magnification.

- Goals of treatment include maintaining length, sensibility, motion, and appearance.
- Most fingertip defects less than 1 cm^2 heal by secondary intention if no bone is exposed; composite grafts heal favorably in children younger than 6 years.
- Defects greater than 1 cm^2 can be grafted with full-thickness skin harvested from the hypothenar eminence.
- Primary closure is performed if adequate soft tissue is present.
- Local flaps are frequently used to cover exposed bone of the fingertip.
- A complication of fingertip injury is hypersensitivity; early desensitization training can minimize this debilitating complication.

Flexor Tendon Injuries

- Arteries, nerves, and bone may also be injured.
- The severed flexor tendon can retract proximally, the superficialis tendon inserts at the base of the middle phalanx, and the profundus lies deep and inserts at the base of the distal phalanx.
- After entering the hand, the tendons pass through fibro-osseous tunnels that are covered by annular and cruciate pulleys.
- The second and fourth annular pulleys are most important in the prevention of bow stringing.
- Flexor tendon injuries are classified into five zones, and treatment is planned based on the zone of injury.
  - Zone I affects only the FDP tendon.
  - Zone II, referred to as no-man s land, is located between the distal palmar crease and the PIP joint crease; it contains the FDS and FDP tendons.
  - Dynamic splinting incorporates active extension and passive flexion of the fingers with protection from hyperextension.
  - Zone III is located between the distal carpal ligament and the distal palmar crease.
  - Zone IV is the area coinciding with the carpal tunnel below the transverse carpal ligament.
  - Zone V is located in the forearm.

Extensor Tendon Injuries

- The subcutaneous location of extensor tendons makes them susceptible to crush, laceration, and avulsion injuries.

- Extensor tendons have been classified into zones; the odd number zones begin at the DIP joint and are located over the joints, whereas the even number zones are located between the joints.
- Extensor tendon repair methods include a figure-of-eight mattress suture or a weaving Kirchmayr suture.
- Early motion can increase tensile strength through collagen remodeling.

Nerve Injuries

- Neurapraxia is the interruption of nerve conduction but with anatomic preservation of all neural elements.
- In axonotmesis, there is axonal injury with wallerian degeneration.
- Neurotmesis is the anatomic disruption of the nerve trunk.
- Spontaneous recovery is impossible without surgical repair.
- Nerve repair is facilitated with the operating microscope.
- Repair is accomplished by an epineural repair.
- Primary repair is carried out for sharp transections.
- The extent of crush or avulsion injuries is often difficult to determine in the acute setting; these injuries may require re-exploration to determine the extent of nerve injury.
- A peripheral nerve regenerates at a rate of roughly 1 mm/day.

Vascular Injuries

- Arterial injuries in the upper extremity can occur by laceration, contusion, avulsion, thermal and blast injury, dislocation, and fracture.
- Repetitive trauma from vibratory tools may lead to thrombosis of the ulnar artery in Guyon s canal; this is referred to as the *hypothenar hammer syndrome.*
- Emboli may lodge in arteries at a vessel branch point, obstructing blood flow.
- Major arterial injuries producing limb ischemia may occur after severe, compound fractures and require artery reconstruction.
- If major arterial reperfusion is established after an ischemia time of 6 hours or longer, edema is likely to ensue, which increases compartmental pressures and the possibility of compartment syndrome; in these instances, fasciotomies should be carried out at the time of surgery.
- Venous injuries in the hand or upper extremity often result from intravenous cannulations that lead to thrombophlebitis;

treatment consists of elevation, antibiotics, and warm compresses.

FRACTURES AND DISLOCATIONS

- Fractures of bones are categorized according to their bony anatomic location.
- Intra-articular fracture-dislocations of small joints require precise articular surface realignment for prevention of traumatic arthritis.

Distal Phalanx Fractures

- Fractures of the distal phalanx are the most commonly encountered fractures of the hand.
- Undisplaced or minimally displaced fractures can be treated with a gutter or thimble splint for a period of 3 to 4 weeks.
- Unstable transverse shaft fractures require fixation with 0.035-inch diameter Kirschner wires.

Mallet Finger

- A mallet finger can result from an avulsion fracture of the attachment terminal slip of the extensor mechanism at the base of the distal phalanx.
- Most closed mallet injuries are managed by splinting the DIP joint in extension, provided the fracture involves less than 30% of the joint surface and is displaced by less than 2 mm.
- Grossly displaced or large intra-articular fragments may require internal fixation with a Kirschner wire.

Jersey Finger

- Jersey finger is an avulsion fracture of the insertion of the FDP tendon into the distal phalanx.
- It occurs after a violent pull of the FDP against resistance, as can occur when a footballer catches onto the jersey of an opponent and forcefully pulls.
- This fracture generally requires open reduction and internal fixation with a mini-screw or Kirschner wires.

Middle Phalanx, Proximal Phalanx, and Metacarpal Fractures

- Phalangeal fractures can be immobilized in finger splints whereas metacarpal fractures are treated in a splint with the wrist in 20 to 30 degrees of dorsiflexion, the MCPJs in

70 degrees of flexion, and the IPJs fully extended; this is termed the *universal position of immobilization* of the hand.

- Gross displacement requires accurate restoration of the articular surface by surgery.
- Rotation can then be maintained by traction through an external device or by fixing the fragments with mini-screws or Kirschner wires.
- Neck fractures are generally due to a combination of axial compression and bending.
- They are also called booby-trap fractures in the middle phalanx and boxer s fracture if involving the metacarpal of the little finger.
- Shaft fractures are caused by bending, torsional, or crushing forces.
- Sometimes, buddy taping the finger to the adjacent unin-jured one suffices; this protects the IPJs and allows collateral ligaments to heal.
- Base fractures are caused by axial forces with or without an associated bending component and may be intra-articular.
- An abducted fracture of the base of the proximal phalanx of the little finger is called the extra octave injury; a special fracture in this category is an intra-articular fracture of the base of the thumb metacarpal, called Bennett s injury.
- An intra-articular comminuted fracture of the base of the thumb metacarpal is known as Rolando s fracture.
- If undisplaced, most of the just-mentioned fractures can be treated by percutaneous pinning with Kirschner wires followed by appropriate splinting.
- Isolated fractures of the bases of middle and ring finger metacarpals do not require splinting because they are immo-bilized quite adequately by other intact metacarpals.
- Complications that may occur after phalangeal or metacarpal fractures include malrotation, malunion, nonunion, and stiff-ness of the digit resulting from tendon adhesions and joint contractures.

Carpal Fractures

Scaphoid Fracture

- The scaphoid is the most common carpal fracture.
- Examination reveals tenderness over the anatomic snuffbox and also over the scaphoid tubercle.
- Initial radiographic examination may not reveal a scaphoid fracture; repeat radiographs obtained in 2 weeks may reveal a fracture.

- The scaphoid receives its blood supply mainly through its distal segment, and proximal fractures may lead to avascular necrosis.
- Displaced fractures require open reduction with screw fixation.

Hook of the Hamate Fracture

- Long-standing hook of the hamate fractures are usually treated with resection of the hook.

Fractures in Children

- Pediatric fractures may alter bone growth by affecting the epiphyseal plate.
- Phalangeal epiphyses are located in the proximal aspect of the bone.
- The metacarpal growth centers are located at the distal aspect of the bone with the exception of the thumb, which has its growth center at the metacarpal base.
- The Salter-Harris epiphyseal classification describes five types of fractures.

Dislocations

- Dislocation is more frequently seen in the PIP joint.
- Dislocation is described based on the position of the distal side in reference to the proximal articular surface.
- Dorsal dislocation is classified into three groups:
  - Type I is hyperextension of the joint with avulsion of the palmar plate; these injuries can be treated by a dorsal blocking splint for 3 weeks.
  - Type II is a dorsal dislocation with rupture of the palmar plate with no contact present between the two articular surfaces; after reduction, if the joint is stable, a dorsal blocking splint prevents recurrence of the dislocation.
  - Type III dorsal dislocation is a fracture-dislocation of the palmar base of the middle phalanx; stability is usually maintained if less than 30% of the articular surface is involved; larger fragments or unstable dislocations require fragment stabilization with wires or pins.
- In palmar dislocation, the condyle of the proximal phalanx often becomes trapped between the central slip and the lateral bands of the finger extensor mechanism; if this trapping occurs, open reduction is necessary.

- After surgery, palmar dislocations should be placed in an extended position, particularly if the central slip is repaired.

Traumatic Joint Instabilities

Gamekeeper's Thumb

- Gamekeeper s thumb results from rupture of the ulnar collateral ligament of the thumb MCPJ.
- The adductor pollicis tendon insertion is interposed between the distal ulnar collateral ligament attachment and the proximal phalanx.
- Instability can occur in the PIP and DIP joints because of collateral ligament and palmar plate tears.
- Most injuries are incomplete and are treated by a protective splint.

AMPUTATION AND REPLANTATION

- Clean-cut or sharp amputations are favorable for replantation.
- Crushing and avulsion injuries are less likely to be salvageable.
- Most replantations should be attempted in children and young adults because these patients have a greater propensity for regeneration of nerves and less propensity for joint stiffness.
- The thumb is always replanted if possible.
- The severed part is cleansed, placed in sterile gauze, placed in a sealed bag, and bathed in ice water until replantation.
- Bone fixation is followed by the repair of flexor tendons, digital arteries, digital nerves, extensor tendons, dorsal veins, and skin.
- Clinical examination remains the most reliable monitoring technique.

NERVE COMPRESSION SYNDROMES

Median Nerve Compression

Carpal Tunnel Syndrome

- Carpal tunnel syndrome is the result of abnormal swelling in the tunnel, which compresses the median nerve.
- The patient experiences pain and numbness in the median nerve distribution, especially at night.
- Synovitis is the most common cause of carpal tunnel syndrome.

- Examination must include the neck, shoulder, and arm.
- Initial treatment of carpal tunnel syndrome is nonoperative and includes a night wrist splint and vitamin B_6.
- If signs and symptoms persist or if there is thenar weakness or atrophy, surgical release is indicated.

Pronator Syndrome

- Compression of the median nerve in pronator syndrome is easily mistaken for carpal tunnel syndrome.
- Sites of compression in pronator syndrome include the pronator teres muscle, the lacertus fibrosus, the FDS muscle fascial arch, and the ligament of Struthers.
- Treatment is surgical release of the deep head of the pronator teres muscle and chiasm of the FDS muscle fascial arch or other sites of compression at the elbow.

Ulnar Nerve Compression

Guyon's Canal

- Compression of the ulnar nerve can occur at Guyon s canal, which is composed of the hook of the hamate, pisiform, pisohamate ligament, and palmar carpal ligament.
- Treatment consists of exploration of Guyon s canal for a space-occupying mass and decompression of the ulnar nerve.

Cubital Tunnel Syndrome

- Compression of the ulnar nerve at the elbow may result in cubital tunnel syndrome.
- It can occur from an abnormal angulation of the elbow; after fracture of the lateral condyle or radial head; or by compression from the ligament of Struthers, intermuscular septum, flexor carpi ulnaris muscle fascia, and anconeous muscle.
- Symptoms include an aching pain with numbness and paresthesias in the ring and small fingers.
- The elbow is in a flexed position, which can elicit or exacerbate the symptoms already present.
- Treatment consists of night splinting with the elbow in the neutral position and avoidance of elbow flexion or direct pressure on the elbow during the day.
- If muscle weakness or atrophy is present, surgical exploration is indicated.

Radial Nerve Compression

- Sites of radial nerve compression include the triangular space in the axilla, the spiral groove in the axilla, the spiral groove in the arm, and the lateral intermuscular spectrum proximal to the elbow.
- More distally, the posterior interosseous nerve, which is the principal motor division, can get depressed near the annular ligament of the radial head or within the substance of the supinator muscle.
- Initial treatment is splinting the arm; and, if this fails, the nerve is surgically decompressed.

Thoracic Outlet Syndrome

- The thoracic outlet is bounded by the first rib inferiorly, the scalenus anterior muscle anteriorly, the scalenus muscle posteriorly, and the clavicle.
- Thoracic outlet compression can be triggered by motor vehicle collisions, sporting injuries, or work activities.
- Symptoms may include pain in the shoulder and tingling and numbness along the ulnar distribution of the hand that usually occur with compression of the lower trunk of the brachial plexus.
- In upper brachial plexus compression, the symptoms may include pain in the side of the face, jaw, or ear associated with paresthesias that radiate down the lateral side of the arm.
- Percussion over the supraclavicular and infraclavicular areas and over the medial arm result in a positive Tinel s sign.
- Passively flexing the neck away from the affected side or arm usually reproduces symptoms.
- Production of symptoms when the head is tilted to the symptomatic side usually signifies compression of the nerve rootlets by osteophytes in and around the foramina of the cervical spine.
- Treatment of thoracic outlet compression is primarily non-operative; physical therapy is implemented to increase the size of the outlet, and activities are modified or curtailed that precipitate the symptoms.
- Persistent symptoms after these measures may require surgical intervention, including cervical rib resection, first rib resection, or scalenectomies.

TUMORS

- Most tumors of the hand are benign; 95% are ganglion cysts, giant cell tumors, epidermal inclusion cysts, hemangiomas, and lipomas.

Ganglion Cyst

- Ganglions are the most common soft tissue tumor of the hand and contain a mucinous fluid that originates from a joint or tendon space.
- About 60% are located over the dorsal aspect of the wrist and usually arise from the scapholunate ligament.
- Palmar wrist ganglions arise between the flexor carpi radialis and the abductor pollicis longus tendons.

Giant Cell Tumor

- Giant cell tumors are the second most common hand tumors; they arise from synovium of the joint or the tendon sheath and are yellow-brown in color.
- Treatment consists of microsurgical excision, removing all the tumor and any discolored synovium from its origin, which may require opening the joint and repairing the collateral ligaments and palmar plate.

Epidermal Inclusion Cyst

- Epidermal inclusion cysts usually result from injury; the epithelial cells become lodged in the subcutaneous tissue.
- They produce keratin, which leads to a cystic lesion of varying size.
- Recurrence after complete excision is rare.

Lipoma

- Lipomas make up 3% of hand tumors.

Pyogenic Granuloma

- Pyogenic granulomas are highly vascular lesions that are friable, bleed easily, and can grow rapidly.
- They occur most commonly on the fingertips and respond to either curettage or simple excision.

Verruca Vulgaris

- Verruca vulgaris are viral warts.

Vascular Malformations

- Congenital arteriovenous fistulas are treated by compression garments.

INFECTION

Paronychia

- Paronychial infection usually results from a penetrating injury to the nail fold.
- The most common causative organism is *Staphylococcus aureus*.
- Early erythema can be treated with antibiotics and hygiene.
- If fluctuation has developed, surgical incision and drainage are indicated.

Felon

- A felon is an abscess in the fibrous septa closed space of the fingertip pad.
- Appropriate treatment is surgical incision and drainage.

Suppurative Tenosynovitis (Acute and Chronic)

- Suppurative tenosynovitis is an infection of the flexor tendon sheath of fingers or thumb; most are caused by *S. aureus*.
- Four cardinal signs may be present: fusiform swelling, a digit held in a flexed position, tenderness over the tendon sheath with palpation, and pain on passive extension of the digit.
- Early cases may respond to nonoperative treatment, including elevation, warm soaks, and intravenous antibiotics.
- Unless improvement is noted within 6 to 8 hours, surgical incision and drainage are indicated.

Deep Space Infections

- The *subaponeurotic space* is an area beneath the extensor tendon on the dorsum of the hand and is dorsal to the interossei fascia; incision and drainage can be carried out by a longitudinal incision between the extensor tendons.

- *Thenar space abscesses* develop in the space palmar to the adductor pollicis muscle fascia and deep to the level of the FDS and FDP tendons of the index finger.
- The *midpalmar space* is located palmar to the third, fourth, and fifth metacarpals and below or dorsal to the flexor tendons of these fingers; surgical incision and drainage are indicated, taking care to avoid injury to the neurovascular structures in the palm.
- The *hypothenar space* is bounded radially by the fascial septum connecting the palmar fascia to the fifth metacarpal and the fascia of the hypothenar muscles ulnarly.

Herpes Infection

- Herpetic infection, or *whitlow,* of a digit is caused by the herpes simplex virus and is frequently seen in health care personnel.
- These lesions can mimic other infections, such as paronychia and felons.
- The diagnosis is made from a potassium hydroxide preparation and Tzank smear.
- Herpetic infections are self-limiting, and treatment is nonoperative; surgical incision and drainage can lead to systemic involvement and possible viral encephalitis.

Bites

- Common organisms are *S. aureus, Streptococcus* and *Bacteroides* species, and *Eikenella corrodens.*
- Most human bites to the hand occur when an individual strikes another person in the mouth with a clenched fist.
- A tooth produces a puncture wound in the skin extending into the MCPJ.
- Surgical exploration, d bridement, and lavage are mandatory in the treatment of these injuries.
- Human bite wounds should not be closed primarily and are treated with penicillin or cephalosporins after surgery.

CONGENITAL ANOMALIES

Syndactyly

- The most common hand anomalies are syndactyly and polydactyly.
- Syndactyly is characterized by webbing between the fingers and is most common between the ring and long fingers.

Polydactyly

- Polydactyly is classified as a duplication of parts, the most common being thumb duplication.

Growth Arrests

- Brachydactyly is a failure of parts or short digits.
- *Radial club hand* occurs when the radius and radial-sided structures are hypoplastic or totally absent.
- Radial club hand can be associated with other anomalies such as thrombocytopenia absent radius syndrome; Fanconi s anemia (cardiac defects); and vertebral defects, anal atresia, tracheoesophageal fistula with esophageal atresia, and radial and renal dysplasia (VATER) syndrome.
- *Ulnar club hand* is a congenital absence or hypoplasia of the ulna and can be associated with other syndromes that tend to encompass musculoskeletal disorders.
- Poland s syndrome often presents with short fingers, hypoplastic breast structures, absent pectoralis muscles, and clavicle deficiencies.

Constriction Band Syndrome

- This syndrome is secondary to intrauterine bands that exert tourniquet-like pressure that can threaten the viability of digits, limbs, and other parts.

Clinodactyly

- Clinodactyly is a deviation of the digit in the radial or ulnar direction; it is usually found at the distal phalanx.

Camptodactyly

- Camptodactyly is a fixed flexion deformity in the anteroposterior plane and is more severe in the small finger at the PIP joint.

TENOSYNOVITIS

De Quervain's Disease

- De Quervain s disease is an inflammation of the synovium of the first dorsal compartment at the wrist, which contains the extensor pollicis brevis (EPB) and the abductor pollicis longus (APL) tendons.

Trigger Finger

- Trigger finger is characterized by snapping or catching during flexion and extension because of inflammation of the tendon or its sheath.
- The usual site of catching of the flexor tendon is the first annular pulley.
- Nonoperative treatment includes blocking MCPJ flexion with a splint and injecting small amounts of lidocaine and corticosteroids into the flexor tendon sheath; injection can be repeated up to three times.
- If this regimen fails, surgical division of the first annular pulley under direct vision is indicated.

Extensor Carpi Ulnaris (ECU) Tenosynovitis

- Inflammation of this tendon may occur after repetitive strain and forms an important cause of the enigmatic ulnar-sided wrist pain syndrome (USWP).
- Diagnosis is made by eliciting tenderness along the ECU tendon and pain on resisted ulnar extension of the wrist.
- Treatment includes splinting and local corticosteroid injection.

Intersection Syndrome

- This is an ill-understood condition characterized by pain and crepitus at the point where the APL and EPB tendons intersect the tendons of extensor carpi radialis longus (ECRL) and extensor carpi radialis brevis (ECRB).
- Initial treatment is by splinting, local corticosteroid injection, and anti-inflammatory medication.
- Refractory cases require surgical excision of involved tenosynovial membranes and local fascial thickening, which is frequently seen.

ARTHRITIS

Osteoarthritis (Primary and Secondary)

- Osteoarthritis is a degenerative joint disease that generally occurs later in life and is seen in 90% of women and 80% of men in their late 70s.
- There is a loss of cartilage and the formation of osteophytes around the margins of the joints.
- Osteoarthritis most commonly affects the DIP, PIP, and first carpometacarpal joints.
- DIP joints develop pain, stiffness, and Heberden nodes, which are osteophytes at the DIP joint.

- In severe cases, resection of osteophytes and arthrodesis, or fusion, of the DIP joint provides the best pain relief and correction of the deformity.
- Osteoarthritis of the PIP joint is frequently associated with joint subluxation and osteophytes that are referred to as *Bouchard nodes.*
- Osteoarthritis also affects the first carpometacarpal (trapeziometacarpal) joint, which is shaped like a saddle; symptoms can initially be treated with a lidocaine and corticosteroid injection, thumb splint, and anti-inflammatory agents.
- Surgical treatment options for chronic osteoarthritis are arthrodesis or arthroplasty.
- Arthrodesis is usually favored in the young manual laborer in whom strength and durability are paramount.
- Arthroplasty uses autogenous or alloplastic materials for joint reconstruction.

Rheumatoid Arthritis

- Rheumatoid arthritis is a chronic, systemic autoimmune disorder of unknown cause that leads to inflammation and hypertrophy of the synovium.

Boutonniere Deformity

- PIP joint boutonniere deformity develops from synovial erosion and attenuation and rupture of the central slip with accompanying palmar migration of the lateral bands; these produce the classic clinical picture of PIP joint flexion with hyperextension of the DIP joint.

Swan-Neck Deformity

- Swan-neck deformity is characterized by MCPJ flexion, PIP joint hyperextension, and DIP joint flexion.
- The classic appearance is radial deviation of the hand at the wrist and ulnar deviation of the fingers at the MCPJs as the proximal carpal row slides ulnarward.
- Surgery is indicated in an effort to avoid progression of the disease to the destructive phase.
- The flexor pollicis longus tendon is the most common tendon to rupture secondary to erosion from scaphoid osteophytes that protrude into the carpal canal.
- Management includes medication, splints, and protected exercises.
- If synovitis has not subsided after 6 months, synovectomy is indicated to prevent joint destruction.

Ulnar Drift

- This deformity occurs typically at the MCPJs and is accompanied by an ulnar subluxation of the long extensor tendons.
- In combination with a radial deviation of the wrist, ulnar drift of the fingers produces a characteristic Z deformity of the hand.
- If seen early, dynamic splinting helps correct the deformity and also decreases synovial inflammation.
- Late cases require surgery.
- If the MCPJs are not eroded or grossly volar luxated, soft tissue realignment suffices.
- Eroded and grossly luxated MCPJs require additional prosthetic replacement.

CONTRACTURES

- Dupuytren s disease is contracture of the palmar fascia extending into the fingers.
- The disease affects the ring and small fingers more commonly and may progress to cause flexion contractures at the MCPJs and IPJs.
- PIP joint contractures are produced by involvement of the spiral band, lateral digital sheath, Grayson s ligament, retrovascular band, and palmar fascia, either singularly or in combination.
- Surgery is reserved for patients with more than 30 degrees of MCPJ flexion contracture or any degree of PIP joint flexion contracture.

Volkmann's Ischemic Contracture

- Ischemic contracture frequently results from compartment syndromes occurring after crushing injuries.
- The ischemia and resultant fibrous contracture of muscle produce finger flexion, which becomes resistant to passive stretching.

CHAPTER 73

GYNECOLOGIC SURGERY

PELVIC EMBRYOLOGY AND ANATOMY

Embryology

Anatomy

External Genitalia

- It is important for the surgeon dissecting the external genitalia to be cognizant of the variability of direction from which the blood supply of the operative field is derived.
- Surgical injury to the pelvic nerve plexus can result in neuropathic pain and diminished sexual, voiding, and excretory function.
- Because of various fascial fusions, infections spreading from the vulva to the anterior abdominal wall do not spread into the inguinal regions or the thigh.

Internal Genitalia

- Ovary.
  - The infundibulopelvic ligament, with the ovarian blood supply, crosses over the ureter as it descends into the pelvis. As the surgeon divides and ligates the ovarian vessels, it is critical that this relationship be identified to avoid transecting, ligating, or kinking the ureter.
  - If there are adhesions between the ovary and the peritoneum of the pelvic sidewall, careful dissection is necessary to avoid tenting the peritoneum with the attached ureter and creating injury.
- Fallopian tubes.
  - The surgeon must be aware of the fragility of the fallopian tube and handle this structure delicately, especially in women wishing to preserve their fertility.
- Uterus and cervix.
  - The size of the uterus is influenced by age, hormonal status, prior pregnancy, and common benign neoplasms.
  - If during a surgical procedure, the surgeon encounters an enlarged uterus, undiagnosed pregnancy must be considered.

- Because the cervical canal is continuous with the vagina, surgical procedures involving the uterus and tubes are considered to be clean-contaminated cases.
- Often, the most prudent way to secure the uterine artery is to expose its origin and place hemostatic clips on the vessel.
- With relatively normal pelvic anatomy, it is unlikely to be subjected to injury; but under circumstances in which the surgeon must dissect the retroperitoneal or paravaginal spaces, this relatively subtle structure can be injured with significant neuropathic residual.
- Vagina.
  - Traumatic lacerations of the vagina are most commonly located along the lateral sidewalls, and the degree to which there is major injury to the vessels can be associated not only with significant evident hemorrhage but with concealed hemorrhage as well.
  - In the absence of an accumulating hematoma, often the best approach to management is a bulk vaginal pack to achieve tamponade.

REPRODUCTIVE PHYSIOLOGY

- Ovarian cycle.
- Endometrial cycle.
- Early pregnancy.
- Amenorrhea and abnormal menses.
  - Patients with chronic anovulation with chronic unopposed estrogen are at risk for endometrial hyperplasia and even endometrial cancer.
  - Histologic diagnosis requires an endometrial biopsy or curettage.

CLINICAL EVALUATION

History

- Age.
  - The young patient may be fertile and sexually active; thus, pregnancy with complications must always be considered.
  - Any postmenopausal woman who presents with uterine bleeding must be presumed to have uterine pathology and have an appropriate evaluation for possible hyperplastic or neoplastic endometrial pathology.
- Pregnancy history.

- Menstrual history.
- Excessive flow (menorrhagia) associated with regular cycles at normal intervals suggest structural abnormalities of the endometrial cavity, most commonly submucous leiomyomas or endometrial polyps. Random or intermittent bleeding episodes during the cycle should prompt consideration of a lesion of the cervix, endometrial hyperplasia, or, occasionally, adenocarcinoma of the endometrium.
- Sexual history.
- Pregnancy must be ruled out in any circumstance in which there is a clinical presentation that is *not inconsistent* with complications of pregnancy.
- Contraception.
  - Patients with an intrauterine contraceptive device (IUD) may have spotting and cramping, but because the IUD increases the risk of endometrial infection and because a disproportionate percentage of pregnancies that are conceived with an IUD are extrauterine, these patients need careful evaluation.
  - Patients with previous tubal sterilization have a 1% to 3% lifetime risk of pregnancy, with a disproportionate number of extrauterine pregnancies.
- Prior gynecologic diseases and procedures.
- History of present illness.
  - Bleeding.
  - Pain.

Physical Examination

- This includes an adequate sense of physical privacy, the continuous presence of a chaperone, a comfortable examination table on which to assume lithotomy position, and patience by the examiner.
- The examiner or the assistant should inform the patient at every step in the process what the next sensation will be.
- Tenderness with cervical motion may be related to traction on the ligamentous attachments, collision of the cervix against a structure in the direction to which the cervix is being displaced, or collision of the fundus against a structure on the opposite side.

Diagnostic Considerations

- Bleeding without pain.
- Bleeding associated with midline suprapubic pain.

- Bleeding associated with lateralized pelvic pain.
- Bleeding associated with generalized pelvic pain.
- Midline pelvic pain without bleeding.
- Lateralized pelvic pain without bleeding.
- Generalized abdominal pain without bleeding.
- Obstipation.
- Flank pain.

Other Acute Clinical Presentations

- Necrotizing fasciitis is a life-threatening infection that can occur in the vulva.
- It is very important that women with risk factors for necrotizing fasciitis who present with a vulvar cellulitis be admitted for intravenous antibiotics and possible surgical treatment.

Pelvic Masses

Ancillary Tests

- Imaging.
- Pregnancy tests.
  - Unless a viable fetus can be detected clinically or by ultrasound, a positive urine test, in the clinical setting that could suggest an ectopic pregnancy, must be followed-up with a quantitative serum radioimmunoassay.
  - A decline in value over a 2-day period is always ominous, and, therefore, demands a clinical decision about intrauterine versus extrauterine failed pregnancy.
  - Progesterone levels less than 5 ng/mL are rarely associated with successful pregnancies.
- Serum hormone assays.
- Cervicovaginal cultures, Gram stain, and wet prep.
- Lower genital cytology.

MANAGEMENT OF PREINVASIVE AND INVASIVE DISEASE OF THE FEMALE GENITAL TRACT

- Preinvasive vulvar squamous lesions.
  - Because appearance can be variable, a 4- or 5-mm punch biopsy should be taken to differentiate dysplasia from an invasive lesion.

- Evaluation of the patient with vulvar dysplasia should include colposcopy of the vulva, vagina, and cervix because 15% to 20% of patients will have dysplasia in more than one of these sites.
- Invasive vulvar squamous lesions.
  - Any lesion with greater than 1 mm depth of invasion requires not only treatment of the primary lesion but also evaluation of the inguinal lymph nodes.
- Melanoma of the vulva.
- Bartholin's gland carcinoma.
  - Unlike squamous cell cancers, lymph node involvement is common and can be bilateral.
- Basal cell carcinoma.
- Paget's disease of the vulva.
  - Paget's disease of the vulva is also associated with coexisting malignancies such as breast, colon, or genitourinary locations. Workup of patients with this diagnosis should include screening for other malignancies.
- Vulvar sarcomas.
- Preinvasive vaginal lesions.
- Invasive vaginal lesions.
  - Evaluation for metastasis should include not only evaluation of the chest, abdomen, and pelvis but also the head and bones.
- Preinvasive disease of the cervix.
- Invasive disease of the cervix.
  - Whether there is a grossly visible lesion or abnormal cytology and abnormal colposcopy, diagnosis requires tissue biopsy.
  - When the diagnosis of cervical cancer is made from a large-loop excision of the transformation zone (LEEP) or a cone biopsy, it is important to determine as accurately as possible the depth of invasion involved. The type of treatment recommended varies significantly based on depth of invasion.
- Treatment of stage IA1 disease.
- Treatment of stage IA2 disease.
- Treatment of stage IB1 disease.
  - It does not necessarily include oophorectomy.
- Treatment of stage IB2 disease.
- Treatment of stages IIA to IVA.
- Treatment of stage IVB disease.
- Treatment of patients with enlarged lymph nodes.
  - Radiation therapy alone cannot sterilize bulky adenopathy.
- Treatment of neuroendocrine tumors.
- Treatment of recurrent disease.

Special Considerations in Management of Cervical Cancer and Treatment Complications

- Inappropriate surgical management.
- One of the most frequent and deleterious errors in surgical management of cervical cancer is failure to recognize the importance of block dissection of the tumor.
- Treatment of the pregnant patient.
- Management of the cervical cancer patient with acute hemorrhage.
  - Do not attempt a surgical resection.
- Management of radiation complications.
  - Biopsies should be avoided because of risk of fistula formation.

Endometrium

- Hyperplasia.
  - In patients with complex atypical hyperplasia who have completed childbearing, hysterectomy is recommended.
- Endometrial adenocarcinoma.
- Endometrial cancer in young women.
- Endometrial sarcomas.
  - High-grade endometrial sarcomas are rare and tend to be aggressive.

Mixed Mullerian Tumors of the Uterus

Management of a Pelvic Mass

- A mass with complex features such as septations, papillations, and solid components is more worrisome.
- CA-125, therefore, should not be checked in the premenopausal patient with a pelvic mass because the false-positive rate is too high. However, in the postmenopausal patient with a pelvic mass and an elevated CA-125, ovarian cancer is diagnosed in 80% of these patients.
- In patients with potential for carcinomatosis, laparoscopy should not be done because of port site metastasis that occurs quickly and can make debulking difficult.
- Patients who have a gonadoblastoma must be evaluated with chromosomes.

ALTERNATIVES TO SURGICAL INTERVENTION

- Dysfunctional uterine bleeding.

- Spontaneous abortion.
  - The need for acute surgical intervention with curettage is wholly dependent on the amount of blood loss and intensity of pain.
- Ectopic pregnancy.
  - Consultation with an experienced gynecologist before initiation is advisable.
- Pelvic infection.
  - The diagnosis of pelvic inflammatory disease (PID) should be made only when the patient has fever, leukocytosis, purulent discharge from the cervix, bilateral adnexal tenderness on gentle palpation, and peritoneal signs limited to the pelvis.
  - This diagnosis must be applied cautiously, because it is stigmatizing and labels the patient, disproportionately among women of color, from lower socioeconomic status, or with counterculture lifestyles.
  - Acute PID, as a polymicrobial infection, is a medical not a surgical disease.
- Functional ovarian cysts.
  - If the event is on the right ovary, the acuity clearly will force consideration of appendicitis, but prior gastrointestinal symptoms, fever, and leukocytosis are rarely present.
  - The surgeon should untwist the ovarian pedicle and directly observe for return of blood flow before considering removal.
- Uterine leiomyomas.
- Endometriosis and endometriomas.

TECHNICAL ASPECTS OF SURGICAL OPTIONS

Surgery for Menorrhagia and Abnormal Uterine Bleeding

- These ablative techniques (rollerball, thermal balloon, hydrotherapy, cryotherapy, microwave) are advanced techniques best reserved for a surgeon with extensive experience in hysteroscopy and the evaluation and manipulation of the endometrial cavity.
- Technique: fractional dilation and curettage.

Potential Complications

- Treatment of Bartholin gland cyst or abscess.
  - Excision of the gland is rarely indicated.
- Cone procedure.

Surgery for Ovarian Cysts

- It is critical to remember that, any time surgery is performed on the adnexal structures, there is a risk of adhesion formation that might inhibit fertility.
- Technique.
  - Ovarian cyst drainage. It is imperative, before considering drainage, that the ovarian cyst is benign and functional in nature.
  - Oophorectomy ± salpingectomy.
  - Ovarian cystectomy.
- Potential complications.

Surgery for the Fallopian Tube and Ectopic Pregnancy

Technique

- Salpingostomy.
  - The tube is not sutured but rather left open to spontaneously heal. This has been shown to improve patency rates and fertility.
- Segmental resection.
- Salpingectomy.

Potential Complications

- Bleeding is a risk both during and after the surgery is completed.

Hysterectomy

- Because of the significant impact of the transvaginal approach on appreciating anatomic relationships, vaginal hysterectomy and laparoscopically assisted hysterectomy should only be performed by an experienced vaginal surgeon.
- Technique.
- Potential complications.
  - It is imperative that these injuries be recognized and repaired intraoperatively, if possible.
- Radical hysterectomy.

SURGERY DURING PREGNANCY

Physiologic Changes

- Cardiovascular system.
  - Pregnancy should be considered a hypervolemic state.

- Respiratory system.
  - Early intervention is mandatory.
- Gastrointestinal tract.
  - Pregnant women should be considered to have a functionally full stomach at all times.
- Coagulation changes.
  - Pregnancy is a hypercoagulable state.
- Renal changes.
  - Asymptomatic bacteriuria should be aggressively treated.

Imaging Techniques

- In patients with abdominal pain, an ultrasound should be considered the first-line diagnostic test.
- Existing evidence suggests that there is no increased risk to the fetus with regards to congenital malformations, growth restriction, or abortion from x-ray procedures that expose the fetus to doses of 5 rads or less.
- It cannot be stressed enough that maternal well-being is of the utmost importance, and appropriate diagnostic procedures should be obtained to facilitate a rapid diagnosis.

Clinical Evaluation during Pregnancy

- Appendicitis.
  - Appendiceal location during pregnancy changes with the upward displacement of the appendix with advancing gestation (Fig. 73–1). Nevertheless, the most common presenting symptom is pain in the right lower quadrant. This presents regardless of gestational age.
  - It is prudent that the clinician make an early diagnosis and proceed immediately with surgical intervention.
- Cholelithiasis.
  - Delay of surgery in patient with cholecystitis may increase perinatal morbidity.
  - Pancreatitis caused by milk-alkali toxicity may be seen in patients with excessive intake of antacids.
- Intestinal obstruction.
- Ovarian masses.
  - If surgery is required for symptoms of torsion or bleeding, every effort should be made to preserve the corpus luteum in the first trimester.

Obstetrical Complications Resulting in Abdominal Pain

- Abruption.

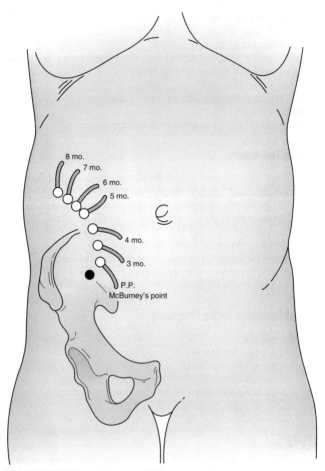

■ **FIGURE 73–1.** Location of the appendix in pregnancy. As modified from Bauer et al, JAMA, 1932, the approximate location of the appendix during succeeding months of pregnancy is diagrammed. In planning an operation, it is better to make the abdominal incision over the point of maximum tenderness unless there is a great disparity between that point and the theoretical location of the appendix. *(From Ludmir J, Stubblefield PG: Surgical procedures in pregnancy. In Gabbe S, Nubyl JR, Simpson JL [eds]: Obstetrics. Normal and Problem Pregnancies, 4th ed. Philadelphia, Churchill Livingston, 2002, p 617.)*

Pregnancy-Related Hepatic Complications

- Hemolysis elevated liver enzymes low platelet (HELLP) is a form of severe pre-eclampsia. It is important that the clinician not mistake this for cholelithiasis or other gastrointestinal pathology. Progression of this disease can result in rupture of the hepatic capsule and maternal death if the diagnosis is missed.
- Trauma.

Common Obstetrical Surgical Procedures

- It is difficult to remove the cervix, especially after a vaginal delivery secondary to dilatation of the lower uterine segment. Only surgeons who are skilled in this procedure should proceed without consultation.

Other Procedures

- An inappropriate repair may result in a rectovaginal fistula.

Pregnancy-Related Specific Computations

CHAPTER 74

SURGERY
IN THE PREGNANT PATIENT

PHYSIOLOGIC CHANGES OF PREGNANCY

- Progesterone and estrogen mediate many of the maternal physiologic changes in pregnancy.
- Elevated progesterone levels and decreased serum motilin result in smooth muscle relaxation.
- During the second and third trimester, the volume of the gallbladder may be twice that found in the nonpregnant state, and gallbladder emptying is markedly slower.
- Cardiac output increases by as much as 50% during the first trimester of pregnancy.
- Up to 10% of patients may experience supine hypotensive syndrome.
- Oxygen consumption increases during pregnancy.
- The decreased $Paco_2$ increases the CO_2 gradient from the fetus to the mother, facilitating CO_2 transfer from the fetus to the mother. The oxygen-hemoglobin dissociation curve of maternal blood is shifted to the right.
- There is an increase in the glomerular filtration rate by 50%.
- Serum creatinine also decreases by the end of the first trimester.
- Increase in plasma volume and red blood cell mass.
- Progressive rise in the leukocyte count.
- Platelet count progressively declines.
- Fibrinogen levels are elevated.

RADIOLOGY SAFETY CONCERNS IN PREGNANCY

- The accepted maximum dose of ionizing radiation during the entire pregnancy is 5 rad (0.05 Gy). The fetus is at the highest risk from radiation exposure from the preimplantation period to approximately 15 weeks' gestation.

ANESTHESIA SAFETY CONCERNS IN PREGNANCY

- The most profound effects on the fetus are related to decreased uterine blood flow or decreased oxygen content of uterine blood.
- Differentiation of the major organ systems occurs during the first trimester of human embryonic development.
- Elective surgical procedures should be delayed until at least 6 weeks after delivery, when maternal physiology has returned to the nonpregnant state and when the impact on the fetus is no longer a concern.

PREVENTION OF PRETERM LABOR

- Gestational age at treatment and severity of the underlying disease are the most predictive indicators of patients at risk for preterm labor.

ABDOMINAL PAIN AND THE ACUTE ABDOMEN IN PREGNANCY

- It is usually not the treatment but the delay in diagnosis and severity of the primary disease process that poorly impact outcomes.

MINIMALLY INVASIVE SURGERY IN PREGNANCY

- Major concerns of laparoscopy during pregnancy include injury to the uterus, decreased uterine blood flow, fetal acidosis, and preterm labor from increased intra-abdominal pressure.
- As the gravid uterus enlarges superiorly, adjustments in trocar placement must be made to avoid uterine injury and to improve visualization.

BREAST MASSES IN PREGNANCY

- Women with pregnancy-associated breast cancer present with a larger primary tumor and a higher risk of positive axillary lymph nodes.
- Any palpable mass that persists for 4 weeks or more should be evaluated.
- Tissue diagnosis is essential.
- Fine needle aspiration (FNA) may be a reliable alternative to core needle or open biopsy.
- Therapy for pregnancy-associated breast cancer is surgical resection.

- In stage I and II cancers, mastectomy with axillary dissection is preferred.
- In patients diagnosed during the late second trimester or later, immediate breast-conserving lumpectomy and axillary dissection followed with radiation postpartum is a treatment option.
- Chemotherapy is indicated for node-positive cancers or node-negative tumors greater than 1 cm.

HEPATOBILIARY DISEASE IN PREGNANCY

- Prompt delivery after diagnosis may prevent progression to fulminant hepatic failure and reduce the risk of fetal death.
- Hepatic hemorrhage or rupture occurs primarily during the third trimester or can develop up to 48 hours after delivery.
- Hepatic hematomas without evidence of ongoing bleeding in hemodynamically stable patients may be managed non-operatively with serial imaging and close monitoring, and these lesions typically heal without intervention.
- Immediate laparotomy with either abdominal packing or hepatic artery ligation reduces maternal and fetal mortality.
- Surgical intervention should be considered as primary management of gallstones in pregnancy.
- The timing of cholecystectomy for biliary colic depends on the gestational age and severity of symptoms.
- The optimal time for cholecystectomy is the second trimester, when the risk of spontaneous abortion and preterm labor are the least.

ENDOCRINE DISEASE IN PREGNANCY

- Pheochromocytomas that remain undiagnosed during pregnancy have a postpartum maternal mortality as high as 55% with fetal mortality also exceeding 50%.
- Surgical resection should be performed before 20 weeks' gestation, when spontaneous abortion is less likely and the size of the gravid uterus does not interfere with the procedure.

SMALL BOWEL DISEASE IN PREGNANCY

- The symptoms of an obstruction are identical to those in the nonpregnant patient and consist of the triad of abdominal pain, vomiting, and obstipation.
- Treatment for small bowel obstruction in pregnancy is identical to that in the nonpregnant patient.
- A lower threshold for operative management is necessary.

COLON AND RECTUM IN PREGNANCY

- Timely and accurate diagnosis is challenging because the typical clinical findings of nausea, vomiting, abdominal pain, and mild leukocytosis may be findings in a normal pregnancy.
- The treatment for suspected acute appendicitis in the pregnant patient is emergent appendectomy.
- Because of the increased risk to both mother and fetus with appendiceal perforation, a negative rate of 30% to 33% is acceptable (see Figure 47–13 from *Textbook of Surgery*, 17th Edition, page 1393, for location of appendix during pregnancy).

VASCULAR DISEASE IN PREGNANCY

- A splenic artery aneurysm of 2 cm or larger should be treated electively because of the increased risk of rupture during pregnancy.

TRAUMA IN PREGNANCY

- Trauma is the leading nonobstetric cause of maternal mortality and occurs in as many as 7% of pregnancies.
- Resuscitation of the fetus is accomplished by resuscitation of the mother.
- The pregnant trauma patient should be placed in left lateral decubitus position.
- Early and rapid fluid resuscitation should be administered even in the pregnant patient who is normotensive.
- The Kleihauer-Betke (K-B) test for the assessment of feto-maternal transfusion is useful after maternal trauma and should be drawn with the initial laboratory tests that include a type and crossmatch.
- The most common cause of fetal death after blunt injury is abruptio placentae.

CHAPTER 75

UROLOGIC SURGERY

KIDNEYS AND URETERS

Anatomy

- The kidneys and associated adrenal glands are surrounded by perirenal fat, which is enclosed in perinephric fascia, known as the *Gerota fascia*.
- The kidney is made up of an outer cortex, a central medulla, and the internal calices and pelvis.
- The blood supply to each kidney is usually through a single renal artery, which is a direct branch of the aorta; variations of the main renal artery and vein are common.
- The renal veins are paired with the arteries, but they contain abundant collateral circulation, thus allowing drainage even if flow through one or more veins is interrupted.
- The right renal vein enters the right lateral aspect of the inferior vena cava directly; the left renal vein usually receives direct branches from the left adrenal superiorly, left gonadal vein inferiorly, and a lumbar vein posteriorly before entering into the vena cava.
- The renal collecting system includes the calyces, the renal pelvis, and the ureter.

Physiology

- The kidneys are responsible for maintaining water and electrolyte balance under normal circumstances; they are also responsible for elimination of waste products and reabsorption of important solutes.
- The kidneys influence blood pressure maintenance and have a key role in the balance of acid-base interactions; additionally, the kidneys function as an endocrine organ as the site of renin production and of vitamin D synthesis.
- Erythropoietin is produced in the renal cortex; the renomedullary interstitial cells of the kidney produce platelet-activating factor.
- The proximal tubule is the site of conversion of calcidiol to calcitriol, one of the most potent stimulators of intestinal calcium absorption and a metabolite of vitamin D_3.

Patient Evaluation

- A complete history and physical examination is an essential initial component in the evaluation of a patient with a suspected urologic disease.
- The frequency, duration, chronicity, and severity of subjective symptoms should be elicited when possible.
- The presence of fever, chills, weight loss, malaise, nausea, or vomiting should be assessed, as well as the presence of any hematuria, pneumaturia, or lower urinary tract symptoms.
- Pain is usually the direct result of urinary tract obstruction or inflammation; renal pain may be felt as a dull, constant ache; alternatively, pain may be sharp and stabbing.
- Pain may be localized to the flank or may radiate from the flank into the lower abdomen, groin, scrotum, or labia.
- The urine should be analyzed for specific gravity, pH, protein, sugar, ketones, red blood cells, white blood cells, bilirubin, nitrites, and leukocyte esterase.
- Gross hematuria of any degree in an adult should never be ignored; it should be regarded as a symptom of urologic malignancy until proven otherwise.
- Hematuria can be distinguished from myoglobinuria and hemoglobinuria by microscopic examination of the centrifuged urine.
- An evaluation of renal function should be determined in all patients with urologic disease by determining the amount of urea or creatinine; serum creatinine level is a better indicator of overall renal function.

Imaging of Kidneys and Ureters

- Conventional plain films and intravenous pyelography (IVP) have historically been the initial imaging procedures.
- IVP remains the mode of choice for visualizing the entire urinary tract.
- Retrograde ureteropyelography allows for visualization of the collecting system and ureter without the need for intravenous contrast administration.
- Ultrasonography is a valuable adjunct in the evaluation of suspected solid or cystic renal parenchymal masses.
- Computed tomography (CT) scan yields unique anatomic and physiologic information and is generally superior to conventional radiographs because of greater tissue contrast resolution.

- Magnetic resonance imaging (MRI) has been useful in the evaluation of a variety of renal disorders; the ability of MRI to generate multiplanar images is an advantage over conventional CT scanning.
- Radionuclide imaging is best suited for demonstrating pathophysiologic changes that result from abnormalities in perfusion and function; estimation of total and split renal function is commonly performed.
- Arteriography permits visualization of the main renal arteries and its branches; its use has steadily declined with the increasing use of CT scans, MRI, and Doppler ultrasound.

Traumatic Injuries

- Renal trauma can be classified as *blunt* or *penetrating*.
- Blunt renal trauma represents approximately 80% of all renal injuries and usually results from injuries occurring during motor vehicle accidents, falls, or contact sports.
- The two most critical factors in determining whether to obtain an imaging study are the presence of shock and gross hematuria; if either is present, the patient should undergo a contrast-enhanced imaging study, which is initially an intravenous pyelogram (IVP) in suspected cases of isolated renal injuries.
- An IVP may demonstrate the presence or absence of two functioning kidneys and the integrity of the collecting system and ureters.
- Nonfunction of a segment or an entire kidney, parenchymal lacerations, and urinary extravasation are among the indications for a CT scan.
- Renal contusions, nonexpanding hematomas, and minor parenchymal lacerations in clinically stable patients are best managed conservatively with hydration and bed rest; some cases of isolated major parenchymal lacerations and select cases with urinary extravasation have been managed conservatively.
- Suspected renal injuries from penetrating trauma should be staged with a contrast-enhanced abdominal CT scan; as many as 75% of these injuries are associated with additional intra-abdominal injuries.
- For most grade 3 and 4 renal injuries, an attempt at repair of the kidney is usually justified.
- Nephrectomy may be the best initial option when there are many associated injuries or massive blood loss.

- In cases of suspected renal injury, every reasonable attempt should be made to adequately stage the injury and confirm the presence of a functioning contralateral kidney.
- In general, nonexpanding and nonpulsatile retroperitoneal hematomas discovered in the absence of a major renal injury should be observed.

Benign Diseases

Infectious

- Pyelonephritis presents with flank pain, fever, chills, and occasionally nausea and vomiting.
- The most common organisms are gram-negative rods, with *Escherichia coli* (*E. coli*) as the most commonly isolated pathogen; others, including *Pseudomona*, *Klebsiella*, and *Proteus*, are also common.
- Acute pyelonephritis usually responds to broad-spectrum intravenous antibiotics.
- Gram-negative sepsis is a serious and potentially life-threatening complication of an untreated urinary tract infection.

Nephrolithiasis

- The prevalence of nephrolithiasis is 2% to 3%; the peak incidence of stone formation occurs in patients between 20 and 40 years of age.
- Risk factors include a diet high in calcium and hyperparathyroidism.
- The most common urinary stones are composed of calcium oxalate and represent up to one third of stones.
- Uric acid stones are also commonly seen; cystine stones are usually seen in families with a history of cystinuria; struvite or "infection stones" develop in patients with urinary obstruction and urinary tract infections.
- Renal colic is the presenting symptom in most patients with symptomatic stones; large nonobstructing renal calculi are usually asymptomatic.
- Radiographic studies include an initial plain kidney-ureter-bladder film; either IVP or a noncontrast CT scan may confirm the diagnosis.
- Treatment of urinary calculi depends on the size, location, and composition of the stones.
- Criteria for intervention include intractable pain, nausea and vomiting, high-grade obstruction, and obstruction associated with infection.

- For symptomatic renal calculi 5 to 10 mm in size, extracorporeal shock wave lithotripsy (ESWL) is the choice of therapy.
- The most common complications are infection, hemorrhage, and arid ureteral perforation with subsequent urine leak.
- Percutaneous nephrostolithotomy is indicated for most renal stones larger than 3 cm; open surgical treatment is performed in only a small percentage of cases.

Benign Renal Masses

- Most simple cystic renal lesions are asymptomatic and benign and require no intervention; a complex cyst is generally considered a cancer until proven otherwise; benign solid tumors of the kidney are encountered occasionally.
- An angiomyolipoma can usually be diagnosed by the characteristic appearance of fat within the lesion on CT scan; they develop in approximately 50% of patients with tuberous sclerosis.
- Oncocytomas are benign renal tumors; the cell of origin is thought to be that of distal renal tubules.

Malignant Diseases

Tumors of the Renal Parenchyma

- Malignant renal tumors are either primary or metastatic.
- Renal cell carcinoma is the most common and accounts for more than 85% of all primary renal cancers.
- Renal cell carcinoma is a relatively rare tumor, representing approximately 3% of all adult malignancies; it usually occurs in adults between the ages of 40 and 60 years.
- Hematuria is the single most common sign, with flank pain and palpable flank mass occurring next most frequently; other common symptoms are fever, anemia, and elevated sedimentation rate.
- Renal cell cancers can present only with nonspecific symptoms such as weight loss, fever, or weakness.
- Renal cell carcinomas often involve the renal vein and vena cava, and may even extend into the right atrium; it metastasizes most frequently to lungs, bone, and brain, in that order.
- Metastatic lesions may appear in both the ipsilateral and contralateral kidney, and late metastasis may occur to the liver.
- Treatment has traditionally been radical nephrectomy; preoperative evaluation should include a chest x-ray and liver function tests.

Tumors of the Renal Pelvis and Ureter

- Tumors of the renal pelvis account for approximately 10% of all renal tumors and approximately 5% of all urothelial tumors.
- Cigarette smoking is strongly associated with an increased risk of development of upper tract transitional cell carcinomas; additionally, analgesic abuse and cyclophosphamide have been associated with an increased risk.
- The most common presenting symptom is hematuria; the work-up usually includes an IVP and urine cytology followed by cystoscopy.
- Patients with low-grade, low-stage lesions do well with either conservative or radical treatment; patients with intermediate or high-grade tumors are best managed with aggressive surgical resection; treatment of high-grade and high-stage tumors is nephroureterectomy with removal of a cuff of bladder at the ureteral orifice.

THE BLADDER AND URETHRA

Physiology

- Bladder dysfunction can be divided into disorders of storage and disorders of emptying.
- The disease processes that produce these disorders can be identified by a combination of urodynamic and radiographic studies.
- *Urodynamic evaluation* is a physiologic study that determines the neuromuscular response to the bladder filling, storage, and emptying; it includes a cystometrogram (CMG) with coordinated sphincter electromyography, urinary flow rate, postvoid residual urine volume, and fluoroscopic cystography.
- The normal bladder should fill to capacity of 350 to 500 ml without a significant increase in pressure or detrusor contraction.

Patient Evaluation

- Symptoms include irritative voiding symptoms such as frequency, urgency, and nocturia; obstructive symptoms include decreased force of stream, intermittent stream, incomplete emptying, and double voiding.
- Dysuria, or painful voiding, may be present; urinary incontinence, including physical stress, urge, and total incontinence, may also be present.

- Hematuria may be initial, terminal, or total; additionally, pneumaturia may signal either a gas-producing infection or a fistula.
- Trauma should be suspected if blood is found at the meatus; this finding indicates that a retrograde urethrogram be done before any instrumentation.

Traumatic Injuries

Bladder Trauma

- Bladder injury may occur as a result of penetrating or blunt trauma; approximately 90% of blunt trauma resulting in bladder perforation occurs in association with an anterior pelvic fracture.
- Bladder perforations may result in either intraperitoneal or extraperitoneal urinary extravasation.
- Traumatic bladder ruptures are often associated with damage to other pelvic and intra-abdominal organs, and concomitant urethral injuries are often present.
- Patients often complain of severe suprapubic or pelvic pain with an inability to void; bladder ruptures almost invariably cause hematuria, and a urethral disruption must be suspected.
- A carefully performed cystogram is the radiographic study of choice for a suspected bladder rupture; if accompanying urethral damage is suspected, a retrograde urethrogram must be performed to exclude a urethral tear *before* catheterization.
- Small extraperitoneal ruptures can be managed with 10 to 14 days of Foley catheter drainage; large extraperitoneal or intraperitoneal bladder ruptures usually require surgical repair.

Urethral Trauma

- Urethral injuries occur more frequently in males than in females because the male urethra is fixed to the pubis by the puboprostatic ligaments and the suspensory ligament of the penis; tearing occurs at these fixed areas.
- Urethral injury should be suspected in patients with blood at the urethral meatus, inability to void, or penile or perineal edema and ecchymosis.
- If digital rectal examination reveals a superiorly displaced prostate gland, a pelvic hematoma with urethral injury must be considered and evaluated.

- Radiographic evaluation should precede urethral catheterization; otherwise, attempts to pass a urethral catheter may convert a simple urethral laceration or incomplete rupture into a complete transection.
- IVP should precede retrograde urethrography or cystography.
- Small, incomplete anterior urethral ruptures with extravasation limited by the Buck fascia are treated by draining with a urethral catheter.
- When extravasation is large, surgical drainage is usually indicated; complete anterior urethral ruptures require primary surgical repair.
- Partial posterior urethral ruptures are treated with suprapubic cystostomy, urethral catheterization, and retroperitoneal drainage; complete posterior urethral rupture is managed with either immediate or delayed surgical repairs.

Malignant Diseases

Benign and Premalignant Bladder Lesions

- Benign lesions of the bladder are relatively uncommon.
- *Leukoplakia* is defined as cornification of a normally noncornified epithelium; it is thought to represent a reaction of normal epithelium to noxious stimuli and is considered a premalignant lesion.
- Cystitis glandularis may appear as a papillary bladder lesion; it is thought to be a precursor of adenocarcinoma.
- *Dysplasia* is a term used to identify lesions that are intermediate between benign and malignant urothelium.

Transitional Cell Carcinoma

- Bladder carcinoma is the fifth most common malignancy in the United States with more than 50,000 new cases being reported annually; it is approximately four times more prevalent among cigarette smokers and is associated with known carcinogens, including rubber and oil refinery workers.
- Patients given cyclophosphamide have up to a ninefold increased risk of bladder cancer development, and analgesic abuse has been associated with a higher risk as well.
- Approximately 90% of bladder malignancies are transitional cell carcinoma; of these, 70% of tumors are papillary, 10% are sessile, and 20% are mixed.
- Of patients with muscle invasive bladder cancer, approximately 80% to 90% have invasion on initial presentation; a strong correlation exists between tumor grade and stage.

- Carcinoma *in situ* (CIS) is a poorly differentiated transitional cell carcinoma confined to the urothelium; it may be found as a solitary or multifocal process and is associated with a poor prognosis.
- Gross painless hematuria is a common presenting sign; approximately 20% of cases may present with only microscopic hematuria.
- Irritative voiding symptoms such as frequency and urgency may also suggest a malignancy, particularly CIS.
- Patients should undergo an evaluation of their upper tracts, cystoscopy, and a urine cytology work-up; transurethral biopsy or resection confirms the diagnosis.
- Management depends on tumor stage; for most superficial bladder carcinomas, transurethral resection of the tumor is often the only treatment required.
- For CIS or high-grade superficial tumors, tumors that involve the lamina propria, and rapidly recurrent tumors, treatment with intravesical chemotherapy agents such as thiotepa or intravesical bacillus Calmette-Guérin may be indicated.
- Bladder surveillance is mandatory and includes cystoscopy and urinary cytology studies every 3 months for the first year, every 4 months for the second year, semiannually in the third year, and annually thereafter.
- In superficial tumors, which progress in stage or fail conservative therapies, and in tumors that invade the bladder muscle, radical cystectomy is usually required.

Adenocarcinoma

- Adenocarcinomas account for less than 2% of bladder cancers; it is the most common type of cancer in patients with bladder extrophy.
- Radical cystectomy with pelvic lymphadenectomy is the treatment of choice.

Squamous Cell Carcinoma

- Squamous cell carcinoma accounts for approximately 6% of bladder cancers in the United States.
- Chronic bladder inflammation, recurrent bladder infections, or bladder diverticula are associated with an increased risk of squamous cell carcinoma.
- Approximately 80% of squamous cell carcinomas in Egypt are associated with *Schistosoma haematobium*.
- The prognosis for squamous cell carcinoma is generally poor; radical cystectomy is the standard treatment.

Urethral Carcinoma

- Urethral carcinoma is the only urologic malignancy that is more common in females than males.
- A patient should be evaluated for urethral carcinoma when a urethral mass is palpable; the treatment of the primary tumor is surgical excision.
- In female urethral carcinoma, the usual presenting symptom is a papillary or fungating urethral mass and hematuria.
- For tumors of the proximal urethral structures, cystectomy with en bloc urethrectomy and anterior vaginectomy along with pelvic lymphadenectomy are usually required.

THE PROSTATE, SEMINAL VESICLES, AND VAS DEFERENS

Benign Diseases

Benign Prostatic Hyperplasia

- Benign Prostatic Hyperplasia (BPH) defines a process of hyperplasia (proliferation in the number of cells) and hypertrophy (enlargement in size of the prostate) associated with voiding symptoms.
- Enlargement of the prostate typically results in a relative bladder outflow obstruction.
- Classic obstructive symptoms are hesitancy in initiating voiding, a decrease in the force of the urinary stream, terminal dribbling, intermittency, and a feeling of incomplete bladder emptying; frequency, urgency, and nocturia are also common.
- Digital rectal examination of the prostate shows palpable enlargement.
- Most patients with BPH who desire treatment are first given medications; they only undergo surgery or other treatment if the medical management fails or is not well tolerated; alpha$_1$-adrenergic blocking agents are the medications most commonly used.
- The surgical removal of obstructing prostatic tissue can be performed by way of either an open or transurethral route.
- More often, the endoscopic route is chosen for the performance of transurethral prostatectomy; an electrocautery loop is used to successively remove prostatic tissue under direct visualization; hemostasis is obtained with electrocautery.

Malignant Diseases

- Carcinoma of the prostate (CaP) is the most common cancer in men in the United States and the second leading cause of cancer death; more than 95% of prostatic cancers are adenocarcinoma.
- The incidence of CaP increases with age, and the disease is more common in blacks than in whites.
- CaP can be identified at autopsy in more than 75% of men older than 80 years; thus, there is a large discrepancy between the microscopic presence of the disease and clinically significant disease.
- Most men with early stage prostate cancer have no disease-related symptoms; obstructive voiding symptoms or hematuria may be present.
- Patients with advanced disease may have pelvic pain, ureteral obstruction, or bone pain from distant metastasis.
- Digital rectal examination is an important method for early detection of prostate cancer.
- Prostate-specific antigen (PSA) is a serine protease enzyme specific for the prostate but is secreted by both benign and malignant prostatic epithelial cells; it may be elevated in men with prostatitis, BPH, or prostate cancer.
- The best imaging test for the prostate is transurethral ultrasound (TRUS); prostatic cancers typically are located in the peripheral zone and may have a hypoechoic pattern.
- Because of its lack of sensitivity and specificity, TRUS is not used as a screening test; it is used to direct prostate biopsy in men with a palpable abnormality of the prostate or an abnormal PSA value.
- Biopsy for detection of prostate cancer is almost always performed by transrectal route.
- The grading of adenocarcinoma of the prostate is based on the degree of differentiation of the tumor; most often, the Gleason grading system is used.
- Tumors with a Gleason score of 2 to 4 are usually considered well differentiated, 5 to 7 moderately differentiated, and 8 to 10 poorly differentiated.
- Staging of prostate cancer defines the local, regional, and distant extent of disease.
- Radionucleotide bone scanning is the most sensitive method for detection of bone metastases.
- Lymph node staging is of critical importance in selecting patients for therapy; CT scanning may show enlarged lymph nodes.

- The optimal therapy for localized prostate cancer is uncertain and a point of continual controversy.
- For men with a life expectancy of less than 10 years, observation alone (watchful waiting) may be appropriate.
- Surgical removal of the prostate or radiation therapy are the most commonly used treatments; 10-year survival statistics are similar.
- Brachytherapy using interstitial implantation is also a valid option, but long-term outcome is uncertain.
- Prostate cancer is a partially androgen-dependent disease; therefore, the primary treatment for metastatic carcinoma of the prostate is deprivation of androgens from the cancer cell by bilateral simple orchiectomy.

THE PENIS

Traumatic Injuries

- Penile injury may result from blunt or penetrating trauma, avulsion, strangulation, burns, and, occasionally, biting.
- Retrograde urethrography is indicated in all cases of suspected urethral injury.
- Blunt penile trauma can result in a contusion or a fracture; hematoma formation is usually small and limited by Buck fascia.
- Management is supportive and consists of analgesics, bed rest, scrotal support, and elevation.
- Fracture of the penis involves rupture of the tunica albuginea of the corpus cavernosum and usually occurs following trauma during erection when the protective thickness of the tunica albuginea is reduced; the patient typically reports pain, detumescence, and rapid penile shaft swelling.
- Concomitant urethral injury occurs in one third of patients, and retrograde urethrogram should be performed; immediate surgical exploration with evacuation of the hematoma and repair of the tunica albuginea is the treatment of choice.
- Penetrating penile injuries may be caused by gunshot or knife wounds.
- Low-velocity gunshot wounds without involvement of the urethra may be cleaned and left open; high-velocity gunshot wounds are associated with significant tissue destruction and usually require surgical management.
- Injuries that involve the urethra or testis require surgical exploration.
- Avulsion injury of the penile skin may be caused by the patient's clothing becoming entrapped in rotating machinery;

small noncircumferential penile avulsions are closed primarily with a full-thickness preputial skin graft or a split-thickness skin graft.

Malignant Diseases

- Five penile lesions have been identified as premalignant: leukoplakia, balanitis xerotica obliterans, Bowen's disease, erythroplasia of Queyrat, and giant condyloma acuminatum.
- Leukoplakia appears grossly as a white plaque; treatment is local excision.
- Balanitis xerotica obliterans presents as white, atrophic, edematous lesions involving the glans penis, prepuce, or both; treatment consists of local excision and topical steroids.
- Bowen's disease typically appears as a solitary, erythematous plaque on the penile shaft.
- Erythroplasia of Queyrat consists of raised, red, velvety, well-marginated areas of the glans penis or coronal sulcus.
- Both Bowen's disease and erythroplasia of Queyrat histologically appear as CIS and may be treated by neodymium-yttrium aluminum garnet (Nd-YAG) laser fulguration, local excision, or topical application of 5-fluorouracil.
- Giant condyloma acuminatum is a large exophytic lesion often grossly indistinguishable from squamous cell carcinoma; local excision is required, often necessitating partial or total penectomy.
- Although rare in the United States, penile cancer is common in men living in hot, humid regions.
- Poor personal hygiene and retained phimotic foreskin have been implicated in the etiology of penile carcinoma; penile cancer is extremely rare in men circumcised at birth.
- Small penile cancers limited to the prepuce can be treated with circumcision alone.
- Partial penectomy is used to treat smaller distal penile tumors.
- Larger distal penile lesions or proximal tumors require total penectomy and perineal urethrostomy.
- If inguinal lymphadenopathy persists or subsequently develops, there is a high likelihood of metastatic lymph nodal disease and ilioinguinal lymphadenectomy should be performed.

THE TESTES

Patient Evaluation

- The most common physical finding of the testicle is a mass.

- Most solid masses arising from the testis are malignant, whereas almost all masses arising from the spermatic cord structures are benign.
- Testicular tumors usually manifest as painless, firm, irregular masses on the surface of the testicle.
- Testicular tumors can be readily distinguished from benign masses arising from the spermatic cord by transillumination and scrotal ultrasonography.
- Testicular torsion is the twisting of the testicle on the spermatic cord, resulting in strangulation of the blood supply and infarction of the testicle; the condition is frequently misdiagnosed as epididymitis.
- Age is the most useful criteria in distinguishing torsion from epididymitis, because torsion usually occurs around puberty whereas epididymitis more often occurs in sexually active men, usually after age 20 years.
- Imaging of the testes and scrotal contents is best performed by sonography; the ability to assess the vascular supply to the testicle makes color Doppler imaging an essential element of sonographic evaluation.

Traumatic Injuries

- A direct blow to the organ may lead to injury.
- A contusion of the testicle presents with pain and a scrotal mass; the mass does not transilluminate.
- A real-time ultrasound examination should be performed; if a fracture has occurred, scrotal exploration should be performed.
- A contused testicle responds best to bed rest, ice, and analgesia.

Benign Diseases

Benign Masses

- Benign testicular masses can be divided into two main categories, with the first being benign fluid collections and the latter being benign solid tumors.
- Fluid collections may be a *varicocele*, *hydrocele*, or *spermatocele*.
- A *varicocele* is a dilatation of the pampiniform venous plexus and internal spermatic vein, with a prevalence of approximately 15%.
- Varicoceles arise most often on the left side because of the more perpendicular insertion of the gonadal vein on this side.

- Patients with sudden onset of a varicocele, a right-sided varicocele, or a varicocele that does not reduce in size in the supine position should be suspected of having a retroperitoneal neoplasm.
- Treatment consists of ligation or occlusion of the ipsilateral internal spermatic vein.
- A *hydrocele* is a fluid collection between the layers of the tunica vaginalis.
- A congenital or communicating hydrocele occurs as the result of persistent patency of the processus vaginalis.
- A noncommunicating hydrocele is classified as reactive (infection, trauma, or tumor) and nonreactive (idiopathic).
- Transillumination is useful for diagnosis; ultrasound is necessary if the testis cannot be deemed normal by physical examination.
- Indications for treatment include discomfort for treatment of the inciting cause and reactive hydrocele.
- A *spermatocele* is a cystic structure filled with fluid containing sperm; physical examination reveals a soft, transilluminating mass separate from and superior to the testis.
- Scrotal ultrasound is sometimes used to confirm the diagnosis.
- The benign solid tumors include *adenomatoid tumors*, *inflammatory pseudotumors*, and *hernias*.
- The most common solid tumors of the epididymis are the benign *adenomatoid tumors*.
- Most adenomatoid tumors are slow growing, firm in consistency, and have a smooth surface; ultrasound is useful to confirm the extratesticular nature of the mass.
- Inguinal *hernias* and associated lipomas may also present as paratesticular masses; physical examination establishes the diagnosis.

Malignant Diseases

- For treatment purposes, two broad categories of testis tumors are recognized: pure seminoma (no nonseminomatous elements present) and all others, which together are termed *nonseminomatous germ cell tumors* (Box 75–1).
- Ninety-five percent of tumors originating in the testis are germ cell tumors.
- Testicular cancer represents the most common malignancy in males in the 15- to 35-year-old age group.
- Germ cell tumors are seen principally in whites; the cause of germ cell tumors is unknown; familial clustering has been observed, particularly among siblings.

Box 75–1. Classification of Testicular Carcinoma

Germ Cell Tumors
Seminoma
    Classic (typical)
    Atypical
    Spermatocytic
Nonseminomatous
    Embryonal carcinoma
    Teratoma
        Mature
        Immature
        Mature or immature with malignant transformation
    Choriocarcinoma
    Yolk sac tumor (endodermal sinus tumor)
Sex Cord-Stromal Tumors
Sertoli cell tumor
Leydig cell tumor
Granular cell tumor
Mixed types (e.g., Sertoli-Leydig tumor)
Mixed Germ Cell and Stromal Elements
Gonadoblastoma
Adnexal and Paratesticular Tumors
Adenocarcinoma of rete testis
Mesothelioma
Miscellaneous Tumors
Carcinoid
Lymphoma
Testicular metastasis

- Orchiopexy performed before puberty may not reduce the risk of germ cell tumors but improves the ability to observe the testis.
- A painless testicular mass is pathognomonic of a primary testicular tumor.
- Testicular sonography is indicated; a radical inguinal orchiectomy with ligation of spermatic cord at the internal ring is required for all patients with suspected testicular tumors.
- Regional metastasis first appears in the retroperitoneal lymph nodes below the renal vessels.
- CT imaging of the abdomen and pelvis, and chest radiography are required; CT imaging of the chest is required if mediastinal, hilar, or lung parenchymal disease is suspected.

- Testicular cancer is one of the few neoplasms associated with accurate serum markers—human beta-chorionic gonadotropin (beta-HCG) and alpha-fetoprotein.
- Alpha-fetoprotein production is restricted to nonseminomatous germ cell tumors (NSGCT), specifically embryonal carcinoma and yolk sac tumor.
- Increased serum concentrations of beta-HCG may be observed in both seminomatous and nonseminomatous tumors.
- Serum tumor marker concentrations are determined before, during, and after treatment and throughout long-term follow-up.
- Increased or increasing concentrations of alpha-fetoprotein, beta-HCG, or both, without radiographic or clinical findings, imply active disease.
- Treatment is based on cell type and stage of the primary tumor.
- Therapy for low-stage (Stage I, IIa, or IIb) seminomas following radical inguinal orchiectomy is irradiation to the retroperitoneal and ipsilateral pelvic lymph nodes.
- Chemotherapy cures more than 90% of patients who have a relapse after radiation therapy; thus, approximately 99% of patients with low-stage seminomas are ultimately cured.
- The rate of cure for patients with NSGCT in clinical Stage I exceeds 95%.
- Twenty percent of patients with Stage I tumors with no lymphatic or vascular invasion or invasion into the tunica albuginea, spermatic cord, or scrotum are discovered to have regional lymph node or distant metastasis.
- Surveillance and nerve-sparing retroperitoneal lymph node dissection (RPLND) are both standard treatment options for this group of patients.
- Patients with Stage II NSGCT are treated initially with either RPLND or chemotherapy.
- In NSGCT, the need for postchemotherapy RPLND is controversial; some groups advocate surgery in patients with initial bulky retroperitoneal disease, whereas other advocate observation rather than surgery in patients with more than 90% shrinkage of retroperitoneal nodes.
- *Leydig cell tumors* make up between 1% and 3% of all testis tumors; the prognosis for Leydig cell tumors following radical inguinal orchiectomy is good because of their generally benign nature.
- *Gonadoblastoma* are rare tumors occurring almost exclusively in patients with some form of gonadal dysgenesis; radical orchiectomy is the first step in therapy; the prognosis is excellent for patients with gonadoblastoma.

- The most common secondary neoplasm of the testis and the most frequent of all testis tumors in patients older than 50 years of age is *testicular involvement by lymphoma*.
- Malignant paratesticular tumors are generally *sarcomas*; rhabdomyosarcoma accounts for approximately 40% of these paratesticular malignant tumors.
- Based on the group, treatment is directed using a therapeutic regimen including surgery, chemotherapy, or radiotherapy.

Index

Note: Page numbers followed by f indicate figures; page numbers followed by t indicate tables.